1 MONTH OF
FREE
READING

at

www.ForgottenBooks.com

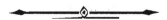

By purchasing this book you are eligible for one month membership to ForgottenBooks.com, giving you unlimited access to our entire collection of over 1,000,000 titles via our web site and mobile apps.

To claim your free month visit:
www.forgottenbooks.com/free24283

ISBN 978-0-483-51025-8
PIBN 10024283

INDEX TO VOLUME XXIV

DENVER MEDICAL TIMES

| Volume XXIV. | JULY, 1904. | Number 1. |

CONSIDERATIONS REGARDING MEDICAL INSPECTION IN THE PUBLIC SCHOOLS.*

By EDWARD JACKSON, M.D.,
Denver, Colo.

We study disease that life and health may be preserved. Medicine began with men already stricken by wound or poison or infection, and the things looked to for their direct relief. It has advanced to warning them of impending danger, whether from pestilence or tainted food or brittle arteries. The line of continued advance is toward development of the greatest possibilities of life and health by knowledge applied to the whole scheme of living. Hygiene understood, taught, practiced, made dominant in the public schools is the next step in this progress.

School hygiene must include attention to actual disease within the schools and provision for its treatment; the immediate suppression of epidemics; the recognition of all physical defects among the pupils, with steps to help secure their correction as far as possible; maintenance of the best sanitary conditions throughout the whole school environment of the child; the training by verbal instruction, exercises and habitual practice of general and individual hygiene; and the inspiring in every scholar the same reverence for health that we seek to instill with regard to patriotism or moral obligation.

Without claiming that this work of fundamental and universal importance is to be done wholly by the medical profession, it is obvious that it must at many points be guided by and founded upon that mass of knowledge which has been and is being laboriously accumulated by the medical profession; and much of which is available from no other source.

---

*Read before the American Academy of Medicine at Atlantic City, N. J., June 6, 1904, as part of a report on Hygiene in the Public Schools, and published here courtesy of the Bulletin of the Academy.

Medical inspection or medical supervision of schools is the chief agency through which our knowledge of vital processes and disease is to be applied. We say medical supervision for mere inspection ending in itself would be a farce. There must be both seeing and doing. Inspection takes value and significance only as it becomes the first step toward modifying what it discovers. But for efficiency the circuit from seeing to doing must be shortened as much as possible. So far as may be the eyes to see, the knowledge to appreciate and the judgment and authority to act should be vested in the same person, and in the immediate future this person will generally be the medical inspector. Generally but not always. Even at the present time the recognition of certain physical defects and the dealing with them is, in many places, left largely or wholly to the teacher; and in some cities the director or teacher of gymnastics is more likely to develop into the true school physician, than is the medical inspector. strictly so-called, therefore, in the present report we desire to call attention to the work to be done, and the ideals to be aimed at without elaborating any detailed system of organization, or distributing the specific duties among the school officers to whom they might be assigned. It is this design that is responsible for this apparent confusion of school inspection and supervision, of using as synonyms medical inspector and school physician, when evidently these terms may be properly used to indicate district officers.

The work of medical inspection in the schools is directed obviously to three purposes: The (A) detection and limiting the spread of contagious diseases. (B) The study of physical defects and other departures from normal health in the scholar, with indication of the remedy. (C) Supervision of the scholar's environment; and to these may be added when we have fully qualified inspectors holding the right relations with other school authorities, (D) some supervision of the instruction regarding hygiene.

The qualifications which this work demands of those who are to carry it on are:

1. *Skill in diagnosis,* the broadest and most difficult department in practical medicine. The diagnosis of disease is some-

thing that cannot be learned in fragments. Only to an extremely limited extent, and then with great uncertainty can any one disease be recognized, except by the person who can recognize all diseases. There are refinements of diagnosis which remain perforce chiefly in the hands of specialists, but every diagnostician knows that each extension of his ability to recognize a new pathological condition increases the certainty and exactness of his diagnosis of every condition. There is no diagnosis which is not differential. The recognition of the condition present demands that a host of other conditions be also borne in mind.

2. At least *outline knowledge of what is required to meet each pathological condition discovered.* Even if medical inspection in the schools dealt merely with contagious diseases, the duty would be well performed only by one who had received the greater part of a thorough medical education. In New York City, where the inspector is not allowed to mention the name of any physician or dispensary to the scholar, or even in general to make the slightest suggestion or criticism of treatment, they have been compelled to give with the exclusion cards full printed directions regarding the management of pediculosis, and to have a corps of trained nurses to send into the children's homes to see that certain skin diseases are efficiently treated.

But the dealing with contagious disease is only of minor importance in school hygiene. It helps greatly to restrict the general morbidity of the community; but affects less the health of actual pupils than do conditions like eye-strain or imperfect general nutrition, that do not exclude the patient from the school room. If the object of school hygiene is the health of the children, almost every morbid condition that may affect the body should be recognized by the medical inspector and the needs of each particular case and the possible ways of meeting them intelligently appreciated.

3. *The medical inspector of schools must have a broad, definite, practical knowledge of hygiene, including the factors which produce disease and those which guard against it.* He must have some special knowledge with regard to the heating. lighting and ventilation of rooms and buildings, the disposal of refuse, disinfection, the general endurance of children and the signs of fatigue. The best medical supervision will go even fur-

ther than this and include an understanding of developmental and corrective physical training.

Enough has been said to indicate that the medical inspector is simply a new specialization in the broad field of medicine. The training of the medical school, the actual treatment of patients, the quickening influence of medical journals and medical societies, are all essential to qualify one for such a line of work. Indeed, the efficiency of the inspector and the value of his work will depend to a considerable extent upon actual personal acquaintance with his colleagues in the medical profession, who practice in the district from which the scholars are drawn. He can only do his best to secure the health of the school, when, with the full advantage of the esprit d'corps of the medical profession, he is free to intrude as a friendly consultant upon any physician from whose families the scholars under his care may be drawn, with a freedom that is only possible to a recognized and friendly member of our profession.

The thing that is required of us as members of the medical profession to-day is a frank, hearty recognition of this new specialty. Recognition of its importance, its scope, the difficulties necessarily encountered by those entering upon it, with the possibilities it offers of useful employment for a certain number of educated physicians, and of benefit to all other branches of the profession and the public at large.

By drawing attention to existing remediable deformities and departures from normal health, there will be created a demand for skilled professional service, of the highest value to the community, and so of direct profit to our profession. The difficulties that have beset other specialists await the medical inspector, sometimes lessened, sometimes increased by the fact that he is working under the authority and in the pay of the general public, but always requiring the same intelligent appreciation of the rights of others, the same avoidance of unfriendly criticism, the same persistent endeavor to maintain a friendly relation that will bear the inevitable friction of contact through unintelligent and fault-finding patients. Let us recognize how much the medical inspector of schools has in common with the rest of us, entitling him or her to full participation in every privilege of our profession. Let us also recognize that if well-qualified for the special work, he or she possesses a certain amount of special knowledge that the mass of the profession cannot lay claim to; and which entitles him to speak with authority in certain situations.

The duties of a medical inspector of schools, or the school physician, may be considered a little more minutely. Inspection which is to guard against contagious diseases depends for its efficiency upon early recognition and prompt action. Anything short of daily inspection of all schools is a very poor protection against acute infectious diseases. The plan which brings before the school physician each morning, every child suspected of acute illness, is the only one that can receive the approval of intelligent sanitarians. The instant dismissal of the child to his home, and the more searching investigation of the case in the home, either by the family physician or the inspector of the health authorities, is probably the most practical way of dealing with the cases of acute infectious disease. Chronic infections, also, must be followed beyond the school room, either through the family physician or the health authorities, or, where it exists, by the staff of school nurses. Something must be done beyond the mere declaration that the child is unfit to attend school if medical inspection is to command the confidence of a practical people.

Acute illness not contagious in character should also be passed upon by the school physician to the extent of deciding whether the interests of the patient demand his exclusion from school. In these cases there is the greatest need for a good understanding between the school physician and the practitioner under whose care the child should properly come.

Chronic diseases and deformities, congenital or acquired, may require more careful investigation; but they allow of more time. Before going into any case minutely the school physician will properly satisfy himself as to whether the disease or fault of development is receiving intelligent attention from some other member of our profession, and if such be the case he should refrain from any investigation of it, except in conjunction with that colleague.

In many chronic cases the school physician should perform another very important function. Through him the practitioner in charge of the case should be able to secure that modification of school routine which the interests of his patient require.

Sometimes it will be a matter of special light or seating, or hours of work in the school; sometimes the arrangement for a special course of physical training or the modification of the course of school instruction to meet the needs of the particular child. But through the school physician we can expect that more and more the individual peculiarities of the scholar shall receive recognition, in the tasks he is put to for the purpose of drawing out and developing his powers. In this direction there is opportunity for original scientific work of great importance. Progressive educators feel keenly that popular machine methods of instruction are defective, and look to those who best understand physiological and pathological processes for guidance and help in their attempts at improvement.

Defects of sight and hearing which directly hamper the child in its school work, and which are liable to arise or increase during school life, should be systematically sought for, at least: once a year, among all pupils. The return of a child to the school room, after exclusion for illness of any sort, should be the occasion for careful examination, which may reveal recently acquired defects of these special senses, but such defects may arise quite apart from illness that would interrupt school attendance.

Even the school physician who may be quite unfitted to give instruction in hygiene, may be able to offer helpful criticism of the teaching of hygiene that goes on in the school. And on this account such teaching should be at least partly under his supervision if he does not take a more active part in it.

There can be no doubt that the medical inspection of schools, like other special work in medicine, will be best done by a distinct class of practitioners who devote their whole time to this and similar work. To have it in the hands of those who are in no way professional rivals will avoid the friction and opposition almost certain to arise where a physician also in private practice is called upon, in his capacity of school physician, to form a medical opinion regarding patients of a fellow practitioner.

This kind of complete specialization is greatly to be desired and in the main aimed at. But in a period of development and transition the most desirable cannot always be attained. In some places it will be possible to have the functions of school physician and health officer combined in one who has withdrawn from private practice. But where a competent school physician can only be found among those actively engaged in practice, one should be chosen largely because he has the respect and confidence of his colleagues, and an unaggressive temper that will help to secure that co-operation which is absolutely essential to the best results.

Special training for the duties of school physician will begin, as has already been indicated, with a complete course in a standard medical college. To this must be added a certain number of years, say three, of general medical practice. We cannot conceive of any other way of acquiring, at the present time, that diagnostic skill which is the first essential in medical inspection of schools. Beyond this there must be a pretty thorough course in hygiene, both personal and public hygiene, including some practical skill in bacteriology.

Courses of the kind required already exist in connection with some of our larger universities and medical schools, although these require some further development before they will fully meet the needs of the school physician. To this should be added a good practical course on physical training, such as is now given in a few of our best institutions, and which should be offered in every one of them claiming the title of college or university.

The current literature of this special department of medicine is already considerable. The appended bibliography includes chiefly the titles of papers that have appeared in English since January 1st, 1903. The periodical literature appearing in French and German is in some respects more extensive and more important. Those who can avail themselves of it will find it brought together in the Index Medicus chiefly under the headings: Hygiene of Person and Hygiene of Schools. In the near future the work of the school physician will doubtless become the subject of special text books.

BIBLIOGRAPHY.

Andrews, F. Paper in opposition to the introduction of Military Drill into Public Schools, J. State M. London, 1904, XII B1-83.

Baker, L. K. Sanitary Legislation Affecting Schools. Cleveland. M. J. 1903, II 571-575.

Bancroft, Jessie H. The Place of Automatism in Gymnastic Exercises. Am. Phys. Educat. Rev. Brooklyn, 1903. VIII, 218-231.

Berry, F. May D. The Education of Physically Defective Children Under the London School Board. Lancet. 1903, II, 17-29.

Beszant, Miss S. B. The Teaching of Hygiene. J. San. Inst. London, 1903-4, XXIV, 788-797.

Boyd, J. J. School Notification of Infectious Disease. Public Health, London, 1903-4, XVI., 94-98.

Brief Statement of the Results Obtained by the Commission of the British Dental Association Appointed to Investigate the Condition of the Teeth of School Children. British Dental J., London, 1903, XXIV, 809-816.

Bracken, C. W. Practical Hygiene in Elementary Schools. J. State M., London, 1903, XI, 314-325.

Bronner, A. On the Importance of Examining the Eyes and Ears of All Children, Not Only Those of the Board Schools. J. San. Inst., London, 190 I., 189-198.

Bryce, P. H. The Eethical Value of Education in Preventive Medicine. Canad. J. M. and S., Toronto, 1903, XII, 1-9.

Burnell, T. The Teaching of Hygiene in Elementary Schools. J. State M., London, 1903, XI, 326-330.

Discussion in Applied Hygiene for School Teachers. J.

Ehinger, C. E. Physical Examination in Normal Schools

Eninger, C. E. Physical Examination in Normal Schools and Public Schools. Am. Phys. Educat. Rev., Brooklyn, 1903, VIII, 237-244.

Emerson, Florence G. Medical School Inspection in Greater New York. Brooklyn Med. J., May, 1904.

Foster, B. Some Problems of Preventive Medicine. Am. Med., Philadelphia, 1903, V, 422-466.

Great Britain. Royal Commission on Physical Training. (Scotland). Report of the . . . 2 V., London, 1903. Neil & Co., 199, p. 1 diag. 648 p. 101.

Groff, G. G. Physiology vs. Hygiene in Our Public Schools. Bull. Am. Acad. Med. (Easton, Pa.) 1902-3 VI, 370-374.

Hall, G. S. Child Study at Clark University; an Impending New Step. Am. J. Psychol. Worcester. 1903 XIV, 96-106.

Hancock, H. Irving. Japanese Physical Training. New York and London, 1904. G. P. Putnam's Sons. 171 p. 19 pl. 12.

Hay, M. Notification of Measles and Whooping Cough. Public Health. London. 1902-3 XV, 382-397.

Hermann, C. The Present Method of Medical School Inspection in Greater New York. N. Y. Med. J. 1903. XXVII, 401-403.

Jackson, E. Testing of Vision in the Public Schools. Colorado Med., Denver, 1903-4 I, 97-102.

Johnson, H. P. Medical School Inspection in the City of New York. Tr. M. Soc. of N. Y. Albany, 1903. 183-189.

Knott, J. Brain Fag, and Its Effects on the Health. N. Y. M. J., 1903. LXXVIII, 986-989.

Little A. Care of the Eyes of the Children Attending Elementary Schools. J. San. Inst., London. 1903-4, XXIV, 814-824.

Lloyd, R. J. The Education of Physically and Mentally Defective Children. Westminster Rev. London. 1903. CLIX, 662-674.

Lydston, G. F. Briefs on Physical Training. Am. Med., Philadelphia. 1903, V, 300, 342, 383, 419, 463.

Mackenzie, W. L. Medical Inspection of Schools and School Children, with Special Reference to the Royal Commission on Physical Training. County and Municip. Rec., Glasg. and Edinb. 1903, I, 486.

Macpherson, J. D. Popular Medical Education, Its Aid in Limiting the Spread of Disease. Buffalo M. J., 1902-3, XLII, 709-722.

Moore, S. G. The Advantages to be Gained by the Teaching of the Elements of Hygiene in Schools. J. State Med., London, 1903, XI, 309-313.

Nesbit, D. M. Warming and Ventilating of Public Schools. J. San. Inst., London, 1903-4. XXIV, 825-833. 3 plans, Idiag.

Newsholme, A. School Hygiene, the Laws of Health in Relation to School Life. New Ed. London, 1903. S. Sonnenschien & Co., VI. 311 p. 12.

Newton, R. C.   Some Practical Suggestions on Physical Education in the Public Schools.   Med. News, New York, 1903, LXXXIII, 1115-1117.

Powers, L. M.   Some Observations made on the Inspection of Schools.   S. California Pract.   Los Angeles, 1903.   XVIII, 292-297.

Putnam, Helen C.   The Desirable Organization for a Department of Hygiene in Public Schools.   Bull. Am. Acad. of Med. (Easton, Pa.)   1902-3, VI, 378-386.

Richards, H.   The Education Bill, and the Sanitary Control of Schools.   Med. Mag. London, 1903, XII, 77-82.

Richards, H. M.   The Sanitary Control of Schools With Reference to the Education Bill.   Public Health, London, 1902-3, XV, 121-136.   Some of the Medical Problems of Public Elementary Schools.   J. San. Inst., London, 1903-4, XXIV, 775-782.

Robertson, J. C.   The Introduction of Military Drill Into Public Schools.   J. State M., London.   1904, XII, 75-80.

Rothwell, Annie.   Hygiene in Elementary Schools, and Its Bearing in Home Life.   J. San. Inst., London.   1903-4, XXIV, 773.

Savage, W. B.   Physical Education, Past and Present.   Am. Phys. Educat. Rev., Brooklyn, 1903.   VIII, 209-217.

Schmidt, H. F.   School Hygiene and the Need of Medical Supervision in All Our Schools.   N. Y. State M. J.   New York, 1904.   IV., 24-28.

Sedgwick, W. T., and Hough, T.   What Training in Physiology and Hygiene May We Reasonably Expect in the Public Schools?   Science, New York and Lancaster, Pa.   1903 n. s., XVIII, 333-360.

Sheard, C.   Infectious Diseases Among School Children.   Can. Lancet.   Toronto, 1903-4.   XXXVII, 621-625.

Sherer, J. W.   School Hygiene of the Eye.   St. Louis. Cour. of Med., 1903.   XXIX, 369-379.

Smith, Alice M.   A Study of School Hygiene, Development of Children and Preventive Medicine.   Am. Med., Philadelphia, 1903.   VI, 743.

Somers, B. S.   The Medical Inspection of Schools; A Problem in Preventive Medicine.   Med. News, Jan. 17, 1903.

Swain, R. L. The Brain of Children and Some Suggestions From the Standpoint of the Physician As to How It Should Be Regarded by the Teacher. Am. Med., Philadelphia, 1903. VI, 950-955.

Todd, F. C. School Sanitation Relative to Sight and Hearing. St. Paul Med J., St. Paul, 1903. V, 274-280.

Tomlinson, J. The Present Methods of Education From the Standpoint of the Physician. Am. Med., Philadelphia, 1903. VI, 196.

Towne, S. R. Medical Inspection of Schools, West. M. Rev., Lincoln, Neb., 1903. VIII, 33-36.

Vaughan, V. C. The Michigan Method of Tteaching Sanitary Science or Hygiene in Public Schools of the State, Bull. Am. Acad. of Med. (Easton, Pa.) 1902-3, VI, 387-390.

Walker, J. R. The Care of the Eyes During School Life. Occidental Medical Times, San Francisco, 1903. XVII, 409-413.

Ward, J. W. Medical Inspection of the Public Schools. Pacific Coast Journal Homeop, San Francisco, 1904. XII, 34-38.

Ward, T. D. The Training of Teachers of Hygiene for Public Schools. Bull. Am. Acad. Med. (Easton, Pa.) 1902-3, VI, 391-409.

Warner, F. The Inadequate Teaching of Hygiene in Public Schools. Columbus M. J., 1903. XXVII, 261, 271.

Wilcox, DeW. G. Further Investigation Regarding the Physical Effects of Regent's Examination Upon School Children. Tr. Homeop. M. Soc., New York, Rochester, 1903. XXXVIII, 65-81.

Wintsch, C. H. Medical School Inspection. N. Am. J. Homeop., 1903. LI, 210-217.

THE ANTI-BACTERIAL SECRETIONS OF THE BRONCHIAL TUBES—PRELIMINARY WORK.

By DANIEL S. NEUMAN, M.D.,

Denver, Colo.

THE PHILOSOPHY OF NATURAL SELF-PROTECTION.

The energy of animal life is expended either in making war or resisting it. "Offense and defense are sciences which the inferior creatures cannot neglect."[1] In life there is no cessation of hostility. The warfare of the internal organs armed with antidotes against the introduction of outside poisons and bacteria, aided at the same time by swift currents of secretion to sweep away micro-organism by the law of gravitation, never ceases.

In all bodies, both animal and vegetable, there is a perfect system of self-protection. In animals the nose secretes a fluid which contains potassium sulphocyanide, besides other substances which have not yet been perfectly separated, and which form a strong antiseptic fluid. Tears possess bactericidal properties. The characteristic fluid produced by one gland or set of glands, is never reproduced by another. The blood itself is not only the great nutritive fluid of the body, but carries different ingredients to different glands, from which each gland individually extracts the particles necessary in its normal functions. "Even in the process of elimination of foreign bodies, the organs possess a power of selecting different substances; for instance, sugar and potassium ferricyanide are eliminated by the kidneys, the salts of iron by the gastric tubules and iodine by the salivary glands."[2]

"The mammary glands are among the most remarkable organs in the economy, not only on account of the peculiar character of their secretion, which is unlike the product of any of the other glands, but from the great changes which they undergo at different periods, both in size and structure." "The formation in the liver and muscles of glycogen from dextrose, and the reverse change, are among the most important. Experiments on animals and autopsies on the human body seem to prove that the pancreas furnishes the blood or lymph with an internal secretion

1. Gosse, the Microscope.
2. Flint, Physioloyg.

necessary either to the normal consumption of sugar in the body or to the control of the sugar output from the liver and muscles. The function of the thyroid appears to be connected with metabolism and when the glands are extirpated or atrophied the subject becomes affected with myexdema and succumbs. The essential secretion of the thyroid is thyroidalbumin, from which thyroidin is obtained. Suprarenal extract is a true internal secretion, and is a most powerful vascular tonic."[2] The sphincter muscles form a good defense for the different cavities of the body.[3]

The fluids of the stomach and intestines are so well and thoroughly known, that I do not consider it necessary to describe them.

The epithelium of the bile passages and the liver tissues are decidedly resistant to the invasion of various micro-organisms.[4]

To sustain the theory of natural self-protection, I will introduce some examples, not only from animal, but also from vegetable life. For instance, a peach stone contains hydrocyanic acid in large quantities, undoubtedly to protect it from the attack of worms and insects. Even certain flowers (wax plant) have been known for ages to give out odors which render them dangerous to life and make them fungi-proof. During the time that the constructive work of plants goes on, there proceeds also a work of disintegration. In the economy of the organism, life and death go hand in hand. The alkaloids, resins and volatile oils are waste products, so far at least as nutritious purposes are concerned; however, they are of the greatest use by offering some protection against animals and destructive fungi.[1] It is well known also that the potato tuber when left to grow exposed to the full sunlight, develops a poisonous principle, solanin, but when the potato is grown normally, i. e., under ground, it is not present except in a very minute quantity in the skin. This process of destructive change is apparently supplied by nature as self-protection from destruction. The leaves of the pitcher plant and Venus-fly plant, entrap insects, and destroy them by secretory fluids.

---

1. Flint, Physiology.
2. Text Book of Chemistry, E. C. Hill.
3. Meltzer.
4. S. Talma.
1. Bastin, Botany.

Bees and wasps have for self-protection an apparatus supplied with secretory glands for preparing and injecting a powerful poison in time of need.

Healthy pigeons' blood has a great bactericidal power, unaffected by previous bleeding of the animal. This power is exercised not only on bacilli, but also on spores.

The rattle-snake would be practically defenseless had not nature supplied it with a deadly poison, which is manufactured in its own body.

The tarantula not only manufactures a deadly poison, but also has an anti-serum produced in its gland, used by the Russians as an antidote.

Take even the defenseless rabbit: nature has so adapted it to its environments by evolution, that in summer its fur is grayish-brown, to match stones, earth and dried grass, and in winter it is white as the surrounding snow. The gall-fly pierces the part of a plant which it selects and injects into the cavity a drop of its corroding liquid and immediately lays an egg or more there. The circulation of the sap is thus interrupted and thrown by the poison into fermentation.[1] M. Virey says, "the gall tubercle is produced by irritation in the same way as an inflammatory tumor in an animal body, by the swelling of the cellular tissue and the flow of liquid matter." In reality, the mechanism of production of the gall tubercle is only secondary, due to the secretion of the antidote against gall-fly poison.

Doderlein isolated from the vaginal secretions the vagina-bacilli and regards them as one of the chief defenses of the genital tract against bacterial invasion from without.

PROTECTION BY IMMUNITY:

Immunity may be classified as follows:

1st. Natural Immunity.

2nd. Acquired Immunity ((by heredity
(" disease
(" accident   Temporary

3rd. Artificial Immunity.

---

1. Riforma Medica, Naples.
2. Gosse.

Some individuals possess immunity to a marked degree, while others exhibit only a very feeble resistance to bacterial organisms. Immunity is never general; it confers protection against all contagious or infectious diseases, but is always special according to the disease, rendering a person perfectly invulnerable to one or the other.[1]

Many animals are less susceptible to infection than others. Some species of animals are naturally immune to certain infectious diseases; they even resist artificial infection.

A good illustration is as follows:

Infusoria and yeast fungi possess a complete immunity from tetanus and diphtheria toxins. [2]The rabbit possesses a marked resistance to tuberculosis. "Buffaloes are not susceptible to experimental tubercular infection." I might as well mention the natural age immunity from chicken-pox, measles, whooping-cough, etc. White men are naturally immune to bubonic plague in comparison to the Mongolians.[1]

Natural immunity is either due to the perfect physiological condition of the body, with its normal secretions and chemical reactions, or to the resisting power of the system developed by evolution.

Immunity acquired by heredity:—Occasionally a person will be found in whose family a certain common infectious disease has not occurred for a generation, although the members of each generation passed through one or more epidemics of that particular disease and took no special precaution to escape it.[2] Negroes and mulattoes enjoy an immunity from certain tropical diseases.[3] Immunity from the paternal side is not as readily transferred as from the maternal side.[4] Vaccinal immunity is sometimes transferred through the placenta.[5] It might be transferred during the nursing period through the milk of the mother.

Climatic immunity:—Persons who have lived all their lives in a yellow fever region are less apt to contract yellow fever, and when they contract it, the disease usually manifests itself in a milder form than it would in a newcomer.[6]

1. Dr. H. B. Weaver.
2. Dr. Gengou.
1. Dr. Prattner.
2. Dr. Wm. J. Class.
3. Dr. W. C. Wells.
4. Dr. O. Lambert Ott.
5. Dr. Beclere Menard.
6. Dr. Wm. J. Class.

Immunity acquired by disease:—The attack of certain diseases confers protection from a subsequent attack of the same disease, or an attack by modification of one disease confers immunity from the original source of modification.

Dr. Lake, from a study among a tribe of Indians, came to the conclusion that Indians who have suffered from scrofula in childhood become immune to tuberculosis in after-life.

Scrofula by itself is modified tubercular disease by involution of the bacteria, which might be due, taking into consideration that bacteria is acid-proof, to the alkalinity of the secretions which destroy by neutralization the waxy-fatty capsules and render them less virulent and severe.

Nature cures typhoid fever by the action of anti-bacterial agents acting upon the specific bacilli. These agents are found in the body cells, the blood and lymphatic apparatuses.

Immunity acquired by accident:—Sometimes immunity to a certain disease may be produced by the development of antitoxins in the body through the·agency of infected food.

Acquired immunity is due to the presence in the body of the specific microbe of some disease in a form sufficiently benign to be tolerated by the host, yet sufficiently active to stimulate the protection of the antitoxins.[1] Sometimes it is due to the reaction between the tissues of the invading body and the enzymes of the host. In some instances the germs undergo modification before their entrance into the body, and become less active by involution and modification of their structures in accordance with the surrounding circumstances; as climate, temperature, etc.

It may be due to transformation of the biological functions of the organisms.

Artificial immunity is due to vaccination, antitoxin serums and accidental inoculations.

Emerich and Low's theory refers to the resisting power produced by soluble chemical substances of the nature of bacteriological enzymes.

Ehrlich's lateral chain theory leads us to the conclusion that immunity depends upon the chemical combination of toxin with antitoxin; for instance, that during neutralization of the toxin

1. Dr. Richardson.
2. Dr. Carbon E. Sudo.

by antitoxin, one molecule of the latter combines with a definite quantity of toxin, forming a double salt.

Temporary immunity is due to the development of antitoxin for a short period, usually a few weeks.

Nuttall first demonstrated the antiseptic properties of the blood serum.

The activity of the serum alone against bacteria, according to Buchner, is greater than when the cellular elements of the blood are present.

Schloger's chemico-cellular theory is that in all animal cells there exists certain antiseptic properties which are increased by the bacterial attacks.

Vaughan claims that the most important protective germicidal agents possessed by the body are the nuclei.

Meltzer believes that the defense of the body against hostile germs is not due to a single tissue or a single function, but to the concentrated action of the independent factors.

LOSS OF RESISTING POWER OF SYSTEM AND AFFINITIES.

Castration both in male and female animals lessens the resistance against infection.[1]

Temperament bears an indirect connection to the resistibility of infection. The state of the general health appears to be connected with the susceptibility to infection.

"Experiments with tetanus and anthrax show that animals treated with alcohol after they have been vaccinated lose their immunity. If treated with alcohol during vaccination, they acquire immunity with difficulty. If vaccination was begun after the treatment with alcohol, it was only successful if the latter was stopped at the beginning of the vaccination." In the case of anthrax it was impossible to immunize animals while they were being treated with alcohol.[2]

Certain cells of the body have a minimum resistance against certain poisons, which is manifested in the case of tetanus poison by a special affinity for the nervous system.[3]

Indians are very susceptible to tuberculosis.

Some certain diseases, as pneumonia and erysipelas, have

1. Dr. Sirleo.
2. Dr. Deleorde.
3. Dr. Deleorde.

the tendency, as after-effects, to leave the patient more susceptible to all infectious diseases.

Immunity acquired in one country against specific infectious diseases might be lost by the climate of another.

The principle of phagocytosis is that the wandering cells of
the animal organism (the leucocytes), possess the property of
taking up, rendering inert and digesting micro-organisms which
they encounter in the blood and other tissues.

Rauschenbach demonstrates that when in the process of co-
agulation fibrin was formed, it was not as a specific product of
the action of the colorless elements of the blood alone, but also
as a result of the combined action between all animal protoplasm
and healthy blood-plasma, and there was always a disintegration
of the leucocytes present.

Hankin and Martin isolated from the spleen and lymphatic
glands a globulin body, which in solution possessed germicidal
properties. Ogota isolated from the blood ferments like globulin.

After long efforts I have succeeded in isolating the enzyme
of the racemose glands of the bronchial tubes. The method I
employ in separating the same is as follows:

I carefully separate the glands and the lining of the bronchial tubes, cut the glands into the smallest possible particles and
then put these into a vessel containing equal parts of water and
glycerin, after which I subject the same to a temperature of from
$35°$ to $40°$ C. for six to seven hours. I then filter the same, after
which I add some hydrochloric acid, and precipitate with alcohol
and hydrate of sodium.

As far as my experiments shows, this ferment has a slight
anti-bacterial action, and has a tendency to dissolve colonies of
tubercle bacilli in culture in from six to ten hours.

ECCLAMPSIA — FORCEPS DELIVERY — RESUSCITATION—COMPLETE RECOVERY.

By WM. H. HEISEN, M.D.,

Denver, Colo.

.The following case presents points of interest as to etiology of ecclampsia, its treatment and the time needed for resuscitation.

The patient, a woman of about 22, two years married, had had one miscarriage and had been having labor pains five hours previous to my seeing her. I found her in a very serious eclamptic convulsion, absolutely unconscious, with intense twitching of muscles and eyes, mouth, and face in general. Eyes wide open, staring towards one side, pupils dilated, violent contractions, especially of arms and legs.

While morphine and chloral hydrate had been used before with no or little relief, chloroform inhalations promptly subdued these spasms and reduced the frequency as well as the intensity of the attacks to the greatest satisfaction.

As the os uteri was hardly passable enough for one finger, the chloroform was continued carefully and in very much diminished doses. In the course of one hour, consciousness partly returned, labors became stronger, and the cervix dilated gradually. Soon the forceps could be introduced and the child was promptly delivered without any incident, within five minutes after blades were inserted. The child fell into my hands limp as a wet rag; there was no pulsation in the cord; the skin of the child was of a death-like pallor. I tied one end of the cord and threw the other end toward the nurse to pinch it until I had time to tie it myself, and asking the attendant to watch the womb, I started at once resuscitation by the Schultz swinging method. This method is described by Schultz himself in Edgar's "Practice of Obstetrics," page 846, as follows:

"The child lying upon its back is grasped by the shoulders, the open hands having been slipped beneath the head. The three last fingers remain extended in contact with the back, while each index is inserted into an axilla, the thumbs lying upon and in front of the shoulders. When the child thus held is allowed to hang suspended, its entire weight rests upon the two fingers in the arm pits. It is now swung forward and upward, the operator's hands going to the height of his own head, the pelvic end of the child rises above its head and falls slowly toward the operator by its own weight, flexion occurring in the lumbar region.

"The thumbs in front of the shoulders compress the chest, while the hyperflexed lumbar vertebræ and pelvis compress the abdomen, and through it the thorax. Finally the three last finfiers on each side compress the thorax laterally. As a result of this manœuvre, when properly done, aspirated secretions flow abundantly from the mouth. The distended heart also feels the compression which forces the blood into the arteries. The child is now swung back into its original position and supported entirely by the fingers in the axilla. The compression of the thumbs and three last fingers is removed. The downward swing elevates the sternum and ribs, while gravitation and the traction of the intestines depress the diaphragm. It is often possible to hear the air rush into the infant's glottis, as it reaches the original position, although this can occur in a cadaver.

"The amplification of the thorax lowers the intra-cardiac pressure. The child should be swung up and down ten times in the space of a minute. The effects of the manœuvre should be as follows: The heart beat increases in frequency, the cadaveric pallor becomes replaced by a rosy hue, and the muscular tonus appears. The child is then placed in a. warm bath and watched.

"If the inspirations are superficial, a momentary dip in cold water is indicated. If the heart action becomes poor the child should be swung again. If prolonged swinging becomes necessary the root of the tongue should be compressed forward, in order to raise the epiglottis and permit the removal of secretions with the fingers.

"In premature children the thoracic walls are often too soft to benefit by the compression of the fingers. In these cases insufflation of air should be practiced."

While this method is a most brilliant and classical one, and in my opinion far superior to other methods, I take exception to a few minor points that need correction in order to avoid errors: First, the upper illustration on page 846 accompanying this description of Schultz's method is wrong, as to relative position to right hand of operator to right shoulder of child, viz: right arm of child should lie in front of operator's index, and between it and thumb of operator, exactly as on left side of body of child.

Second, the "flexion occurring in the lumbar region" part of the foregoing description is insofar incorrect, as the flexion of body of child, after its upward swinging, especially in the case under discussion, where absolute limpness had taken the place of muscular tonus, occurs not only in the lumbar region, but all along the spine, from cervical to sacral region.

The down and upward swinging of the child, unless the figure of the operator is either too tall or too short, gives this method a singular simplicity and uniformity of time, pressure and weight, which places it unquestionably ahead of any rival one. One needs no assistant or preliminaries for executing this method, each up and down swinging motion requires the same number of seconds, the same combination of manual and gravity pressure. Besides the alternate reversion of the course of gravitation of the blood adds another valuable factor to the total of direct or reflex impulses, that other methods are short of.

There had been nothing in the least to indicate that there was any reasonable hope or encouragement for an attempt at resuscitation, and if I should give now an explanation why I went to this task with so much haste and energy I could not give any at all. The fact is, I continued these swinging motions for about two or three minutes, until bloody mucous and phlegm oozed out of nostrils and mouth, which, to gain every possible atom of time, I sucked with my mouth out of nostril and mouth of child, and at once resumed the swinging motions, after I had obtained not the least reflexes from slapping the buttocks or from hot and cold water ablutions to chest. After another lapse of five minutes, I noticed a short gasp from the mouth of the child. but another hot and cold water stimulation, and slapping produced no visible effects or reflexes. The earthen pallor indeed seemed to become even more distinct. The discoloration and limpness seemed to be even more intense than ever, and it appeared to me to be really absurd, to continue my efforts for resuscitation. However—after another few minutes of swinging, I felt a faint but distinct gasp, and subsequently an abrupt expansion of the chest under my thumbs. Another hot and cold water

douche produced no visible effects whatever, but a hard slapping
of butt produced a grimace, without a cry, however. After three
minutes' more swinging I felt distinct gasps for breath, and now
and then a stronger expansion of chest. The stethoscope held
to the heart revealed now distinct heart beats. Another few minutes' work along the line restored perfect physiological functions
of the child, normal color of the skin, respiration, pulsation and
prompt response to influences of temperature and pain. Mother
and child made a complete recovery and have remained in that
condition since, which is one month at this writing.

The particular points of interest in the case are the etiology
of the eclamptic fits, their prompt response to treatment, their
disappearance through chloroform inhalation and the successful
resuscitation of an apparently hopeless case after an unusually
long time of and vigorous efforts at reviving.

Inquiring into the history of the woman, I learned that a
week or so previous to her confinement, this woman while sitting at the window, saw an automobile with its crowded occu-
pants apparently doomed to a fatal collision with an electric car.
The sight of the imminent wholesale destruction of life so upset
her mind as to momentarily unbalance it and cause her to rave in
the wildest fashion for an hour or more. The family history of
the woman being otherwise absolutely negative, there is no doubt
in my mind as to this incident being responsible for the subsequent eclamptic attacks, during the impending delivery. I
would, therefore, call these series of eclamptic fits latent, reflex
convulsions, the nervous impact traveling along the optic nerve
to the nerve center and thence being switched over to the motor
ganglia and to their respective motor nerves. On account of the
intensity of the causative nervous shock or impact, a comparatively large number of motor centers were affected directly or indirectly.

The supposition is also manifest, that the excitability of the
nerve centers and the subsequent effect on the motor ganglia and
nerves, having once been established, every following impulse is
more apt than ever to produce corresponding disastrous results.

As in physics, the same maxim rules here: the stronger the
causative impulse, the stronger the resulting effect, or in this
case the greater the nervous shock the greater the ensuing con-

vulsions (motor spasms). Of as much if not greater interest, is the motto to be derived from the successful experiment of the prolonged resuscitation:

Never relax or stop your efforts of resuscitation for at least 30 minutes of uninterrupted and persistent work, since the case under consideration occupied me very nearly 30 minutes, to be finally successful after hope had been given up more than once.

With this lesson before our minds, many of us may have cause for regret not to have persisted longer in our efforts of resuscitation in the past, in spite of an absence of any material encouragement at the start or any visible improvement during the first ten or fifteen minutes of incessant work.

THE USE OF THE TRIAL CASE IN CORRECTING ERRORS OF REFRACTION, OR OBJECTIVE OPTOMETRY.

By EMMA J. KEEN, M.D.,
Denver, Colo.

All general practitioners, especially those practicing in small towns or country places, should be able to fit glasses for ordinary cases of hypermetropia, myopia, simple astigmatism and presbyopia, if for no other reason than to keep patients out of the hands of the optician, and in the hands of those, whom it is hoped, have their eyes upon the welfare of the patient and not on the excessive price they are to obtain for a pair of glasses, and will refer patients whose error of refraction is beyond their knowledge to correct or office equipment, to a competent oculist. Few general practitioners wish to spend time or money on the instruments which we use in making our objective examinations, i. e., the ophthalmometer, ophthalmoscope and retinoscope, instruments which require much time and experience to be able to use correctly in diagnosing errors of refraction. Therefore I shall take up the correction of errors of refraction with the trial case only. With the proper knowledge of the use of the trial case almost all errors of refraction excepting compound, mixed astigmatism and those slight errors against the rule, which are very important but very likely to be overlooked by one not accustomed to refraction work, can be corrected without difficulty, but a definite way must be followed.

Astigmatism is the most important error, and should be corrected first, unless a spherical hyperopic error reaches 5 or more dioptres, or in myopia it reaches 8 or more dioptres with slight astigmatic errors. In these cases vision must be brought up sufficiently so that the eye will recognize any change in vision when a weak cylinder is added.

I always begin my test by putting on the *weakest plus* glass, and gradually work up. By so doing any liability of causing spasm of accommodation will be avoided, and if spasm is present can in the majority of cases be overcome. (Spasm can be avoided also by correcting both eyes at the same time. Some oculists use strong plus glasses to blur vision and gradually decrease to avoid spasm.) Use a plus cylinder if the lines on the clock dial indicate astigmatism, i. e., if some lines are seen plainer than others, remembering that the lines seen plainest correspond with the meridian of greatest error and the axis of the cylinder used must be placed at right angle to the plain meridian. Use plus spheres if no astigmatism is shown, because we have not used any of the objective methods and do not know what our error is.

Minus glasses should not be tried until plus glasses have been given a thorough trial, because in hyperopia of low degree patients often accept minus if tried first. Minus glasses tend to excite spasm of accommodation, the thing we must avoid, and it is not an indication that a patient is myopic because minus glasses are accepted. The eye instinctively makes an effort to overcome minus glasses, thus producing artificial myopia and causing spasm of accommodation which minus glasses partially or wholly correct, thus the apparent improved vision.

First place your patient 20 feet from the test card (Snellen's) and clock dial (Green's) ; correct astigmatism first; always begin the trial with plus 0.12D or 0.25D lenses and increase gradually, for reasons mentioned above, remembering to place axis of cylinder at right angle to lines seen plainest on clock dial. (Most cases of hyperopic astigmatism will accept cylinders at or near 90° and most cases of myopic astigmatism at 180°. (When the vertical meridian of the cornea or any meridian within 45° of the vertical meridian is more curved than a meridian at right angle, we have astigmatism with the rule; if the opposite condition is present, we call it astigmatism against the rule.)

Place lenses in trial frame as follows:

(1) Plus cylinder lenses axis 90°, and change to any meridian within 45° to find if vision is improved at any point, but as stated above, most hyperopes accept a cylinder at 90° alone.

(2) Add plus spheres.

(3) Minus cylinder at right angle to plus cylinder glasses, if vision is not made perfect by plus cylinder alone and plus spheres are not accepted in addition.

(4) Spherical glasses in addition first plus then minus, to find if adding to or taking from correction made will improve vision.

(5) If astigmatism is not present try plus spheres, and if not accepted, minus spheres, and prescribe in all corrections the strongest plus and the weakest minus that the eye will accept when not under a cycloplegic, and you will rarely need to use atropine or scopolamine when the above method is properly used.

Simple presbyopia is the primary error of refraction and requires little skill or judgment to correct. It will require about a plus 0.50D for each 5 years beyond 40, but these eyes you will seldom be called upon to fit because the glasses they get of the optician give them satisfaction.

Therefore you should always look for an astigmatic error in a presbyope who consults you; also remember that the patient may have been a hyperope or myope, and correct all errors for distant vision first, then add the plus glasses that will enable the patient to read Jaeger No. 1 at 8 inches, and he can easily read it at a more distant point to suit himself.

The above method is followed in the clinic of Dr. Edward A. Davis, of New York, where I used it, and later in my own private and clinic practice with satisfaction, having had to resort to a cycloplegic only in cases in which I have found a marked ciliary spasm.

Prophylaxis of Lockjaw.—The consensus of expert opinion is that autitetanic serum is an effective prophylactic and is much less effective in the cure of the established disease. Bearing on this fact, Nocard observed 275 animals of various species, all of which had been wounded, accidentally or surgically, and subjected to tetanic infection. These animals were given antitetanic serum at once, with the result that not a single case of tetanus occurred among them. On the other hand, of 55 traumatized animals that had been exposed to tetanic infection, every one developed the disease. Dr. Joseph Hughes, a prominent veterinary surgeon of Chicago, has used the serum as a prophylactic in over 500 cases following surgical and accidental wounds, and not a single case of tetanus developed. The serum is harmless to the human being, and it has been proposed to immediately inject it in every case of traumatism of a suspicious character, hoping in this way to prevent the subsequent development of tetanus. With the specific remedy should be combined the open treatment of all wounds, however insignificant, in which from the nature of the surroundings there is any risk of tetanic infection.

Revaccination.—Jenner and other leading inaugurators of vaccination believed firmly that the protection afforded by vaccination would be perpetual. Thomson deserves credit for overthrowing this delusion and for establishing the identity of varioloid in the vaccinated with variola in the unvaccinated. The revaccination movement, beginning in 1824, was furthered by the European epidemics of smallpox that then raged up to 1833, in which the relative immunity of the revaccinated stood out in marked contrast to all others, and emphasized the necessity of revaccination—an experience that has been confirmed in every subsequent epidemic. The establishment of the practice of revaccination did much to turn the balance in favor of primary vaccination, and the English "Blue-Book of Vaccination" (1857), collated by the general board of health from 542 leading medical authorities of the world, was a triumphant scientific vindication of Jenner's great discovery. The only question left in doubt was as to the transmission of syphilis and other diseases by humanized lymph.

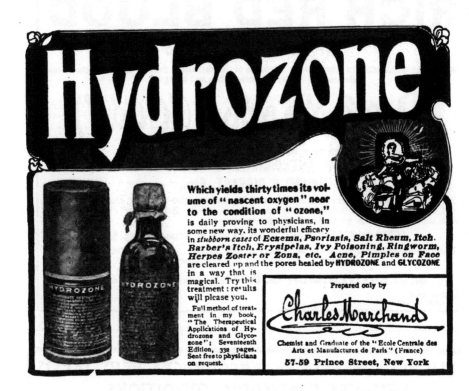

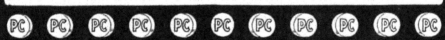

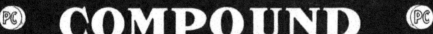
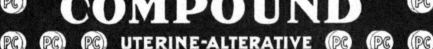

DENVER MEDICAL TIMES

THOMAS H. HAWKINS, A.M., M.D., EDITOR AND PUBLISHER.

COLLABORATORS:

Henry O. Marcy, M.D., Boston.
Thaddeus A. Reamy, M.D., Cincinnati.
Nicholas Senn. M.D., Chicago.
Joseph Price, M.D., Philadelphia.
Franklin H. Martin, M.D., Chicago.
William Oliver Moore, M.D., New York.
L. S. McMurtry, M.D., Louisville.
Thomas B. Eastman, M.D., Indianapolis, Ind.
G. Law, M.D., Greeley, Colo.

S. H. Pinkerton, M.D., Salt Lake City
Flavel B. Tiffany, M.D., Kansas City.
Erskine M. Bates, M.D;, New York.
E. C. Gehrung, M.D, St. Louis.
Graeme M. Hammond, M.D, New York.
James A. Lydston, M.D., Chicago.
Leonard Freeman, M.D., Denver.
Carey K. Fleming, M.D., Denver, Colo.

Subscriptions, $1.00 per year in advance; Single Copies, 10 cents.

Address all Communications to Denver Medical Times, 1740 Welton Street, Denver, Colo.
We will at all times be glad to give space to well written articles or items of interest to the profession.
[Entered at the Postoffice of Denver, Colorado, as mail matter of the Second Class.]

EDITORIAL DEPARTMENT

THE ROCKY MOUNTAIN INTERSTATE MEDICAL ASSOCIATION.

The next meeting of this truly intermountain society, which occurs September 6 and 7, 1904, at Denver, bids fair to surpass previous gatherings. Each year its purposes, as stated, "The promotion of medical interests in the West, and the fostering of good fellowship among its members" are becoming more fully recognized.

The coming meeting is the sixth in the history of the organization, previous conventions having been held in Cheyenne, Denver, Salt Lake City and Butte, Montana.

While the practice of medicine in its broadest sense is essentially the same without reference to geographical locality, yet none will doubt but that certain pathological conditions, therapeutic results, etc., are known to vary under diverse conditions of climate and altitude, such as are found in the tropical as compared with temperate zones, and in this country the coast and middle states contrasted with the mountainous districts. The interchange of experiences, therefore, within the jurisdiction of this society constitutes an important and unique factor of its success.

The territory represented includes the states of Arizona, Colorado, Idaho, Montana, New Mexico, Utah and Wyoming.

A splendid program is promised, and all members of the regular profession are invited to attend.

The officers for the current year are: H. D. Niles, Salt Lake, President; Robt. Levy, Denver, and T. J. McKenzie, Anaconda, Mont., First and Second Vice-Presidents; Donald Kennedy, Denver, Treasurer; Henry LaMotte, Salt Lake, Recording Secretary; Geo. A. Moleen, Denver, Corresponding Secretary.

MORBID EFFECTS OF COAL-TAR PRODUCTS.

Sajous *(Monthly Cyclopedia of Practical Medicine)* criticises the use of antipyrin and similar antipyretics under the following paragraph—introductions: Antipyrin promptly causes marked vasoconstriction. The vasoconstriction, both of the arteries and veins, may be sufficiently marked to obstruct the circulation in, and cause engorgement of, the capillaries. Very large doses in subjects whose adrenal system is abnormally sensitive, may cause sufficient vasoconstriction of the arteries and veins to greatly reduce their caliber. The arterial blood in the capillaries is then exposed to the reducing action of the surrounding tissues sufficiently long to become transformed into venous blood, thus causing cyanosis. When the adrenal system is unable, owing to congenital, acquired or temporary susceptibility, or an organic lesion of its component parts, to withstand the violent stimulation to which antipyrin subjects it, the functions of the adrenals may suddenly cease under the influence of even small doses of the drug, and the symptoms of adrenal failure appear. Antipyrin, in the stage of depression, reduces the temperature by causing adrenal insufficiency. The resulting dilatation of the great central vascular trunks causes depletion of the peripheral capillaries, and the internal temperature is thus raised, while that of the surface is lowered. Antipyrin should not be used during toxemias, especially when fever is present. It only acts as an antipyretic by causing excessive hyperemia of the adrenals—a condition exposing the patient to general collapse, even when small doses are administered.

HISTORY OF SMALLPOX.

Smallpox seems to have been indigenous in Hindustan from the most ancient times. The old Brahman mythology recognized a special divinity for this disease, and inoculation of human virus for immunization was practiced by their skilled priests with religious rites. Smallpox, according to the national records, invaded China twelve centuries before Christ. The early spread of Islam within and without Arabia was accompanied by epidemics of variola. It had already appeared in Egypt about 544 A. D. The malady was introduced into Southern Europe near the end of the sixth century. The first accurate description of the disease was by the celebrated Arabian physician Rhazes in 925.

The Crusades did much to make smallpox general. About the year 1000, when Europe in terror was expecting the Day of Judgment and the end of the world, smallpox raged as never before or since. The afflicted crowded the churches, whither the bishops brought their sacred relics. "The crowd increased," says Michelet, "and so did the pestilence; and the sufferers · breathed their last on the relics of the saints."

The smallpox penetrated to Iceland in 1241, and exterminated the Norman colony on the west coast of Greenland. It gained entrance to America with the Spanish conquerors, and wrought fearful havoc among the aborigines. In 1633-34 the smallpox in Massachusetts swept off both colonists and Indians in large numbers. In 1682, says Packard, the ship which brought Wm. Penn to this country lost thirty of its company by smallpox on the voyage. According to Toner, in the eighteenth century there were eight important epidemics in Boston, three in New York and Philadelphia, and five in Charleston.

As often "It is darkest just before the dawn," smallpox was the dominant pandemic of the eighteenth century, accounting in England for one-tenth of the total mortality. Two-thirds of the pauper blind were made so by this horrid sickness. About 30,000 people died annually of the disease in France alone. In America, as an extra inducement, negroes advertised for sale were frequently stated to have had the smallpox.

Smallpox spared neither the peasant in his hut nor the monarch on his throne, and to the survivors it bequeathed ugly scars and blindness and other lasting defects. In a grim humor of despair the proverb took shape, "From smallpox and love but few escape."

Variolation. In the third decade of the eighteenth century the oriental preventive method of variolation, or direct inoculation from smallpox subjects, began to be practiced in Europe, as was also the exposure of healthy persons to mild cases of the disease—a very uncertain procedure. Variolation, as practiced in India, consisted in scarifying the outer surface of the arm and forearm, followed by the application of cotton compresses impregnated witih year-old virus. The method was introduced into England by Lady Montague, wife of the English ambassador at Constantinople.

June 27, 1721, only two months after the introduction of inoculation into England, Dr. Boylston, of Boston, successfully inoculated his only son and two negro servants. In the same and the next year, says Hutchinson, the doctor and others inoculated 286 persons, with only six deaths; while in the same period 5,759 took the disease the natural way, and of these 844 died. Dr. Boylston and Cotton Mather, who supported the former, were for a time unmercifully persecuted, and the House of Representtaives passed a bill prohibiting inoculation under severe penalties, but it never became a law. Franklin, at first an active opponent, became later a strong advocate of this prophylactic practice. Against popular prejudice and official opposition, the practice of inoculation spread gradually to the other colonies.

Falling largely into the hands of charlatans, the procedure was often followed by fatal consequences—the mortality in the latter half of the.eighteenth century was about one in 300—though on the whole the results from inoculation were better than trusting to the chances of the natural disease. Inoculation as a prophylactic measure passed in general quickly out of use after Jenner's discovery of vaccination, first published in 1798. Variolation is still practiced in India, China and Algeria.

Vaccination. Vaccinia (vacca, a heifer), or cowpox, appearing on the udders of milch-cows, was long known to be communicable, not only in the bovine species, but to human beings as well. The protective effect of accidental vaccinia against variola, as observed in milkmaids and others, was a popular conviction among country people, but received little attention from the medical fraternity until Jenner opened their eyes to the facts. The first person, probably, to perform intentional protective vaccination was Benjamin Jesty, a Gloucestershire farmer, who, in 1774, inoculated his wife and two sons with cowpox. Thirty-eight years later these three persons were found to be still immune to variolous inoculation.

Edward Jenner (1749-1823), a practicing physician of Berkely in Gloucestershire, began in 1768 to test the correctness of the popular belief in the prophylactic value of vaccinia. For thirty years he continually experimented along this line, and when he gave to the world the results of these researches the efficacy of vaccination was proved absolutely. In 1796 he was the first to inoculate with the virus of humanized vaccinia, inoculating a boy with virus from accidental cowpox in a milkmaid. In 1798 he inoculated another boy with bovine virus from a case of original vaccinia. The humanized virus from this boy was then inoculated from one person to another five times, and in each and every case subsequent variolation tests were negative. Only after these most complete proofs did Jenner publish, in 1798, his epoch-making "Inquiry Into the Causes and Effects of the Variolæ Vaccinæ, Known by the Name of the Cow-pox," and recommended vaccination as a safe and sure prophylactic against smallpox.

Jenner's publication naturally elicited widespread attention, both in England and on the Continent, and his doctrines were quickly confirmed by the most extensive series of tests, so that within a very few years the preventive practice of vaccination spread throughout the entire civilized world. The first of many public vaccination institutes was founded in London in 1799.

The very marked and permanent decrease in variola that ensued in districts where vaccination was thoroughly carried out, led a number of governments to make this procedure obligatory on all their subjects. Bavaria blazed the path by an exemplary vaccination law enacted in 1807, and executed faithfully with most gratifying results, throughout the century. England, the cradle of vaccination, did not make the vaccination of children compulsory till 1867. Outside of Italy, no national government controls the manufacture and sale of vaccine.

Vaccination was introduced into the United States in 1800, and has been enforced at various times by state and municipal governments, but there has been no national law on the subject. The first person vaccinated in America was Daniel, the young son of Dr. Benjamin Waterhouse, Professor of Medicine in Harvard College. The virus, obtained from England, was inoculated July 8, 1800, with successful results. Dr. Waterhouse was foremost in introducing the new method in this country, against much ridicule and misrepresentation.

Following the universal interest in vaccination, there came a general apathy of reaction, which was favored by the marked malignancy of the epidemics of smallpox during the third decade of the nineteenth century. Up to this time it was believed that the immunity conferred by vaccination was perennial, and many held the mistaken notion that varioloid was a separate disease. At the same time considerable active opposition to vaccination arose among a certain class of minds not yet extinct.

Statistics of Smallpox: A statistical comparison best shows the change that vaccination, even though imperfectly carried out, has wrought upon the world. Ninety-five per cent. of all the inhabitants of Europe in the eighteenth century had smallpox, according to the universal testimony of contemporary writers. Wernher states that in non-epidemic years smallpox caused 8% (now 1% or less) of the total mortality; in epidemic years, one-half. It ranked next to pulmonary phthisis as the chief cause of death. In London the mortality from variola per million of population from 1660 to 1810 was 2,040 to 5,020. The rate in the period of 1831-53 was 830; 1854-71, 388; 1872-82, 262, and 1883-92, 73 per million. In 1721 in Boston, then a town of only 11,000 population, 6,000 people were sick with smallpox, and of these 850 died. At the same rate there might be today 30,000 or 40,000 deaths annually from variola in Boston. The only great epidemic of smallpox in Massachusetts during the nineteenth century was in 1872-73, when the mortality from this disease amounted to less than one-tenth of one per cent. of the living population. During the first decade after the introduction of revaccination, the yearly average of variola mortality per 100,000 in Berlin was only 1.16; Hamburg, .74, and Dresden, 1.03. In the same period the laxly vaccinated city of Paris showed a mortality from the same cause of 26.24 per 100,000; St. Petersburg, 35.82; Vienna, 64.9, and Prague, 147.9. From 1893 to 1899 inclusive, counting the German mortality from smallpox as the unit, Switzerland had an average comparative mortality from this cause of 30; England, 35; Belgium, 97; Holland, 176, and France, 293. Until the beginning of the nineteenth century the average annual mortality from smallpox in Prussia was 3 in 1,000. Since compulsory vaccination it has been about .03 per thousand. In Porto Rico for ten years prior to the American occupation the deaths from smallpox averaged 621 annually. Governor Henry issued an order in 1899 for universal vaccination. The result has been a reduction to one or two deaths a year from variola.

OBJECTIONS TO VACCINATION.

Every light has its shadow, and all great truths have had their opponents and detractors. There are not wanting civilized people to-day who still believe the earth is flat. So vaccination was at its inception attacked with all the fury of little minds, and with the records of the past century altogether in its favor, some individuals are yet found so biased against scientific facts and principles as to oppose and evade vaccination.

The same over-pious scruples that viewed the use of chloroform in labor as a direct infraction of divine command, construed vaccination and other preventive measures as a crime against the Deity who sent the plagues upon mankind to chasten them for their sins. Political demagogues pandered to the prejudices of the multitude by inveighing against the trespass upon personal liberty which compulsory vaccination would imply. In this way they set the despotism of the individual above the public weal, and the prejudice and caprice of parents and guardians before the welfare of innocent children. The would-be funny cartoonist ridiculed the subject by representing vaccinated persons as developing horns and other bovine characteristics.

Finical people found fault with vaccination as being a brutalizing and unnatural contamination with unclean products of animal metabolism. The most inane pseudo-scientific objection to vaccination, however, was the fanatical doctrine that variola is a beneficial life process necessary to purify the human race in general from the "congenital acrimony of their humors." Impressionable individuals have been most agitated against vaccination by the fear of physical degeneration (scrofula, rachitis) or of specific contagion (syphilis, erysipelas, tetanus) transmitted through the vaccine virus. There is absolutely no proof of the existence of the former danger, and the likelihood of contracting a contagious disease from vaccination with a pure virus and a proper technique, is so remote as to be a negligible quantity. The recent outbreak of acute and fatal tetanus in Camden, N. J., following vaccination, was proved by the period of incubation (19 to 23 days) to be due to secondary infection on account of lack of cleanliness in the care of the wound.

EDITORIAL ITEMS.

Portland, Oregon, selected as next place of meeting of A. M. A.

Dr. McMurtrie, of Louisville, Kentucky, elected president of American Medical Association.

Medicine in Japan.—Japan, says the *Medical Standard*, has 31,000 physicians and eight medical schools.

Albuminuria of Pregnancy.—According to De Lee's rerearches, 79 per cent. of women have albuminuria during labor.

Clavus.—Thornton treats corns by the nightly application of salicylic acid, ten grains to two drams of cerate.

Periodic Headaches.—These forms (*Alkaloidal Clinic*) are generally relieved by picrotoxin, grain ¹⁄₁₄₄ every two to four hours, or three times a day.

Stench of Cancer.—To control the fetor Thornton directs to wash every two hours with a solution of eight drops of formalin in a pint of hydrogen dioxide water.

For Hepatalgia.—The paroxysms are relieved (*Alkaloidal Clinic*) by glonoin and atropine, grain ¹⁄₂₅₀ each, every five minutes in hot water until face is red.

Uterine Bleeding.—The persistent oozing (*Alkaloidal Clinic*) that follows puerperal hemorrhages may be checked by hamamelin, grain ½ to 1 every hour or two.

For the First Stage of Pneumonia.—℞ Ext. digitalis gr. ¼; pulv. ipecac. comp. gr. ii: A pill every two or three hours.— Shoemaker.

Passive or Hypostatic Congestion of the Lungs.—℞ Ergotini gr. 1-3; ext. digitalis gr. ¼; pulv. ipecac comp. gr. ii: A pill every three or four hours.—Shoemaker.

For Sale.—The instruments, Books and furniture belonging to the late Dr. Crocker, of Littleton, Colorado; also horse, physician's buggy, light phaeton, harness, etc. Office to rent, situated in the best location in the town. Mrs. F. B. Crocker, Littleton Colorado.

Pulmonary Embolism.—Anders recommends absolute rest of body and relief from distressing symptoms; atropine and morphine for pain and dyspnea; and special etiologic treatment.

Hemoptysis Due to Wound.—Heath employs turpentine inhalations from a handkerchief; ice internally and externally; venesection; and lead acetate or gallic acid.

For Callosities.—Cantrell advises to apply for 48 hours an ointment of salicylic acid, one dram to the ounce of cold cream. Curette and renew the application night and morning for several days.

Cardiac Disease With Accelerated Pulse.—℞ Ext. verat. vir. fl. m. i; ext. ergotæ fl. m. iv; acidi sulph. arom., m. iv; aquam q. s.: A half teaspoonful well diluted every half hour as long as needed.—Howe.

Syphiloderma Tuberculosa.— Lydston directs to apply locally a solution of five or ten grains of mercuric chloride to the ounce of compound tincture of benzoin or collodion, in addition to the general treatment.

Pneumorrhagia of Pulmonary Agoplexy or Bright's Disease.—Anders advises absolute rest in the horizontal posture, the internal and external use of cold, and cardiac stimulants with onset of collapse.

Aneurysm.—In early cases Osler advises absolute rest and very low diet with restriction of fluids, avoidance of constipation and straining, and the administration of potassium iodide ten to twenty grains three times a day.

Ferrosol.—This new remedy, says the *Medical Critic*, is a double saccharate of ferrous oxide and sodium chloride. It is a clear, dark brown liquid, and is used in anemia and chlorosis in doses of one teaspoonful three times a day.

Potent Medicines.— Although the number of proprietary medicines, outside of the standard preparations of the pharmacists and those in the pharmacopeia, (*Dietetic and Hygienic Gazette*) is estimated at 50,000, they are said to be decreasing in number.

Rupture of Aneurysm or Erosion of a Blood Vessel.—The bleeding in these cases may be sudden and profuse, welling up through the nose and mouth, or slight and protracted. Keep the patient alive, says Osler, in hopes that a sufficient thrombus may form. Encourage cough while bleeeding is profuse, and give no opium.

Verruca Necrogenica.—For dissection wounds and similar localized septic sores, Bulkley advises the use of a fifty per cent. salicylic acid paste, or repeated cauterization with acid nitrate of mercury. Thorough erasion with the curette is necessary in some cases.

Treatment of Glanders.—Shoemaker says sustain with food, stimulants and large doses of tincture of iron and quinine; use solution of mercuric chloride locally; cleanse nasal cavities frequently and cauterize lesions thoroughly, followed by suitable soothing applications.

Interlobar Pleurisy.—Copious and repeated hemorrhages may occur, though the patient is not tuberculous. If evacuation of pus is incomplete, as shown by persistence of fever and symptoms of infection, Dieulafoy states that prompt surgical intervention is indicated.

The Biggest Man in the World.—An editorial note in the May number of *Medicine* refers to the recent death of Thomas Longley, a Dover citizen, who was over six feet in height, 70 inches around the chest, 85 inches around the waist, and weighed 664 pounds.

Ferropyrine or Ferripyrine.—This local hemostatic (*Medical Critic*) contains 64 per cent. of antipyrine and 36 per cent. of ferric chloride. It is an orange-red non-hygroscopic powder, soluble in water or alcohol. It may be used pure or in 20 per cent. solution.

Injury to the Cervical Spine.—Perfect rest, says Herbert W. Page, is the chief consideration. Asepsis for wounds is in order, and hot flannels or linseed poultices for sprains. Ice locally—and ergot or gallic acid internally are indicated for hemorrhage.

Passive Pulmonary Congestion.—Hamamelis is claimed to be almost a specific for venous hemorrhage. Bruce uses venesection, leeching or cupping and purging, and does not try to check the bleeding from the lungs. Hare recommends digitalis and similar remedies for slight hemoptysis from a weak right heart.

Abrams asserts that morphine is the best remedy, along with rest iu bed and gelatin by the mouth.

General Paresis. Although the outlook for paretics is almost hopeless, Osler advises large doses of potassium iodide in syphilitic cases. They do best with careful nursing and the orderly life of an asylum. Bromides are useful in sleeplessness and epileptiform siezures.

A New and Powerful Poison, The fuming liquid, oxide of cacodyl (*Medical Age*), has recently been combined with the radical cyanogen, producing cyanide of cacodyl, a white powder, melting at 33° and melting at 140°. On exposure to air this substance gives off a slight vapor, the inhalation of which is instant death.

"The First Gun in the Public Warfare Against Tuberculosis". Portland, says the Oregon *Medical Sentinel,* has taken a step which, when completed, will place her in the front rank of cities upon the Pacific slope in the matter of sanitary progress and education. This is the establishing of a free sanatorium for the open air treatment of consumptives.

How Brains Grow. Marchand (*Clinical Review*) asserts that the weight of the human brain at birth doubles in the first nine months of life, and trebles before the end of the third year, after which the rate of increase is much lessened. In men the full brain-weight is attained at from 18 to 20 years; in women, at 16 to 18 years.

Treatment of Tetanus..—Senn says: Prevent by treating small wounds with great care antiseptically; remove any foreign bodies; inhalation of chloroform for excruciating pain; morphine and atropine hypodermically, or chloral hydrate and potassium bromide each 19 or 20 grains every three or four hours; bodily and mental rest in quiet, dark room; liquid food sipped through elastic tube; warm baths grateful in chronic cases.

Active Pulmonary Congestion.—Hare recommend ergot for capillary hemorrhage, and small doses of aconite for hypertrohied heart. To relieve hyperemia of the mucosa Osler advises rest in bed and seclusion; light unstimulating diet; no alcohol; ice to suck; small doses of aromatic sulphuric acid and salts freely if bleeding protracted; opium freely for cough; aconite when much vascular excitement.

Bleeding Lungs.—In the ordinary hyperemic form of hemoptysis Babcock gives syrup of Ipecac in moderate doses until slight nausea is produced, also phosphate of codeine for cough, and a mild saline aperient. When the hemorrhage is profuse, from rupture of an artery in a cavity he injects hypodermically $\frac{1}{60}$-$\frac{1}{40}$ grain sulphate of atropine, and proceeds as above. The subsequent treatment of both varieties includes absolute rest, light, unstimulating diet; ipecac, codeine and salines p. r. n.

Cardiac Insomnia. Characteristic of this type, according to an editorial in the Journal of the *American Medical Association*, is to fall asleep readily and in a short time awake suddenly, usually with a sense of fear and slight oppression of the chest and almost always palpitation. Relief of such sleeplessness, says Feilchenfeld, will usually be afforded by free evacuation of the bowels and moderation in diet, especially in the last meal of the day.

Rheumatic Abdominal Pain.—S. Vere Pearson (quoted in *Medical Record*) says this pain is nearly always about the upper half of the abdomen. It is said to be "inside", yet it does not go through to the back nor travel round the trunk. It is of short duration but recurs, and is not associated with nausea or vomiting nor with the taking of food. The treatment is that of acute rheumatism, chiefly salicylates.

Melanoma. This rapid, malignant affection is characterized by multiple—iron-gray to blackish, soft or firm, rounded papules, tubercles or nodules and fungoid or pultaceous ulcers. There may be general melanosis. It often starts from a wart or mole. By way of treatment J. A. Fordyce states that arsenic may be tried internally and hypodermically, and bandaging and emollient applications should be used for painful infiltration of hands and feet.

Brain Tumor. C. E. Beevor recommends tonics and cod-liver oil in tubercular cases; a thorough course of mercury and potassium iodide in syphilitic cases: surgical operation when diagnosis can be made of cortical or subcortical growths, and sometimes even for deeply seated tumors to relieve pressure and agonizing headache even when growth cannot be removed; morphine, indian hemp, chloral and ice to head chief remedies for relieving pain.

Heatstroke or Sunstroke.—Bartholow employs ice to the head and friction of the surface with ice; also the cold wet pack or cold bath. Anders directs to remove clothing, lay patient on bed, cover with a rubber blanket and sponge with ice water, or lay a piece of ice on the belly and rub another piece over rest of body, using at same time brisk rubbing of surface; watch temperature and stop cold applications when it falls to 101°, applying cold again as it rises; free venesection for consecutive meningitis.

Disseminated Sclerosis. Hammond has praised barium chloride, one grain t. i. d., and tincture of hyoscyamus, one or two drams morning, noon and night; also a mild primary current passed through the brain anteroposteriorly and laterally and through sympathetic nerve; induced current for paralysis and contractures; cod-liver oil, iron and strychnine if general health materially impaired; highly nutritious food; a glass or two of wine daily; avoid excitement, mental labor and excessive physical exertion; passive exercise in open air always beneficial.

The Chloride Reduction Treatment of Parenchymatous Nephritis.—F. Widal and A. Javal (*International Clinics*) have shown by careful clinical tests that edema and albuminuria increase with the amount of common salt in the food and diminish or disappear on cutting out this condiment as much as possible. By observing this precaution they were able to give considerable variety to the diet. Even with 400 grams of dark meat, 500 grams of bread and 1000 grams of potatoes, all unsalted, edema was removed and albuminuria decreased at will.

Spinal Meningitis.—In pachymeningitis we should treat the cause (caries, pus collection, etc.), and resort to rest, the actual cautery, sedatives and tonics. For leptomeningitis Gowers advises perfect rest and quiet; dry or wet cupping or leeching along spine at onset, followed by local application of cold in traumatic or hemorrhagic cases and heat in others; morphine, chloroform, belladonna or atropine for pain and spasm; chloral and bromide for insomnia; for cases due to cold, hot air or vapor bath at onset, or warm bath followed by moist pack for several hours; open bowels freely; oleate of mercury rubbed in along spine; blisters or repeated sinapisms when disease subsiding; iodides, iron, quinine and strychnine in chronic stage.

Treatment of Lupus Vulgaris.—Stelwagon recommends nutritious food, fresh air and outdoor exercise; cod-liver oil, potassium iodide, iron and quinine; cauterization with lunar caustic, or ointment of two drams pyrogallin with one dram lead plaster and five drams cerate of resin applied for a week or two alternately with poultices; or ointment of arsenous acid gr. xx with 60 grains of red sulphide of mercury to the ounce of cold cream, spread on lint and renewed daily for three days, followed by poultice and simple dressing; or galvanocautery or repeated linear or punctate scarifications (followed by simple salicylated ointment), or erosion with curette (followed by pyrogallol ointment), or excision if patches quite small.

The Pan-American Congress.—The next meeting of the Pan-American Congress will be held in Panama the latter part of December. The Pan-American Congress meets every three years. It was started by Dr. William Pepper of Philadelphia, Dr. C. A. L. Reed of Cincinnati, Dr. Albert Vander Veer of Albany, and Dr. H. L. E. Johnson of Washington. The first meeting was held in Washington in September, 1893, the second in Mexico, in 1896, the third was to have been held in Venezuela in 1899, but was given up on account of the war in that country. The place of meeting was changed to Cuba, but had to be postponed until 1901 on account of the fever there. These meetings have always been well attended, and it is thought that Panama will be an interesting place for the convention.

Treatment of Acute Myelitis.—Gower's method may be summarized as follows: Hot bath followed by sweating and counter-irritation at onset when due to cold; if considerable paralysis already present, give perfect rest on face or side with plank back-rest; leeches, wet or dry cupping, hot fomentations, mustard plaster or hot water bags; nutritious but stimuliating diet; free purgation if constipation; nitrous ether and tincture of digitalis as diuretics; ergot of use in hemorrhagic form; extreme cleanliness and care to avoid bed-sores (cotton-wool, water bath; regular catheterization when either simple retention or overflow of incontinence; iron, quinine and arsenic when disease has become stationary—also electricity and massage for atrophied muscles.

Treatment of Meningitis.—This varies with the cause. The otitic form demands surgical measures. Antiphlogistics and counter-irritation are generally of value. In leptomeningitis infantum Angel Money advocates the daily inunction of blue ointment into the back of the neck. For the simple and cerebrospinal types he advises absolute rest in a quiet, dark room, well ventilated at 60° to 65°; keep bowels regularly open by simple means or saline purges; digestible, nutritious diet; ice bags or cold applications to the shorn scalp; bromides, chloral, hyoscyamus, paraldehyde, sulphonal, opium, injections of morphine or cocaine; leeches behind ears if great heat of head; iced or effervescing drinks to relieve vomiting; calomel or gray powder till gums are touched; iodides and mercury to promote absorption in later stages and subacute and chronic cases.

Multiple Neuritis.—Says Gowers: Discover and remove special cause; rest in bed and careful feeding; warm fomentations over any tender nerves at outset; cocaine hypodermically over seat of pain; wrap tender limbs in cotton wool (may be covered with oiled silk); warm bath for 15 or 20 minutes daily; prevent habitual postures leading to deformities; mercury may be tried whenever pain and tenderness of larger nerve-trunks prominent; during acute febrile onset of alcoholic form give potassium citrate, nitrous ether and tincture of cinchona, with a little digitalis if pulse feeble; sodium or potassium salicylate when due to cold; quinine for malarial cases; in toxemic forms give tincture of iron m. xx-xxx 3 or 4 times a day; in subacute and chronic cases, iron, quinine and small doses of strychnine; in chronic cases, also potassium iodide and arsenic (continuously in small doses) cod-liver oil, massage and electricity.

Acute Anterior Poliomyelitis.—Archibald Church recommends salicylates or mercuric chloride in the early febrile stage; faithful employment of hot applications or mild sinapisms to spine; keep child lying on side or face with affected limbs thoroughly enveloped in cotton wool; systematic use of galvanic electricity to paralyzed muscles when active process has come to a standstill (about a fortnight)—taking care not to alarm child or unduly fatigue muscles; also local frictions, salt baths, warm wrappings and massage. In the active stage Henry M. Lyman gives solution of antipyrin with tincture of aconite, and evacuates bowels thoroughly with 1-10 grain calomel every hour, giving full dose of castor oil if overloaded. Codeine phosphate is given after the evacuation to relieve pain and restlessness; baths and sponging only when agreeable; chloral and bromides if convulsions. In stage of convalescence use good food and small doses of strychnine and arsenic, daily bathing of affected limb with hot water followed by massage, and electricity for ten minutes daily.

Uremia.—Bartholow advocates the vapor bath and hot water pack to excite the skin and promote free diaphoresis. When diaphoresis and catharsis fail in promptness or efficiency, Anders employs venesection; also the intravenous injection of physiologic salt solution in cases of profound weakness threatening collapse.

Tubercular Hemoptysis.—Fraenkel directs to calm patient and soothe cough, for which purpose codeine is preferable to morphine. Have patient rest in bed. Give digitalis for rapid, feeble heart. Use ice-bag on precordium. Antipyrin or phenacetin may be given occasionally to produce quiet and euphoria. Ligation of the extremities and infusion of saline solution are resorted to in critical cases. Solis-Cohen recommends turpentine and calcium chloride internally. Flick uses nitroglycerin, ½ drop of one per cent. alcoholic solution every half hour. Karl Von Ruck gives sufficient apomorphine to produce emesis, as the best and quickest sedative. Ringer advises the spinal hot water bag to the cervical or upper dorsal vertebræ. Anders praises oil of erigeron in 5 minim capsules every two, three or four hours. Hare gives one-fourth grain morphine hypodermically as a routine measure;; small, frequent doses of aconite if profuse bleeding produces collapse; chloral to quiet the circulation, allay cough and induce sleep; and a small ice-bag over the affected bronchial vessel. Kenworthy recommends suprarenal extract, three grains every half hour for three doses. When cough accompanies, Scarpa prescribes 15 grams each of the tincture and fluid extract of hydrastis with 0.3 to 0.45 gm. codeine, the dose being 20 to 25 drops t. i. d. For mere spitting of blood Brasher recommends the fluid extract of geranium maculatum, five to ten drops every two hours.

Editorial items continued on Page 59

BOOKS.

PROCEEDINGS OF THE AMERICAN MEDICO-PSYCHOLOGICAL AS-
SOCIATION AT THE FIFTY-NINTH ANNUAL MEETING, held
in Washington, D. C., May 12-15, 1903.

Among the many able papers in this volume we note one by
Dr. J. E. Courtney, of Denver, being a "Report of a Case of
Cerebral Lues."

ELECTRO-DIAGNOSIS AND ELECTRO-THERAPEUTICS. By Dr.
Toby Cohn, Nerve Specialist of Berlin. Translated from
the Second German Edition and edited by Francis A.
Scratchley, M. D., of New York. With eight plates and
thirty-nine illustrations. Cloth, 280 pages. Price, $2.00.
Funk & Wagnalls Company, New York and London.

This is the authorized translation of the most popular German manual on the diagnosis and cure of disease by electricity.
The work is designed for students and practitioners who know
little or nothing of the subjects treated; hence the author begins
with primary facts and takes nothing for granted. The principles and technique of electro diagnosis are presented in a clear
and simple manner, sometimes in the way of object lessons. All
that is of positive value in electro-therapeutics is placed before
the reader, with careful directions as to modes and methods of
use. The eight anatomical plates are reproductions of the German originals, and have coverings of transparent paper on which
are indicated the points of application of the electric current.

TUBERCULOSIS AND ACUTE GENERAL MILIARY TUBERCULOSIS.
By Dr. G. Cornet, of Berlin. Edited, with additions, by
Walter B. James, M. D., Professor of the Practice of Medicine in the College of Physicians and Surgeons (Columbia
University), New York. Handsome octavo volume of 806
pages. Philadelphia, New York, London: W. B. Saunders & Company, 1904. Cloth, $5.00 net; Half Morocco,
$6.00 net.

This is the seventh volume to be issued in Saunders' American Edition of Nothnagel's Practice. The vital importance of
the subject is manifest to all. The work of Professor Cornet is
complete and exhaustive from every standpoint, and is quite up
to date. It is a pleasure and satisfaction to be able to get an
immediate comprehensive view of any point concerning the disease, by referring to the full and orderly index. Besides this, a

bibliography of tuberculosis covering ninety pages is appended for consultation purposes. The text is clearly and interestingly written, and, like other members of the series, the book presents a handsome typographic appearance. Physicians of the Rocky Mountain region would do well to procure this volume at least of Nothnagel's great work.

DISEASES OF THE INTESTINES AND PERITONEUM. By Dr. Hermann Nothnagel, of Vienna. The entire volume edited, with additions, by Humphrey D. Rolleston, M. D., F. R. C. P., Physician to St. George's Hospital, London, England. Octavo volume of 1032 pages, fully illustrated. Philadelphia, New York, London: W. B. Saunders & Company, 1904. Cloth, $5.00 net; Half Morocco, $6.00 net.

This is the eighth volume in Saunders' American Edition of Nothnagel's Practice. The remaining three volumes are in active preparation for early publication, probably before the end of the year. The present book is by Nothnagel himself, and is characterized by the thoroughness and practicality of this famous clinician. The English editor has performed his task with much care, and has made many important additions. Peritonitis and appendicitis receive an exhaustive discussion commensurate with their clinical importance. The plates are of great diagnostic value. The work is in every way a safe and reliable guide.

EPILEPSY AND ITS TREATMENT. By William P. Spratling, M. D., Superintendent of the Craig Colony for Epileptics at Sonyea, N. Y. Handsome octavo volume of 522 pages, illustrated. Philadelphia, New York, London: W. B. Saunders & Company, 1904. Cloth, $4.00 net.

This work is the first complete treatise on epilepsy during the present generation. It represents the practical experience of the author for ten years as Superintendent of the famous Craig Colony for Epileptics at Sonyea, New York. There has been marked progress of late years in the knowledge and treatment of this important nervous disease, all of which is fully portrayed in the forelying volume. Treatment is discussed with the ripe wisdom of a well-rounded and thorough knowledge of the subject. The phases and stigmata of the disease are fully illustrated, mostly from photographs. For those who wish to know what there is to learn about epilepsy, this is the book.

OBSTETRIC AND GYNECOLOGIC NURSING. By Edward P. Davis, A. M., M. D., Professor of Obstetrics in the Jefferson Medical College and in the Philadelphia Polyclinic. 12mo volume of 402 pages, fully illustrated. Second Edition, thoroughly revised. Philadelphia, New York, London: W. B. Saunders & Company, 1904. Polished Buckram, $1.75 net.

Prof. Davis is well fitted to write this book for nurses, and he has taken pains to make the text simple, practical and complete. He tells the nurse not only what to do and how to do it, but also what not to do. The second edition of the work has been carefully revised throughout, and considerable new matter has been added. It is instructively illustrated.

CLINICAL TREATISES ON THE PATHOLOGY AND THERAPY OF DISORDERS OF METABOLISM AND NUTRITION. By Dr. Carl Von Noorden, Physician in Chief to the City Hospital, Frankfort A. M. Authorized American Edition, translated under the direction of Boardman Reed, M. D. Part IV. *The Acid Autointoxications.* Price, 50 cents. New York: E. B. Treat & Company. 1903.

In this brochure the authors (Drs. Von Noorden and Mohr) consider the forms of self-poisoning due to acetone, diacetic acid and oxybutyric acid, occurring in diabetes and other diseased conditions. They have gone into the subject very thoroughly. Some old theories are finally disproved, and many new facts with definite clinical bearings are educed. The volume will well repay a careful perusal.

THE MOTHER'S MANUAL. A Month to Month Guide for Young Mothers. By Emelyn Lincoln Coolidge, M. D., Visiting Physician of the Out-Patient Department of the Babies' Hospital, New York. Illustrated. New York: A. S. Barnes & Company. 1904.

This tasteful little volume tells what the baby does and what should be done for it up to the seventh year. The text is replete with little practical points of prophylactic importance, which the young mother has generally been forced to learn by sad experience. The book shows no evidence of faddism, and can be safely recommended to mothers by the family physician.

CLINICAL TREATISES ON THE PATHOLOGY AND THERAPY OF DISORDERS OF METABOLISM AND NUTRITION. PART V. CONCERNING THE EFFECTS OF SALINE WATERS (KISSINGEN, HAMBURG) ON METABOLISM. By Prof. Carl Von

Noorden, Frankfort, and Dr. Carl Dapper, Bad Kissingen. Price 50 cents. New York: E. B. Treat & Company, 1904.

This brochure is of considerable practical value since, on scientific evidence, it sets to rest a number of disputed points regarding the use of saline waters. The text consists largely of clinical reports, and the accompanying laboratory findings. The authors conclude that in many cases of gastric disorder, particularly gastric catarrh, the use of saline mineral waters leads to an active and permanent increase in the production of hydrochloric acid, while, on the other hand, many cases accompanied by hyperacidity (particularly in nervous dyspepsia) are likewise benefited by drinking these waters. The administration of the waters does not call for any particular diet.

THE PRACTICAL MEDICINE SERIES OF YEAR BOOKS, comprising Ten Volumes on the Year's Progress in Medicine and Surgery. Issued monthly. Volume V. *Obstetrics.* Edited by Joseph B. De Lee, M. D., Professor of Obstetrics, Northwestern University Medical School. Price of this volume, $1.00; of the series, $5.50. April, 1904. Chicago: The Year Book Publishers, 40 Dearborn street.

The compiler has covered the ground fully and impartially; in the more practical subjects collating the views of many authors side by side. Particular attention has been given to diseases of the puerperium, both for the mother and the babe.

SELECTIONS.

SANATORIUM.—Great plains open air sanatorium.   Dr. John Fewkes, Superintendent, Lamar, Colorado.

A WONDERFUL REMEDY.—J. G. Steiner, A. M., M. D., Knoxdale, Jefferson county, Pa., says: "Satyria is a wonderful remedy. It has not disappointed me in any trial, but to the contrary is the best preparation of all remedies in its class. Have accomplished wonders in cystitis, gonorrhœa, suppression of urine and impotency."

ALETRIS CORDIAL.—Where hysteria is the result of uterine troubles, aletris cordial Rio, combined with celerina, is an excellent remedy.

SEMINAL EMISSIONS AND GENERAL WEAKNESS.—
    ℞   Tr. Nux Vom.............2 drachms
       Satyria...............q. s. 8 ounces
  M. Sig. Teaspoonful four times daily.

SOMETHING TO CONSIDER.—After many trials of a remedy that has previously given you satisfaction, have you ever experienced a time when results seemed to fail? You evidently presumed that your old standby had lost its efficacy, when in reality, if upon investigation, you will many times find that your patient is taking a worthless substitute and not the genuine product. Dysmenorrhœa, that most painful affliction of women, readily responds to treatment with Hayden's Viburnum Compound, and as this well-known remedy is always uniform in composition, uniform good results follow its administration. All reputable products are imitated, which is the best evidence of the value of the original preparation, therefore, where pain is manifest. it is important that the genuine Hayden's Viburnum Compound be administered.

HOW TO AVOID PRESCRIBING OPIUM AND MORPHINE.—Dr. N. B. Shade of Washington, D. C., in an article published in the *Medical Summary* refers to many unfortunate effects of prescribing opium and morphine. intimating that the depressing after-effects of the administration of these drugs more than offsets the temporary good accomplished by their use. He mentions a very prominent congressman whose life, in his opinion, was cut short by the administration of morphine hypodermically in the case of pneumonitis. Dr. Shade states that he still prescribes morphine, but very seldom, as he finds it much safer to use papine. Papine, in his opinion, possesses all the desirable qualities of opium with the bad qualities eliminated. Some of the brightest minds of the present age are now being devoted to the development of a therapy in which the primitive bad effects of many important drugs are eliminated. Where the therapeutic action of morphine is desired, it would seem to be a safe procedure to give papine a trial.

GOOD AND SEASONABLE.—A word about some remedial preparations which the busy practitioner will find always useful, particularly at this season of the year, will no doubt be of interest. First, we will mention the old time-tried antikamnia and salol tablet, so useful during the hot weather, when even the "grown folks" load up their stomachs with the first offerings of the season. Hare says: "Salol renders the intestinal canal antiseptic and is the most valued drug in intestinal affections." The anodyne properties of antikamnia in connection with salol render this tablet very useful in dysentery, indigestion, cholera morbus, diarrhœa, colic, and all conditions due to intestinal fermentation. Then the "triple alliance" remedy so well and favorably known by its self explanatory title, namely: "Laxative Antikamnia and Quinine Tablets." To reduce fever, quiet pain, and at the same time administer a gentle tonic-laxative, is to accomplish a great deal with a single tablet. Among the many diseases and affections which call for such a combination, we might mention coryza, coughs, and summer colds, chills and fever, biliousness, dengue and malaria with their general discomfort and great debility.

We cannot overlook our old friend, the antikamnia and codeine tablet. The efficacy of this tablet in neuroses of the larynx is well known, but do all of our doctor friends know that it is especially useful in dysmenorrhœa, utero-ovarian pain and pain in general caused by suppressed or irregular menses? This tablet controls the pain of these disorders in the shortest time and by the most natural and economic method. The synergetic action of these drugs is ideal, for not only are their sedative and analgesic properties unsurpassed, but they are followed by no unpleasant after-effects.

AN OBSTINATE CASE OF GOUTY ECZEMA.—By E. Foucault, M. D. (Paris). History. Patient, Mr. F., aet. 49, well nourished, no family history of gout, had dieted for years (on advice of dermatologists whom he had consulted in Europe and in this country, for his skin affection). He had a previous attack of acute gout a year before. There was some tendency to obesity and varicose veins. He was suffering from a severe attack of gout and I put him on the usual treatment, viz: colchi-sal capsules in full doses for the first three days (16 capsules daily), and recommended him to reduce the dose to four capsules daily, as soon as the severe pain and inflammation around the articulations, were removed.

Saline purgatives were prescribed to be continued for a week at least. He responded nicely to this treatment on the third day, when I recommended him to continue the colchi-sal in doses of four capsules daily for a week and to take four during one day each week for some time, to prevent a return of the symptoms. My patient on this occasion, showed me his arms and chest which were almost raw and so covered with old scars, that it was almost impossible to say from what form of skin disease he was suffering. These scars he complained came from the intolerable itching, owing to the heat of the bed clothes, which compelled him to scratch himself in the night. This condition he had long come to look on as a part and parcel of his daily cross, for while at times, he was less troubled than others, he was never free from it and he despaired of a cure, since all treatments had failed to relieve him permanently. Severe diet seemed to be the only effective method of getting relief.

Since he had seen so many well known authorities, who must have recognized the gouty nature of the eczema, I hardly expected to be more fortunate and I prescribed simply solutions of bicarbonate of soda to be applied and a little zinc ointment to the abrasions caused by the scratching. A week later, my patient came to my office, delighted at what he called my "cure." The irritation had entirely left him for the first time in 26 years and up to date of writing (which is eight months since he began to take colchi-sal), there has been no return of the gouty eczema. His skin is free from redness or even signs of urticaria, but during this period, he has had two slight attacks of gout in the big toe, which however did not last long. The patient continues to take four capsules of colchi-sal one day of each week.

EDITORIAL ITEMS.— Continued.

Cerebral Pneumonia.—The ataxic apex pneumonia of drunkards, with marked cerebral symptoms, is treated by Anders with hydrotherapy, including the ice cap; arterial stimulants and morphine.

Lacerating Injury of Brain Tissue.—Charles C. Allison advocates the ice cap; mercurials and morphine or bromides; and a dark, quiet room. No operative interference should take place until shock has been combatted and reaction secured, unless there is excessive hemorrhage.

Injury to the Cervical Spine.—Perfect rest, says Herbert W. Page, is the chief consideration. Asepsis for wounds is in order, and hot flannels or linseed poultices for sprains. Ice locally —and ergot or gallic acid internally are indicated for hemorrhage.

Spinal Apoplexy.—Gowers advises absolute rest on face or side; scarify beside the spine opposite seat of pain, allowing blood to flow freely; follow this with application of ice and administration of ergotin; move bowels freely; sedatives usually required for pain.

Traumatic Fever.—Frederick S. Eve advises drainage, cleanliness and avoidance of tension; remove sources of irritation and pain if possible; aconite early;· quinine or sponging with tepid water or the bath for excessive fever; cinchona when hectic, the result of exhausting discharges.

Traumatic Asphyxia.—The institution of artificial respiration, in conjunction with oxygen inhalations *(Journal of American Medical Association)* is of most service immediately after the release of an individual who has been subjected to forcible compression and presents livid or cyanotic discoloration of the face and neck.

The Rhythmical Pulsating Pain of Renal Colic.—Angelo Signorelli (quoted in *Medical Record*) calls attention to the rhythmical pulsating pain, which he considers peculiar to this affection, which is present only during the violent colic and which is due to increase of tension in the arteries obstructed by the calculus.

Saline Enemata.—MacCallum (*Journal of American Medical Association*) has studied the effect of saline purgatives and diuretics, and finds that the sodium salts are safest and most effective. The premature expulsion of saline enemata, owing to the peristaltic effect of the sodium chloride, can be prevented by the addition of a small amount of calcium chloride, which is in general inhibitory to the action of sodium salts.

Management of Apoplexy.—Anders advises to keep quiet as possible in the recumbent posture with the head somewhat elevated and clothing loose around neck; ice bag to head and hot bricks or hot water bottles to feet; sinapisms to back of neck or other parts of body; venesection if pulse full, strong and incompressible and face congested; one or two drops of croton oil by mouth—also an enema; liquid food for several days.

Value of Olive Oil in Gastrointestinal Diseases.—Cohnheim (quoted in *Journal of American Medical Association*) has found olive oil effectual in relieving and curing gastrectasia not due to an organic obstacle, and even in organic and relative stenosis it proves a valuable lubricant. He gives a wineglassful half an hour or an hour before meals, two or three times a day. The remedy is of no benefit in purely nervous or hysteric gastric affections.

Practical Method of Destroying Snake Venom.—It is positively established, says L. Rogers (quoted in *Medical News*) that potassium permanganate will destroy *in vitro* nearly its own weight in every class of snake venom. Brunton and Fayrer advise ligation above the inoculation, then incision of the wound, followed by the rubbing in of pure crystals of the salt. Brunton has devised a lance surrounded by a sheath in the base of which permanganate crystals are kept, the whole outfit being easily carried in one corner of the vest pocket.

Bacteriologic Diagnosis of Typhoid Fever.—Ruth and Rider *(Journal of American Medical Association)* place the bacteriologic examination of the blood above even the Widal reaction. They say that Eberth's bacillus can be found in from 80 to 90 per cent. of the cases, most frequently from the second to the fifth day, a much earlier date than the agglutination test. The skin of the forearm is sterilized, a vein rendered prominent, and by means of a sterile aspirator needle, blood is withdrawn, and inoculated into a tube of blood serum or agar, and after from 24 to 48 hours in an incubator the bacillus is identified by its cultural and morphologic peculiarities. The use of plate cultures is recommended as an aid in the identification of the colonies, and an additional safeguard against contamination of the cultures.

Sterilizing Catgut.—Weller Van Hook *(Medical News,* May 14) has used the Elsberg method for two years with great satisfaction. Select raw, rough, unbleached material. Soak for a week in pure ether or a mixture of one part chloroform and two parts ether. Wind on glass spools in single layers. Soak for three days in aqueous solution of chromic acid 1:1000. Boil for twenty minutes in water to which, while boiling, chemically pure ammonium sulphate has been added until the crystals cease to dissolve. Wash the catgut for half an hour in cold water. Place the spools in a solution of corrosive sublimate, one part in 1000 parts of 95% alcohol. Should the material become infected, it may be reboiled. The use of the ammonium sulphate depends on the principle that organic substances are insoluble in the fluids by which they are precipitated from their solutions.

Fetal Nutrition.—J. Veit (quoted in *Obstetrics, Practical Medicine Series)* explains the special blood changes in pregnant women as due to deportation of chorionic villi and interaction of these with the red and white blood cells. Using the hemolytic method of Ehrlich, he finds there is formed syncytiolysin and hemolysin, producing a solution of hemoglobin and syncitial protoplasm in the blood serum. The nourishment of the child depends on the absorption of albumin dissolved in the serum, and the loss of substance due to dissolution of chorion epithelium is replaced by syncitium growth. This balance of exchange may be disturbed, as when too many chorionic villi are deported. Then hemolysis produces hemoglobinemia, albuminuria, hemoglobinuria and less syncytiolysis. When too little chorionic epithelium is received, the pregnancy changes are less marked, and on these differences may depend certain abnormal nutritional conditions of the fetus and diseases of pregnancy.

Age and Smallpox.—The age incidence of smallpox has been markedly altered by the general practice of vaccination. In the 18th century 95% of the deaths from this plague were in children under ten years. Of new-born children one-third died of smallpox in the first year—one-half before the fifth year. In Massachusetts during twelve years, 1888-99, the variola mortality of children in the total population constituted 26% of the total deaths from this cause, but no vaccinated children under ten years died of smallpox. A parish priest in London has recently issued a sermon-pamphlet beginning with these words: "In the town of Gloucester there is a beautiful cemetery, and in one corner of the cemetery there are the graves of no less than 280 little children, all under ten years of age, all of whom died seven years ago when a terrible attack of smallpox visited that town. Of these 280 children who died of smallpox, 279 were unvaccinated, and only one was vaccinated."

Points on Taking Temperature.—The carefully taken records of Burton-Fanning and Champion *(International Medical Annual)* show that the rectal temperature is on an average 0.4° higher than that of the mouth, 0.6° higher than the groin, and 0.9° higher than the axilla. In healthy men a very slight amount of movement only is required to produce an appreciable rise in the mercury, while with more exertion they noted a rise of as much as $3\frac{1}{2}°$. These fluctuations can be reliably observed only in the rectum. The exercise reaction is not peculiar to tuberculosis, but usually exceeds that of health or other diseases. The authors note the frequency of a distinct rise of temperature during the six days preceding menstruation in 18 out of 34 women

under treatment for, pulmonary tuberculosis. They recommend
keeping the mouth closed on the thermometer for ten minutes,
particularly after breathing cool air with parted lips, exercise en-
tailing rapid respiration, or the contact of cold with the outside
of the cheeks. They also found that certain drugs raised the oral
temperature, presumably by dilating the capillaries. Thus, the
sucking of a menthol lozenge for half a minute caused a rise
of 1.6°.

Knopf on Tubercular Homoptysis.—His treatment comprises absolute rest and reassurrance; small pieces of ice to suck
or small sips of ice water; morphine or atropine by injection, or
hydrastis canadensis; bags of morseled ice, or a piece of coarse
linen wrung out of cold water and folded triangularly (renewed
as warmed), placed over pectoral region of apices; hypodermic of
ether, digitalin or caffeine if much shock, or rectal irrigation with
hot saline solution; venous ligation of lower or upper limbs near
trunk, loosening bands every half hour or so; hot water bag to
feet; ergot or gallic acid (dose, ten grains) and iced drinks continued for some time after hemorrhage stopped. He advises deep,
quiet respirations every 30 or 60 seconds in an hour or two after
an acute attack of hemoptysis has subsided, to hasten complete
cessation of bloody expectorations; also outdoor life and respiratory exercises or pneumatic cabinet treatment and careful administration of saline cathartics, for chronic bloody expectoration due
to congestion of respiratory organs.

Compulsory Vaccination.—The imperial German law, put
in force April 1, 1875, requires the vaccination of every child
before September of the year following its birth, and revaccination of all the inhabitants every twelve years. It has been executed with exceptional thoroughness, and the results have been
most striking, lowering the death rate from smallpox of 262.67
per 100,000 inhabitants in 1872 to a general average of 1.91 per
100,000 in the years 1875-86. No other nation has enforced
compulsory vaccination so completely and continuously, and at
the present time Germany is the only country that enjoys comparative immunity from variola. The disease has indeed become
almost exotic, nearly all the cases occurring on the borders of

the empire in persons who have crossed from neighboring territory. In 1899 the total deaths from smallpox in 185 German towns with a population of nearly 16,000,000 was only four. In the same year 116 French towns with a population of 8,500,000 showed a mortality from smallpox of 600. Out of only 28 deaths in the whole empire from smallpox, 14 occurred in unprotected infants under two years of age. It should be remembered that variola was formerly reckoned a disease of childhood, as measles is now.

Smallpox Pandemics.—The rather passive public aspect to the use and need of vaccination was changed to one of active interest by the European smallpox pandemic of 1870-73, due chiefly to the Franco-Prussian war. In the French army vaccination had been greatly neglected, and revaccination was unknown. The German recruits, on the other hand, had been generally vaccinated in childhood, and were revaccinated on entering the service. The results of this difference in prophylaxis were that the mortality of the French was nearly fifty times that of the Germans, with twice as many deaths to the total number of cases. The German field army, numbering over a million men, had, during the year of the war and the pandemic, 4,991 cases of smallpox with 297 deaths, a death rate of 5.97%. The total number of cases of the disease in the French army is unknown, but was enormous, causing a death loss of 23,469 men. At the same time the German soldiers succumbed to other diseases often in greater numbers than the French troops, notably so from dysentery and typhoid fever. That this great difference regarding variola was due solely to vaccination and revaccination, is shown by the mortality records of Berlin (population in 1871, 826,341), then only partially vaccinated. In this city of less people than were in the German army there occurred 5,508 deaths from smallpox—nearly twenty times the number in the more exposed but thoroughly vaccinated army.

Hemoptysis of Systemic Origin.—In vasomotor affections adrenal substance, five or ten grains every two or three hours, is useful. The common arteriosclerotic type is remedied with nitroglycerin. Pulmonary syphilis requires mercurials and potassium iodide. Salicylates are specific in those cases of frequent occurrence in the subjects of lithemia and rheumatism. Neurotic cases, says, Mays, should be given strychnine in progressive doses, beginning in adults at 1-32 grain four times a day, and gradually increasing to limit of tolerance; rest is also a vital factor. Suggestive treatment, aided if need by electricity, is the best for hysterical cases. In hemophilic subjects Ochsner advises to lessen tendency to bleeding by giving four to six whites of eggs thrice daily. For anæmic subjects Bartholow prescribes nux vomica with syrup of iron and phosphates of quinine and strychnine. Hemophila with pulmonary tuberculosis and frequent hemoptysis is treated by Knopf with a saturated solution of potassium iodide, five drops in milk increased gradually to fifteen drops three times a day. In the black hemoptysis of infectious fevers quinine, strychnine, alcoholics and other remedies are indicated to counteract the toxemic infection. Alcoholic cases of hemoptysis are treated by Mays with tincture of capsicum, one-half to one dram every hour or two in water, with strychnine and morphine, and suppositories of asafœtida in large doses.

Denver and Gross College of Medic

Medical Department University of Denver

EDMUND J. A. ROGERS, A.M., M.D.,
Professor of Surgery.

THOMAS H. HAWKINS, A.M., M.D.,
Professor of Gynecology and Abdominal Surgery.

EDMUND C. RIVERS, A.M., M.D.,
Professor of Ophthalmology.

ROBERT LEVY, M.D., Secretary.
Professor of Laryngology, Rhinology and Otology.

HENRY SEWALL, PH.D., M.D.,
Professor of Physiology.

WILLIAM H. DAVIS, M.D.,
Professor of Dermatology and Venereal Diseases.

CHARLES B. LYMAN, M.D.,
Professor of Fractures and Dislocations.

WILLIAM J. ROTHWELL, M.D.,
Professor of Medicine.

JOHN M. FOSTER, M.D.,
Professor of Otology.

CAREY K. FLEMING, M.D.,
Professor of Gynecology and Abdominal Surgery.

FRANCIS H. McNAUGHT, M.D.,
Professor of Obstetrics.

LEONARD FREEMAN, B.S., A.M., MD.,
Professor of Surgery.

HORACE G. WETHERILL, M.D.,
Professor of Gynecology and Abdominal Surgery.

JOSIAH N. HALL, B.S., M.D.,
Professor of Medicine.

CHARLES A. POWERS, A.M., M.D.,
Professor of Surgery.

CHARLES F. SHOLLENBERGER, M.D.,
Professor of Pediatrics.

HOWELL T. PERSHING, M.Sc., M.D.,
Professor of Nervous and Mental Diseases.

EDWARD C. HILL, M.Sc., M. D.,
Professor of Chemistry and Toxicology.

HERBERT B. WHITNEY, A.B., M.D.,
Professor of Medicine.

HORACE G. HARVEY, A.B., M.D.,
Professor of Fractures and Dislocations.

SHERMAN G. BONNEY, A.M., M.D., Dean,
Professor of Medicine.

MOSES KLEINER, M.D.,
Professor of Therapeutics.

GEORGE B. PACKARD, M.D.,
Professor of Orthopedic Surgery.

T. MITCHELL BURNS, M.D.,
Professor of Obstetrics.

WALTER A. JAYNE, M.D.,
Professor of Gynecology and Abdominal Su

CHARLES B. VAN ZANT, M.D.,
Professor of Physiology.

CARROLL E. EDSON, A.M., M.D.,
Professor of Therapeutics.

MELVILLE BLACK, M.D.,
Professor of Ophthalmology.

JAMES M. BLAINE, M.D.,
Professor of Dermatology and Venereal Di

WILLIAM C. MITCHELL, M.D.,
Professor of Bacteriology.

DAVID H. COOVER, M.D.,
Professor of Ophthalmology.

SAMUEL B. CHILDS, A.M., M.D.,
Professor of Anatomy.

JAMES H. PERSHING, A.B.,
Professor of Medical Jurisprudence.

JOHN A. WILDER, M.D.,
Professor of Pathology.

SAMUEL D. HOPKINS, M.D.,
Professor of Nervous and Mental Diseases.

PHILIP HILLKOWITZ, B.S., M.D.,
Professor of Pathology.

WILLIAM C. BANE, M.D.,
Professor of Ophthalmology and Otology.

Four years' graded course. Sessions of eight months each. 23d Annual Sessions begins September 15, 1903. Matriculation fee, $5.00. Tuition fee, $100.00. Well-equipped laboratories in all departments and excellent clinical advantages in dispensary and hospitals.

The climate of **COLORADO** offers many advantages to students whose health compels them to leave the east

Catalogue on application.

Sherman G. Bonney, A.M., M.D., Dean

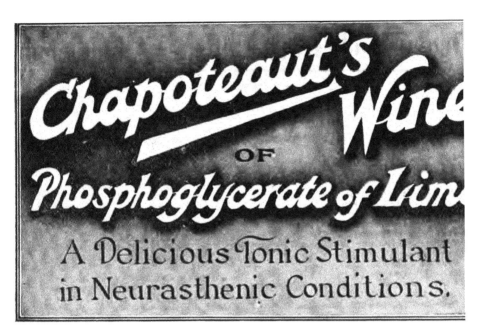

Agents: E. Fouger

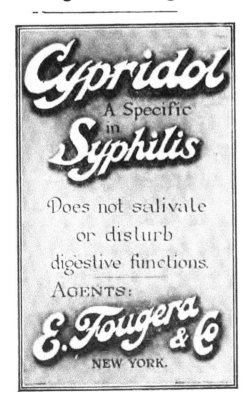

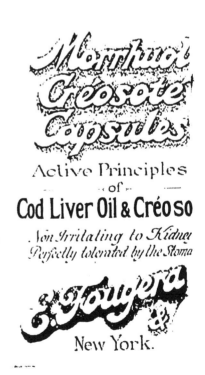

DENVER MEDICAL TIMES

Volume XXIV.   AUGUST, 1904.   Number 2.

NORMAL OBSTETRICS.

THE OBSTETRIC ANATOMY OF THE BONY PELVIS.
CHAPTER ONE.

BY T. MITCHELL BURNS, M. D.,

Denver, Colo.

Prof. of Obstetrics, The Denver and Gross College of Medicine.

The Obstetric Bony Pelvis includes, besides the ossa innominata, the sacrum, and the coccyx, the last two lumbar vertebræ.

The Static Pelvis is the bony pelvis. The Dynamic Pelvis is the pelvis in the living subject in labor (soft, mobile and active).

THE BONES OF THE PELVIS.

THE SACRUM (PLURAL, SACRA).

The Sacrum is wedge-shaped. The promontory is the projection formed by the anterior superior border of the body of the sacrum. The first transverse line (linea transversa) may project sufficiently to be mistaken for the promontory. The curvature of the sacrum varies, being generally well marked, rarely nearly straight.

THE COCCYX (CYGES).

The Coccyx, tail or "crupper bone," is triangular in shape. Anomalies of its apex, or lower end, are deviation forward, backward or laterally, and bifurcation. Ankylosis of the coccyx to the sacrum occurs between the 45th and 50th year. In those who have not given birth to children or who sit much, as dressmakers or equestriennes, it may be earlier. Horseback riding is given as the cause of the frequency of the low forceps operation in England.

THE OS (SL) INNOMINATUM (A).—THE ILIUM (A).

The Ilium presents a crest which is S-shaped. The anterior end of this crest is directed forward and inwards and is called the anterior superior spinous process; the posterior end is called the posterior superior spinous process, and is represented by a dimple in the surface of the skin. About one inch below the anterior superior spinous process, and separated from it by a notch, is the anterior inferior spinous process. The same distance below the posterior superior process, and separated from it by a notch (which lies close to the sacrum in the articulated pelvis), is the posterior inferior spinous process.

THE PUBIS (ES).

The Pubic Spine is the prominence on the upper border of the pubic bone about three-fourths of an inch from the pubic joint.

The Pubic Crest is a ridge on the upper border of the pubis between the public spine and the public joint.

The Pectine Pubis is the sharp ridge on the upper border of the pubis between the pubic spine and the ilio-pectineal eminence.

The Ilio-pectineal Eminence is the large eminence on the upper surface of the union of the horizontal ramus of the pubis with the ilium (or on the horizontal ramus of the pubis near its union with the ilium.—Jewett.)

The Pubic Arch and Angle are made by the union above of the inner or lower borders of the two descending rami of the pubes.

THE ISCHIUM (A).

The Tuberosity of the Ischium is the broad, rough eminence on which the body rests in sitting.

The Spine of the Ischium is a very well marked spine projecting into the pelvic cavity from about the middle of the posterior border of the ischium.

The Great Sacro-Sciatic Notch is between the spine and tuberosity of the ischium.

The Lesser Sacro-Sciatic Notch is between the spine and the tuberosity of the ischium.

THE PELVIS AS A WHOLE.

The True Pelvis, small or lower pelvis, is that part of the pelvis below the brim (or the ilio-pectineal line).

The Brim (or margin) of the true pelvis consists of the ilio-pectineal lines, the anterior superior border of each wing of the sacrum, and the promontory.

Each Ilio-pectineal or Innominate Line consists of the ridge just below the iliac fossa, the ilio-pectineal eminence, the pectine pubis, the pubic spine and the crest of the pubis.

The term Pelvis alone signifies the whole pelvis or the true pelvis.

The False Pelvis is composed of the two lumbar vertebræ, the wings of the ilia, and is completed in front by the abdominal wall.

The True Pelvis consists of the sacrum, coccyx, ischia and the portion of the ilia below the innominate line.

THE SUPERIOR STRAIT.

The Superior Strait, inlet or isthmus (of the pelvis) is the opening into the true pelvic cavity from above.

It is bounded by the brim. (Anatomically this is correct, but obstetrically it is anteriorly a little lower than the anatomical brim because of the projecting in of the upper part of the posterior surface of the pubic bones.)

Its shape is like a heart.

Its axis extended upward would strike the navel, downward the coccyx. (The downward extension of this axis illustrates the direction in which traction should be made when the forceps are used at the inlet.)

DIAMETERS.

The Anterior-Posterior:—The Anatomical Conjugate extends from the promontory to the union of the posterior and superior surfaces of the pubic joint and measures $4\frac{1}{4}$ inches.

The Obstetric Conjugate extends from the promontory to a point on the posterior surface of the pubic joint nearest the promonotory, a point about one-fourth of an inch below the upper surface of the pubic joint.

The Oblique Diameters extend from one ilio-pectineal eminence to the opposite sacro-iliac joint, and measure five inches each.

The First Oblique Diameter extends from the left ilio-pectineal emience to the right sacro-iliac joint. It is called the first oblique because the long diameter of the head more often passes down through this oblique than through the opposite oblique, i. e., because it is first in frequency of use.

The Second Oblique Diameter is the opposite one, extending from the right ilio-pectineal eminence to the left sacro-iliac joint.

It is called second because second in frequency of use. (The first oblique is also called in France, Germany and America the right oblique, being named after the right sacro-iliac joint, but as in England it is called the left oblique, after the left ilio-pectineal eminence, the terms first and second oblique are preferable.)

The Transverse Diameter extends from the points on the ilio-pectineal lines which are farthest aprt. It measures 5¼ inches.

The Largest Diameter of the Inlet then in the bony pelvis is the transverse, 5¼ inches. This is not the case in the dynamic pelvis.

The Antero-Posterior Diameter is increased by extension and superextension of the lower extremities. Walcher's position is the dorsal position with superextension of the lower extremities effected by having the buttocks on the edge of the bed or table and the lower extremities falling downward.

THE INFERIOR STRAIT.

The Inferior Strait, or outlet, is the opening out of the pelvis cavity below.

It is bounded by the sub-pubic ligament in front, by the tip of the coccyx posteriorly, and laterally by the rami of the pubis and ischium, by the tuberosity of the ischium and by the great sacro-sciatic ligament.

Its shape is like a lozenge or a diamond with the edge of the figure rounded off.

Its Axis extended upward would strike the promontory; extended downward would strike the anus.

DIAMETERS.

The Antero-Posterior extends from the sub-pubic ligament to the tip of the coccyx and measures 3¾ inches, but as normally the coccyx recedes whenever there is any pressure from above, its practical length is 4½ inches, making it the *longest diameter of the outlet* in the normal bony and also in the dynamic pelvis.

The Oblique Diameters extend from the junction of the descending ramus of the pubis and the ascending ramus of the ischium of one side to about the middle of the great sacro-sciatic ligament of the opposite side. Because of the yielding of the sacro-sciatic ligaments, the average length of the oblique diameters is not given, but it is well to remember that the oblique diameters are greater than the transverse, and may be greater than the antero-posterior provided the coccyx does not recede.

The Transverse Diameter extends between the nearest points on the two ischial tuberosities and measures 4¼ inches.

The Antero-Posterior Diameter of the Outlet is increased by flexion of the thighs onto the abdomen.

THE PELVIC CAVITY.

The Pelvic Cavity is in the space in the pelvis between the superior and inferior straits.

It is bounded in front by the bodies of the pubes, laterally by the horizontal and descending rami of the pubis and the ischium and the part of the ilium below the innominate line, and posteriorly by the sacrum and coccyx.

Its shape is somewhat cylindrical or barrel like. The depth of its walls vary; in front at the pubic joint it measures 1¾ inches, laterally from the brim to the tuberosity 3½ inches, and posteriorly from the promontory to the tip of the coccyx 5 inches. (The distance following the curvature of the sacrum is about 5½ inches, but this is not the depth.)

Its Axis:—Between the superior strait and a plane drawn backward from the subpubic ligament parallel with the plane of the inlet, i. e., to the middle of the second sacral vertebræ, it is straight and parallel with the axis of the inlet. From this subpubic plane to the inferior strait it is curved, representing the arc of a circle, which if extended beyond the outlet would reach the navel. This whole curve from the subpubic plane to the navel is called the Curve of Carus. The direction of this axis illustrates how traction should be made when the forceps are used. If the head is at the inlet, the traction should be first downward and backward towards the coccyx to correspond with the straight part of the canal, then downward and forward to correspond with the curvature of the lower part of the cavity.

DIAMETERS.

The Diameters of the Pelvic Cavity are larger than those of the straits, but their lengths vary considerably in different planes.

The Antero-Posterior is longer than that of the inlet, because of the curvature of the sacrum, and is longest between the subpubic ligament and the middle of the second sacral vertebra.

The Transverse Diameter above is as long as that of the inlet, but it diminishes from above downwards.

The Medium Strait or Obstetric Outlet is the narrowest part of the pelvic cavity. It is situated between the subpubic ligament, the lower end of the sacrum and the spines of the ischia. Its antero-posterior diameter, from the subpubic ligament to the end of the sacrum, measures 4½ inches, and the transverse diameter between the spines of the ischia measures 4 inches.

The so-called Inclined Planes of the Pelvic Cavity are not really planes, but the curved surfaces of the lateral walls of the pelvic cavity. They are four in number, two anterior and two posterior. The anterior inclined planes each consist of the side wall of the pelvic cavity between the pubic joint and a line drawn from a point on the ilio-pectineal line half way between the ilio-pectineal eminence and the sacro-iliac joint to the spine of the ischium. The posterior inclined planes each consist of the side wall of the pelvic cavity between the posterior boundary of the anterior plane and the medium line of the sacrum. These planes are concave from before backwards, and the anterior, the larger, slopes downward and forward towards the median line, i. e., towards the pubic joint; the posterior slopes downward and backward towards the median line of the sacrum. Hence, an end of an ovoid object, like the fetal head, tends to pass forward as it enters an anterior inclined plane, and backwtrd as it enters a posterior plane.

THE PELVIC JOINTS.

The Pelvic Joints are limited in motion, except the sacro-coccygeal. Next in freedom of motion comes the joint between the last lumbar vertebra and the sacrum, then the pubic joint, and lastly the sacro-iliac joint. Pregnancy, by infiltration, increases the motion of the pelvic joints, and during pregnancy the pubic joint can be felt to move by placing the index finger beneath it while the patient stands first upon one foot and then upon the other. In symphysiotomy during pregnancy the sacro-iliac joint can be safely separated sufficiently to allow the pubic joint to spread 3 inches.

The pubic joint contains a central disk of cartilage, but no synovial fluid; the sacro-iliac joint has no central disk of cartilage, but may possible have a little synovial fluid.

THE PELVIC LIGAMENTS.

The ligaments of the Sacro-Iliac joint are much stronger behind than those in front. Hence, in symphysiotomy they allow separation of the joint in front, but prevent it posteriorly.

The Great Sacro-Sciatic ligament is attached by its broad end to the posterior surface of the wing of the sacrum and by its narrow end to the tuberosity of the ischium. This ligament converts the lesser sacro-sciatic notch into a foramen.

The Lesser Sacro-Sciatic ligament is attached to the lateral border of the coccyx, and then comes together like a fan and is attached to the spine of the ischium and converts the great sacro-sciatic notch into a foramen.

The Subpubic Ligament is nearly half an inch in depth and is very dense. The other pubic ligaments, superior, anterior and posterior, are thin.

THE OBLIQUITY OF THE PELVIS.

The obliquity, inclination or position of the pelvis means the angle which the pelvis forms with the rest of the vertebral column. For convenience it is estimated by the angle which the plane of the inlet forms with the horizon, an angle on the average of about 55 degrees. (This obliquity is due to the anterior portion of the last lumbar vertebra, the first sacral vertebra and the intervening cartilage being thicker in front than behind, and to the manner in which the ilia join the sacrum.) It can be increased by superextension of the thighs, which is assisted by placing a firm object, such as a compressed pillow, under the small of the back. It is diminished by flexion of the thighs, which is assisted by a firm object under the sacrum.

By remembering that the promontory is 3½ inches above the upper surface of the pubes, an idea of the amount of the average pelvic obliquity is obtained, and also where the fingers should be passed to reach the promontory or the fundus of the uterus through the abdominal wall.

CAUSES OF DIFFERENCES IN PELVES.

The Causes of Difference in Pelves are the character of the genitals, male or female, well or poorly developed, muscular development and heredity or race.

THE DIFFERENCES BETWEEN THE MALE AND THE FEMALE PELVIS.

These can best be remembered by considering what changes

in the male pelvis would make it possible for the fetal head to pass through it, viz., increase of the diameters of the inlet by making the projection of the promontory less marked, and by further separation of the ilia; increase of the cavity by increased curvature of the sacrum and further separation of the ischial spines; lessened depth of the cavity (to diminish the time of passage); increase of the outlet by further separation of the tuberosities of the ischia; increased obliquity of the pelvis to make the axes of the uterus and pelvis correspond; and lessened thickness of the bones to make them more elastic and not heavier than those of the female pelvis. (The increase in the curvature of the lower end of the sacrum seems to be an exception to the above, but this is probably of value in directing the fetal head towards the vulvar orifice, and the setting back of the whole sacrum more than compensates for the bending forward of the lower end.) The alæ of the ilia are made more flaring in the female to give rest for the pregnant uterus.

THE RACIAL CHARACTER OF THE FEMALE PELVIS.

The form and size of the female pelvis depends upon the race, or rather on the conditions of nutrition and activity. Pelvic deviation from the normal Caucasian type consists in a relative elongation of the antero-posterior diameters. Thus in the Australian the outline is nearly circular and in the Bush woman the antero-posterior exceeds the transverse diameter. The pelvis of the Laplander is small.

(To be continued.)

AN OUTLINE OF HEMATURIA.

BY EDWARD C. HILL, M. D.

Medical Analyst and Microscopist; Professor of Chemistry and Toxicology in the Denver and Cross College of Medicine.

Reacts to chemic tests for hemoglobin and shows red corpuscles under microscope—swollen and more spheric in alkaline urine; crenated and shrunken in dense, acid urine—reduced to shadows if long in urine. One to 1,500 makes urine smoky; one to 500 bright red; chocolate brown if much acted on by urine.

Hematoidin crystals show previous hemorrhages—always present in chronic abscess of kidneys and often in vesical tuberculosis or cancer. Intermittent hematuria (considerable albumin and rise of temperature) usually gives history of gout, ague or intermittent chyluria.

RENAL.

Amount usually slight, well mixed with urine, which is generally smoky—spectroscope shows methemoglobin absorption bands; microscopic blood casts, red blood cells more or less fragmented, faded or decolorized; urine usually acid; local uneasiness, heat or vague dull pain; often sudden appearance and disappearance of attacks.

General treatment: Turpentine in emulsion 10 m. to a dram every 3 hours, with due regard to possible strangury.—Lydston.

Alum waters or alum iron, 10 gr. well diluted every 2 hours.—McNutt.

Rest in bed; liquid diet (preferably milk and buttermilk); diluent drinks; open bowels; if bleeding moderate and persistent give ergot in full doses (5 gr. ergotin hourly) or turpentine (3 drops in mucilage emulsion every hour for 6 or 8 hours) or oil of erigeron (5 m. in emulsion every hour) or gallic acid (gr. x every hour); if bleeding profuse, give full dose of morphine and empty bladder with catheter, followed by irrigation with hot astringent antiseptic solutions (silver nitrate 1 :2000 or carbolic acid 1 :200 or fluid ext. hydrastis ounce to pint).—White and Martin.

If obstruction of bladder, wash out with large-eyed catheter and boric acid solution; after the bladder is free from clots, employ silver nitrate 1 :10000 to 1 :500 carefully; if catheter fails, perform supra-pubic or perineal cystotomy.—*Am. Text-Book of Surgery.*

℞ Tinct. ferri chlor. m. xxx; tinct. digitalis m. xv; aquam menth. pip. q. s.: An ounce every 4 hours.—Aitken.

A teaspoonful of fluid ext. ergot every hour or two.—Bartholow.

Ergot extremely effective after more acute symptoms of nephritis have subsided.—Dickinson.

Hamamelis in venous hemorrhage.

Calcium chlorid best hemostatic, 15 gr. every 3 hours.—Moullin.

Simple nephrotomy with gauze drainage in acute inflammatory cases tending to suppression.

Sprains and Contusions: May be large, regular clots.

Treatment: Ergotin hypodermically; ice bag over lumbar region; strap side with long strips of adhesive plaster applied as for fractured ribs and apply broad roller bandage holding compress of gauze or cotton over kidney; exploratory lumbar incision if bleeding severe and persistent.—White and Martin.

Wounds.

Treatment: Lumbar or abdominal incision; ligature, packing or nephrectomy.—White and Martin.

Overheating or Overexertion: Lifting or racing; may be even small blood or granular casts.

Passive Hyperemia: Urine porter-colored; from heart weakness, pressure on (tumors, fecal impaction, pregnancy) or torsion of veins or spasm of arterioles, or tight lacing.

Treatment: Ice bags or bladders over kidney; lying on belly; alum whey ad libitum.—Reginald Harrison.

Cardiac Passive Congestion: Active saline catharsis and free administration of cardiac stimulants, digitalis, strychnin and alcohol.—McNutt.

Passive Hematuria with Debility: Turpentine in 1-10 m. dose.—*Flint's Encyclopedia.*

Recumbent posture and saline aperients; cantharides, turpentine, camphoric acid worthy of trial; in obstinate cases expose kidney, split capsule or perform acupuncture or nephrotomy.—Belfield.

Active Renal Hyperemia: May result from chilling of skin.

Treatment: Hot bath or vapor bath, diaphoretics and saline cathartics.

Nephritis: Particularly the acute, suppurative and chronic interstitial varieties.

Acute digitalis with potassium citrate; cupping or leeching.—N. S. Davis, Jr.

Treatment: Scarlatinal: Gallic acid and ergotin.—Hatfield.

Chronic Nephritis: Mercury or iodids in syphilitic.

Renal Calculus: Colicky pains on affected side; bleeding increased by movement, diminished by rest; diurnal frequency of urination.

Treatment: Recumbent posture; full doses of acetate of lead and opium, or ergot, gallic or tannic and dilute sulphuric acid; cold to loins or dry cups.—Osler.

Renal Tuberculosis: Bleeding slight, at long intervals; tubercle bacilli in sediment and general symptoms; murky polyuria and nocturnal frequency; pain as in stone; many monoculear and but few polynuclear leucocytes.

Malignant Growths: Pronounced and recurrent (apparently causeless) hematuria, more profuse at night; tumor; cachexia; may be tumor fragments; no leucocytes; large clots in cancers.

Treatment: Renal tumors: Renal puncture for simple cysts, hydronephrosis, and hydatid cysts; nephrotomy for cases where puncture fails, pyonephrosis, suppurative nephritis and pyelonephrosis, tubercular kidney and calculous disease; nephrectomy where puncture fails or would be useless, in certain neoplasms of kidney, for fistulæ and for degenerated kidney.

Iron alum (dose 1 or 2 gr. or more) as a palliative.—Henry Morris.

Cysts: Spongy tumors (usually bilateral) in renal region: rarely echinococci.

Floating Kidney: Very mobile reniform tumor slipping back into loin; bleeding usually slight and diminished by rest.

Embolism: Sudden bleeding with dyspnea and irregular action of heart.

Thrombosis of Renal Veins: Injuries, tumor, abscess, puerperal fever.

Rheumatism and Gout: Irritating excess of normal salts.

Treatment: Gouty: Turpentine, 10 drops every 2 hours in emulsion with acacia and cinnamon water.—McNutt.

Abundance of distilled water, to which may be added sodium phosphate, a teaspoonful to the pint.

Uric Acid Infarctions in Infants: Red sand on diapers; crying.

Chronic Endarteritis: Hard, tortuous pulse and high blood pressure.

Cardiac Hypertrophy.

Alcoholism: May be nephralgia simulating calculous pain.

Hemic Dyscrasiae: Hemorrhage profuse but clots rare;

scurvy, purpura, hemophilia, leukemia, congestive stage of malaria.

Treatment: ℞ Acidi gallici gr. iv; acidi ulph. dil. m. viii; tinct. opii deod. m. viii; infusum digitalis q. s.: Tablespoonful every 4 hours.—Druitt.

Malarial hematuria usually refractory to quinin; often promptly arrested by turpentine.—Wm. T. Belfield.

Severe Acute Infections: Scarlet, relapsing, typhus and yellow fevers, smallpox, diphtheria, septicemia, malaria, cholera, rarely syphilis; acute renal congestion.

Treatment: Keep bowels active with Rochelle or Epsom salts; drink water freely; hot baths or vapor baths for not more than 10 minutes; 4 gr. caffein citrate in water every 3 or 4 hours. —*Gould and Pyle's Cyclopedia.*

* *Irritant Drugs:* Turpentine, cantharides, carbolic acid, quinin, salicylic acid, potassium chlorate.

Treatment: Camphor in 2 to 5 gr. doses.—Ringer.

Vicarious Hematuria: Suppressed menstruation or hemorrhoidal flow of blood.

Morbus Maculosus.

Endocarditis.

Intestinal Catarrh of Infants.

Parasites: Endemic in tropics; distoma, bilharzia hematobia, filaria, strongylus gigas; psorospermiasis (sporozoa).

Treatment: Turpentine or oil of male fern.—Healey.

Reflex Inhibition: Acute abdominal affections.

Sudden Release of Intra-abdominal Pressure: Removal of large tumor.

Angioneurosis of Neuropaths: Unilateral and pretty constant; may come on after excitement; no casts or crystals; neurasthenia and secondary anemia. Rhubarb, strawberries or gooseberries may excite bleeding.

Treatment: Try tonics and cold baths; these failing, simple nephrotomy cures.—Harris.

Rickets and Scurvy: Young children.

PELVIC.

Blood well mixed with urine; may be small molds of calices; hemorrhage usually unilateral, as shown by cystoscopy, segregator or ureteral catheterization; tailed, columnar epithelium.

Pyelitis: Nearly always secondary to gravel or obstruction of lower tract.

Pelvic Calculus: Pain in loin increased by motion and radiating down ureter; crystals in freshly voided urine; a few "washed-out" blood corpuscles usually present in intervals.

Treatment: One-half dram each of fluid extract ergot and tinct. krameria every 2 or more hours.—Bartholow.

Glycerin in doses of 1½ to 4 oz. diluted with an equal part of water, repeated a number of times (caused passage of stone in 6 to 36 hours in 31 cases out of 85).—Hermann.

Piperazin solution, made fresh daily and continued for a long period—12 gr. in a pint of water after each meal.—Thornton.

Pelvic Tuberculosis: Slight hemorrhage; tubercle bacilli in sediment, best obtained by ureteral catheterization.

Vascular Tumors, especially Renal Cancer: Recurrent, with tumor and some cachexia; may be large clots.

Echinococci Cysts: Characteristic hooklets in urine.

Hydronephrosis: Fluctuating tumor, varying in size.

URETERAL.

Long, thin, earth-worm-like clots, with renal colic in passing (sometimes also from renal or pelvic hemorrhage); hematuria may alternate with normal urine when passage stopped.

Impacted Renal Calculi: Excruciating, griping pain in direction of ureter, passing into thigh and genitals.

Treatment: Morphin hypodermically and hot bath; surgical interference if repeated attacks or hydronephrosis or partial or complete suppression or fever, hectic, and pus in urine.—White and Martin.

Ureteritis: Palpation shows vesical end of ureter swollen and tender.

Wounds.

Treatment: Incise and suture.

Blocking from Movable Kidney: Dietl's crises of pain, vomiting and collapse.

VESICAL.

Large, irregular-edged, scarlet blood clots at end of micturition; urine often alkaline; blood brighter (may be dark brown if alkaline) and less well mixed with urine (settles quickly) than in renal form; if bladder is washed out with borax solution and more fluid injected, it will come away bloody; spectroscope shows oxyhemoglobin absorption bands (methemoglobin in cystic retention and decomposition) ; considerable accompanying mucus.

Vesical Calculus: Nearly normal blood at end of painful micturition; sudden involuntary stoppage of stream relieved by change of posture; sounding and bimanual palpation reveal cause; urine turbid, often offensive.

Treatment: Removal through intact urethra, through vaginal incision or by suprepubic or perineal cystotomy.—Kelly.

Cystitis of Vesical Neck: Like stone as to symptoms, but sounding and palpation negative.

Severe Acute Cystitis: Slight amount of fresh red blood with great pain and tenesmus.

Treatment: Ulceration: Irrigate bladder with water at 105°, gradually raised to 120°.—Reginald Harrison.

Inject diluted fluid extract or distilled extract of hamamelis. —Butler.

Benign Vesical Growths, commonly Papilloma: Profuse, (blood cells fragmented in clot) recurrent, early hemorrhages; endoscopy shows tumor; may be villous fragments in sediment.

Treatment: Inject silver nitrate solution daily for 4 to 5 months, then every other day for 6 months more, and finally every third day for a time—strength of solution at first 12 gr. to 4 oz. of warm water acidulated with a little free nitric acid, and gradually increased as patient becomes tolerant.—Herring.

Remove growth if practicable; empty bladder of clots with large catheter or by incision and permanent drainage; inject 5% solution of gelatin in 0.7% sodium chlorid solution, removing and reinjecting till bleeding stopped.—Nouges.

Vesical Carcinoma: Marked, persistent, late hemorrhages; bimanual examination and cystoscopy; microscopic examination of curettings or fleshy shreds passed spontaneously.

Treatment: Hot injections of alum 4 dr. to pint, hydrastis 2 oz. to pint, or acetanilid 5% solution; if clots, aspirate through catheter or litholopaxy evacuating tube; permanent catheterization if bleeding persists.—White and Martin.

Tumors producing retention: Eradicate by dilated urethra,

vaginal incision, suprapubic incision, symphyseotomy or cystect-
omy.—Kelly.

Varicose Bladder: Often associated with piles; may be
periodic bleeding alternating between rectum and bladder; retention of urine common in men; blue, congested vessels easily
seen with cystoscope—may be encrusted with phosphates.

Treatment: For mild cases galvanocautery may be introduced through speculum and used over several small areas; in
severe cases dilate urethra to admit No. 15-18 speculum and tie
several of large venous trunks by means of a fine curved needle
on a fixed handle carrying fine silk and a little instrument pronged
like a pitchfork to afford a point of counterpressure within bladder, or incise through anterior vaginal wall, evert veins at neck
of bladder and tie them with fine silk.—Kelly.

Passive Congestion of Vesical Veins: From pregnancy, portal obstruction or cancer.

Blader Dilation: Due to hypertrophied prostate or weakness of advancing age; may follow sudden emptying of the bladder; usually combined with a catarrhal condition of the mucous
membrane.

Ulceration of Bladder: Simple, gonorrheal, syphilitic or tubercular; blood, pus, connective tissue and columnar epithelium
of bladder; cystoscopy; light odorless urine and persistent post-
scrotal pain with tuberculosis.

Treatment: Vesical Tuberculosis with Bleeding: Curet tubercular area through endoscope, remove detritus with ½ strength
Thiersch solution and establish drainage through urethra with a
twist of gauze folded in gutta percha tissue; subsequent antiseptic irrigations of boric acid injections, of iodoform emulsions and
thorough local application of silver nitrate, 80 gr. to ounce every
4 or 5 days for 2 weeks using sodium chlorid as a corrective),
then flushing out cavity with sodium salicylate solution a dram
to the pint.—J. O. Polak.

Irritating Drugs: By mouth or urethra.

Parasites: Particularly distoma hematobia; endemic in
tropics.

Treatment: Oil of turpentine and male fern in 15 m. doses
with 5 m. chloroform and tragacanth mixture every morning;
also bicarbonate of potassium internally; inject into bladder

every second or third day 5 oz. tepid water containing 20 or 30 gr. of potassium iodid.—Harley.

Trauma: Instrumentation or external injury; previous inflammation or varicose veins predispose.

Treatment: Wounds: Injection of hot astringent antiseptic solution (4% solution of antipyrin) with internal administration of ergotin; packing or ligature if severe and persistent.—White and Martin.

Scurvy, Purpura, Hemophilia: Frequently after emptying bladder with catheter.

Arteriosclerosis: Hard, tense pulse; senility.

Fatty and Amyloid Degeneration of Vesical Lining.

Irritation of Uric Acid, Phosphates or Prostatic Concretions: Cystoscope shows shining deposit.

Treatment: Removal of deposit by irrigation with boiled water and use of curet or catheter under cystoscopic inspection.

PROSTATIC.

Appears chiefly toward or at end of micturition (sometimes at beginning); first urine may contain clotted fusiform molds of prostatic sinuses; endoscopy shows lesion.

Causes: Chronic prostatic hypertrophy (seldom profuse unless adenoma complicates); prostatitis and prostatocystitis (enlarged, hot and tender prostate); passive congestion of prostate and vesical neck (usually mornings after stool); tuberculosis; new growths; ulcerated surface of third lobe; stone.

Treatment: Profuse with Retention: Evacuate blood by means of catheter and syringe, and keep bladder empty by means of retained catheter; if blood cannot be removed this way, use perineal or suprapubic cystotomy; if bleeding persists try pressure above pubs with compressess.—White and Martin.

Moderate from Prostatitis and Prostatocystitis: Balsams combined with diluents and rectal use of opium.—White and Martin.

Hot baths, leeches and hot fomentations; saline cathartics and alkaline diuretics.—Lydston.

Passive Congestion: Perineal counter-irritation; cold sitz baths; cholagogue laxatives and removal of urethral contractures; ergot, hamamelis, turpentine.—Lydston.

Hypertrophied Prostate: Opium as a sedative; calcium chlorid; ice continuously over pubes, against perineum and in rectum; if catheter is needed for retention, wash out interior with cold water or with diluted tincture of matico or tincture of hydrastis; in exceptional instances of very profuse bleeding, perform suprapubic cystotomy, clear out coagula and stop bleeding with hot water or actual cautery, or by inserting catheter and plugging around it with iodoform gauze.—Mansell Moullin.

℞ Tinct. Belladonnæ m. viiss; potass. acetat. gr. xv; aquam menth. pip. ad.   Take t. i. d.—Guiteras.

SEMINAL VESICULAR.

Usually small amount; pink semen.

Causes: Gonorrhea; tubercle (terminal hemorrhage with painless gleet, frequent urination and tubercular nodules forming fistulas); malignant diseases.

URETHRAL.

Bright blood; from anterior urethra passed at beginning of micturition and during intervals, or can be stripped out; from posterior, usually slight, at beginning or end of micturition or both, sometimes clotting (long, thick).

Causes: Acute gonorrhea (pus containing gonococci); neoplasms (sounding and endoscopy); urethral chancroid or chancre (history, inspection, palpation); chronic posterior urethritis (slight, recurrent hemorrhage at end of micturition, with tenesmus; may be profuse after coitus or exertion; often with stricture or localized patch of diseased membrane following old gonorrhea); tuberculosis; irritating injections; trauma (accidental or surgical); caruncle (cockscomb tumor).

Treatment: Inject a little ice water into urethral canal.—Reginald Harrison.

Apply ferric chlorid solution to granular or papillary patch; check increased discharge with protargol.—J. F. Dobson.

VULVAR, VAGINAL AND UTERINE.

Readily excluded by catheterization; blood corpuscles slightly, if any, altered.

A MODEL ACT TO PROTECT THE PUBLIC HEALTH
AND REGULATE THE PRACTICE
OF MEDICINE.

To THE MEDICAL PROFESSION OF THE STATE OF COLORADO.

Gentlemen: The following draft of a medical registration law is based upon my observation and study of the statutes of other states and countries, together with the practical experience gained in the administration of the Colorado medical law. It is not supposed that different legislative committees can or will agree upon a bill to be presented to the approaching legislature that follows my draft in detail. However, that the rights and views of all may be recognized, changes can be made which will not sacrifice the basic principles and essential features upon which this Act is drawn that will enable us to agree. Such a plan must be pursued because it is an absolute necessity for success. We must settle our differences out of the assembly halls. With this understanding it is hoped that no member of the medical profession will "knock" the medical bill that is offered for passage, simply because some feature does not agree with his ideas. Concessions from the ideal must be made, for reasons not necessary to explain. Remember, one medical man as a "knocker" can do more to thwart the enactment of a new medical law than twenty workers can assist in its passage; that a half loaf is better than none; and that those in charge will endeavor to unite upon the very best measure possible.

Therefore, let everyone throughout the state awaken to the duty he owes his profession in securing the passage, not only of a proper practice act, but in assisting the legislative committees and executive council of the Legislative League in their efforts to improve the other statutes in which medical men should take the deepest interest. Our lunacy law is disgraceful, the coroner system is obsolete and totally lacking justification of its perpetuation, and our public health statute is defective to a marked degree. If anything is to be done we must have the united support of the profession. Our labors are onerous at best, and we need all encouragement possible.

Trusting that we shall receive the support and assistance we need—and we need it now (don't wait until after the legislature is elected and convened), I am

Respectfully,

S. D. VAN METER,

Ch. Com. on Public Policy and Legislation.

A MODEL ACT TO PROTECT THE PUBLIC HEALTH AND REGULATE THE PRACTICE OF MEDICINE.

BY S. D. VAN METER, M. D.

Denver, Colo.

Creation and Composition Of Board. SECTION 1. A board is hereby established to be known by the name and style of the State Board of Medical Examiners. Said Board shall be composed of nine practising physicians of known integrity and judicial ability, who shall be graduates of medical schools of high educational requirements, and who shall have been engaged in the active practice of their profession within the state for a period of five years.

(A board so constituted provides for one composed of educated, competent physicians, and does not raise the question of sectarianism. Such a board could with propriety be designated by other statutes to be the proper tribunal to pass upon the qualifications of medical experts, as commissioners in lunacy, etc.)

Board. How Appointed. SEC. 2. The Governor shall, as soon as practicable after this Act shall have become a law, appoint nine physicians possessing the qualifications specified in Sec. 1 of this Act, to constitute the members of said Board. Said members shall be classified by the Governor that the term of office of three shall expire in two, three in four, and three in six years from date of appointment. Biennially thereafter the Governor shall appoint three members to serve for the term of six years, and he shall fill vacancies in the membership of said Board as soon as practicable. The appointments of all members of said Board shall be made from a list of nominations furnished the Governor by the incorporated State Medical Societies, which have a bona fide licentiate membership of ————. Each society of such membership and standing shall be entitled to send three (3) nominations for each position to which an appointment is to be made.

(This allows the profession to nominate the timber, from which the most obtuse governor could hardly go far astray in making appointments. As most states elect a new governor every two years, it will be further seen that the same one would have to be elected three times before he could change the personnel of the board, except by resignation or death.)

Organization of Board.

SEC. 3. Said Board shall biennially elect a President, a Vice-President, and a Secretary-Treasurer from their membership; and they shall from time to time adopt such rules and regulations as they shall deem necessary for the performance of their duties. They shall also adopt a seal, which they shall affix to all certificates issued by them.

(Needs no comment, other than to call attention to the simplicity of construction for the necessary provision of organization.)

General Requirements of Applicants to Practice Medicine.

SEC. 4. Anyone wishing to practise medicine, who has not heretofore been licensed in this state, shall make application to said State Board of Medical Examiners, through the Secretary-Treasurer thereof, upon the form adopted by said Board, and shall present himself to such members as may be designated by the Board to conduct his examination, and submit himself to the examination defined in Sec. 7 of this Act. If such examination shows the applicant to be qualified to practise medicine, then the Board shall issue a certificate to that effect, and this certificate shall be a license to said applicant to practise medicine in this state. All such applicants shall furnish the State Board of Medical Examiners with satisfactory evidence of good moral character.

(This section provides for the admission of all persons wishing to practise the healing art to apply for license, and consequently gives the Examining Board control or jurisdiction over all who claim to be doctors of medicine, irrespective of therapeutical belief. It further provides for the production of *satisfactory* evidence of moral character.)

Authority of Board.

SEC. 5. Said Board shall have authority to administer oaths, to summon witnesses, and to take testimony in all matters relating to its duties. Said Board shall issue satisfactory evidence of qualification. Such certificates shall be signed by the President and attested by the Secretary-Treasurer. It shall be the duty of the Secretary-Treasurer, under the direction of the Board, personally or by deputy to aid in the enforcement of this Act, and in the prosecution of all persons charged with violating any of its provisions.

Duties of Secretary-Treasurer.

(This section provides for the authority of the Board to sit as a quasi-judicial body, and designates the Secretary-Treasurer, or his deputy, as the officer of the law whose duty it is to enforce the Act—a most essential feature of a practical law.)

Fees. Part to Be Returned If Application Is Refused.

SEC. 6. There shall be paid to the Secretary-Treasurer of the State Board of Medical Examiners by each applicant for a license a fee of Twenty-five Dollars ($25.00), which must accompany the application. Two-fifths of the fee shall be returned to the applicant in case the Board shall refuse to grant him a certificate.

(Some objection may be raised to the size of the fee provided for in this section. It is none too large, however, as the labor involved in investigating and examining applicants to determine their qualifications, when properly done, is far greater than is ordinarily supposed. Two-fifths of the fee is returned when license is refused, as there is no expense of engrossing certificate. This in reality should not be done, but to retain the full amount of fee gives room for unjust criticism, on the ground that the Board would refuse a license to induce a second application.)

Style of
Examinations.

SEC. 7. Examinations of applicants for license to practise medicine shall be made by said State Board of Medical Examiners according to the method deemed by it to be the most practicable and expeditious to test the applicant's qualifications.

What Subjects.

The subjects of written, oral, or clinical examinations shall be as follows:—Anatomy, physiology, chemistry, toxicology, pathology, surgery, obstetrics and symptomatology (exclusive of materia medica and therapeutics.)

Duty of Making Investigation of Applicant's Credentials and Consideration of Same in Conducting Examinations.

The credentials of applicants relating to their general reputation, preliminary education and courses of study they have pursued; degrees they have received; number of years they have been engaged in the lawful practice of medicine; their experience in general hospitals, medical departments of the Army, Navy and Public Health and Marine Hospital Service; licenses granted to them by other states and countries; and their experience as teachers of medicine, shall be given due consideration by the Board in conducting its examinations.

Power of Board to Grant a License Without Examination When Convinced of Applicant's Qualification.

Upon investigation of an applicant's credentials the Board may, when convinced that an applicant is qualified to practise medicine, grant him a license thereon without further examination.

(Sec. 7 provides for a sufficient number of branches for examination ample to test an applicant's educational qualifications. None of these branches should raise the question of medical sectarianism.

It further provides for the due consideration of an applicant's credentials, in deciding the question of his qualification, and permits of the wide discretionary power on the part of the Board necessary in the equitable treatment of the many different classes of applicants. It does not encumber the Board, however, with specific detail as to what it shall accept as evidence of qualification, and permits of examining any applicant, when not satisfied of his qualification, by the method deemed most practical and expeditious.)

Record of
Certificates.

SEC. 8. Every person who shall receive a certificate from said State Board of Medical Examiners shall have it recorded in the office of the recorder of deeds of the county in which he resides, and shall likewise have it recorded in the counties to which he shall subsequently remove for the purpose of practising medicine. The failure on the part of the holder of a certificate to have it recorded within ninety (90) days after its date of issue, shall render the certificate null and void.

rder of
ds' Record.

SEC. 9. The recorder of deeds shall keep for public inspection, in a book provided for the purpose, a complete list and description of the certificates recorded by him. When any such certificate shall be presented to him for record he shall stamp or write upon the face thereof a memorandum of the date when such certificate was presented for record.

(Sections 8 and 9 provide for a county record of licenses, something necessary for the practical operation of a registration law, owing to the difficulty and loss of time in making inquiry of the Secretary of the license board.)

wer of Board
Refusing and
voking
rtiflcates.

SEC. 10. The State Board of Medical Examiners may refuse to grant, or may revoke, a certificate or license to practise medicine in this state, or may cause a licentiate's name to be removed from the record in the office of any recorder of deeds in the state upon any of the following grounds, to-wit:—The employment of fraud or deception in applying for a license, or in passing the examination provided for in this Act; the conviction of a crime involving moral turpitude; habitual intemperance in the use of ardent spirits, narcotics or stimulants; unprofessional or dishonorable conduct; the procuring or aiding or abetting in procuring criminal abortion; the obtaining of a fee on the assurance that a manifestly incurable disease can be permanently cured; the betrayal of a professional secret to the detriment of a patient; causing the publication and circulation of an advertisement of any medicine or means whereby the monthly periods of women can be regulated, or the menses, if suppressed, can be re-established; causing the publication and circulation of an advertisement relative to any disease of the sexual organs. Any person charged with the violation of any of the foregoing grounds or provisions of this Section shall be furnished with a copy of the complaint and shall have a hearing before said Board in person, or by attorney, and. witnesses may be examined by said Board respecting the guilt or innocence of said accused. Said Board may at any time within two years from the refusal or revocation of a license or certificate, or cancellation of registration under this Section, by a majority vote, issue a new certificate or a license to the person affected, restoring to him all the rights or privileges of which he had been deprived by said Board. Any person so restored shall pay to the Secretary-Treasurer a fee of Ten Dollars ($10.00) on issuance of such new certificate.

(Section 10 is a most important one, as it provides for that most necessary requisite of refusal and revocation of license for those established causes that should forfeit anyone's right to practise medicine. No provision is made for appeal to the courts because it is understood that such privilege is an inherent right of citizenship, and any Board abusing the power of refusing or revoking a license under this Section could be handled severely by the applicant affected by such abuse. Provision for an appeal has the objection of acting as an invitation for applicants who have been refused, or licentiates whose licenses have been revoked, causing endless and unnecessary trouble, when no abuse of the power has been participated in by the Board.)

finition of
t Consti-
m the
ctice of
edicine.

SEC. 11. Any person shall be regarded as practising medicine, within the meaning of this Act, who shall in any manner hold himself out to the public as being engaged within this State in the diagnosis and treatment of diseases or injuries of human beings; or who shall suggest, recommend, or prescribe any form of treatment for the intended palliation, relief or cure of any physical or mental ailment of any person, with the intention of receiving therefor, either directly or indirectly, any fee, gift or compensation whatsoever; or who shall maintain an office for the reception, examination and treatment of any person suffering from disease or injury of body or mind; or who shall attach the title of M. D., Surgeon, Doctor, or any other word or abbreviation to his name, indicative that such person is engaged in the practice of medicine as hereinbefore defined.

(A section constructed as the foregoing permits of no equivocation and covers the practice of medicine by any system so thoroughly, that it is inconceivable how anyone who is treating the sick or injured could evade the law.)

What Constitutes a Violation of This Act. SEC. 12. If any person shall hold himself out to the public as being engaged within this State in the diagnosis and treatment of diseases or injuries of human beings; or shall suggest, recommend or prescribe any form of treatment for the palliation, relief or cure of any physical or mental ailment of any person, with the intention of receiving therefor, either directly or indirectly, any fee, gift or compensation whatsoever; or shall maintain an office for the reception, examination and treatment of diseased or injured human beings; or shall attach the title of M. D., Surgeon, Doctor, or any other word or abbreviation to his name, indicative that he is engaged in the treatment of diseased or injured human beings, and shall not theretofore have received, and shall not then possess, in full force and virtue, a valid license to practise medicine under the laws of this State, shall be deemed to be practising medicine without complying with the provisions of this Act.

(The foregoing Section, while apparently a duplication of Sec. 11, is desirable, as it aids in simplifying criminal procedure. It relieves the State of the necessity of finding some one who has been treated by the accused and who is willing to testify. This kind of evidence is most difficult to obtain, and such difficulty has prevented successful prosecution more often than all other technical formalities of procedure combined. It is rare that a pa-

tient who has been gulled by a quack can be prevailed
upon to further expose his gullibility, and perhaps his
physical or mental ailment by appearing as a witness,
unless he be prompted by revenge, which always detracts
from his qualities as a witness.)

**Does Not
Prohibit
Gratuitious
Service, Army
and Navy
Surgeons or
Licensed
Physicians from
Other States.**
SEC. 13. Nothing in this Act shall be construed to
prohibit gratuitious service in case of emergency, nor
shall it apply to commissioned surgeons of the United
States Army, Navy or Public Health and Marine Hos-
pital Service, while so engaged, nor to regularly licensed
physicians in actual consultation from another State or
Territory, nor to regularly licensed physicians actually
called from other States or Territories to attend specified
cases in this State.

(The purpose and justice of the provisions of Sec. 13
are so manifest that they need no comment.)

**Penalty for
Practicing
Without
License.**
SEC. 14. Any person practising medicine in any of
its departments, in this State, without complying with the
provisions of this Act, shall be punished by a fine of not
less than Fifty Dollars ($50.00), nor more than Three
Hundred Dollars ($300.00), and by imprisonment in the
county jail for not less than Ten (10) Days nor more
than Thirty (30) Days.

(The question of penalty for practising without a
license is one that deserves careful consideration. If too
severe it often prevents conviction, whereas if too light it
does not deter those who may desire to disobey the law
from doing so. From the experience of the author the
best solution of the question is to be found in imposing
both a fine and imprisonment, as provided in Sec. 14.)

**Penalty for
Giving False
Evidence.**
SEC. 15. Any person presenting or attempting to
file as his own the diploma or certificate or credentials of
another, or who shall give either false or forged evidence
of any kind to the State Board of Medical Examiners, or
any member thereof, in connection with an application for
a license to practise medicine, shall be deemed guilty of
a felony, and upon conviction thereof shall be punished
by imprisonment in the state penitentiary for a term of

not less than Three (3), nor more than Ten (10) Years, at hard labor.

(The inexcusable crimes of perjury and forgery in securing a license to practise medicine deserve and permit a severe penalty, hence this Section, and the provision for a greater penalty for such crimes than that of practising without a license.)

Disposition of Fees and Maintenance of Board.

SEC. 15. All fees received by the State Board of Medical Examiners, and all fines collected by any officer of the law under this Act shall be paid to the Secretary-Treasurer of said Board, who shall at the end of each and every month deposit the same with the State Treasurer; and the said State Treasurer shall place said money so received in a special fund to be known as the fund of the State Board of Medical Examiners, and shall pay the same out on vouchers issued and signed by the President and Secretary-Treasurer of said Board upon warrants drawn by the Auditor of State therefor. Said moneys so received and placed in said fund may be used by the State Board of Medical Examiners in defraying its expenses in carrying out the provisions of this Act. At the end of every biennial period, if there shall remain in said fund any balance, said balance shall be transferred to the general revenue fund of the State. The Secretary-Treasurer of said Board shall keep a true and accurate account of all funds received and all vouchers issued by the Board; and on the first day of December of each year he shall file with the Governor of the State a report of all receipts and disbursements for said Board for the preceding fiscal

Per Diem of Members.

Salary of Secretary.

year. Members of the said Board shall receive a per diem for the time during which they shall be actually engaged in the discharge of their duties; and the Secretary-Treasurer shall receive an annual salary; said per diem and salary to be fixed by the Board.

(The foregoing Section, taken in connection with the size of the license fee, makes ample provision for the maintenance of the Board. When a Board is dependent upon legislative appropriation it is too frequently the case that its work is forced to a standstill for lack of funds.)

Place and Time
of Meeting. SEC. 17. The State Board of Medical Examiners shall meet in the City of ——————— on the first Tuesday of January, April, July and October of each year, and at such other times and places as may be found necessary for the performance of their duties.

(The provisions of this Section need no comment.)

The especially good features of such an Act may be briefly summarized as follows:

1st.—Unquestionable constitutionality.

2nd.—Nonsectarian Board.

3rd.—Subjects of examination limited to those upon which all schools agree. This solves most practically the objectionable feature of separate boards for each school. Number of subjects, however, are adequate to determine most thoroughly an applicant's educational qualifications.

4th.—Wide discretionary power of Board in examinations, and in granting, refusing or revoking licenses. Board may use any method they deem most practical in arriving at a decision of an applicant's qualifications. Such power enables a Board to extend reciprocity when and where it should be, without being compelled to by statute.

5th.—Unequivocal definition of what constitutes "the practice of medicine" and "practising medicine without a license"—absolute essentials in the practical administration of a medical practice Act.

[In our next issue will be published an argument by Dr. Van Meter in support of the essential features and principles upon which the foregoing act is drawn.—ED.]

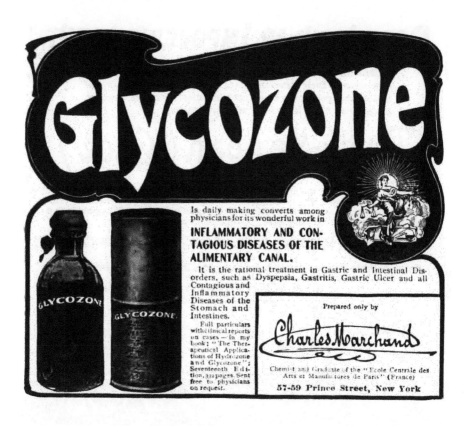

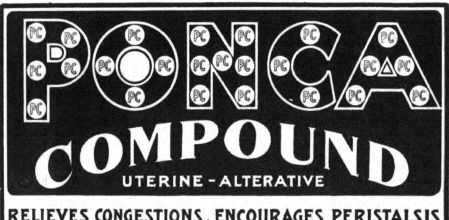

DENVER MEDICAL TIMES

THOMAS H. HAWKINS, A.M., M.D., EDITOR AND PUBLISHER.

COLLABORATORS:

Henry O. Marcy, M.D., Boston.
Thaddeus A. Reamy, M.D., Cincinnati.
Nicholas Senn, M.D., Chicago.
Joseph Price, M,D., Philadelphia.
Franklin H. Martin, M.D., Chicago.
William Oliver Moore, M.D.. New York.
L. S. McMurtry, M.D., Louisville.
Thomas B. Eastman, M.D., Indianapolis,Ind.
G. Law, M.D., Greeley, Colo.

S. H. Pinkerton, M.D., Salt Lake City
Flavel B. Tiffany, M.D., Kansas City.
Erskine M. Bates, M.D:. New York.
E. C. Gehrung, M.D, St. Louis.
Graeme M. Hammond, M.D, New York.
James A. Lydston, M.D., Chicago.
Leonard Freeman, M.D., Denver.
Carey K. Fleming, M.D., Denver, Colo.

Subscriptions, $1.00 per year in advance; Single Copies, 10 cents.

Address all Communications to Denver Medical Times, 1740 Welton Street, Denver, Colo.
We will at all times be glad to give space to well written articles or items of interest to the profession.
[Entered at the Postoffice of Denver, Colorado, as mail matter of the Second Class.]

EDITORIAL DEPARTMENT

YELLOW FEVER.

The frightful "Yellow Jack," endemic for the past century in the focal zone of the West Indies and the Mexican shores and on the coast of Guinea, may soon be extirpated by sanitary science.

America, according to Toner, suffered no less than 37 severe epidemics of yellow fever in the 18th century. The last extensive outbreak in this country was in 1878, when the disease prevailed in Louisiana, Mississippi and Alabama. The first certain appearance of yellow fever in what is how the United States is recorded in Winthrop's History of New England as occurring in 1647, under the title of the Barbadoes Distemper. In 1699 a malignant epidemic of yellow fever in Philadelphia caused 220 deaths. In the summer and autumn of 1702 the "great sickness" caused 570 deaths in New York. Philadelphia's terrible visitation in 1793, so vividly described by Benjamin Rush and Mathew Carey, put a stop to all business and friendly intercourse, drove a third of the inhabitants into the country, and rigid quarantine was enforced against the fleeing citizens by other cities. From the 1st of August to the 9th of November, says Packard, there had been 4,030 interments in the burial grounds of Philadelphia, almost entirely from yellow fever. In Havana up to 1889 the average number of deaths from yellow fever for 45 years was 751, and in 1857 2,058 died of the pest. From 1889 to 1901 the mean number of deaths from the fever in Havana from April 1 to February 1 was 457. During the same period of 1901-02 there were only five deaths from this cause, and the city has been free from the pest since August, 1901. There were 301 deaths from yellow fever in 1900, in spite of the fact that the sanitary condition of Havana was much better than ever before, and that every means was used to destroy the fomites, until recently considered the chief infective agent.

On March 1, 1901, by order of Governor-General Wood, the work of destroying mosquitoes was begun, with an immediate decrease in the number of attacks and deaths from yellow fever. No attention was paid to the destruction of fomites.

Finlay, of Havana, in 1881, suggested that the infection of yellow fever might be propagated by mosquitoes. Within the past two years Drs. Reed, Carroll, Lazear and Agramonte demonstrated the carrier relation of stegomyia fasciata, by allowing mosquitoes to feed on yellow fever patients and then on non-immune persons. Unfortunately Dr. Lazear and also Dr. Myers of the British Commission fell victims to these experiments—martyrs of science far more worthy of renown than any of war's heroes seeking to slay and despoil. The bacillus x of Sternberg (1888) and the bacillus icteroides of Sanarelli (1897) found in about 50% of fresh cadavers of yellow fever victims, are said by Reed and Carroll to be secondary invaders and varieties of the hog cholera bacillus.

Of 17,000 Havana houses examined by the "mosquito corps" during January, the larvæ were found only in 411, whereas if a similar inspection had been made the year previous, larvæ would have been discovered in nearly every instance. Our lately acquired knowledge of yellow fever has had its legitimate effect upon quarantine. Surgeon-General Wyman, of the U. S. H. M. S., has ordered that healthy non-immunes on board a vessel from a yellow fever port, need not be detained longer than the time required to make five days from the port in question.

THE CITY.

, Paving streets and courts keeps the soil free from impurities. Asphalt is the most sanitary pavement. Stone roads form much dust and mud, and wood is generally too pervious.

Streets should not be less than 1½ times in width the height of the houses abutting thereon, so as to furnish sufficient air-flow.

There should always be open spaces between the backs of buildings.

In the smoke nuisance there is for the community as a whole more expense than saving, aside from its injurious effects on the health, and particularly the lungs. This nuisance can be abated somewhat by the use of petroleum, coke and anthracite in place of bituminous coal, and by the consumption of smoke. To insure the smokeless combustion of soft coal, wide grates, boilers high above the fire, and artificial stokers can be employed.

Dust is a great danger in city streets, being the chief medium, perhaps, of infections. In Los Angeles successful experiments have been made in substituting the oiling of roads for watering. Oiled roads are said by Longden to be free from dust in summer and mud in winter, requiring only two or three applications of oil the first season. About sixty barrels of kerosene oil per mile were used the first time for a road twelve feet wide, and forty barrels the second time.

Public conveyances need more sanitary attention. Compressed air is a good cleansing agent for railway cars; formaldehyde is perhaps the best disinfectant. The board of health of St. Paul compels all street cars to be disinfected every night.

Isolation is the only means of checking contagious diseases in crowded towns, and special hospitals and conveyances should be provided for the subjects of these maladies. Isolation is especially indicated during malignant epidemics. Removal of patients to special hospitals minimizes the risk of infection to the remainder of the household and the community; the other members of the family can proceed with their regular occupation or education, and there is better control and nursing generally than in the homes of the poor. Smallpox spreads to surrounding buildings, and should not be treated in the same hospital with other infectious diseases, but at a considerable distance from aggregations of population. The disinfecting building should be divided in two parts, with the only communication through the disinfecting machine in the wall between the two rooms. The hospital accommodations of a city should consist of at least one bed for every thousand of population. . The really modern hospital has impervious floors, smooth walls and inclined planes in place of stairs and elevators.

The water supply of towns and cities should be constantly sufficient, that is, a minimum of 25 gallons per head daily in a municipality with sewers and water closets; 14 to 20 gallons without these; five to ten gallons additional per head if there are manufactories using large quantities of water. Soft water is probably the best, and there should not be more than two or three grains of vegetable matter per gallon. Hard waters possibly favor the onset of arteriosclerosis.

The water supplies of towns generally need to be stored and filtered in reservoirs with a capacity for from one to three months. These reservoirs ought to be clear of trees and of refuse castings. The filters are usually made of a layer of sand about three feet thick, sustained on a bed of gravel. According to Koch, they should not filter more than 3.94 inches per hour. The experience of larger cities is in favor of continuous sand filtration, after leaving in subsidence reservoirs one to four days. Intermittent sand filtration is not so efficient. Mechanical filtration with coarse sand and alum is open to objections from both sides—free sulphuric acid is sometimes evolved, or there may be failure to precipitate germs because of the lack of bases in the water. According to Geo. M. Kober, mechanical filters at the most have reduced the death rate from typhoid 26%; sand filtration, 78.5%.

The constant plan of delivery is much better than house storage of water. If house cisterns cannot be dispensed with, they should be well made of slate, stoneware or galvanized iron, be readily inspected and drained, and overflow pipes should always end in the open air. Contamination by foul air, dust or soakage must also be avoided. If the water supply is cut off at intervals, or if leakages take place in street mains, foul air or dirty liquids may be sucked in. The same insuction sometimes occurs from sewer pipes into water pipes laid in the same trench. High pressure increases the freshness of water. Dirty house water is to be carried out by trapped pipes opening outside the house over a grating in connection with a trapped inlet or gully into larger pipes or sewers.

Excreta in towns and cities should not be allowed to soak into the earth or remain near dwellings. Old middens and cesspools are veritable nuisances. There are three general methods of removing human excreta. The dry plan, or earth closet system, consists in the daily removal (pail system) along with dry earth or ashes, and is unsuited to large towns or cities. In the pneumatic system, employed largely on the Continent, the excreta are sucked through pipes into a central reservoir by an air pump. The water system is generally utilized in this country, and is the best for health and comfort. There should be separate impermeable pipes for the house sewage. There should likewise be a siphon-trap always containing water near the junction of the house drain and the common sewer; an inlet opening from the outside air to the house drain on the outside of the siphon-trap; and an outlet pipe from the farther end of the drain to above the roof.

Sewer deposits are prevented by egg-shape sewers, easily inspected and cleaned, a regular flow of water and periodic flushing. Sewers are best ventilated by numerous openings with tall shafts at the dead ends.

An inexpensive plan of sewerage disposal is to filter by intermittent filtration on properly prepared and drained ground. In septic tanks the sewage is subjected for 24 hours to the liquefying action of anerobic bacteria, and is then passed through coke breeze or other filters. The plan is uncertain and troublesome. London sewage is treated with lime and sulphur iron, and the sludge is sent out to sea.

Destructor furnaces for dry refuse are making rapid progress. The garbage should be gathered daily from the galvanized iron receptacles. The waste heat produced may be utilized for converting the contents of pail closets into dry manure or to generate steam in boilers to drive electric lighting machinery. Clinkers from the furnace may be ground in a mortar mill and be converted into bricks or concrete. The kitchen fire is the best place for most food scraps and much other organic refuse.

CREMATION.

Cremation obviates all risk of infection from dead bodies. Sir Henry Thompson thus tersely states the problem of disposal of the dead: "Given a dead body: to resolve it into carbonic acid, water and ammonia and the mineral elements rapidly, safely and not unpleasantly."

Cremation alone fulfils all these requirements. The only objection which reason and science offer to this model process is that which Bunge has put forward, namely, the diminution of the total fixed terrestrial nitrogen. Any medico-legal defects could be overcome by a better system of death registration, with the production of two medical certificates and a voucher to the effect that the deceased desired cremation. Mortuary chapels are a fitting adjunct to crematoria, and corpses should be removed to them within 36 hours after death. In a properly constituted apparatus the average body is converted into three pounds of ashes in 1½ hours. Three hundred and one bodies were cremated in 1900 at the Woking crematorium in London. According to Klein, the organism largely concerned in the destruction of the human body in the soil is the anerobic bacterium, bacillus sporogenes cadaveris. Decomposition is indefinitely delayed in clay soils, and the dead body may be converted into soap-like adipocere. Deep cracks may form in such a soil in dry weather. Cemeteries should be as far as possible from dwelling houses—a minimum of 200 feet. They should have a dry, porous soil in a site well ventilated and well planted. Perishable coffins should be used, and brick graves disallowed. Deep interment delays decomposition.

CRAB ALLEY, April 30th, 1904.

MISTER HAWKINS, *Editor.*

My Dear Mr. Hawkins:

Say Hawkins I was in a doctor shop the other day and found in your paper an account of a Denver Methodist preacher gettin his spinal column squeezed back into place by Dr. F. A. B. of the B. I. of Osteopathy.

Now say, Hawkins, I aint no Methodist preacher in no Denver suburb and I aint likely to be but Ive had somethin crawlin up my umbilicus fur a month and I was a wunderin if that might be my spinal column out of place. I never knowed a spinal column got legs when it was out of place but, say Hawkins, you'd think I had all the spinal columns in Colorado, why say honestly Ive caught moren a million of them gettin out of place. Ive given up hope of ever keepin the turnal thing together any more.

A preachers spinal column cant have any more joints than this wanderin thing has yung uns. Now do you suppose that if I was to go to this doctor he could catch that queen bee spinal joint? Im just as willin as a Methodist preacher in Asbury Church or any other church to testin on his success. Ive taken Peruna and had my picture in the paper along side of congress-men and preachers, and I can approve of the Eddie Boks and the *Laides' Home Journal* article on spiritual comfort for the closet shelf. Ive signed Francis Murphy's pledge but I dont like these pregnant spinal columns out of place either in a Methodist preacher or a Janitor of an Equestrium Emporium, speshul rates to transhunts.

EZRA SWIPES.

A PRELIMINARY ANNOUNCEMENT.

ROCKY MOUNTAIN INTERSTATE MEDICAL ASSOCIATION.

Which occurs at the Brown Palace Hotel, Denver, Colo., September 6 and 7, 1904. All papers limited to twenty minutes and discussions to five. Titles reaching the secretary later than August 15, will not appear upon the program. The following have been received and are hereby recognized:

Grant, W. W., Denver: Complications and Sequelæ of Appendicitis.

Baldwin, S. C., Salt Lake: Hip Joint Disease.

Munro, John C., Boston: Report of Cases of Operation Upon the Lung.

Fairchild, D. S., Des Moines; Pregnancy Complicated by Tumors of the Uterus.

Mayo, Chas. H., Rochester, Minn.: Peritoneal Tuberculosis.

Arneill, Jas. R., Denver: Hyperchlorhydria, A Common Expression of Neurasthenia and Allied Conditions.

Hall, J. N., Denver: Report of Eight Cases of Pernicious Anemia.

Ewing, A. C., Salt Lake: Typhoid Fever.

Stover, Geo. H., Denver: X-Ray Treatment of Urethral Caruncle.

Kerr, A. A., Salt Lake: Ectopic Pregnancy.

Stemen, Geo. C., Denver: Shock.

Hill, Edw. C., Denver: The Chemistry of Drug Action.

Fleming, C. K., Denver: Title not registered.

Adams, Frank C., Sacramento:

One and one-fifth fare for the round trip in Colorado has been obtained and proportionate concessions for outside states are expected.

A banquet will be held on the evening of the first day. Tickets will be $2.00. All desiring to attend are requested to notify the secretary on or before Monday, September 5, in order that reservations may be made.

Address all communications and titles to

GEORGE A. MOLEEN,

Corresponding Secretary.

Mack Block, Denver, Colorado.

THE MEDICAL MAN'S VACATION.

The opinion lately expressed by a financier, noted for personal economy, that vacations are needless and not beneficial to health, has aroused a considerable amount of interest in the matter. Not that the views of the New York millionaire are considered seriously, but because the time for taking holidays has come and the subject is always worthy of discussion. No one really thinks that vacations are unnecessary evils, and that a cessation from work and a change of air and scene are not for the good of toilers. The majority of people will continue to take an annual holiday, and furthermore will derive benefit therefrom to body and mind. All dwellers in great cities require a temporary respite from the noise and turmoil of the crowded streets, and a period of rest or distraction from the exciting or monotonous routine of daily business. There are indeed some who by reason of their poverty are unable to get away from the town, but are doomed from year's end to year's end to exist among wretched surroundings, compelled by an unhappy fate to labor unceasingly. No one, however, who knows the inhabitants of the tenement districts, will not say that a stay in the country would do them good. In fact, it may be laid down as an axiom that to those who live in modern towns, a vacation is more or less of a necessity. This statement may be made with greater truth of members of the medical profession than those of any other class.

The recommendations as to holidays are widely different. Some advise a long holiday, others a short holiday two or three times a year. One lays stress upon the importance of fresh air and a change of scene, another holds the view that sight-seeing should be strictly eschewed, while yet another will assert that two or three weeks in bed is the most sensible manner of spending a vacation. Lastly, there is the crusty exponent of materialism, who thinks that the vacation idea is entirely a weariness to the flesh and a vexation of spirit, a needless expense for no adequate return, and a grave mistake in most respects. *Quot homines tot sententiae.* In such jeremiads there is undoubtedly a substratum of' truth, insomuch as vacations seldom come up to the expectations, and some are total failures. Nevertheless, although perhaps the ideal holiday is seldom or ever found, it does not alter the fact expressed before, that a yearly vacation is needed by every worker, and by no worker more than by the medical man.

The medical profession is, on the whole, the least holiday-making of all the professions. Not a few medical men are literally wedded to their profession; indeed, sometimes the knot is so tightly tied that they never sleep away from home, and when in bed usually have one ear open for the night bell. A great number of practitioners are perforce slaves to work and must content themselves with a week's or, at the longest, two weeks' vacation in the course of the year. The general practitioner, especially in the country, has the greatest difficulty in leaving his practice even for a short time. He and his patients are on terms of such intimate relationship, that, if, when the vacation time has come, those whom he has known for years are grievously sick, he is unwilling to leave them, and if he does go, departs with almost as great reluctance as he would leave a member of his own family under like circumstances.

With regard to the kind of holiday suitable to the medical man, it would be presumption to advise as well as an impossible task. Men's tastes differ as widely as their appearances, while the tastes of their wives and daughters, who must be considered, differ even more widely. In a general way, however, it may be said that the town doctor will be happier and better "far from the madding crowd" in the sweet seclusion of a country retreat. But, although it is well to regard country life from its picturesque and romantic aspect, the matter-of-fact side of the question must not be overlooked. The beauties of rural scenes and of idyllic dwellings are too often the masks which conceal all kinds of evils. The moss and ivy-covered cottages in the woods is frequently but a whited sepulcher. Its drains are defective, its water impure,

and its overhanging creepers and surrounding woods and under-
growth are the home of malaria-bearing mosquitoes, and keep the
health-giving sunlight from its inmates. Such points should not
be neglected when choosing a place in which to spend the summer vacation.

The country doctor, upon the theory, or fact, that a change
of life and scene is the best way to spend a vacation, should visit
the haunts of his busy fellowmen. Perhaps there is no more
healthful and pleasant mode of taking a holiday for the country
practitioner than attending the meetings of the American Medical Association and of State and County Medical Societies.
Such a meeting, for instance, as that which has recently taken
place in Atlantic City afforded unbounded opportunities for instruction and amusement to the medical man. At these gatherings he meets and can listen to men eminent in the profession;
men from all countries and of world-wide reputation. Such com-
munion is of inestimable advantage in many ways; he receives
new ideas, and some of the rust which has gathered upon him in
his necessarily somewhat contracted sphere of life is rubbed off.
Over and above these advantages, the mixing in the social life
of his equals, denied him to a great extent when at home, tends
to enlarge his views. The unaccustomed stir and bustle of the
town or of the pleasure resort stimulate his faculties, dulled by
the monotonous routine of his daily toil, and elevate his entire
being, so that he goes back to his work like a giant refreshed.
The feminine part of his family can also participate in the social
amusements which are a part of present-day medical meetings
with equal benefit.—*Medical Record,* July, 1904.

Spastic Constipation.—The most characteristic sign, according to Singer *(Practical Medicine Series)* is the powerful contraction of the rectal sphincters on inserting the fingers. Avoid
all irritants, especially cathartics. Warm oil enemata and warm
compresses to the abdomen are recommended. Belladonna suppositories are most valuable. The author has had good results
from the introduction of conical bougies in the knee-elbow position, beginning with a small size and gradually increasing.

EDITORIAL ITEMS.

For Rachitis.—A. Jacobi advises fresh air, nourishing mixed diet, outdoor exercise, cold baths, iodides and cod-liver oil.

Epistaxis of Fevers.—Ergot is useful when there is weakness, with cold sweating and blue skin.

Slight Epistaxis.—Suck ice, put ice on the back of the neck, and inject into the nostril ice water, alum water or a solution of tannic acid.

For Xeroderma Pigmentosum.—A. W. Brayton curettes the morbid growths and applies Fowler's solution locally to prevent recurrence and further extension of the malignant process.

For Arthritic Purpura.—Fox advises rest, ergot, and iron and quinine at the close. Osler recommends arsenic in full doses and sodium salicylate with discretion.

A Hematinic Anti-Rheumatic.—Peabody prescribes 10 gr. salicylic acid, 5 gr. iron pyrophosphate and 1 gr. sodium phosphate in a tablespoon of water every two hours.

Nosebleed in Children.—A. Rosenberg directs to tampon to stop bleeding; cocainize and cauterize with chromic acid to prevent repetition.

Treatment of Keloid.—In slight cases Bazin uses oil of cade frictions every other day; also iodine and potassium iodide internally in barley water.

For Xeroderma Pigmentosum.—A. W. Brayton curettes the morbid growths and applies Fowler's solution locally to prevent recurrence and further extension of the malignant process.

Referred Pain in Cholelithiasis.—Murphy states that in about one case in ten this pain is referred to the left subscapular region, and in one case in five to some other portion of the left side.

Cider Vinegar.—Our so-called pure cider or wine vinegar, says James W. Ward *(Dietetic and Hygienic Gazette)*, is often made from grain and burnt sugar; sometimes shavings and molasses.

False Tapeworm.—Salisbury *(Practical Medicine Series)* calls attention to the fact that certain residues passed after eating bananas may closely resemble tapeworm, especially the dwarf variety.

Once and No More.—The *Clinical Review* says: "So rarely does herpes zoster ever occur in the same patient that it may be quite safely stated to one who has suffered that it will never affect him again."

Rheumatism in Children.—A Roosevelt Hospital prescription is the following: ℞ Acidi salicyl. gr. x; sodii bicarb., potassi bicarb. aa. gr. viiss; syrupi limonis m. xv; aquam q. s.: A dessertspoonful to a ten-year old child.

Obstinate Rheumatism.—For refractory cases of acute, subacute or chronic rheumatism Hare uses 15 gr. potassium iodide, 4 m. wine of colchicum root, and compound syrup of sarsaparilla q. s.: A dessertspoonful t. i. d. after meals.

Pain of Burns.—Washing soda is found in every house *(International Journal of Surgery)*, and a saturated solution of this substance allays the pain of burns probably better than any other immediate application.

Persistent Furunculosis.—Cantrell praises arsenic sulphide, 1-100—1-25 grain t. i. d. Brocq has used successfully creamy brewer's yeast, a dram or more at each meal—obtained fresh every day in summer—every other day in winter.

Jaundice and Hepatic Colic.—According to Murphy *(Medical News)*, jaundice due to gallstones is always preceded by colic, whereas jaundice due to malignant disease or catarrh of the ducts with infection is never due to colic.

Vomiting and Hepatic Colic.—The relief that follows vomiting depends on its relaxing effect, favoring the dropping back of the stone into the gall-bladder. This relief is so marked that a diagnosis of gastralgia is made by the physician in the large majority of cases.

Dengue—"Breakbone fever" was originally described as a distinct disease in 1824. It was first recognized in this country in 1826, at Savannah. Other widespread epidemics occurred in the Mississippi Valley and along the southern seaboard in 1848, 1854 and 1873.

Green Stools of Infants.—To distinguish the cause, whether polycholic or microbal (Le Sage's colon bacillus), Levi-Sirugue states that if acid to litmus bile coloring matters are present, whereas if neutral or alkaline the color is due to the action of bacteria.

For Acute Bursitis.—Herbert L. Burrell recommends rest to part, uniform pressure and cold applications, together with aspiration if effusion and swelling do not diminish. If pus is present open sac freely, curette out and pack to secure obliteration of cavity by granulation.

American Neurological Association.—The American Neurological Association meets at St. Louis at the Planters Hotel instead of in the World's Fair grounds as originally planned. The sessions will last from 9 a. m. to 1 p. m. daily. A general invitation to attend it is extended to the medical profession.

Muscular Rheumatism.—Fever (rarely exceeding 102°) is present in one-third of all cases. Pain is much increased by muscular contraction. For acute cases Anders recommends morphine hypodermically; hot anodyne applications; salicylates; ironing with a hot flatiron over flannel; acupuncture for lumbago.

Hemorrhage After Tonsillotomy.—One may apply a solution of tannic acid or any of the suprarenal liquids, or full strength turpentine. Mackenzie recommends six drams of tannic acid and two drams of gallic acid to the ounce of water: Sip and swallow one-half teaspoonful at short intervals.

Age and Herniae.—It is held *(Clinical Review)* that 90 per cent. of herniæ of children under three years of age can be satisfactorily cured, in time, by proper general attention and mechanical means. After the seventh year of life, however, it is the exception for a cure to be effected by mechanical appliances.

Gas Phlegmon.—In emphysematous cellulitis, says Joseph C. Bloodgood, if recognized early before much destruction of tissue, try ice incisions with immediate continuous bath treatment. If the general symptoms of infection are not relieved at once, or if the infection is recognized late, amputate immediately.

Ambrosin.—This is a white, odorless, tasteless, colloid substance extracted by Otto Scherer *(Journal of Michigan State Medical Society)* from the pollen of ragweed. From physiologic experiments, the writer regards ambrosin as the exciting principle in the causation of hay fever in subjects whose constitutional condition predisposes to this neurosis.

To Abort Boils.—Shoemaker recommends cold, wet applications. Oehme covers the affected spot well with a coating of collodion containing one-half to two grains of salicylic acid to the dram, repeating the application two or three times within twelve hours. Lassar uses yeast poultices, and Cantrell employs ichthyol in a 50 per cent. ointment.

A California Medical College.—Dr. Walter Lindley, the editor of the *Southern California Practitioner,* has recently been elected Dean of the Medical College of the University of Southern California. This Los Angeles school is now entering its twentieth session. Dr. Lindley was one of the organizers of the school and is Professor of Gynecology in that institution.

Passive Hematemesis.—This is characterized by debility, relaxed vessels and impoverished blood. The bloody vomitus is darker than in the arterial form. Bartholow recommends Monsel's solution, one or two drops well diluted with ice water, or small doses of opium; also the following prescription: ℞ Olei terebinth. m. xi: ext. digitalis fl. m. iv; mucilag, acaciæ m. xv; aquam menth. pip. q. s.: A teaspoonful every three hours.

Cholecystic Tperesthesia.—In all varieties of medicine infection and calculous obstruction, says Murphy, *(Progressive Medicine),* the gall-bladder is hypersensitive, as shown by deep palpation just below the right ninth intercostal cartilage. When pressure is made at this point the patient is unable to take a deep breath. This hypersensitiveness is absent in obstruction due to neoplasm, torsion, flexion or adhesions.

Solution of Calcareous Opacities.—To promote the solution of calcareous deposits in the cornea, Mazet (quoted by Jackson) has used with success instillations two or three times a day of aqueous solutions of lithium benzoate, gradually increasing from 2.5 to 10 per cent. in strength. Though lithium compounds are of no account when given internally, one can conceive that their local use might be of distinct value.

Cheap Jellies.—Jellies costing eight cents a pound, says James W. Ward *(Dietetic and Hygienic Gazette),* represent the bulk of all the jellies manufactured. Only that sold at 16 cents or more is pure, and to the others glucose and apple juice are added

Editorial Items continued on Page 106

BOOKS.

DISEASES OF THE NOSE AND THROAT.—By D. Braden Kyle, M. D., Professor of Laryngology and Rhinology, Jefferson Medical College, Philadelphia; Consulting Laryngologist, Rhinologist and Otologist, St. Agnes' Hospital. Third edition, thoroughly revised and enlarged. Octavo volume of 669 pages, with 175 illustrations, and 6 chromo-lithographic plates. Philadelphia, New York, London: W. B. Saunders & Company, 1904. Cloth, $4.00 net; Sheep or Half Morocco, $5.00 net.

We have had occasion heretofore to commend this work for its thoroughness and practicality. The author founds treatment firmly on pathology. His therapeutic statements are definite and precise. Symptomatology and diagnosis are fully considered. He places more stress on the chemistry of altered secretions than on the accompanying bacteria, which are usually of secondary origin. In the present edition the most important additions and alterations relate to hay fever, septal deformities, keratosis, influenza, paraffin injections and the use of the x-rays in treating carcinoma. The text is profusely and beautifully illustrated, and is quite up-to-date.

A TEXT-BOOK OF MECHANO-THERAPY (Massage and Medical Gymnastics). For Medical Students, Trained Nurses, and Medical Gymnasts. By Axel L. Grafstrom, B. Sc., M. D., Attending Physician to the Gustavus Adolphus Orphanage, Jamestown, N. Y. Second edition, revised, enlarged, and entirely reset. 12 mo of 200 pages, fully illustrated. Philadelphia, New York, London: W. B. Saunders & Company, 1904. Cloth, $1.25 net.

The second edition of this useful little work has been entirely rewritten, reset and very much enlarged. It contains seventeen new illustrations and two new chapters, on pelvic massage, and massage of the eye, ear, nose and throat respectively. The text is clear and practical, and the book is of real value as a textbook for students, trained nurses and medical gymnasts and as a reference book for the general practitioner. The cuts are distinctly helpful in grasping easily the technique of the various methods.

MATERIA MEDICA FOR NURSING. By Emily A. M. Stoney, Superintendent of the Training School for Nurses in the Carney Hospital, South Boston, Mass. Beautiful 12 mo volume of 300 pages. Second edition, thoroughly revised. Philadelphia, New York, London: W. B. Saunders & Company, 1904. Cloth, $1.50 net.

The value of this compendium to nurses is evidenced by the demand for a second and carefully revised edition. The main body of the text is taken up with the consideration of the materia medica in alphabetic order. The author's statements are clear and accurate. The appendix contains considerable useful information on poison emergencies, doses, weights and measures, etc.; also an extensive glossary of terms used in materia medica and therapeutics, with a miscellaneous list of the newest drugs.

PROGRESSIVE MEDICINE. Volume VI, No. 2. A Quarterly Digest of Advances, Discoveries and Improvements in the Medical and Surgical Sciences. Edited by Hobart Amory Hare, M. D., assisted by H. R. M. Landis, M. D. June 1, 1904. Six Dollars per annum: Lea Brothers & Company, Philadelphia and New York.

The present volume comprises a profusely illustrated section on surgery of the abdomen, including hernia, by William B. Coley; a careful resume of Gynecology, by John G. Clark; a full and scientific discussion of advances in diseases of the blood, diathetic and metabolic diseases, diseases of the spleen, thyroid gland and lymphatic system, by Alfred Stengel; a concise review of the year's progress in ophthalmology, by Edward Jackson. The selections and comments of the section editors render this volume, like others of the series, thoroughly instructive and reliable.

PRACTICAL MEDICINE SERIES OF YEAR BOOKS.—Comprising Ten Volumes on the Year's Progress in Medicine and Surgery. Volume VI. General Medicine Edited by Frank Billings, M. S., M. D., and J. H. Salisbury, M. D. Price of this volume $1.00; of the series, $5.50. May, 1904. Chicago: The Year Book Publishers, 40 Dearborn Street.

In our opinion this is the best volume yet published in the Practical Medicine Series. The editors have chosen for the most part important clinical subjects and have treated these subjects in a most practical way. The sections on diseases of the stomach and intestines are especially instructive. The medical practitioner who does not avail himself of the aid of this or some similar work is hardly doing his whole duty to himself and his patients.

THE OPHTHALMIC YEAR-BOOK. A Digest of the Literature of Ophthalmology, with Index of Publications for the Year 1903. By Edward Jackson, A. M., M. D., Emeritus Professor of Diseases of the Eye in the Philadelphia Polyclinic; President of the American Academy of Ophthalmology and Oto-Laryngologist; Ophthalmologist to the Denver County Hospital, St. Anthony's Hospital and Mercy Hospital. Denver. Royal octavo; 260 pages.

Dr. Jackson's book seems to us a distinct advance in the literature of special year-books. He gives a critical digest of the most important ophthalmic literature of the past year, with impartial comments and in sufficient detail to be of actual value in practice. One is surprised to learn that, "The literature bearing on Ophthalmology grows by some 20,000 to 30,000 pages each year." Hence the justification for this ophthalmic year-book, aside from its intrinsic merits, and masterly presentation of each subject. The latter portion of the volume includes a list of books and monographs for 1903, and also an extensive and presumably complete catalogue of journal articles, along with page references as to this work. The index is a model one. The book is of an excellent mechanical makeup, and comes from the press of the Reed Publishing Company, Denver. The illustrations are 45 in number, modern and original, in addition to a fine colored frontispiece. We are certain that this year-book will prove of real service to ophthalmologists. It is to be procured from the Herrick Book and Stationery Company, of this city.

THE SURGERY OF THE HEART AND LUNGS. A History and Resume of Surgical Conditions Found therein, and Experimental and Clinical Research in Man and Lower Animals, with Reference to Pneumonotomy, Pneumonectomy and Bronchotomy, and Cardiotomy and Cardiorrhaphy. By Benjamin Merrill Ricketts, Ph. B., M. D. Octavo; 510 pages. Price in cloth, $5.00; half leather, $7.00. The Grafton Press, New York, 1904.

This work has the great merit of dealing with a comparatively new subject in an original and exhaustive manner. The historical compilation and chapter bibliographies are also very complete and satisfactory. In addition to the clinical records and remarks on technique, the author briefly discusses his experimental researches on the heart (19 cases) and the lungs (50 cases) of dogs. There seems little doubt that the domain of operative surgery in the chest will be considerably widened within a few years, to the benefit of all concerned, and the author of this book deserves considerable credit for opening up the way in such a lucid and systematic manner. The text is beautifully illustrated with 87 full-page plates of pathologic and microscopic specimens, in addition to a colored frontispiece plate. Although of special use to progressive surgeons, physicians likewise would find the book of frequent service, particularly in the diagnosis of thoracic conditions requiring surgical intervention.

INTERNATIONAL CLINICS. A Quarterly of Illustrated Clinical Lectures and Especially Prepared Original Articles on Treatment, Medicine, Surgery, Neurology, Pediatrics, Obstetrics,

Gynecology, Orthopedics, Pathology, Dermatology, Ophthalmology, Otology, Rhinology, Laryngology, Hygiene and other topics of interest to students and practitioners. By leading members of the medical profession throughout the world. Edited by A. O. J. Kelly, A. M., M. D., Philadelphia. Volume II. Fourteenth Series. 1904. Philadelphia: J. B. Lippincott Company.

The present volume contains a new departure in that more than one-third of the text is taken up with a symposium on the diseases of warm climates. This section, comprising nine articles, is authoritative and most instructive, and is handsomely illustrated with plates and other figures. The intestinal lesions of uncinariasis, as shown in the colored plate, bear considerable resemblance to those of typhoid fever. Among the papers in the section on treatment, that of Walter L. Bierring, on "The Significance and Treatment of the Gastrointestinal Form of Arteriosclerosis," is noteworthy for its originality and practical value. "Neurotic Asthma" is the title of an interesting contribution by William H. Katzenbach. The amply illustrated clinical lecture by J. Torrance Rugh, on ankylosed joints and their non-operative treatment, will appeal with special force to surgeons.

THE DOCTOR'S LEISURE HOUR. Facts and Fancies of Interest to the Doctor and His Patient. Charles Wells Moulton, General Editor. Arranged by Porter Pavies, M. D. Octavo; 352 pages. Price in cloth, $2.50; half morocco, $4.00. 1904: The Saalfield Publishing Co., Chicago, Akron, New York.

This book has a pleasing appearance, which does not belie the interest and entertainment to be found within. Though composed in the main of witty and humorous sketches drawn from contemporaneous literature and the pages of good authors, yet there is much information of real value—considerable indeed that should serve as an antidote to Eddyism and other forms of quackery. The arrangement of the text under such section headings as "The Student," "The Professor," "The Prescription," etc., is a good idea, albeit along the line of a Methodist hymnal. The work is illustrated with four plates. No more suitable book, we think, could be on the practitioner's waiting-room table; to while away the time for impatient patients. The present volume is the first of a series called the "Doctor's Recreation Series," to be published in monthly succession. The undertaking is a large one and deserves a cordial support on the part of the medical profession.

SELECTIONS.

INTESTINAL PARASITES.—We have just issued the second of the series of twelve illustrations, of the Intestinal Parasites, and we will send them free, to the physicians on application.— Battle and Co.

NEPHRITIS.—℞ Satyria Liquid, teaspoonful three times daily. One Satyria Tablet morning and night.

CELERINA.—Brainfag, from worry, overwork or excesses of various kinds, is quickly relieved by the use of celerina, in teaspoonful doses three times a day.

SANMETTO.—Dr. J. L. Waffenschmidt of Cincinnati, Ohio, who graduated from Miami Medical College in 1872, writing, says: "My experience with Sanmetto has been pre-eminently satisfactory in all cases of irritable conditions of the urinary organs, and I prescribe it with a feeling of certainty of good results in catarrhal conditions of the pelvic organs and atonic conditions of the sexual glands. In cystitis, spermatorrhea, enuresis and loss of sexual power it is par excellence."

LISTERINE.—As an antiferment, to correct disorders of digestion, and to counteract the intestinal putrefaction processes in the summer diarrheas of children, Listerine possesses great advantages over other antiseptics in that it may be administered freely, being non-toxic, non-irritant and non-escharotic: furthermore, its genial compatibility with syrups, elixirs and other standard remedies of the materia medica, renders it an acceptable and efficient agent in the treatment of diseases produced by the fermentation of food, the decomposition of organic matter, the endo-development of fetid gases, and the presence or attack of low forms of microzoic life. An interesting pamphlet relating to the treatment of diseases of this character may be had upon application to the manufacturers of Listerine.—Lambert Pharmacal Co., St. Louis.

A SEASONABLE ITEM.—Bruises, sprains and abrasions consequent upon tennis, golf, mountain climbing and other out-door sports are prevalent at this season. Infected wounds are frequent and disabling. Country life also brings the results of contact with poison-ivy, poison-oak and the various venomous insects with their characteristic weapons of offense. In all these cases the physician's first thought should be Antiphlogistine. It reduces inflammation of all sorts better and more quickly than any other application, while for poisoned wounds and dermatitis venenata it is almost a specific.

GLYCOGEN IN DIABETIC ALBUMINURIA.—(From *Monthly Cyclopedia*, April, 1904.) The writer calls attention to the value of glycogen in the treatment of diabetic albuminuria. He recalls the fact that last year he was led to conclude that the hepatic cell in diabetics seemed to have lost the power of fixing glycogen in its cytoplasm. His researches have since been confirmed by Monier, of Liege. This brings to mind the fact that Frerichs many years ago, having obtained·by trocar from a diabetic patient a parcel of hepatic tissue, ascertained microscopically the absence of glycogen in the hepatic cell. Albuminuria is a grave complication of diabetes and requires active treatment. Unfortunately, this symptom and diabetes are, as it were, antagonistic, the former requiring a milk diet, or at least a diet rich in hydrocarbons; the second, on the contrary, demanding a diet from which are excluded as much as possible starches and sugars. Again, considering the condition of the kidneys in diabetics, certain remedies now used, antipyrin and other toxics, cannot be employed. The writer found that the methodic use of glycogen seemed to avoid this difficulty, and mentions a number of cases with charts to sustain his point. The dose administered began, as a rule, with one gramme (15 grains) in the course of the day. —M. Laumonier *(Bulletin General de Therapeutique*, January 15, 1904.)

HAY FEVER.—For years the malady known as hay fever has been the theme of many an able discussion. Its etiology, pathology, prophylaxis and treatment often have been the subject of study and experiment by physicians, and also by intelligent laymen. The disease has been described as a catarrhal affection of the conjunctivæ and the mucous membrane of the respiratory tract, characterized by an anual recurrence at about the same date in a given case. Another view is that the disease is a neurosis, and that the local symptoms (rhinorrhea, sensory disturbances, etc.) are due to vasomotor paralysis. The most conspicuous symptoms of hay fever are a burning and itching sensation in the nasal region and between the eyes; violent paroxysms of sneezing; a copious discharge of serum and liquid mucus from the nasal passages; profuse lacrimation; now and then, febrile manifestations; frontal headache, and in not a few cases, some asthma. The diagnosis having been established, the subject of prevention and treatment is of the utmost importance. It would be utterly useless and wearisome to attempt to review the list of remedies and the methods of treatment that have been proposed for this disorder. The interests of physicians and patients will best be served by a recital of facts respecting the most successful mode of treatment known at this time. A glance at the list of symptoms and a brief consideration of the pathology of hay fever lead to the immediate conclusion that the chief indications are to check the discharge, allay the irritation that gives rise to the paroxysms of sneezing, reduce the turgescence of the nasal mucosa and relieve the stenosis. The only single remedy that meets these indications is Adrenalin, as represented in Solution Adrenalin Chloride and Adrenalin Inhalant. By stimulating the vasomotor supply it contracts the arterioles, and thus promptly and efficiently relieves all the annoying symptoms referable to vasomotor paralysis. By its powerful astringent action upon the mucous membrane, which it blanches completely in a few moments, it controls symptoms referable to a catarrhal inflammation of that structure. Indeed the results that have been accomplished with Adrenalin in this field alone are really remarkable and of the utmost importance. Parke, Davis & Co., who market Solution Adrenalin Chloride and Adrenalin Inhalant, have prepared a very complete treatise on the topic, which contains more information than is to be found in the average text-book. They will cheerfully mail a copy of the booklet to any physician applying for it.

Illuminating Gas Poisoning.—In the *Medical Record* of July 9, W. Gilman Thompson gives a clinical study of ninety comatose cases of carbon monoxide poisoning, a large proportion of which were treated at the New York Presbyterian Hospital in the service of himself or his colleagues. Of these ninety cases, many suicidal in intent, 73 recovered and 17 died. The writer calls attention to the gas stove as being more dangerous than the illuminating burners. He is convinced that besides the deoxidizing effect on the blood of carbon monoxide, it has some specific toxic influence upon the central nervous system. Leucocytosis is both high and persistent, the polymorphonuclear cells predominating, and increases with the gravity of the condition. An eccentric though moderate fever is present in nearly all instances, commonly preceded and followed by subnormal temperature. The pulse is disproportionately rapid. Convulsions occur in about seven per cent. of all cases. Coma lasting even four or five days is not invariably fatal. The results of combined phlebotomy (a pint when pulse permits) and saline infusion (at least 1500 c.c.) justify the prompt and thorough employment of these measures. In a large percentage of fatal cases the cause of death may be referred to cerebral congestion or hemorrhage.

EDITORIAL ITEMS.— Continued.

in increasing quantity as the price goes down, until the eight cent
variety hardly contains a trace of the fruit after which it is named.
Some jams and jellies are made from bullock's blood as a base,
with coloring matter, gelatin, starch, rotten fruit and vegetables.

Mastoid Abscess.—Clarence J. Blake makes a preliminary
incision from above downward one-half inch back from insertion
of auricle and following its curve. He bares the bone of periosteum and searches the bone for perforation, congestion or softening, opens at this point by means of chisel, gouge and mallet or
drill. He then removes dead tissue thoroughly from the cavity
by means of a sharp curette, flushes surface of wound with hot
water, and applies a simple baked dressing.

Suppurative Arthritis.—Pick advises careful support of limb
on splint from first, and he says to evacuate pus at once and provide free drainage, or aspirate if the effusion is passive without
pain or redness. Amputation may be necessary if joints become
disorganized. Anders recommends aromatic sulphuric acid or
atropine (gr. 1-120) and agaricine (gr. $\frac{1}{8}$-$\frac{1}{4}$) at bedtime for
sweating. Antistreptococcic serum has sometimes led to imme-
diate improvement.

Acute Arthritis or Epiphysitis of Infancy.—In the treatment
of this very serious disease J. Pickering Pick says: Keep limb
at rest on splint in early stage, when one or two leeches are often
useful; immediate antiseptic evacuation of pus (if possible before it reaches joint), free drainage by strips of gutta percha
tissue, use of splint to prevent deformity and of liquor cinchonæ
and brandy to support strength; appropriate mechanical support
for displacement if epiphysis becomes detached.

"Mother Marks."—Nevus vasculosus is characterized by one
or several bright red to purple, level or raised vascular plexi, fading into the normal skin, showing a transient pallor on pressure.
In size they range from a pinhead to the palm. They are usually
about the head or face and are congenital. By way of treatment
American Text-Book of Surgery advises ligation by passing a
pin under the mass and throwing a single or double ligature
around the tumor below the pin; or excision may be practiced.

Severe Epistaxis.—DaCosta recommends a nasal plug of absorbent cotton saturated with a solution of one part of gelatin in sixteen parts of normal salt solution. In obstinate venous hemorrhage Thornton prescribes ten to twenty drops of fluid extract of hamamelis in water every hour. In hemophiliac cases calcium chloride may be given in the dose of two or three grains four or five times daily. In these cases Osler recommends ergot internally, and says that ice, tannin and gallic acid may be tried before resorting to plugging.

The Chicago Drovers Journal.—We very seldom notice journals out of our special line of work, but this journal is of special interest to us, because it is managed and edited by Mrs. Goodall. The juornal has been a success in every particular, and especially a financial success, and shows what a woman can do. Those physicians particularly interested in agriculture and stock growing could not do better than to read this journal, for the paper is kept fully abreast of the times and the general issues of the day are discussed.

Moles.—Nevus pigmentosus appears as· brown or black, linear, irregular or roundish spots of· hyperpigmentation and sometimes hypertrophy or hairiness. The lesions vary from a pinhead in size to a large area. Though often congenital, they occur on the backs of hands and toes from recurrent chilblain, and the linear form from nervous defects. Hardaway recommends electrolysis for small moles, and excision in the case of extensive growths. He cautions against the use of mild caustics and other teasing methods. Fox applies a drop of nitric acid carefully on the flat nevus, and cuts off the warty nevus with scissors or knife.

Diagnosis of Tophi in the Ear.—According to the investigations of Wilhelm Ebstein (quoted by the editor of the *Medical Record*), true tophi may be hard and sandy or soft, yielding a milky juice on puncture. They are sometimes, says Garrod, smaller than a pinhead, and again larger than a split pea. They generally have a pearly appearance, and usually lie on the borders of the helix. True tophi differ from other nodules in the ear in being seated in the subcutaneous tissue, and not in the cartilages themselves, and, most important of all, in containing uratic contents.

Influence of Fatigue in Causing Organic Ocular Disease.—
Nettleship, says Jackson, has come to attribute greater influence
to fatigue and overwork, local and general, than to more directly
mechanical agencies in the production of organic disease of the
retina and choroid, particularly intraocular hemorrhage. He
cites a series of nine cases in which the effects of fatigue were
quite striking. Myopic and senile eyes are especially liable to
suffer from fatigue. Influenza and similar depressing conditions
appear to render the eye more susceptible to the evil effects of
overuse.

Acute Osteomyelitis.—Roswell Park charges to lose no time
in making incisions sufficiently long and deep, and then by means
of suitable instruments (bone drill and chisel) open interior to
relieve tension and remove septic products. Scrape entire pus-
containing cavity, disinfect with hydrogen peroxide, cauterize
with zinc chloride, and pack, leaving wound open. If neighboring joints appear infected, explore, and if pus is found, open
freely, wash out and drain. If the parosteal veins are found filled
with septic thrombi, open them so far as exposed and remove contents. When there is total necrosis of the shaft, remove completely all dead and dying tissue.

Treatment of Carbuncle.—Thornton prescribes nuclein,
14-15 grains in tablets t. i. d. Manley employs a hypodermic injection of pure carbolic acid into and about the affected area—one
to three drops in early stages, 15 to 30 drops in the suppurative
stage. Hardway says: Keep up strength of patient; morphine
usually needed to secure rest; good hygiene; nutritious, easily
digested diet; alcoholic stimulants and tonics; crucial incision
through entire thickness and width of infiltration, followed by
thorough removal of necrotic masses with sharp spoon and scissors, and application of moist antiseptic dressings, to be changed
daily.

Bleeding Gums.—Osler recommends in scurvy the juice of
two or three lemons daily and a varied diet with plenty of fresh
vegetables. When the stomach is much disordered, small quantities of scraped meat and milk may be given at short intervals,
and lemon juice in gradually increasing quantity. A bitter tonic
or the steel and bark mixture is of service. Permanganate of
potassium or dilute carbolic acid is the best mouth wash. Pen-

cil the swollen gums with a tolerably strong solution of silver
nitrate. In the infantile form give fresh cow's milk and a teaspoonful of meat juice or gravy with a little sieved potato, also
a little orange or lemon juice in water.

Statue to Dr. William Elias B. Davis.—The statue will be
made by G. Moretti, who was the designer of Vulcan (the Colos-
sus iron man which represents the Birmingham district at the St.
Louis Exposition) and will be in bronze, 7½ feet high, standing
upon a granite pedestal 9½ feet high. Signor Moretti is now
making a marble bust of Dr. Davis in Alabama marble. The
plaster cast is a very fine likeness. He has made an indemnity
contract to have the statue ready by the first of December next
that it may be unveiled at the coming meeting of the Southern
Surgical and Gynecological Association.—*Editorial from the
Alabama Medical Journal, May, 1904.*

Mississippi Valley Medical Association.—The thirtieth annual session of the Mississippi Valley Medical Association will be
held at Cincinnati, Ohio, October 11, 12, 13, 1904, under the
presidency of Dr. Hugh T. Patrick, of Chicago. The headquarters
and meeting places will be at the Grand hotel. The annual ora-
tions will be delivered by Dr. Wm. J. Mayo, of Rochester, Minn.,
in Surgery, and Dr. C. Travis Drennen, of Hot Springs, Ark.,
in Medicine. Request for places upon the program, or information in regard to the meeting, can be had by addressing the Secretary, Dr. Henry Enos Tuley, Louisville, Ky., or the Assistant
Secretary, Dr. S. C. Stanton, Masonic Temple, Chicago, Ill. The
usual railroad rates will be in effect.

Erythema Nodosum.—This is characterized by few, symmetric, roundish, more or less elevated, hard or soft, elastic, nut-
sized nodes, bright red or ecchymotic and changing color like a
bruise. They appear suddenly and in crops on the arms, tibiæ
or back of hands and feet, and are accompanied by pain, tenderness and burning sensations, and perhaps rigors, malaise, vomiting and arthralgia. It is for the most part an affection of rheumatic young women. In its treatment Stelwagon advises relative
or absolute rest and unstimulating diet; intestinal antiseptics,
quinine and saline laxatives; and the local application of lead
water and laudanum.

Acute Rheumatoid Arthritis.—This differs from acute articular rheumatism in the fact that it does not migrate from joint to joint and in the absence of local redness. In its management Anders advises a generous dietary, systematic warm bathing, abundance of fresh air, properly regulated physical exercise; iron and cod-liver oil; arsenous acid (gr. 1-30) and sodium iodide (10 to 15 drops of saturated solution) in milk an hour after food; hot mineral spas; cold compress wet with narcotic agent and covered with oiled silk if joints inflamed; thorough and systematic massage to reduce swelling and rigidity; also Swedish movements.

Hemorrhage After Tooth Extraction.—Among the measures recommended for this condition are, firm plugging of the cavity with antiseptic cotton, plain or saturated with liquor ferri chloridi, local use of chromic acid crystals; and application on cotton of tannin, suprarenal extract or antipyrin, or two parts of chloroform in one hundred parts of water. In the case of "bleeders" we may apply a crystal of subsulphate of iron, or use a cotton pledget soaked in Monsel's solution or a solution of lunar caustic in water. For these cases Osler advises absolute rest and compression, followed by styptics if these fail; iron and arsenic during convalescence.

Gonorrheal Arthritis.—Superheated air relieves pain and diminishes effusion into joint. Anders advises absolute rest of limb on splint; ichthyol or belladonna ointment, followed by firm bandaging or immobilization in plaster of paris dressing (anesthetic necessary in acute cases); in chronic forms remove effusion (if present), swelling and stiffness, using massage and passive movements, themocautery and blisters; careful attention to urethral or vaginal condition. If the effusion is purulent and gonococcal Bloodgood directs to open the joint at once and irrigate with 1:1000 mercuric chloride (prevent absorption by Esmarch bandage on limb), then close wound unless a very virulent case; aspirate first if effusion contains a few gonococci but is only slightly cloudy, employing arthrotomy in 24-48 hours if no relief.

Treatment of Synovitis.—Joseph Ranoshoff directs to curtail inflammation by rest and suspension of limb at nearly a right angle, placing part on a proper splint and using an elastic bandage over one or two thicknesses of gauze, or applying ice-bag and lead water and laudanum. To remove products of inflammation when acute stage has passed, make repeated use of blisters and hot iron, methodical massage followed by elastic compression, and potassium iodide internally. Aspiration of joint by oblique puncture should be done after two or three weeks if the effusion continues. When one or two aspirations have failed, inject into joint cavity two or three drams of five per cent. solution of carbolic acid through a large trocar. In suppurative cases use efficient drainage at earliest possible moment. Prevent deformity by keeping limb in a proper position from the very beginning. Restore function by passive movements and massage.

For Bleeding from the Nose.—Adrenalin chlorid (1:10,000) or similar preparations, applied locally on cotton, is one of the most certain remedies. Aconite is recommended in plethoric persons, especially when the bleeding is due to arterial excitement or passion; pulsatilla has been employed for vicarious hemorrhage at the menstrual period. Salicylates, says S. Phillips, are specific against rheumatic epistaxis. Waugh recommends the injection of chromic acid, five grains to the ounce of water. Alonzo Clark injects a solution of one dram persulphate of iron in four to six ounces of water. Hutchinson directs to immerse hands and feet in water as hot as can be borne. H. D. Didama gives a grain or more of opium, repeated if necessary in two or three hours. Wm. P. Northrup irrigates the nasal cavity with cold water, or applies an absorbent cotton plug saturated with hydrogen peroxide or an iron solution.

Dust and Rheumatic Pains.—Robert Hessler *(Fort Wayne Medical Journal Magazine,* June) says that all of us constantly meet with patients complaining of rheumatic pains and aches, with more or less lassitude, headache and backache, with a bad taste in the mouth and perhaps also nausea, sore throat and frequent urination. In some individuals these pains tend to localize, particularly in the region of an old sprain. These so-called cases of rheumatism are commonly attribted to "catching cold," but according to Dr. Hessler's observations, they are really due to the inhalation of infective dust. They are most prevalent after high, dry winds, and on the approach of cold weather with attendant confinement in close rooms. The writer cites two men who are in perfect health while on the farm, but invariably begin to grow feverish and to complain of pain and aching when they come to town on a dusty day, though not on wet days. May it not be that much of our prevalent muscular rheumatism here in Colorado is really a dust infection?

Pain in Appendicitis.—Moullin *(Progressive Medicine)* calls attention to the fact that, since the abdominal organs are largely insensible to pain, its absence is no proof that appendicitis does not exist. The first feeling of pain, usually referred to the umbilicus, is due to a drag upon the posterior abdominal wall by peristaltic action in the cecum or appendix, particularly when adhesions are present. If the pain lessens without general improvement, the inflammation has spread to the muscular coat of the bowel and lessened the peristaltic action. Local pain depends on the spread of inflammation from the appendix to the cellular tissue, and usually develops before the umbilical pain entirely ceases. If severe, the inflammation is widespread or intense. Besides deep tenderness, there is often marked cutaneous hyperesthesia, the sudden cessation of which without amelioriation in the general symptoms suggests gangrene and immediate operation.

Leprosy.—The lepra of Bible times included some forms of syhpilis and psoriasis as well as leprosy proper. Leprosy was contracted by the Crusaders in the Orient, and it has been calculated, says Park, that in the fifteenth century Europe had no less than 19,000 lepers. The disease is endemic in Japan, Norway, Mexico, Cuba and the Sandwich Islands, where there are 909 lepers at the Molakai settlement. In China and Japan, according to Hirsch, people of mixed blood are more frequently affected than Caucasians. There are estimated to be about 30,000 lepers in the Philippines. Leprosy, unknown in France twenty years ago, is now very prevalent in Brittany. There are some 200 lepers on the island of Teneriffe, and about thirty in Canada, including a number of Chinese in British Columbia. A recent report of the Secretary of the Treasury shows 278 known cases of leprosy in the United States, 155 being in Louisiana, and 145 American-born—the majority at large. From the days of the cry, "Unclean! unclean!" the segregation of lepers has been the rule, although the disease is but slightly contagious. A retreat for lepers is suggested in the arid Southwest or on some island in the Gulf of Mexico or on the Pacific coast.

DENVER MEDICAL TIMES

Volume XXIV.   SEPTEMBER, 1904   Number 3.

A CASE OF SPLENO-MEDULLARY LEUKEMIA CURED BY THE X-RAY.

By THOMAS B. EASTMAN, M.D.,

Indianapolis, Ind.

My object in making this report of the subjoined case of spleno-medullary leukemia, at least symptomatically and temporarily cured by the X-ray, is to add to the already numerous reports of such cases which before the advent of the X-ray treatment were relegated to the list of incurables and left to their fate after a more or less indifferent treatment by arsenic, quinine, etc. It is well known that cases of spleno-medullary leukemia often show marked improvement with or even without treatment by the ordinary methods only to suffer relapse and eventually die. Therefore, when the X-ray treatment was advocated, doubt was very properly expressed as to the permanency of the improvement or cure. While it is yet too early to lay any claim to permanency of cure, nevertheless not a few of these cases remain well after nearly a year has elapsed since treatment was begun, and particularly is this true of those cases where it has been possible to reduce the spleen to a size approximating the normal.

In the writer's case the spleen gradually grew smaller and the patient's general health steadily improved notwithstanding the fact that during the course of treatment the condition of the blood would at times improve and then fall back to a much less satisfactory condition, only to improve again until at the present writing, the blood is normal and has been for some time. The writer believes that the reduction of the spleen to a size at least approaching normal is a *sine qua non* in these cases, as in those cases which he has observed where death finally resulted, the spleen could not be materially reduced. In short the blood count is not always an infallible index of the patient's condition or of the prospect of cure.

On June 19th, 1903, I was asked by Dr. W. M. Heward of Grass Creek, Indiana, to see with him a case of tumor of the abdomen. On arriving at the bedside, I found a young man twenty-one years of age, thin, pale and giving every evidence of profound exhaustion. He gave a history of being quite well up to the time he had spent several months in a lumber camp in Arkansas, where malaria was prevalent. Sometime before he left the camp, he noticed on the left side under the short ribs an enlargement which gradually grew in size until when I saw him the tumor occupied the entire left abdomen from a point on the level of the ensiform cartilage to Poupart's ligament and extending two inches to the right of the umbilicus through its entire inner border.

There was pain and tenderness over the mass; the notch could be distinctly felt. The pulse was 110 and full in volume. The apex beat of the heart was heard an inch above the normal point. There was œdema in the feet. He had had nose bleed. He was very short of breath. There were few gastrointestinal symptoms. He complained of headache and was so dizzy that he could not stand alone. His temperature was 100.6. Having no means at hand for examining the blood, I made a provisional diagnosis of spleno-medullary leukemia and put him on arsenic, quinine and tonics. There was no improvement.

On reading the report of a case of spleno-medullary leukemia cured by Senn by the X-ray I determined, after having had the young man examined by Dr. Frank B. Wynn, to give this treatment a trial.

An early blood count showed the following: Red cells, 3,000,000; white cells, 1,110,000. Differential count: Myelocytes, 11%; eosinophiles 2%, normoblasts were present in small number, averaging about two such cells per field, No. 7 Leitz lens. A few erythroblasts were seen, polymorpho-nuclears 67%, lymphocytes 18%. In cover glass preparations this blood presented a picture not to be mistaken. The ratio of whites to red, about one white to every three red cells, the presence of large numbers of myelocytes, the presence of a large number of esinophile cells and nucleated red blood cells fully confirmed the clinical diagnosis of leukemia of the spleno-medullary variety.

Without receiving any treatment whatever other than the X-ray treatment, he began to improve. A medium vacuum tube was used over the region of the tumor and the ends of the long bones ten minutes daily. The condition of his blood improved. There was marked decrease in the size of his spleen.

The patient desiring to be nearer home, the treatment was continud by Dr. J. P. Hetherington of Logansport. About the fifteenth week of treatment, the blood count did not seem so favorable as it had earlier in the treatment, although the spleen continued to diminish in size and the patient's condition to improve. At the end of five months he was working in a lumber camp near his home. At the present time the spleen is not more than one-fifth larger than normal and the blood count is normal. He is apparently in perfect health.

NORMAL OBSTETRICS.

THE OBSTETRIC ANATOMY OF THE PELVIC SOFT PARTS.

CHAPTER II.

BY T. MITCHELL BURNS, M. D.

Denver, Colo.,

Professor of Obstetrics, The Denver and Gross College of Medicine.

THE OPENINGS OF THE PELVIS AND STRUCTURES CLOSING THEM.

1. The superior strait is not closed but slightly encroached upon by the ilio-psoas muscles and the external iliac vessels.

2. The inferior strait is closed by the pelvic floor.

3. The great sacro-sciatic foramen is closed by the pyriformis muscle. (Through this foramen also pass the great sacro-sciatic, internal pudic and gluteal nerves and vessels.)

4. The lesser sacro-sciatic foramen is closed by the obturator internus. (Through this foramen also pass the internal pudic vessels and nerves.)

5. The obturator foramen is closed by the obturator membrane (and through it pass outward the obturator vessels and nerves).

The oblique diameters are the longest because the soft parts, the ilio-psoas muscles, lessen the transverse diameters half an inch and do not really affect the oblique.

The ilio-psoas muscle has its origin from the tranverse processes of the lumbar vertebræ and the iliac fossa. It fills in the space on each side of the promontory over the wing of the sacrum. It traverses the ilio-pectineal line on the ilium to the outer side of the ilio-pectineal and then passes downward to be inserted into the lesser trochanter of the femur. When the ilio-psoas muscles contract they flex the thigs upon the trunk, or if the thighs are fixed the trunk is flexed upon the thighs. If the muscles are very well developed and act very strongly, they may so encroach upon the inlet during labor as to interfere with the entrance of the head.

The external iliac vessels and nerves are situated just internal to the ilio-psoas muscles in the following order, from without inwards, nerve, artery and vein, (N. A. V.) They are not pressed upon in normal labor, but may be in case of contracted pelvis or abnormally large head.

The pyriformis muscle is fan-shaped, has its origin by digitations on the anterior surface of the. wing of the sacrum between the sacral foramina and is inserted into the upper surface of the great trochanter.

The internal obturator muscle arises from the internal surface of the obturator membrane—the rim of the foramen, and the surface of the ischium posterior to the foramen; passes through the lesser sacro-sciatic foramen to be inserted into the upper surface of the great trochanter.

THE PELVIC FLOOR.

The pelvic floor, or pelvic diaphragm, is a muscular, elastic, connective tissue structure, which closes the outlet of the pelvis. Its function is to support the pelvic contents and to be capable of great distention, as for exit of the fœtus, and subsequent retraction. This is rendered possible by the large amount of elastic tissue, by the fact that all the tissues on one side, instead of being inserted into bone and by its openings.

The ilio-psoas, the internal obturator and the pyriformis muscles, together with the pelvic floor, form a cushion for the fetal head and trunk as they are passing through the pelvis.

The openings or perforations in the pelvic floor are the urethra, the vagina and the rectum. When not in use these canals are closed by the apposition of their walls.

The divisions of the pelvic floor are the anterior and posterior perineal regions formed by a line (the bis-ischiatic line) drawn between the anterior borders of the ischial tuberosities. (Heath.)

THE LAYERS OF THE PELVIC FLOOR FROM WITHIN OUTWARDS.

1. The pelvic peritoneum.
2. The subperitoneal cellular tissue.
3. The fascia of the upper surface of the levator ani and coccygeus muscles—the recto-vesical.
4. The levator ani and coccygeus muscles.
5. The fascia of the lower surface of the levator ani and coccygeus muscles—the anal.
6. The deep perineal fascia (only in the anterior perineal region).
7. The superficial perineal fascia (deep layer only in the anterior perineal region).
8. The skin.

The pelvic peritoneum, beginning at the promontory, passes downwards in front of and attached to the sacrum and rectum until opposite the external os of the cervix, then it turns forwards and upwards over the posterior surface of the vagina, uterus and broad ligaments, then downwards over uterus and broad ligaments until opposite the internal os of the uterus, where it turns forwards and upwards over the bladder to the abdominal wall, to which it is attached about one and a half inches above the pubes—the site varying, being sometimes $2\frac{1}{2}$ inches above the pubes.

The folds and pouches of the pelvic peritoneum are the broad, the round, the utero-sacral and the utero-vesical ligaments or folds and the utero-sacral and the utero-vesical pouches.

The utero-sacral pouch, or the cul de sac of Douglas, is formed by the peritoneum dipping down in between the utero-sacral ligaments. It is bounded in front by the upper part of the cervix and vagina, laterally by the folds of peritoneum formed by the utero-sacral ligaments, and posteriorly by the rectum.

The subperitoneal cellular tissue is also called the subperitoneal connective tissue. It follows the course of the peritoneum, lying between it and the fascia of the side wall of the pelvis and the muscles of the pelvis, and then spreads to all the structures below the peritoneum so that "no pelvic organ is without more or less of the cellular or musculo-cellular covering except the lower two-thirds of the urethro-vaginal septum, which is scarcely within the pelvis." (Savage.)

It consists of muscular, fibro-elastic and connective elements in proportion exactly according to the physical relations it has with the organs it encloses or sustains. (Savage.)

Its functions are to hold in place all the other soft parts of the pelvic cavity and to fill up the space between the organs, as between the lower part of the bladder and uterus and the folds of the broad ligament. (Savage.)

The pelvic fascia, beginning at the pelvic brim, is a continuation of the iliac and transversalis fasciæ. From the brim to the tendinous arch, it is attached to the periosteum of the side wall of the pelvis, except where it covers the internal surface of the pyriformis muscle, the sacral plexus and the upper half of the obturator internus muscle. (Its inner surface is covered by the subperitoneal cellular tissue.) The "tendinous arch," or "white line," is a thickening of the fascia at the origin of the levator ani muscle, and extends from the lower part of the posterior surface of the body of the pubis, about ½ inch from the pubic joint, to the spine of the ischium. (It is called the "white line" because in dissecting after the obturator externus is removed this tendinous arch looks like a white line through the obturator membrane.) At the "white line" the fascia gives off two layers, one to cover the upper surface of the levator ani and coccygeus muscles, called the recto-vesical fascia, and another to cover the under surface of these muscles, called the anal fascia. Below the "white line" the fascia continues down, covering the lower half of the obturator internus muscle, and is then attached to the periosteum of the side wall of the pelvis, running down to the tuberosity of the ischium (being attached posteriorly as far back as the great sacro-sciatic ligament and anteriorly as far as the rami of the ischium and pubis, passing beneath the origin of the levator ani muscle to the apex of the pubic arch.) (Godlee, Heath.) (The fascia of the upper surface of the levator ani and coccygeal muscles, the recto-vesical fascia, is prolonged as a sheath to the bladder, vagina and rectum, forming the two anterior and two lateral ligaments of the bladder.)

The levator ani muscle arises from the lower part of the posterior surface of the body of the pubis (about $\frac{1}{2}$ inch from the pubic joint), the tendinous arch and the spine of the ischium; then with its fellow of the opposite side it passes from before backwards and downwards like a collar or sling, including the urethra, vagina, perineum and rectum, and becomes attached to the side of the perineum, the rectum and the median raphe between the rectum and coccyx. Its relations are above the recto-vesical fascia, below the anal fascia; posteriorly (border), coccygeus muscle; and anteriorly (border), triangular space separating its edge from the muscle of the opposite side and giving passage to the urethra and vagina. The function of this muscle is to support the lower end of the rectum and vagina and the bladder, especially during efforts at expulsion. (It elevates and inverts the lower end of the rectum after it has been protruded and everted during the expulsion of the feces.) When it contracts it carries the vagina, rectum and coccyx forwards and upwards, so that the vaginal axis is nearly parallel with the plane of the inlet and the vaginal orifice is nearer the subpubic ligament. (It also acts as a muscle of forced respiration.) The thickness of this muscle varies, but the average is about $\frac{1}{4}$ inch. Its inner edge, running antero-posteriorly, can be felt, with varying distincness, just within the vagina like a double band.

The coccygeal muscle, triangular in shape, arises by its apex from the spine of the ischium, then it passes downwards and backwards to be inserted by its base into the lateral border of the coccyx. Its relations are above (internally), the recto-vesical fascia, below (externally), the anal fascia, anteriorly (border), the levator ani muscle; and posteriorly (border), the lesser sacro-sciatic ligament, which separates it from the pyriformis muscle. The function of this muscle is to assist the levator ani muscle in pulling the coccyx forwards and upwards after it has been pushed backwards during defecation or parturition. (If the coccygeus muscle of one side acts alone it tends to pull the coccyx to one side, *i. e.*, in the lower animals to wag the tail.)

The perineal· fascia consists of the deep and superficial layer in the anterior perineal region and of only the superficial layer in the posterior region. (These layers are variously named by different·authors, but the names used in this description will be the simplest and those that correspond best with the same layers in the male. It seems that general anatomists and special anatomists, such as gyencologists and obstetricians, have different names and descriptions for the same structures.)

The deep perineal fascia, or triangular ligament, resembles that of the male, but is not quite so strong, because of the large opening for the vagina; it is composed of a strong process of fibrous tissue; it is triangular in shape (if the opening caused by the vagina is not considered), stretches across the pubic arch and is attached to the rami of the pubis ad ischium of each side (behind the crura clitoridis); closes the front part of the pelvic outlet on each side (for about 1½ inches); (is not present in the posterior perineal region); is perforated by the urethra (about 1 inch from the pubic joint); is divided by the vagina in the median line; is continuous anteriorly with the subpubic ligament, posteriorly with the deep layer of the superficial perineal fascia as it passes around the transversus perinæi muscle and laterally with the rami of the pubis and ischium and the obturator fascia; and is divided into two layers.

The two layers of the deep perineal fascia are separated in front by the subpubic ligament, united behind where they pass around the transversus perinæi to join the deep layer of the superficial fascia.

[The deep layer arises from the internal obturator fascia a little above its attachments to the pubic arch, the superficial layer arises from the inner edge of the pubic arch.]

[The structures between the two layers of the triangular ligament are, starting in front, the subpubic ligament, the dorsal vein of the clitoris, the membranous portion of the urethra, the compressor urethræ (constrictor vaginæ) muscle, the glands of Bartholin and their ducts; the pubic vessel and dorsal nerve of the clitoris; the artery of the bulbi vestibuli; and a plexus of veins. (Gray and according to Heath, the deep transverse muscle and the artery of the clitoris.)]

[There is no deep perineal fascia in the posterior perineal region, as the deep fascia ends at the transversus perinæi muscle, where it is continuous with the deep layer of the superficial fascia as mentioned above.]

The deep layer of the superficial perineal fascia is present only in the anterior·region, and while not as strongly marked as in the male, it has the same connections. It is a continuation of the deep layer of the superficial fascia of the groin and is attached on each side to the front of the rami of the pubis and ischium nearly to the tuberosity, where it makes a turn round the transversus perinæi muscle to join the deep perineal fascia.

Owing to the position of the vulva, this fascia becomes continuous with the sheath of the vagina and is divided into two parts, called the pudendal or vulvo-scrotal sacs of Broca.

The superficial layer of the superficial perineal fascia is the same as the superficial fascia of the general body, except that it contains much fat, forming the labium. (Heath.) It is present in both the anterior and posterior perineal regions.

THE ISCHIO-RECTAL FOSSA.

The ischio-rectal fossa is a rather large space shaped antero-posteriorly like an anvil with the point forwards, transversely like a triangle. It is situated between the rectum and the ischium, is one inch in breadth and two inches in depth and deepest posteriorly, and is bounded in front by the pubis and triangular ligament (limited in front by the junction), behind by the gluteus maximus muscle and the great sacro-sciatic ligament, internally by the anal fascia, externally by the obturator fascia and its continuation on the tuber ischii, above by the white line, below (superfiicially) by the superficial fascia between the anus and the tuber ischii. (Boundaries after Heath.)

THE PERINEUM.

The perineum is the keystone of the pelvic floor. It is pyramidal in shape and consists of muscular, elastic, connective and adipose tissue. It is situated between the ischia, the integument, the rectum and vagina. It extends upward between the rectum and vagina half the length of the vagina. The length of its external surface, *i. e.,* the tegumental surface from the anus to the vaginal orifice in the non-pregnant is about one inch, but in labor during the exit of the head it stretches often to five inches. (Jewett says six inches.) When the levator ani (Burns) transversus perinæi, sphincter ani and sphincter vaginæ muscles act together through their attachment to the central point of the perineum they convert the perineum into a fixed point of support and render it tense. (Gray.) If one of these muscles is torn there is a gap in the perineum, the fixed point of support is broken, the keystone is destroyed, the pelvic diaphragm cannot be rendered tense and the pelvic contents sag more or less.

THE SUPERFICIAL MUSCLES OF THE FEMALE PERINEUM.

Transverse Perinei.   Sphincter Vaginæ.

Erector Clitoridis.   Sphincter Ani.

The superficial muscles of the female perineum resemble those of the male, except that they are smaller and that the two portions of the central muscle, the sphincter vaginæ (the bulbo-cavernosus), corresponding to the accelerator urinæ, are separated by the vulva. (Heath.)

The transversus perinei is a narrow tendinous muscle arising from the fore part of the inner surface of the tuberosity of the ischium and is inserted into the central line of the perineum. (If one of these muscles is torn in a laceration of the perineum, a gaping of the tear occurs.)

The sphincter vaginæ (or bulbo-cavernosus), analogous to the accelerator urinæ in the male, arises from the central tendinous part of the perineum and passes forward on each side of the vagina to be inserted into the sides and superior surface of the corpora cavernosa of the clitoris. Its action is to constrict the vaginal orifice and by its superior slip over the dorsal vein, to assist in the erection of the clitoris. (Gray.) (This muscle is not mentioned by Heath.)

The erector clitoridis [ischio-cavernosa (Heath)] arises from the inner surface of the tuberosity and ramus of the ischium, just posterior to the attachment of the crus clitoridis and thickens a little as it passes forward to be inserted into the sides and under surface of the crus clitoridis. It causes erection of the clitoris by compressing the veins of the crus clitoridis. (Gray.)

THE DEEP MUSCLES OF THE FEMALE PERINEUM.

Compressor urethræ.

Transversus perinei profundus.

These muscles resemble to deep muscles of the male, but the compressor urethræ does not form a sheath for the urethra as in the male.

[The compressor urethræ (the constrictor urethræ, the constrictor vaginæ, the ischio-bulbous, Guthrie's muscle), arises from the ascending ramus of the ischium from the ischio-pubic junction of the rami or higher according to Gray—This is true in the male—and according to Heath it originates also from the central part of the perinuem). It passes forward to be inserted, according to Gray, by its anterior fibers into the muscles of the opposite side in front of the urethra, middle fibers (largest) into the side of the vagina, and by its posterior fibers into the central tendon of the perineum. According to Heath it is inserted into the bulbous portion of the clitoris. [It is probable that this great variance by these two authorities is due to the difficult of dissecting this muscle in the female because of its thinness and the liability of getting some of the fibers of the superficial muscles mixed with it, or the frequent variation of the muscle.]

The deep transverse muscle is generally merely the lower portion of the preceding muscle (Heath). (The posteriod fibers as given by Gray.) It arises from the ascending ramus of the ischium, and in the perineum is inserted or rather unites with its fellow of the opposite side.]

THE DIVISIONS OF THE PELVIC FLOOR IN RELATION TO LABOR.

These are the anterior or pubic segment and the posterior or sacral segment. All the structures in the pelvis anterior to the axis of the vagina, including the anterior vaginal wall, are included in the anterior segment, and all structures posterior in the posterior segment. During labor the posterior division is pushed down because the presenting part is driven against this portion of the pelvic floor; the anterior division normally retracts upward as there is no pressure against it, and by being not so elastic it is pulled upwards by the retraction of the uterus.

ARGUMENT SUPPORTING THE PRINCIPLES UPON WHICH "A MODEL ACT" IS DRAWN.

BY S. D. VAN METER, M. D.

Denver, Colo.

It is presumed that no one claims the existence of a law enacted to regulate the practice of medicine, which satisfactorily accomplishes the purpose of such Acts. With such inefficiency of the medical Acts there is little wonder that even among those eminent in the profession so many have become apathetic and unwilling to lend assistance in the support, enforcement, or amendment of such laws. We are at once confronted with the necessity of analyzing the cause of such failure if we desire to offer any intelligent solution of the trouble. Attempt such analysis and we immediately discover there is no one cause responsible for the inefficiency of the registration Acts, but many interdependent causes, so complex and far-reaching in effect, that he who thinks the task of offering a perfect solution of the problem an easy one dreams of an Utopia never to be fully realized.

In offering this paper I trust no one will assume that the author opines he has solved the problem, nor that the word "model," as used in the title, is to be construed to mean "ideal." He only hopes that by pointing out the weak points or defects in the existing laws, responsible for their admitted failure, some good may be done towards the correction of such inefficiency; and the removal in a measure of the present disgraceful condition of medical licensure in this great Republic, whose very name is synonymous with "progress."

Before considering in detail the defects of our laws it is. well to review their origin, authority and purpose. Briefly stated, their origin comes from the desire of the people to regulate by state authority all professions and trades for the protection of its citizens from incompetency and fraud. The authority for such laws is clearly and unquestionably derived from the general police power of the constitution, under several admitted heads, but especially, according to Black, of a state's right to enact laws for "The protection and promotion of the public health." Their purpose has already been expressed in speaking of their origin, but it is well to repeat it, as the public is prone to the idea that medical registration laws are for the protection of the medical profession, and not the public. This idea, I regret to say, is entertained by many poorly informed members of the profession, and it has often served as one of the most formidable obstacles in the way of securing the much-needed reform in our present defective statutes. From a careful study of the defects in our registration laws, and the causes of their failure to accomplish their purpose, I have concluded that the chief causes of such failures are:—

First: Material defects in statutory construction.

Second: Professional and social conditions that have a deterring influence in the proper administration of such Acts.

The foremost in importance of the first class are:

First: Provisions that raise the question of constitutionality.

Second: Ambiguous diction, especially in defining what constitutes the practice of medicine.

Third: Failure to invest examining boards with proper discretionary power, particularly in granting and revoking licenses.

Fourth: The recognition of sectarianism in medicine.

In considering the causes that fall under the first heading it is unnecessary to call attention to all the provisions of medical statutes that have been assailed as unconstitutional. Fortunately the superior courts have been inclined to be very liberal in rendering decisions favorable to the constitutionality of the provisions attacked. A review of the cases that have failed to go beyond the nisi prius courts shows that many prosecutions have failed because of the court's belief that certain provisions were either unconstitutional, or their constitutionality was debatable. The provision that has been most frequently attacked is that of requiring an applicant for license to practise medicine, to possess a diploma conferring the degree of doctor of medicine, before admitting him to examination. The attack is generally made on the plausible ground that it is injecting within an Act a subject or purpose not clearly defined in its title, viz., an attempt to regulate medical education as well as the practice of medicine. This, of course, can be answered by the argument that by regulating medical education you indirectly protect the public health, and regulate the practice of medicine. However, with the full power to pass upon the educational and moral qualifications of all applicants, such prerequisite requirements are not necessary. My personal belief is that the attendance upon a full graded course of didactic and clinical teaching is absolutely essential for proper qualification of a licentiate in medicine; and boards, as a rule, should consider applicants unqualified who have not pursued a course of instruction equal to that prescribed by our best medical institutions, prior to conferring the degree of doctor of medicine. The fact, however, that occasionally a man may otherwise become qualified, places those who have not received their doctorate, in the tenable position before the courts of pleading that they feel themselves qualified to practise their profession; that they recognize the justice of the registration law in requiring of all practitioners a high standard of educational and moral qualification; and that they stand ready and willing to submit to the examination of the board as a test of their qualifications, but that the statute renders it impossible for them to take such examination. This position is almost always a specious one. Nevertheless, it catches the ear of many courts. It places the license boards in the false position of being the representatives of that newspaper scarecrow, "A Medical Monopoly." When the courts see that a statute gives the board full power to examine applicants and be the absolute judges of their qualifications, they are prone to lean to the opinion that statutes requiring a medical diploma as a prerequisite to examination not only provide for a standard of educational and moral qualification, but prescribe in addition how such qualifications are to-be obtained. This at least has a semblance of class legislation, which is something we should be extremely careful to avoid if we expect the support of public opinion in enforcing any law, and especially those under consideration. It must be admitted that the power granted examining boards, by statute, is limited to deciding the question of an applicant's educational and moral qualifications to take medical charge of the sick and injured, therefore it behooves us to consider well the advisability of any prerequisites, other than citizenship, before admission to examination; although the courses of instruction, medical and preliminary, should be considered in deciding the question of qualification. Admitting that the statutory provision of a diploma as prerequi- ·

site to examination is perfectly constitutional, it certainly, from a practical point of view, is most unwise, for reasons just cited, particularly as it prevents successful prosecution of those who attempt evasion of the law. It is a well-known fact that no bar association in this country requires any prerequisite degree before admission to examination for license to practise law, and if the legal profession feel it is wrong to establish such a precedent we certainly can afford to do likewise. This same specious plea that has caught the ears of so many of our courts, is a most formidable weapon in the hands of that horde of charlatans who seek to become legalized practitioners of medicine by surreptitious methods when they enter our legislative lobbies. By surreptitious methods is meant the passage of acts ostensibly regulating the practice of their claimed peculiar system of healing, but which in reality give the votaries of such cults full power to judge of the educational and moral qualification of their followers, who, when so licensed, secure a legal standing equal to that of the regularly licensed physician. The sage of Kirksville, the nineteenth century reincarnation of Cagliostro, never could have secured legal recognition in so many states, for Osteopathy—that rankest of medical frauds ever perpetrated upon a supposedly educated and enlightened people—had our registration laws permitted any one, whether he had a diploma or not, to come up for examination upon the disputed scientific medical branches. It is true that the study of these branches alone is wholly insufficient to qualify any one in the practice of medicine, but they are ample in affording an examining board the opportunity of testing an applicant's general scientific education; which when considered in connection with his record of preliminary and scientific courses of instruction, is all that is necessary to arrive at an intelligent conclusion as to whether or not he possesses the educational and moral qualifications entitling him to a license. Many eminent men in the medical profession have felt that by granting such charlatans the privilege of taking state board examinations we would be lowering the dignity of the profession, and be recognizing them in their claims as a new school of medicine. That such a stand is unwise cannot be questioned. These impostors, on the one hand, profess to be practitioners of a new school of medicine when catering to the ever ready-to-be-gulled-public, while on the other hand, when being prosecuted for prac-

tising medicine without a license claim that they are not practising medicine, because they administer no drugs, and therefore
are not amenable to law. They have, by legislative acts, in some
seven or more states, gained a legal standing as osteopathic physicians, and for no other reason than the unwise statutory provision in the registration law of those states, requiring all applicants to possess a medical diploma prior to admission to examination. This provision is laudable in intent, but unnecessary
in practice, and as has been clearly shown, most harmful in results. It must be admitted that such a statutory provision has a
salutary influence in improving medical education, but *that*
should be regulated by a separate law providing for proper preliminary education, strict matriculation requirements, capable
disinterested (financially) faculties, efficient graded courses of
clinical and didactic teaching, and general supervision by the
state of its medical institutions.

Another provision so frequently attacked on the ground of
unconstitutionality is that of providing that in the appointment
of members of examining boards, a certain number shall be from
different schools. The unconstitutionality of such a provision
can hardly be considered debatable in face of confirmatory rul-
ings of the superior courts. That it is perfectly just, proper and
necessary to have school representation cannot be questioned, if
the number of subjects for examination are increased to those
branches upon which there is honest difference of opinion; but
when the subjects are limited to those scientific branches upon
which all schools agree, it becomes unnecessary. Furthermore,
when we consider that if one or more schools are recognized by
statute, it establishes the precedent that others should be accorded
the same recognition, which perpetuates the disgrace of sectarianism in medicine. The result of following such a rule would
become ludicrous, as there are today some fifteen sects in existence claiming to be distinct schools of medicine.

Passing next to that general defect of so many registration
acts, viz., ambiguity of diction, it reuires no argument to sustain
the claim that this cause alone has been responsible for more failures in the enforcement of medical laws than all others combined.
The most casual investigation of prosecutions for practising
medicine without a license reveals that in almost every case the
defense offered is that the defendant was not practising medicine

within the meaning of the statute. Very frequently they claim that the section defining what constitutes the practice of medicine should be so construed as to make its essential feature the administration of drugs. Such an idiotic interpretation needs no rebuttal in this audience, but too much stress cannot be laid upon the necessity of amending the section defining the practice of medicine by legal phraseology so free from ambiguity that the most obtuse court could not interpret the meaning other than that "of holding one's self out to the public as being engaged in the diagnosis and treatment (irrespective of system) of diseased or injured human beings."

In considering the third heading of statutory defects responsible for the failure of medical laws in accomplishing their purpose, viz., limitation of discretionary power of examining boards in the granting and revocation of license, the only position that can be taken in favor of the limitation of such power is that when too much authority is given there is danger of its abuse. Gentlemen, is there among you a man who would set even an intelligent mechanic to work and insist on placing restrictions upon him as to how he should use his tools? Is it to be supposed that dishonest boards are likely to be appointed? If so, does any one think for a moment that any restriction will insure the proper administration of the law, be it good or poor? No, let the profession pay more attention to the selection of the members of our examining boards, invest them with discretionary power, and hold them responsible for the trust imposed upon them, and many of the failures alluded to will be done away with.

Of the last enumerated defects responsible for the inefficiency of our statutes, viz., the recognition of sectarianism in medicine, too much cannot be said if it be fruitful in making the profession forget the senseless bitterness existing between the different schools. That arch enemy to science, *ignorance,* is responsible for the dogmatism and empiricism in medicine; and they in turn for the conception, birth and development of sectarianism. The innate tendency of human nature towards self-justification, and too little of that spirit of free masonry which makes us willing to recognize the possibility of error on our part and that others have a right to disagree with us, have in the past been sufficient to keep it alive. The educated men of the different schools are beginning to realize the ridiculousness of sectarianism. No well qualified physician of any school at the present time professes adherence to any dogma. This being the feeling among the profession, why should the state perpetuate sectarianism by providing separate registration boards, or insisting that different schools should of necessity be represented on such boards? It has been shown that by dispensing with those branches of examination upon which there is room for honest difference of opinion the question of necessity for a school representation is done away with. The sooner, therefore, that the educated progressive element in the medical profession comes to an agreement that the state should require members of its examining boards to be men of honesty, integrity, judicial ability and scientific education, irrespective of their therapeutical beliefs, the better it will be for the cause of efficient, equitable and practical registration laws.

There are many other defects in our medical license acts conducive to failure in accomplishing their purpose, among which may be enumerated:—Penalties not in proportion to public sentiment, or too small to deter those desirous of disregarding them; the lack of a provision for a special prosecutor, and the complicated forms of prosecution, all of which should be given due consideration in drafting a registration act.

The professional and social conditions that have a deterring influence upon the successful administration of medical laws, as well as their amendment by legislative enactment, are numerous. Many of them are of a personal nature, and consequently require a delicacy in treatment which naturally makes one reticent to speak freely. Inasmuch as what I have to say relative to such conditions is spoken with no other intent than that of trying to correct evils that are detrimental to the profession, it is hoped no offense will be taken by any one present. The first to which I would call your attention is the absolute lack of interest the medical profession manifests in securing the appointment of examining boards. Why? They are like the busy citizen, too much occupied to take any interest in the nomination and election of the officials of his government, but ever ready to damn the inefficiency of public service. I hear one say, the appointment of examining boards should be left to the medical profession. Such a plan would work well, and does where there is a united medical profession, but we cannot, under conditions existing in this country, claim that any national or state medical body represents the united medical profession. Under the liberal and equitable reorganization of the A. M. A. that organization is the largest and most representative medical body in this country, and it is to be hoped that the time will come when the executive, the legislative, and the judiciary branches of the government will recognize that association as representing the medical profession of the land. So long as we attempt to regulate the practice of medicine by state authority the appointing power must of necessity rest in the chief executive of the state, unless by legislative act it be delegated to some one else. It could hardly be reposed in any other than a state medical association, and that never will be practical so long as there exist several state associations of equal legal status, notwithstanding their numerical or scientific difference. Therefore, until the profession succeeds in burying sectarianism, it is better and more practical to allow the appointing power to rest with the chief executive of the state. This conclusion does not remove the culpability of the profession, individually and collectively, in its lack of effort to influence the Governor in making wise appointments. In my opinion the best solution of the problem would be to allow each State Medical Society possessing a reasonable bona fide resident licentiate membership to nominate an appropriate number of candidates for the positions to be filled. This would furnish the Governor a list of suitable men, from which he could make no great mistake in his appointments. He would gladly welcome a plan which would rid him of the annoyance of listening to the petty differences and bickerings of the partisan delegations from the different medical sects, who too often by their action give good reason for just condemnation of our profession by the public. It would also prevent the possibility of those aspirants for membership on examining boards who have no idea of the duties of the office, but think because they are of the same political faith as the Governor, they could have the honor of appointment. We may well ask why this lack of interest on the part of the profession, and we at once come back to the original problem of the recognized failure of the laws to accomplish their objects, although the natural preoccupation of medical men—who so often neglect their own business affairs—must not be forgotten. When the profession sees that in most of the States the laws impose unnecessary burdens upon the legitimate practitioner, without preventing the most atrocious and outrageous practice of the quack, it is not to be expected it will manifest much interest in perpetuating such laws. It is this dissatisfaction that has given rise to the organization of "The American Confederation of Reciprocating Examining and Licensing Boards." The purposes and objects of this Confederation are praiseworthy, but it is to be regretted that the energy put forth in trying to obviate the unjust burdens imposed upon the legitimate practitioner by statutes requiring universal technical examination of all applicants for license, has not been spent in modifying our statutes so as to give boards the proper discretionary power in deciding by any rational means the question of an applicant's educational and moral qualifications to practise medicine; whether it be by examination, reciprocity in state licenses, diploma, or the consideration of credentials in general. The enactment of statutory provisions to govern and control the proper recognition of state licenses is unwise, unless made possible in a general way for administration by the board. Any attempt to provide for all contingencies is likely to thwart the whole purpose of the provision, inasmuch as simplicity in statutory construction adds strength, whereas detail weakens and limits the range of applicability. All the good that can ever be accomplished by reciprocity provisions can be achieved by the enactment of a section giving the right to grant licenses without examination to those applicants who have, by the presentation of properly authenticated credentials, convinced the examining board of their educational and moral qualifications.* Such a plan removes those unnecessary burdens imposed by laws requiring universal technical examinations, without withdrawing the right of a board to examine any applicant by the method they deem proper whenever they are not satisfied as to his qualifications.

Another factor that plays an important role in thwarting the enforcement of medical laws, is the indisposition on the part of the profession to assist in prosecuting those who disregard the law. The State seldom receives any help from physicians unless something in the case directly affects them in their practice. Complaints filed under such conditions do more harm than good because the courts immediately recognize that a spirit of revenge, instead of the proper one of seeing the law enforced, has actuated

---

*See Section 7. "Model Medical Registration Act," appended hereto.

the complaint. This always gives the most guilty culprit a practical defense, and serves to perpetuate the idea wrongfully promulgated by the secular press, that the medical profession seeks the enactment and enforcement of such laws for their own selfish and pecuniary benefit.

The little restraining influence that our state and postal acts accomplish in preventing obscene medical advertising, and the widespread brazen announcements of professional abortionists, is so small that it amounts to nothing. The explanation of this disgrace upon our country lies, to a great extent, in the general inoperability of those statutes due to the defects already cited, and for which the profession are in a great measure responsible. Not all the blame should rest here, however. We must admit that many physicians, for supposed policy's sake, often wink at the heinous crime of abortion, when they should discharge their Hippocratic oath by condemning this awful sin, which, with its kindred practices, has caused the fall of nations in the past, and now bids fair to repeat such history in this and other countries. The owners of the newspapers are the men who are most to blame for this evil. Many of these inconsistents profess in one column their adherence to all that is good, and yet permit, for no other reason than the treble price paid for such advertisements, the publication of the most flagrant, immoral, yes criminal, matter, side by side with editorials on honesty, morality and integrity. I have often wondered if the owners of our newspapers had any sons and daughters, and if so, could it be possible that no spark of the love and admiration of purity and virtue remained in their character; and in case there was, how they appeased their consciences when they were instrumental in producing reading matter that no man of any pride or respect for self or family would want his children to read, much less appear in a paper they knew he controlled. The tolerance of such vile advertising, and the tacit endorsement of many of the profession of the widespread practice of criminal abortion, has already established in the minds of thousands of people that such practices are but little wrong. Something should be done to check it. Race suicide by criminal abortion staring us in the face on every side, and the sad picture of thousands of innocents being constantly added to the legion of dipsomaniacs by the aluring advertisements of medicines whose principal ingredient is poor whiskey, are grave questions of the

era, for the American people to consider. It is the duty of the
medical profession, who appreciate the importance of these dangers that menace our nation, to show their loyalty by making
war against them, just as much as it is the duty of every able-
bodied man to shoulder arms against an invading foe. Actuated
by the base desire for gain, the newspaper men stoop to the depths
of infamy in furthering the nefarious business of the quack, who
is worse than the most notorious highwayman. The latter robs
the unfortunate of his money, while the former, in addition to
robbing, takes advantage of that perturbation of judgment that
accompanies disease, even among those of highest intellect, and
by deception and incompetency, wrecks both body and mind of
his victims. It can truthfully be said that the press is in league
with the professional abortionist of the country. Without access to the advertising space of the papers these murderers of the
unborn could not thrive, and the owners of the newspapers
throughout this broad land have much to answer for, as abettors
of this terrible crime. Money! Money! is at the bottom of it all.
How can they retain any self-respect as editors, journalists and
moulders of public opinion, and be in league with the abortionist
and patent medicine man? The powerful influence of the press,
then, stimulated by the pecuniary benefit derived from dishonest
and dishonorable co-partnership with men worse than cut-throat
outlaws, is the greatest social condition that prevents the medical
laws, state and national (postal), from accomplishing their purpose. Cognizant of the unrighteous ground upon which they
stand, they are ever mindful not to oppose the enactment or enforcement of medical laws, upon the plea that they cut down their
receipts from criminal advertisements; but assume the hypocrit-
ical position of posing as sponsor for a poor public threatened
with a medical monopoly worse than the Inquisition itself. To
be absolutely just, however, it must be said that a few of our
prominent editors are manly enough not to allow pecuniary gain
to prevent them from exposing the evil of charlatanry. Foremost
among these few is to be mentioned Mr. Edward Bok, editor of
the *Ladies' Home Journal.* His recent editorial entitled, "The
Patent Medicine Curse," although containing nothing not already
known to the medical profession, is an expose of the evil consequences of this well-named "curse," and, appearing in such a
magazine as the *Ladies' Home Journal,* should strike terror in
the camps of the impostors who are behind this nefarious evil.
Mr. Bok cannot receive too much praise for his stand in this matter. The list of patent medicines, whose principal ingredient is
alcohol, that appears in the above mentioned article is so instructive I have copied it in full. It cannot be republished too often—
in fact it should be printed in every journal in the land at regular

intervals—to refresh the memory of the forgetful, and to catch
the eye of those who failed to see it in former issues:

"THE ALCOHOL IN 'PATENT MEDICINES.'

"The following percentages of alcohol in the 'patent medicines' named are given by the Massachusetts State Board Analyst, in the published document No. 34:

	Per cent. of alcohol (by volume).
Lydia Pinkham's Vegetable Compound	20.6
Paine's Celery Compound	21.
Dr. William's Vegetable Jaundice Bitters	18.5
Whiskol, 'a non-intoxicating stimulant'	28.2
Colden's Liquid Beef Tonic, 'recommended for treatment of alcohol habit'	26.5
Ayer's Sarsaparilla	26.2
Thayer's Compound Extract of Sarsaparilla	21.5
Hood's Sarsaparilla	18.8
Allen's Sarsaparilla	13.5
Dana's Sarsaparilla	13.5
Brown's Sarsaparilla	13.5
Peruna	28.5
Vinol, Wine of Cod-Liver Oil	18.8
Dr. Peter's Kuriko	14.
Carter's Physical Extract	22.
Hooker's Wigwam Tonic	20.7
Hoofland's German Tonic	29.3
Howe's Arabian Tonic, 'not a rum drink'	13.2
Jackson's Golden Seal Tonic	19.6
Mensman's Peptonized Beef Tonic	16.5
Parker's Tonic, 'purely vegetable'	41.6
Schenck's Seaweed Tonic, 'entirely harmless'	19.5
Baxter's Mandrake Bitters	16.5
Boker's Stomach Bitters	42.6
Burdock Blood Bitters	25.2
Green's Nervua	17.2
Hartshorn's Bitters	22.2
Hoofland's German Bitters, 'entirely vegetable'	25.6
Hop Bitters	12.
Hostetter's Stomach Bitters	44.3
Kaufman's Sulphur Bitters, 'contains no alcohol' (as a matter of fact it contains 20.5 per cent. of alcohol and no sulphur)	20.5
Puritana	22.
Richardson's Concentrated Sherry Wine Bitters	47.5

Warner's Safe Tonic Bitters......................... 35.7
Warren's Bilious Bitters............................ 21.5
Faith Whitcomb's Nerve Bitters...................... 20.3

"In connection with this list, think of beer, which contains only from two to five per cent. of alcohol, while some of these 'bitters' contain ten times as much, making them stronger than whiskey, far stronger than sherry or port, with claret and champagne way behind."

How can these wrongs be righted? Never entirely, any more than sin can be purged from man by human methods. But, as good and proper laws have changed the rough frontier into the quiet, law-abiding community, so can we in time do much to decrease the evils that our medical laws intend to accomplish. We must, however, recognize the errors of the past, and do all in our might to profit by seeing they do not happen again. Let the profession unite politically, so far as decent medical legislation is concerned, and with a united front it will not take long to restore the respect that should be accredited the title of "Doctor of Medicine." We must further recognize the necessity of purging from our social and scientific bodies, by rigid enforcement of our society law, members who forfeit their right to membership, if we ever expect recognition by the state or society, much less retain such recognition as a representative body of the medical profession.

These, gentlemen, are my views upon the present status of our medical laws, the reasons they fail, the correction of which is essential if we ever expect them to accomplish their purpose. They are based upon several years' experience in an honest attempt to administer one of the weakest statutes in the country, viz., Colorado, which, in my opinion, has a right to claim but two essential features in its registration law, and those poorly defined. Passed in 1881 and practically unamended since that date, it is not surprising that it is obsolete. Some good may come after all to repay us for the mortification it has imposed upon us in the years of struggle experienced in vain attempts to change it. We can see the failures of the more recent statutes and avoid such errors, in the hope that we may get a Governor in 1905 who is not an Eddyite.

That you may know how I should want an "Act to regulate the practice of medicine to protect the public health" to read, were it my duty to administer it as its executive officer, the following "Model Act," with explanatory notes, is appended. That it would have to be altered so as not to conflict with the constitutions and criminal codes in some states is of course admitted, but the essential features could be adhered to without changing its justice, equity or operability.

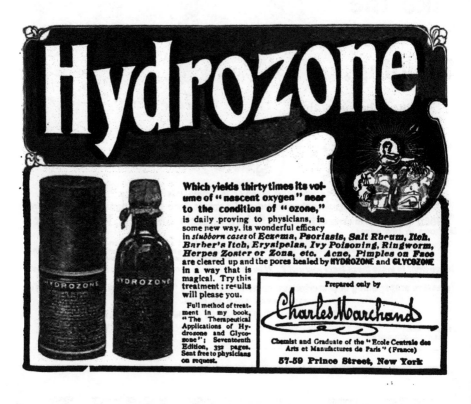

DENVER MEDICAL TIMES

THOMAS H. HAWKINS, A.M., M.D., EDITOR AND PUBLISHER.

COLLABORATORS:

Henry O. Marcy, M.D., Boston.
Thaddeus A. Reamy, M.D., Cincinnati.
Nicholas Senn, M.D., Chicago.
Joseph Price, M.D., Philadelphia.
Franklin H. Martin, M.D., Chicago.
William Oliver Moore, M.D.. New York.
L. S. McMurtry, M.D., Louisville.
Thomas B. Eastman, M.D., Indianapolis,Ind.
G. Law, M.D., Greeley, Colo.

S. H. Pinkerton, M.D., Salt Lake City
Flavel B. Tiffany, M.D., Kansas City.
Erskine M. Bates, M.D:. New York.
E. C. Gehrung, M.D, St. Louis,
Graeme M. Hammond, M.D, New York.
James A. Lydston, M.D., Chicago.
Leonard Freeman, M.D., Denver.
Carey K. Fleming, M.D., Denver, Colo.

Subscriptions, $1.00 per year in advance; Single Copies. 10 cents.

Address all Communications to Denver Medical Times, 1740 Welton Street, Denver, Colo.
We will at all times be glad to give space to well written articles or items of interest to the profession.
[Entered at the Postoffice of Denver, Colorado, as mail matter of the Second Class.]

EDITORIAL DEPARTMENT

TRAUMATIC HEMORRHAGE.

John Parmenter states that ligation is the simplest, safest and best method in general. Torsion is valuable in plastic surgery; four or five complete turns suffice for large vessels. Deep suturing is indicated where the end of the vessel cannot be caught up or is in dense, unyielding tissues. Pressure by long continued digital compression, by clamped forceps for 12 to 48 hours or by gauze or other dressings may be necessary in regions (rectum, vagina, nose, medullary canal, socket of tooth, wound of deep palmer or plamtar arch, etc.) where other means cannot be readily employed. Coaptation of the edges of the wound by sutures is especially useful where the skin is vascular, as in the scalp or scrotum. Styptics, such as persulphate and perchloride of iron, alum, tannin, gallic acid, silver nitrate, vinegar, cocaine, chloroform and water (one dram to pint), turpentine, antipyrin (five to twenty per cent. solution), or mixed solutions of antipyrin and tannin of fifteen per cent. strength—if too strong may cause necrosis and sloughing of tissues. Hot water irrigations (120-150° F.) are of great service upon extensive raw surfaces or in cavities which ooze. The actual cautery at a dull red heat is a powerful hemostatic when applied for a few moments to the bleeding point. Cold in the form of air, ice water or ice cold compresses, acts better in arterial than in venous bleeding. Elevation of an amputated stump for the first few hours after operation, stops oozing from veins and capillaries. Acupressure and acutorsion are now rarely employed.

FOOD.

Adequate nutrition is absolutely essential to physical efficiency. The stunted human life of dire poverty is exemplified by perhaps one-fourth the population of the older countries of the world.

The daily quantity of calories required to keep the healthy adult human machine in good working order has been reckoned at from 3,000 to 6,000, much more being needed when at hard muscular labor than when at rest; also from one-eighth to one-fourth less in summer than in winter.

An excess of protein food above the amount necessary to repair tissue waste is burnt up into urea without serving any useful end, but overtaxes the liver and the kidneys, causing functional or organic disease of these organs. Excess of carbohydrates is stored up as adipose tissue, and may predispose to diabetes mellitus. An excess of fats deranges digestion and overworks the liver, causing diarrhea and skin eruptions. Foods containing nuclein, whether animal or vegetable, give rise to uric acid and its congeners.

The most healthful and economic diet is one so balanced as to nitrogen and carbon (1 to 15) that there is no excess or lack of either. If a person were to live on lean beef alone, two or three kilograms daily would be required to get enough of nonnitrogenous elements; and of potatoes (2%) alone, eight kilograms would be needed to furnish enough nitrogen.

In regard to vegetarianism, W. Gilman Thompson affirms the universal experience has been that while this practice may keep a man in apparent health for some time, it eventually results in a loss of strength and general resisting power against disease. He adds further, "The recent epidemic of esoteric Buddhism has induced some persons to adopt vegetarianism, but few adhere to it strictly or for long."

In a natural state taste should govern nutrition, but when the former is perverted the latter also becomes deranged. The ordinary diets in different climates depend chiefly upon the food supply. Oils and fats are especially indicated in cases of neurasthenia and malnutrition. Fats and carbohydrates are more needed by the young, on account of their greater activity. Soft foods that require no chewing favor early decay of the teeth. Most people in this country eat too much and too fast, and draw the blood from the stomach immediately after eating for the brain and the muscles. If each meal were to consist of only three or four articles of food, or if, like children, we ate the best first, and so did not tempt the appetite to our undoing, there would be fewer dyspeptics and in general a longer lease of life.

Animal foods are generally more rapidly and completely digested than vegetable foods. Oysters, clams and mussels are very nutritious and more digestible than meats. Surgeons are coming to see the advantages of a protein diet, which obviates a distended gut, prior to abdominal operations. The rotting of game until it is "high" aids digestibility by the corrosive action of sarcolactic acid, but it is a dangerous usage. Uncooked meat it liable to give rise to trichiniasis or tapeworm. In 505 unselected necropsies Williams found trichinas by microscopic examination in the muscles in 27 cases, though none of the subjects had died of this disease.

Mother's milk is the ideal food for the human infant. Soft-cooked eggs are digestible and very nutritious, but need to be quite fresh, since they undergo putrefaction readily. Cheese contains about twice as much protein as does meat, and when thoroughly masticated is an excellent food. Meat extracts are stimulants to digestion, but contain very little nourishment. Oats, beans, peas and lentils are rich in nitrogen, and, though less digestible, can take the place of meat in subjects of the uric acid diathesis. Too fresh or poorly baked bread forms in the stomach a putty-like glutinous mass, on which the gastric juice can have little action. Potatoes and other tuberous garden products

often cause flatulence and constipation. . Raw, "green" vegetables, such as lettuce and water cress, have occasionally given
rise to typhoid fever when not very carefully washed.

Dextrinized cereals are becoming deservedly popular as
breakfast foods, but most of them need to be cooked three or
four times as long as directed. Nuts are especially rich in fats,
and hence are quite nutritious, but must be well masticated. The
seeds and organic acids of ripe fruits have generally a laxative
action. If too green or over-ripe, they are likely to set up cholera
morbus; the same is true of melons and cucumbers. Condiments
increase the flavor of other foods, and stimulate absorption and
the flow of secretions, but must be used moderately, lest they irritate and inflame the mucous membrane.

Common salt is the primary source of the hydrochloric acid
of gastric juice, and since hypochlorhydria obtains in three-
fourths of all cases of functional indigestion, many dyspeptics
find prophylactic relief from eating largely of salted meats, salt
crackers, etc. The phosphates are likewise very important salts,
being present largely in fish, ham, legumes and on the surface of
the kernels of cereals. A deficiency of vegetable carbonates in
the blood causes the corpuscles to break down, and is probably a
factor in scurvy.

WATER.

At least three pints of water should be drunk daily by the
average adult, in addition to what is present (50-60%) in the
solid food. A lack of water to flush the sewers of the body leads
to constipation, malassimilation, melancholy and many obscure
aches and pains. Water is best taken mostly between meals,
so as not unduly to dilute the digestive juices. A glass of ice
water taken at a meal drives the blood from the stomach and
delays digestion at least an hour.

Among the diseases produced by impure water are dyspepsia and diarrhea, if too much sulphates or from sewage or from
warm storage; and dysentery, typhoid, cholera, yellow fever and
entozoal diseases, from the specific germs or larvæ. Very hard

waters may predispose to the formation of calculi and possibly to goiter.

Shallow wells are most liable to originate specific infectious diseases, and they should not be tolerated in a city, nor in the country nearer than 100 feet to a cesspool, privy or barn. A shallow well in fact drains a circular area whose radius is equal to the depth of the well. The area of drainage obviously is increased in dry weather. The water of deep wells, particularly those with casings, are generally safe from bacterial contamination, but often contain an excess of mineral matter. Rain water collected from roofs is notoriously impure. The purest natural water is that from snow falling on mountains. The usual source of hydrant water is from ponds, lakes and rivers. It is very important that such water is not contaminated with sewage. Ice water is always purer than the water from which it was formed, but may still contain dangerous germs and their products.

The sanitary chemical analysis of water is an indirect method of testing for bacteria, by establishing the presence or absence of their pabulum and products. The total solids left on evaporation should not exceed 40 grains per gallon, and the organic and volatile matters in this sediment ought never to reach 50%. Unless the source of the water is near salt deposits, an excess of chlorids indicates the presence of sewage. Increase above the normal of oxygen-consuming power points to animal or vegetable pollution. Ammonia represents the first change in the natural putrefactive decomposition of nitrogenous substances, the second and third products being nitrites and nitrates, their pathological import diminishing from first to third. More than six parts of phosphates in 10,000,000 should be regarded with suspicion.

The poisonous metals rarely or occasionally found in drinking water include barium (from dye works), arsenic, copper, chromium, zinc and lead. Solution of the last named metal is favored by softness of the water, by the presence of nitrites and nitrates, excess of carbon dioxid, peaty acids or free sulphuric acid formed by oxidation of iron pyrites. One-tenth grain of lead per gallon of water may produce plumbism. It is well to avoid using internally water which has stood over night in the pipes.

The taste and appearance of a water is no criterion of its fitness for drinking purposes; the most clear and sparkling waters may be deadly in their germ contents. A green coloration of small quantities of water indicates a high degree of vegetable contamination. Dark brown globular masses may come from sewage. Foul odors accompany hydrogen sulphid or putrefaction of animal matters. Saprophytic organisms in running water eventually destroy typhoid and other specific germs.

Ordinary household filters for drinking water are a delusion, and need to be cleansed every day or two in boiling water, lest the germs form dense cultures in them. The filters of bisque and compressed kieselguhr prevent the passage of all known germs. In case of the slightest doubt, however, as to the absolute purity of any given drinking water, the only safety lies in using the water boiled or distilled. Faucet filters may be utilized for removing coarse suspended matters before boiling.

MILK.

Cow's milk is frequently about the only nourishment taken by infants and invalids. It is these very classes that are least able to withstand the ill effects of impure foods, hence the vital importance of securing pure, wholesome market milk.

Each city board of health should have a set of printed rules for dairymen to follow in the location of their buildings, food and water supply for the cattle, the care of the stables, cleanliness of the employees, cows and utensils, and the preservation of the milk up to the time of delivery. The milk should be strained through fine wire gauze, absorbent cotton and cheese cloth, be thoroughly aerated and cooled at once to 45° F. or lower, being kept at such temperature (without addition of ice) in covered vessels in the milk room. Mixing of morning and evening milk should be prohibited, and the milk when delivered ought never to be more than 18 hours old. Flint glass jars, surrounded by ice or ice water, are useful for the retail trade.

Thirty-one states have laws referring to milk for urban use, and nearly all large cities have some special regulations to prevent the sale of impure, skimmed or adulterated milk and milk from diseased cows. Three per cent. of fat is the usual minimum standard. The number of non-pathogenic bacteria per cubic centimenter ought generally to be less than 10,000—specimens containing as many as 50,000,000 germs in each c.c. are occasionally encountered.

In many instances no attempts are made to enforce sanitary conditions about dairies. Licensure helps somewhat to raise the standard, but still better is the system of certificates based upon examinations made by some appointive committee, which should include four experts, a physician, a veterinarian, a bacteriologist and a chemist. Public collective reports of the inspection of dairy farms are useful, especially in small cities.

A commission has been appointed by the New York Medical Society to investigate the character of milk obtained from various dairies and to supervise the methods of transportation. A certificate is furnished to those dealers who comply with certain specified requirements, namely, that the acidity must not exceed 3%, the milk must not contain over 30,000 bacteria per c.c., and butter fat must reach 3.5%. There was a prompt and decided improvement in the milk, and Crandall states that probably more has actually been done during the past year to improve the milk supply than in any previous year. Sour or souring milk is liable to produce gastrointestinal catarrh. Epidemic or summer diarrhea causes about one-fourth of all deaths from zymotic diseases. For the young infants its mother's milk is ordinarily the best protection against bowel complaints. The baby should be nursed regularly and not too frequently. It is often thirsty when it cries, and should be given plenty of boiled water at frequent intervals. Milk does not quench thirst, and nursing too often excites dyspepsia. The young baby should be held in arms only while being nursed or having its toilet made.

The second summer is for good reasons a time of dread to most mothers, in regard to the "summer complaint." To be effective prophylactic measures must begin with the first warm weather. After milk, the first addition to the diet list should be some form of cereal gruel, barley agreeing with most children, but oatmeal is indicated when there is constipation. Dextrnized gruels may be used when the ordinary preparations disagree. Toast and crust are better than soft bread. Baked potatoes are much more digestible than boiled ones. The green vegetables are good for the blood, but must be thoroughly screened. The initial origin of serious summer complaints is generally some indiscretion in diet, particularly pastries and uncooked fruits.

Improper feeding of cows, as with brewery refuse, renders the milk unfit for use. Disease of the udders may cause pseudo-diphtheria or tuberculosis. Many epidemics of typhoid, foot and mouth disease, diphtheria and scarlet fever have been associated with the milk supply. Of 330 such outbreaks analyzed by G. M. Kober, 295 were recorded by English and American authorities, which goes to prove that the Continental method of boiling milk before using has its advantages.

Pasteurization, or heating the milk at 70° C. for a half hour, destroys nearly all pathogenic organisms, but not spores. It is claimed to interfere less with the digestibility and nutritious properties of milk than does boiling. In warm weather milk should be kept in the refrigerator until each portion is needed for use.

To The Editor:

The American Medical Society for the Study of Alcohol and Other Narcotics was organized June 8, 1904, by the union of the American Association for the Study of Inebriety and the Medical Temperance Association. Both of these societies are composed of physicians interested in the study and treatment of inebriety and the physiological nature and action of alcohol and narcotics in health and disease. The first society was organized in 1870, and has published five volumes of transactions and twenty-seven yearly volumes of the *Quarterly Journal of Inebriety,* the organ of its association. The second society began in 1891, and has issued three volumes of transactions and for seven years published a *Quarterly Bulletin* containing the papers read at its meetings. The special object of the union of the two societies is to create greater interest among physicians to study one of the greatest evils of modern times. Its plan of work is to encourage and promote more exact scientific studies of the nature and effects of alcohol in health and disease, particularly of its etiological, physiological and therapeutic relations. Second, to secure more accurate investigations of the diseases associated or following from the use of alcohol and narcotics. Third, to correct tne empirical treatment of these diseases by secret drugs and so-called specifics and to secure legislation, prohibiting the sale of nostrums claiming to be absolute cures containing dangerous poisons. Fourth, to encourage special legislation for the care, control and medical treatment of spirit and drug takers. The alcoholic problem and the diseases which center and spring from it are becoming more prominent and its medical and hygienic importance have assumed such proportions that physicians everywhere are called on for advice and counsel. Public sentiment is turning to medical men for authoritative facts and conclusions to enable them to realize the causes, means of prevention and cure of this evil. This new society comes to meet this want by enlisting men as members and stimulating new studies and researches from a broader and more scientific point of view. As a medical and hygienic topic the alcoholic problem has an intense personal interest, not only to every physician, but to the public generally in every town and city in the country. This interest demands concentrated efforts through the medium of a society to clear away the present confusion, educate public sentiment, and make medical men the final authority in the consideration of the remedial measures for cure and prevention. For this purpose, a most urgent appeal is made to all physicians to assist in making this society the medium and authority for the scientific study of the subject. The secretary, Dr. T. D. Crothers of Hartford, Conn., will be pleased to give any further information.

EDITORIAL ITEMS.

A good opening in Colorado Springs for sale at a very reasonable figure. Address Denver Medical Times, 1740 Welton St.

State Medical Society.—The Colorado State Medical Society will hold its next annual meeting on October 4, 5 and 6, at Denver. Titles of papers should be sent to me not later than September 10th. This meeting promises to be one of the most interesting in the history of the Society, and your presence and help will be a factor very much appreciated, so make up your mind to attend every session. "Something doing every minute."

J. M. BLAINE, Sec'y.

Mississiypi Valley Medical.—The next mreting of the Mississippi Valley Medical Association, October 11, 12, 13, 1904, at Cincinnati, Ohio.

Pan-American Medical Congress.—The Fourth Pan-American Medical Congress, which was to have convened the latter part of December this year at Panama, has been postponed until the first week in January. This was done at the request of many physicians who propose to attend it, as they desired to be at home with their families during the Christmas holidays.

Leech Bites.—When it is time to stop the bleeding, says Ringer, wipe the wound dry and apply lunar caustic locally.

Tubercular Night Sweats.—When other remedies have failed Hare tries pilocarpine hydrochlorate, grain 1-60–1-30 at a dose.

Vicarious Menstruxtion.—When occurring from the stomach Waring states that small doses of ipecac are very effective.

Summer Complaint. — Ia protracted cases (*Alkaloidal Clinic*) give freshly pressed grape and other juices to prevent scurvy.

Phthisical Hyperidrosis. — Thornton prescribes piperidin guaiacolate, five to twenty grains, given in capsules an hour before expected sweat.

Uricidin.—This granular anti-rheumatic salt, according to Bastedo, contains the sulphate, chloride and citrate of lithium and other salts.

Uresin.—This sythetic, says Bastedo, is a double citrate of lithium and urotropine, which is used to diminish uric acid excretion and dissolve gravel.

Chloroform as a Preservative.—The *Alkaloidal Clinic* calls attention to the fact that the addition of a dram of chloroform to a gallon of an aqueous solution will keep it almost indefinitely from spoiling.

Alcohol and the Leucocytes.—Rubin (quoted in *Journal of American Medical Association*) has found that alcohol exerts a negative chemotaxis and leads to hypoleucocytosis, thereby reducing resistance to infection.

For Irritable Conditions of Larynx.—A mixture of equal parts of compound tincture of benzoin, wine of ipecac and a five per cent. solution of cocaine, used as a spray (*Clinical Review*), will very readily relieve a cough due to any irritation of the larynx.

Varicose Veins of Pregnancy.—Lusk advises to regulate the bowels and wear an elastic stocking. The patient should always be provided with a compress and bandage, which she should be taught to apply in case of a sudden emergency.

Operations on the Head.—In these cases Roswell Park puts in a gauze tampon to fill the tumor cavity for 48 hours. Antipyrin in five per cent. watery solution may be used as a spray or to saturate tampons. The old-fashioned small serrefines, properly sterilized, are useful to secure vessels which cannot easily be tied.

Melena Neonatorum.—E. P. Davis recommends tannin in syrup of rhatany. Tyson advises absolute rest with head low, feeding with a teaspoon; uniform warmth—incubator best at 89.6°F.; ergotin hypodermically, one grain every six hours, or gallic acid by the mouth in a one-grain dose.

Scrofulous Ulcers.—Jackson advises treatment of the local lesion on surgical principles; regulated diet and hygiene; cod-liver oil, iron, hypophosphites and other tonics; iodoform ointment, aristol or mercurial ointment or lotions for pustular scrofula.

Bellyache.—A very bad intestinal colic (*International Journal of Surgery*) may simulate an attack of peritonitis. In the first you can move the abdominal wall over the intestinal mass, whereas in the second the wall is rigid.

Infantile Scorbutic Melena.—Wm. P. Northrup says give fresh milk and orange juice, and if old enough potato; general supportive treatment in advanced cases—a few drops of brandy well diluted at intervals of one to four hours; abundance of fresh air; cod liver oil; albuminate or peptonate of iron.

Intestinal Hemorrhage.—Butler recommends tannin and aromatic sulphuric acid. Shoemaker gives five grains of gallic acid in a dram of glycerin every half hour or hour until relieved. For passive hemorrhage, Bartholow has found tincture of iodine, one to two drops frequently repeated, of great service.

Secondary Hemorrhage.—Never delay or temporize, says C. B. Keetley. Try firm, uniform pressure, with perfect rest (splints sometimes useful), elevation and fixation and vascular sedatives. These means failing, use actual cautery, styptics, acu-pressure, ligature or amputation.

Night Sweats from Weakness.—In cases due to debility resulting from acute diseases, such as typhoid, Coston gives camphoric acid, 20 to 30 grains dry on the tongue and washed down with water or milk an hour before sweating is expected to begin. He says the dose need not be repeated ordinarily for several days.

For Scrofula.—Van Harlingen recommends cod-liver oil, iron and iodine internally; occasional doses of calomel or gray powder at bedtime, followed by a saline in the morning; bitters and mineral acids if appetite fails; locally a mild zinc ointment—iodoform powder or ointment for ulceration; curettage when disease is extensive.

Zinc Sulphocarbolates.—J. A. Burnett (*Regular Medical Visitor*) recommends this drug locally in some skin diseases, as an injection in leucorrhea, and as a gargle in sore throat and diptheria. The strength of the solution ranges from one to twenty grains (usually about three grains) to the ounce of water.

Cutaneous Horns.—Hardaway removes the excrescence with knife, scissors or by electrolysis, and cauterizes its base to prevent recurrence. Unna recommends the frequent application by the patient of a solution of fifteen grains of paraformaldehyde and eight minims of castor oil in five drams of collodion.

Hematemesis and Melena from Hepatic Cirrhosis.—Bruce advises rest in bed; morphine hypodermically if patient is nervous and anxious; rectal feeding only; no medication by mouth for four hours—then give mixture of sulphates of sodium and magnesium with alum and dilute sulphuric acid every four hours for at least 24 hours.

Veratrol.—Dimethyl-pyrocatechin, $C_6H_4(OCH_3)_2$, is a clear, mobile liquid soluble in alcohol, ether and fatty oils. It closely resembles guaiacol, but is more irritating, and is used externally. Bastedo states that it has been applied with good results in intercostal neuralgia and epididymitis. Diluted with olive oil it is recommended as an abdominal application in tuberculous peritonitis.

For Sweating Feet.—Fox directs to remove cause (circulatory or nervous); wear socks soaked (and dried) in boric acid and changed twice a day; also powder with salicylic acid three parts, starch ten and talcum eighty-seven parts, or apply diachylon ointment on linen twice a day for a week without washing parts— scales off and leaves new skin dry and soft.

Seborrhea Sicca.—Jackson instructs to remove crusts with olive oil or grease, and apply sulphur, a dram to the ounce of sweet oil, cotton seed oil or vaselin, well rubbed in every night for a week. Then wash with soap and water, and reapply the ointment every other night, gradually lengthening interval each week till treatment is used only once a week.

Seborrhea Oleosa.—Jackson directs to dab ether on part; wash with soap and water; powder with sulphur and starch, or use a three per cent. solution of resorcin in alcohol and water; and give general tonic treatment. Fox tells us to rub with a soft linen cloth wet with ether, then apply a lotion of zinc sulphate three parts, sulphurated lime three parts, alcohol ten parts, and rose water one hundred parts.

Senile Gangrene.—Wyeth envelops the affected part in cotton batting and oiled silk or protective, and places it in a comfortable position. He gives nutritious food, cardiac stimulants and opium. No operative procedure is justified until there is a well defined line of demarcation established, unless septic absorption threatens safety of patient. Amputation, high up, is Park's advice.

Cholera Infantum.—In the initial stage Thornton prescribes two grains of magnesium sulphate and ⅛ minim of dilute sulphuric acid in a teaspoonful of water every half hour. He also employs gentle injections of a large quantity of tannic acid solution (five grains to the pint of water) into the colon by means of a fountain syringe and a soft rubber catheter.

To Control Bleeding from Fractured Ribs.—H. H. Mudd directs to carry a pouch of gauze through the bleeding wound into cavity of thorax and stuff with small strips of gauze to form a knob, which can be pulled firmly against inner thoracic wall. The blue-black welling-up from wounded lung tissue can be controlled, says Dennis, with a tampon, absolute rest and large doses of opium.

For Pigmented Nevi.—Cohn (*Therapeutic Review*) treats these deformities successfully with 30 yer cent. hydrogen peroxide solution. A drop of this is applied on the affected area by means of a glass rod and allowed to dry, then covered with zinc oxide plaster. The treatment is repeated daily on fresh portions of the pigmented area. A complete cure requires from two to four weeks.

Enlarged Bronchial Glands.—H. B. Whitney (*American Medicine*) deduces some useful clinical points in reference to manubrial percussion dulness. He concludes that a limited area of defective resonance at the left of the manubrium is significant of enlarged bronchial glands, especially when taken in connection with the history of a dusty occupation, chronic cough and physical signs of bronchitis.

Chronic Obstruction of Rectum or Upper Bowel.—Harrison Cripps advises gradual dilatation with coniform bougies six inches in length. Pass them once daily and leave in for five minutes to an hour or more, increasing the size every third or fourth day, provided no pain is excited by the increase. Keep in bed or in the recumbent posture during the first few weeks. To prevent, retraction the patient must be taught to pass the bougie once or twice a week.

Hemorrhage from Small Intestine.—Hare says this accident is best combated by taking small pieces of ice by the mouth, and by the use of Monsel's salt (subsulphate of iron), three grains every half hour or oftener in pills hard enough to reach intestine without decomposition. Tannic acid in large amount may be given in solution or pill form if Monsel's salt is not obtainable.

For Syphilitic Ulcers.—Ointments of iodoform, mercury or its oleate, citrine and white precipitate are all of service in different cases, says Lydston. Occasional stimulation with silver nitrate or acid nitrate of mercury may be required. When phagedena is present, use Ricord's paste, bromine, the actual cautery or potassio-tartrate of iron.

Temporary Measures for the Relief of Bleeding from External Wounds.—These, says Parmenter, include digital compression, when the wound is superficial: hemostatic forceps—a few minutes application usually effects permanent closure in small arteries; and tourniquets—must be used with caution and dispensed with as soon as the vessel can be isolated and closed.

For Ulcerative Gastritis.—A milk diet with bismuth salts and silver nitrate are useful. Hemmeter insists on absolute rest in bed. When the hemorrhage is copious and persistent, he gives a hypodermic injection of 20 or 30 minims of ergotol, and places an ice-bag over the epigastrium. If the pain is severe he injects $\frac{1}{4}$ grain of morphine. No food should be given by the mouth for three days, but instead, nutrient enemata of eggs, milk, salt, claret and flour.

Wounds of the Abdominal Wall.—M. H. Richardson advises exploration and careful cleansing and suture if the viscera are not injured. The wound may be sutured immediately unless sepsis is feared—then drain with a strand of gauze. Ligation, tamponage or excision of the wounded organ may be demanded in extreme cases. Extravasation requires repair of rent or, if that is impossible, drainage with general peritoneal cleansing.

Anidrosis.—Partial or complete absence of normal perspiration, with harsh, dry skin and often eruptions, depends on severe diarrhea, diabetes, cancer, Bright's disease, paralytic dementia, advanced tuberculosis (hot, dry, emaciated), fevers or faulty innervation (trophoneurosis) or scaly, dystrophic or atropic skin diseases. It is one-sided in facial hemiatrophy. Belladonna, mineral acids and many other drugs diminish perspiration. One should treat the original disease, says Louis Heitzmann, and stimulate the sweat glands by the ingestion of hot water and the use of hot baths, massage and jaborandi or pilocarpine.

Bleeding Piles.—Boas directs to promote peristalsis by a suitable diet. Treat anal region, after defecation, with a solution of tannin or alum on a cotton wad, or with the ascending douche. If an enema is necessary, use a soft sound and avoid glycerine, salt and other irritants. Use gentle purgatives only in extreme cases. To control hemorrhage persisting in spite of normal feces, give a dram of fluid extract of hamamelis t. i. d. for four weeks, then twice a day for a month. In case of severe hemorrhage, give a powerful dose of opium and tampon bleeding spot with gauze, following after arrest for three days with a dose of castor oil.

Raynaud's Disease.—This vasomotor syndrome is characterized by symmetric local syncope (skin white, waxy, hard), followed by asphyxia (skin swollen and blue) and dry or moist, black gangrenous spots with vesicles on parts having the poorest circulation. There is initial numbness or asleep feeling, succeeded by acute burning pain in the congestive stage. and complete anesthesia with gangrene. The treatment, according to Nancrede, comprises the use of the continuous descending current; warmth, protection of parts, local anodyne applications, massage and administration of nitroglycerin before gangrene has taken place; ordinary treatment of gangrene.

Treatment of Sprains.—Joseph Ransohoff resorts to absolute rest by means of splints, which can be removed daily if required. Elevation and suspension of the affected limb at a right angle will often relieve the pain at once. Hasten absorption by compression with an elastic bandage. Cold applications, lead and opium wash, solution of ammonium chloride and opium, or an ichthyol ointment is useful to relieve pain. After the acute symptoms subside, restore joint function by methodical application of passive movements and massage. In the severest forms, when the intra-articular effusion is not absorbed by this treatment, the joint must be aspirated. Blisters and ignipuncture are often of service in obstinate cases.

Dysenteric or Syphilitic Intestinal Ulceration.—Hare directs to wash out first the colon and rectum with pure water or with a saline or soapy liquid. Then inject carefully with a fountain syringe styptic solutions (two to four ounces for rectum) of alum (10 grains per ounce), Cupric sulphate (5 grains per ounce) or tannin (20 grains per ounce of water and glycerine); or use curative injections of silver nitrate, copper sulphate or potassium chlorate (10–15 grains per ounce).

Umbilical Hemorrhage.—E. P. Davis advises pressure with antiseptic cotton, on which iodoform has been freely sprinkled. This failing, pass a needle armed with a silk ligature beneath the vessels, and tie securely; or pass two surgical pins beneath the bleeding tissues at right angles to each other, and loop a ligature around the pins. Ellis mentions collodian and plaster of Paris; mineral acids and astringents, and cholagogues. In morbus maculosis Osler recommends external warmth, camphor, and ergotin hypodermically. For bleeding cord Davis directs to strip and ligate in several places.

Treatment of Moist Gangrene. – Try to prevent, says Park, by equalizing pressure (water bed); protect skin or stimulate and toughen it with alcohol and astringent lotions, frequent changes of posture, attention to heart, and by watching toes or fingers of bandaged limbs. When gangrene is established, remove dead and dying tissue. Amputate at nearest point of election above injury in acute trauma. For frost-bite amputate at some distance above line of demarcation. In the diabetic form amputation must be high, if done at all.

Tympanic Hemorrhage.—Bleeding from the ear, with ruptured drum head, may take place because of a foreign body, contrecoup or direct injury. By way of treatment Clarance J. Blake advises gentle inflation of the middle ear; and careful cleansing of meatus with a dry, cotton-tipped probe, or if necessary aseptic or antiseptic syringing. After cleansing place ruptured edges in contact and close ear with cotton, cautioning the patient to avoid blowing his nose for at least 48 hours.

Morvan's Disease.—In glossy skin, or analgesic whitlow, the skin, particularly of the fingers, is thickened, hairless, faintly red,

Editorial Items continued on Page 160

BOOKS.

THE GAZETTE POCKET SPELLER AND DEFINER.—English and
Medical. Second Edition, New York: Gazette Publishing
Co., 503 Fifth avenue.

This neat and handy vest pocket volume is the only one of
the kind in which common English and medical words are enclosed within the same cover, though in different sections. The
English words are defined chiefly by their synonyms, and have
attached in parentheses the usual endings of tense, etc. The medical lexicon is quite full, considering limited space, and embraces
all the new words. Each word and its definition are given in a
single line. The second edition contains nearly a thousand new
words. The book has clear type and a flexible cover. We recommend it to medical students for the English as well as its medical
contents.

PHYSICIAN VERSUS BACTERIOLOGIST.—By Prof. Dr. O. Rosen-
bach, of Berlin. Authorized translation from the German,
by Dr. Achilles Rose: Funk & Wagnalls Company, New
York and London. 1904.

The author has a heavy, if somewhat blunt, lance, with which
he goes full tilt against our most approved theories of patho-
genesis, the practice of orotherapy, etc. He makes free use of
italics to emphasize his thrusts, which are inclined to sarcasm,
when directed against ultrascientific laboratory workers. Although we cannot agree with the general trend of Dr. Rosen-
bach's wholesale indictments, yet we think he has done a commendable work in showing forth by contrast the clinical side of
the practice of medicine, the role of the human soil compared to
the pathogenic plant, etc. Some of the chapters, as the "Care of
the Mouth in the Sick" and "Constitution and Therapy," are
particularly well worth reading.

A TEXT-BOOK OF HUMAN PHYSIOLOGY.—By Albert P. Bru-
baker, A. M., M. D., Professor of Physiology and Hygiene
in the Jefferson Medical College; Professor of Physiology
in the Pennsylvania College of Dental Surgery; Lecturer
on Physiology and Hygiene in the Drexel Institute of Art,

Science and Industry. Octavo, 699 Pages, with Colored Plates and 354 Illustrations. Price $4.00. Philadelphia: P. Blakiston's Son & Co., 1012 Walnut Street. 1904.

The author has had an active teaching experience of twenty years. He is commendably conservative in his statements, and endeavors to emphasize the practical bearings of physiological facts. His manner of presenting a subject is clear and full, and the book has all the advantages of a one-man production. About one-third of the text is devoted to the nervous systems. The book is amply and instructively illustrated, the plain and colored diagrams being particularly noteworthy. On the whole it is a work that should prove acceptable both to teachers and to students.

A REFERENCE HANDBOOK OF THE MEDICAL SCIENCES.—Embracing the Entire Range of Scientific and Practical Medicine and Allied Science, by Various Writers. A New Edition, Completely Revised and Rewritten. Edited by Albert H. Buck, M. D., New York City. Volume VIII. Illustrated by Chromolithographs and Four Hundred and Thirty-five Half-Tone and Wood Engravings. New York: William Wood & Co. 1904.

This is the last volume of the "Reference Handbook," the consecutive numbers of which have been got out with commendable dispatch, considering the magnitude of the work. Among the articles in the present volume worthy of special mention are the following: "Urine," by Alfred C. Croftan; "Vaccination," by Samuel W. Abbott; "Pathology of Veins," by Alfred Scott Warthin; "Vital Statistics," by Samuel W. Abbott; "Water," by William P. Mason; "Bacteriological Technique," by F. G. Novy; "Gigantism," by Albert George Nicholls; "Hemolysis," by H. Gideon Wells; "Prescription Writing," by Edward Curtis; "Protozoa," by Henry B. Ward, and "Yellow Fever," by Juan Guiteras.

The articles on protozoa, bacteriologic technique, Asiatic cholera and vaccination are illustrated with beautiful plates. Nearly 200 pages of this final volume is taken up with the general index. The completed series now furnish to medical practitioners a most exhaustive and satisfactory work of reference.

TRANSACTIONS OF THE WESTERN SURGICAL AND GYNECOLOG-
ICAL ASSOCIATION. Thirteenth annual meeting held at Denver, Colo., December 28 and 29, 1903.

The last meeting of this vigorous young society was held in
Denver, and was distinctly a success. Among the twenty-five
valuable papers here reproduced, we notice one each from Grant,
Freeman and Wetherill. The officers for 1904 are: President,
Charles H. Mayo, Rochester, Minn.; First Vice-President, H. D.
Niles, Salt Lake City; Second Vice-President, L. L. McArthur,
Chicago; Secretary-Treasurer, B. B. Davis, Omaha.

Treatment of Typhoid Fever.—Osler's method may be summarized as follows: Feed at stated intervals throughout the day
three pints of milk in 24 hours, always diluted with water, lime
water or aerated waters—if milk not digested, substitute whey or
buttermilk or some mutton or bee broth, albumen water, barley
gruel or beef juice; cool water freely; alcohol when weakness
marked, fever high and pulse failing—8 to 12 ounces of brandy in
24 hours a moderate amount; bath at 70°F for 15 or 20 minutes
every third hour, if temperature above 102½°, sponging head
during bath and rubbing limbs and trunk thoroughly—food and
stimulants after bath; lukewarm baths or tepid or cold sponging
or cold pack in private practice when Brand method impracticable; turpentine stupes for abdominal pain and tympanites; long
rectal tube or turpentine enema for meteorism; for diarrhea,
starch and opium enema or bismuth and Dover's powder; enema
every third or fourth day for constipation; for hemorrhage, absolute rest, restricted diet, ice freely and full doses of acetate of lead
and opium; for progressive heart weakness, alcohol, strychnine
hypodermically, digitalis and hypodermic injections of ether; for
nocturnal restlessness, Dover's powder.

SELECTIONS.

TRAYS.—Any one desiring a beautiful souvenir of the World's Fair may secure the same by writing to the Antikamnia Chemical Company, St. Louis, Mo.

ALCOHOLIC AND DRUG ADDICTIONS—Dr. George E. Pettey has opened a retreat in Denver, at 1939 East Evans avenue, with Dr. John H. McKay physician in charge.

Physicians are requested to visit the retreat and satisfy themselves as to the character of the institution and facilities for taking care of patients suffering from alcoholic or drug addictions.

A SCOTCH DOCTOR'S OPINION.—*The Quarterly Journal of Inebriety*, so well and favorably known through the instrumentality of its brilliant and philanthropic editor, T. D. Crothers, A. M., M. D., quotes the following statement in reference to pain relieving remedies, from one of Great Britain's noted medical men, Dr. John Stewart Norvell, Resident Surgeon, Royal Infirmary, Edinburgh: "Antikamnia Tablets are a remedy for almost every kind of pain, particularly for headaches, neuralgias, and neuroses due to irregularities of menstruation. They act with wonderful promptness; the dosage is small, two tablets. The undesirable after-effects so commonly attending the use of other coal tar analgesics are entirely absent and they can therefore be safely put into the hands of patients, for use without the personal supervision of the physician."

ALETRIS CORDIAL.—When the menses are suppressed from exposure or from colds, wet feet, the result of emotional excitement, or febrile conditions, if not complicated with organic change, but by a mere passive congestion, Aletris Cordial Rio is a very reliable remedy. It is an emmenagogue, not abortifacient.

UTERINE INFECTION, GLYCOGEN.—Geo. W. Tobias, M. D. Patient had two hard chills and was delivered of a dead 3½-months fœtus in the early morning of March 26th. The placenta was retained and her temperature soon went to 104½.

She refused to have the curette used. She is young, and this being her first experience, was very nervous. I concluded to allow her to have her own way a few hours, until the nervous condition subsided somewhat. This put the patient in a comfortable condition for a curetage, which was well borne, the case ending nicely without further accident. It appeared to me that glycogen possesses also hemostatic properties.—New York.

NERVOUS HEADACHE.—For headaches, superinduced by nervousness, Daniel's Conct. Tinct. Passiflora Incarnata, when taken in teaspoonful doses, gives complete relief. Its sedative properties overcome the abnormal tension and permit rest. It has demonstrated its efficiency especially in weak women, whose nerves are overwrought and whose conditions approach the hysterical. Besides removing the pain and anguish, Passiflora strengthens the entire system, acts as a general tonic, as well as calmative, and thus promotes the continued health of the patient. It is most valuable in the treatment of all nerve disorders and the various diseases that result from them.

CHOREA AND ANEMIA.—By Roshier W. Miller, M. D., Lecturer on Nervous and Mental Diseases, University College of Medicine, Richmond, Virginia. In the etiology of chorea, nothing is noted relative to anemia. It is simply accounted as an accompanying symptom of the condition. Medical literature emphasizes the relation between rheumatism and chorea, with anemia as an important symptom. After observation of several cases, I am strongly of opinion, however, that anemia as a causative factor is worthy of investigation.

Anemia of toxic origin presents pathological conditions which favor the production of choreic affections. It is true that simple anemia is, as a rule, of secondary origin, and, viewed in this light, it may be argued that if chorea arises, it is the result of the primary and not of the secondary conditions—thus agreeing with the admitted etiology. This argument, however, will not satisfactorily explain those cases of chorea which arise remotely from the primary condition, but recently from the secondary effects.

I submit cases in which symptoms, treatment, and recovery seem to intimate at least a possible relation between anemia and chorea.

Case I.—A female child of eight years gave a history of typhoid fever eight months prior to my visit. According to the moother's statement, the child had made a quick and good recovery, gaining rapidly in weight and exhibiting the energy of her former life. Six months later she became irritable and pale, with pain in her arms and legs, which condition was soon followed by gastric disorders and irregular spasms of the muscles of the face. Simple anemia was in evidence from objective and subjective symptoms alone, but was unquestioned in the light of the results obtained from blood examination—the red blood element being present to the extent of barely 3,000,000 red corpuscles per c. m.

This case was treated with two teaspoonfuls of pepto-mangan (Gude) and two drops of Fowler's solution, three times a day. After gastric symptoms had abated somewhat, two raw eggs per day were added to the diet. The patient was discharged in five weeks, completely recovered.

Case II.—A female child of ten years of age; gave history of malaria (a well-defined case of intermittent fever) one year previously. The pallid condition of the child induced the mother to solicit my aid. Upon examination, I found slight choreaic movements which had escaped the mother's eye, though she did admit that the child "could not sit still very long at a time," and "was constantly working her fingers." The blood examination revealed no plasmodium. The red cells were reduced to 2,800,-000 per c. m., with a proportionate decrease of hemoglobin.

Pepto-mangan (Gude) alone was employed in doses of two drams in a glass of milk three times a day. The blood examination four weeks later showed red cells present to the amount of 3,900,000 per c. m., at which time I dismissed the case completely recovered.—*Vir. Med. Semi-Mo.*, May 13, 1904.

EDITORIAL ITEMS.— Continued.

or violaceous, smooth and shining as if varnished, and often fis-
sured. There is burning pain preceding and accompanying the
muscular atrophy, anesthesia (except touch) and diminished or
absent tender reflexes. The affection arises from nerve degeneration, and disappears slowly and spontaneously. By way of treatment Stelwagon mentions protective applications.

Perforated Ulcer of the Foot.—In this spontaneous degenerative mutilation we see an indurated, usually painless sinus
leading down through the center of a corn-like formation. The
most common site is over the articulation of the metatarsal bone
with the phalanx of the first or last toe. Absolute rest and antiseptic and stimulating applications are advised by Stelwagon.
Even amputation is not always successful in stopping the course
of the disease.

Hemophilia.—"Bleeders," says Sidney Coupland, should lead
a regular life, avoiding excitement and excess. They should have
a rather dry diet with considerable white meat, and plenty of open
air exercise. The greatest care should be exercised to avoid mechanical injury. Give every month or oftener a mercurial
followed by sodium sulphate, which should also be given once
every week. To arrest external hemorrhage use perchloride of
iron as a styptic application; ice bags to joints when effusion; and
pressure to check bleeding from cuts.

Treatment of Acute Dysentery.—Anders recommends a diet
of milk and light animal broths; castor oil or saline purge at
onset, if scybalous masses still passing; every hour or two a powder containing $2\frac{1}{2}$ grains each of Dover's powder and salol and 20
grains of bismuth subnitrate; vigorous employment of supportive
measures; alternate daily hot to warm astringent (one to two per cent.
tannin, or silver nitrate one-half grain per ounce) and antiseptic
(one to two per cent. salicylic acid) bowel irrigation in gradually
increasing quantity, with hips well elevated—may be preceded by
cocaine suppository or solution, or starch and laudanum enema.
Locally hot fomentations, light poultices and turpentine stupes
often afford much comfort.

Cooking.—Badly prepared food causes disease and drives men to drink. Fried articles are especially indigestible. Vegetables are better steamed than boiled, in order to retain their special virtues. A loaf of bread is not sterilized throughout by baking. Every girl should be taught how to cook plain food well, at home as well as in the special schools. Even if she should not do this work after marriage, she would not then be at the mercy of the cook or baker for her daily bread.

Treatment of Tubercular Anthritis. — Conservatism, says Joseph Ransohoff, is the keynote. Fresh air, suitable diet and cleanliness are important, and prolonged rest in bed is of great service. Guaiacol or creasote may be given internally, and the modified tuberculin treatment is worthy of trial. Local rest to the joint is secured by compression retentive dressings. Traction is very serviceable at the beginning. The author recommends direct injections (three to twenty during two months to a year) into the joint of zinc chloride solution (saturated or 50 per cent.), or undiluted balsam of Peru, or one dram to two ounces of sterilized iodoform solution. Use the aspirator if the joint is so much distended with fluid as to cause tension and severe pain.

Treatment of Acute Gastritis.— Besides removal of the cause, Anders recommends sinapisms locally, followed by warm linseed poultices. large draughts of warm water, or large, when due to errors in diet—followed by a purge of soda and calomel (⅛ grain every hour for six doses), and this by a saline laxative (two hours after last dose of calomel). Now give the stomach rest for 24 hours, when pancreatized milk or milk boiled with lime water may be given at stated intervals — rectal alimentation if nausea and continued vomiting, prohibiting use of milk by the mouth. Give morphine in small doses hypodermically at intervals of twelve hours for nausea, pain and restlessness. Creosote with bismuth or cocaine is. also useful in constant nausea. Mineral acids should be given well diluted when local symptoms have mostly subsided, and later with bitter vegetable tonics.

The Administration of Iodides in Tertiary Syphilas.— White and Martin give the iodide of potassium in 5-grain doses t. i. d., increasing by five grains every third day until the disease symptoms disappear or toxic symptoms supervene. They administer the drug about an hour after meals in a half glass of water or milk, with essence of pepsin if the stomach is disturbed. Tannic acid may be added to the prescription if griping pains are produced. Gottheil, in gummatous cases, gives 100 to 500 grains daily of the drug, preferably in milk after meals, the patient lying down for a time and using a sinapism over the stomach if required. When the potassium salt is not well borne, he substitutes sodium or rubidium iodide. In late, obstinate and chronic lesions he has found an intramuscular injection every five to fifteen days of three to ten minims of a sterilized ten per cent. suspension of calomel in albolene a useful adjuvant measure.

Treatment of Cholelithiasis.—Morphine says Anders, should be given at the onset, $\frac{1}{3}$–$\frac{1}{4}$ grain every hour till relief follows (chloroform inhalations till the morphine has taken effect), or one grain of codeine every hour by the mouth; also prolonged hot baths and hot applications over the liver. Use heat externally and stimulants hypodermically for shock of syncope; and 15 minim doses of spirit of chloroform every half hour for nausea and vomiting. To remove stones, give olive oil (followed with lemon juice), four to six ounces by the mouth, or one to two tablespoonfuls of glycerine every three or four hours; or the free use of pure water rendered alkaline by three per cent. sodium bicarbonate or borate; or sodium phosphate, sodium cholate or oxgall. Surgical treatment may become necessary.

For Contusions.—J. Pickering Pick advises perfect rest and complete immobility of joint by the application of a splint. Elevate limb and apply cold assiduously by means of evaporating lotions, (10 to 20 per cent. in sterilized glycerine or olive oil). When there are many fibrinous shreds, make a free aseptic incision and irrigate thoroughly with saturated boric solution before making iodoform injection. Use rest and compression for hydrops; these failing, aspirate and inject carbolic acid or iodoform. Operative treatment is often needed—free incision into joint and erasion of tubercular foci by cutting instruments, followed by introduction of sterilized iodoform and closure of articular wound by deep sutures, and cutaneous wound in ordinary way. Resection should be reserved for correction of residual deformity. In

Hope, fresh air, rest and Scott's Emulsion are the greatest remedies for consumption. Scott's Emulsion will always bring comfort and relief—often cure.

SCOTT & BOWNE, Chemists, 409 Pearl St., New York.

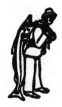

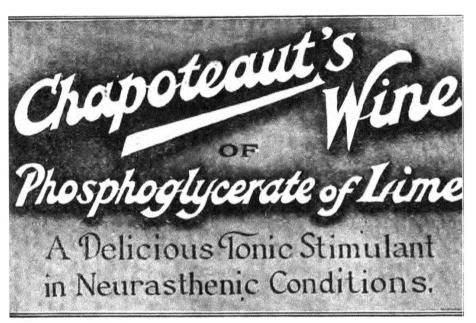

Chapoteaut's Wine OF **Phosphoglycerate of Lime**

A Delicious Tonic Stimulant in Neurasthenic Conditions.

Agents: E. Fougera & Co., 26-30 N. William St., N. Y.

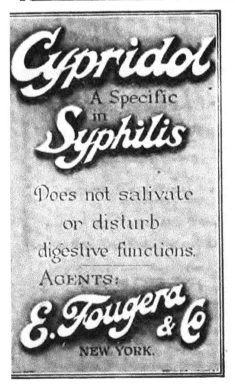

Cypridol A Specific in **Syphilis**

Does not salivate or disturb digestive functions.

AGENTS:

E. Fougera & Co

NEW YORK.

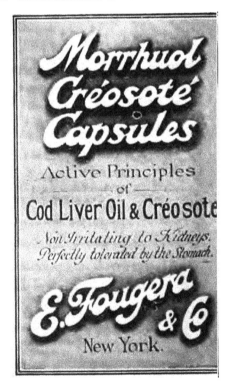

Morrhuol Créosoté Capsules

Active Principles of Cod Liver Oil & Créosote

Non Irritating to Kidneys. Perfectly tolerated by the Stomach.

E. Fougera & Co

New York.

severe cases of bones of wrist, amputation often affords the quickest and safest road to recovery.

Penetrating Wounds of Joints.—Says Joseph Ransohoff: Secure primary union through prevention of infection by cleansing and irrigation of joint cavity with a slim1:0001 ubte solution, leaving in a silkworm-gut strand for drainage if there is much oozing, and closing wound by sutures, dressing joint aseptically and keeping it at rest. With the first evidence of septic infection make a free incision for removal through drainage (rubber tubes of considerable caliber) of contents of diseased joint and antiseptic management of joint interior. In traumatic suppurative arthritis keep limb in most desirable position for probable ankylosis. Primary excision or even amputation may be indicated in complicated trauma. Gunshot wounds require thorough aseptic exploration and removal of the missile, foreign bodies and loose spicules; and atypical resection with ample facilities for drainage or formal excision if both epiphyses are injured. Amputation is rarely necessary.

General Treatment of Ulcers.—Says Roswell Park: Use constitutional measures for scurvy, syphilis, glanders, leprosy, tubercle, etc.; physiologic rest to part. A healthy healing ulcer needs only protection. If there is excessive discharge, use a simple absorbent dressing with enough antiseptic material to prevent putrefaction. Sluggish ulcers may be stimulated with silver nitrate or zinc chloride. Continuous immersion in hot water should be utilized when practicable for foul ulcers; or apply absorbent cotton soaked in brewer's yeast and covered with oiled silk. When granulation is at a standstill in a comparatively recent ulcer, use the sharp spoon or curette. Excision of the entire affected area under an anesthetic is requisite for old and chronic ulcers; follow with skin grafting. For all specific infectious ulcers use the knife, scissors and sharp spoon, followed by thorough cauterization with the actual cautery, nitric acid, bromine or zinc chloride,

Hemorrhage of Gastric Ulcer.— Ewald advises absolute physical and mental rest and avoidance of all irritation to stomach; small pieces of ice or tablespoonfuls of ice-cold tea or ice-cold fluid peptone solutions. If patients are not known to take milk well, give on first day solutions of grape sugar, which is replaced by some bouillon made of meat peptones, taken very cold, or cold thin gruels of barley or oatmeal; or use nutritive enemata. Inject into region of stomach one or two syringefuls several times a day of solution of 2½ parts ext. secalis cornuti (Ph. Ger.) in five parts each of glycerine and water; morphine may be added if patient is much excited. Wash out stomach repeatedly with ice-cold water when the hemorrhage cannot be controlled in any other way. If collapse symptoms appear, give a hypodermic injection of camphor and ether (one to six), or enemata of wine and egg or peptones, as also hot applications to extremities. When death threatens from anemia, use transfusion of blood or infusion of salt solution.

Treatment of Epistaxis.—Bishop says: Keep head upright and compress nostrils or apply cold (ice bag) to nose or back of head and spine. Use locally powdered alum and tannin in powder or on tampons; ten per cent. solution of cocaine on a cotton pledget, packed firmly between the bleeding point and the opposite wall; antipyrin in three per cent. solution or in powder; liquor ferri perchloridi. If simpler measures fail, resort to tampons: Squeeze out a long strip of cloth ⅜ inch wide from a saturated aqueous solution of tannin, and carry one end into nose with forceps or probe, packing in remainder firmly to completely fill the cavity. If this anterior tampon fails, plug also first posterior nares with Bellocq's canula threaded with a long string, to which, after introducing through nasal cavity, a pledget of cotton or lint is tied and drawn into posterior nares—fasten protruding string back of ear with adhesive plaster—remove packing after a day or two.

Acute Articular Rheumatism.—Anders' treatment may be summarized as follows: Sick room well ventilated at 65°-70°; light flannel garments and sheet; liquid diet, particularly milk; sodium or ammonium salicylate, gr. x every two hours during first day, or until pain and other local features have disappeared —then at longer intervals—larger doses if fresh exacerbations occur; salicin gr. x every hour, increased to gr. xv, sometimes efficacious and always agrees; salophen in daily dose of one dram (gr. xv every 4 hours) almost a specific—may be substituted for sodium salicylate if latter produces gastric disturbances; sodium bicarbonate or potassium citrate in all cases in sufficient doses to

The amily axative

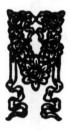

alifornia ig Syrup ompany

an Francisco, California.

Louisville, Ky.
New York, N. Y.

The ideal, safe, family laxative, known as "Syrup of Figs," is a product of the California Fig Syrup Co., and derives its laxative principles from senna, made pleasant to the taste and more acceptable to the stomach by being combined with pleasant aromatic syrups and the juice of figs. It is recommended by many of the most eminent physicians, and used by millions of families with entire satisfaction. It has gained its great reputation with the medical profession by reason of the acknowledged skill and care exercised by the California Fig Syrup Co. in securing the laxative principles of the senna by an original method of its own, and presenting them in the best and most convenient form. The California Fig Syrup Co. has special facilities for commanding the choicest qualities of Alexandria senna, and its chemists devote their entire attention to the manufacture of the one product. The name "Syrup of Figs" means to the medical profession "the family laxative, manufactured by the California Fig Syrup Co." and the name of the company is a guarantee of the excellence of its product. Informed of the above facts, the careful physician will know how to prevent the dispensing of worthless imitations when he recommends or prescribes the original and genuine "Syrup of Figs." It is well known to physicians that "Syrup of Figs" is a simple, safe and reliable laxative, which does not irritate or debilitate the organs on which it acts, and, being pleasant to the taste, it is especially adapted to ladies and children, although generally applicable in all cases. Special investigation of the profession invited.

"Syrup of Figs" is never sold in bulk. It retails at fifty cents per bottle, and the name "Syrup of Figs," as well as the name of the California Fig Syrup Co., is printed on the wrappers and labels of every bottle.

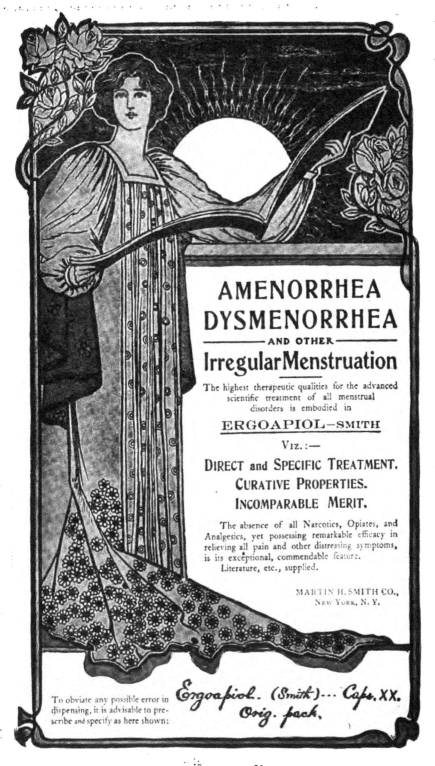

AMENORRHEA
DYSMENORRHEA
—— AND OTHER ——
IrregularMenstruation

The highest therapeutic qualities for the advanced
scientific treatment of all menstrual
disorders is embodied in

ERGOAPIOL–SMITH

Viz.:—

DIRECT and SPECIFIC TREATMENT.
CURATIVE PROPERTIES.
INCOMPARABLE MERIT.

The absence of all Narcotics, Opiates, and
Analgesics, yet possessing remarkable efficacy in
relieving all pain and other distressing symptoms,
is its exceptional, commendable feature.
Literature, etc., supplied.

MARTIN H. SMITH CO.,
New York, N. Y.

To obviate any possible error in
dispensing, it is advisable to prescribe and specify as here shown:

Ergoapiol. (Smith)... Caps. XX.
Orig. pack.

keep urine slightly alkaline; potassium iodide and colchicum should be tried in cases that drag on after acute stage is over; wrap joints in cotton batting of flannel; methyl salicylate may be applied locally; then envelop joint in gutta percha tissue and flannel bandage; cold baths for hyperpyrexia; keep in bed for a week after pain gone and temperature normal; iron during convalescence, with massage and hot water or warm baths for persistent stiffness and swelling; iron, quinine and cod-liver oil in addition to usual anti-rheumatics, and change to warm climate for subacute cases.

Gastrointestinal Arteriosclerosis.—Walter L. Bierring *(International Clinics)* states that the gastric symptoms of this disease type includes anorexia, hypochlorhydria, delayed proteid digestion, mucous vomit, occasionally hemorrhagic, and gastralgia, altogether sometimes closely simulating gastric cancer. The intestinal symptoms are chiefly enteralgia, constipation and meteorism, often localized and simulating obstruction. These symtoms are due to ischemia of the abdominal vessels. The evidences of arteriosclerotic changes in other tissues, as claudication, stenocardia, albuminuria, glycosuria and sclerosis of palpable peripheral arteries should be taken into account in forming a diagnosis. Excessive peristalsis, as by purgatives, and too great taxation of the digestive function, predispose to thrombosis in these cases. The treatment in brief embraces a rational and strict regime; potassium or sodium iodide, 3 to 5 grains t. i. d. with 5 grains of sodium bicarbonate and a stomachic bitter; small meals (milk, fresh vegetables, animal food sparingly), eating slowly and drinking before or after meals; no alcohol or tobacco; mild aperients; for the heart, a few doses of nitroglycerin or a long course of strychnine; tepid baths of short duration, with friction of skin; regular, moderate exercise in good air, always stopping short of fatigue; avoidance of emotional disturbances and of exposure to extremes of heat and cold; warm clothing; a bright, genial climate.

Asiatic or Indian Cholera.—This dread disease has been indigenous since remote times in India, but was unknown to the ancient Greeks and Romans. The delta of the Ganges has been the starting point of every pandemic. Cholera first appeared in

Europe in 1823, at Astrakhan on the Caspian, but was cut short
by a cold winter. Again in 1826 an epidemic in India spread
gradually into Europe, arriving at Paris in the spring of 1832,
and in the same year was carried to America by Irish emigrants,
reaching its climax in 1837-38. A third pandemic was most
prevalent from 1853 to 1855; and a fourth in 1865-66 and
1872-73, since which latter date there has been no outbreak in
the United States. The fifth great epidemic, 1887-92, raged
chiefly in Asia and Egypt, being spread by way of the Indian pilgrims to Mecca. It caused many deaths in Spain, Chili and Ar-
gentina, and threatened North America. In 1892 the disease invaded Russia from Persia and was carried westward to Paris,
Havre and Hamburg. In the latter city from August 16 to
November 12, 19,956 fell sick with cholera, and of these 8,605
died. Comparing Hamburg, then supplied with unfiltered water,
with closely connected Altona, with filtered water, we find that
the number of cases of cholera per 10,000 population was 256
for the former place and 35 for the latter. Many of the residents
of Altona, moreover, worked in Hamburg, and doubtless contracted the disease there. From Hamburg as a center of infection, cholera broke out in 267 other towns and cities, though with
much less fury as a rule. In 1893-95 localized outbreaks occurred
in Germany, Turkey, Africa, Western Asia, Brazil and the La
Plata States, and great epidemics continued in Russia. More
than a thousand deaths from cholera took place during the past
winter in Calcutta, where stupid religious customs and prejudices
make efficient sanitation well nigh impossible. In the month of
March alone 1,129 deaths from cholera occurred in the Hedjaz,
over half of these being in the "Holy City" of Mecca, whither
the unwashed multitudes of Moslem pilgrims congregate from all
parts of the Eastern Continent. The disease is again raging in
parts of China. The word cholera, as used by old European medical writers, signified simply a condition accompanied by pain,
vomiting and diarrhea, and was applied till 1817 to what is now
termed cholera nostras. The spirillum of Asiatic cholera was
discovered by Koch in 1883.

Treatment of Acute Peritonitic.—Anders directs to secure
perfect quiet in a comfortable position, and give four to six
ounces of pancreated milk every two hours — rectal alimentation

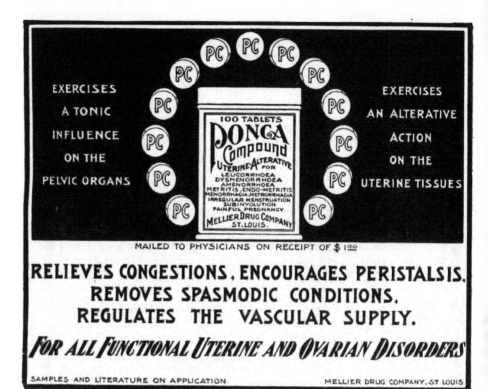
CONTENTS.

INDEX TO ADVERTISERS.

if the stomach is intolerant. Give a saline purgative in concentrated solution, one or two drams every two or three hours, to maintain several copious serous discharges daily. If the patient is robust with a full, tense pulse, give one-half grain of calomel every hour until purgation, then salines. When collapse symptoms not due to perforation occur, use opium in moderate doses. When perforation or abscess is known or even suspected to be present, make a prompt laparotomy, followed by the free use of salines. Locally one may apply twenty or thirty leeches to abdomen at onset, if the patient is strong. When there is not much meteorism apply t. i. d. an ointment of one part each of ung. ichthyol and ung. hydrargyri and two parts of ung. belladonnae. Turpentine stupes or injections containing turpentine (two drams each of turpentine and oxgall to four ounces milk of asafetida and six ounces of warm water), or the long rectal tube, may be used for tympany. Opium is useful for pain; chipped ice sprinkled with brandy. for thirst; small quantities of carbonated waters or iced champagne or one-drop doses of creasote, for vomiting.

—24—

Local Hyperidrosis.—This derangement of excretion is usually most marked on the palms, soles, genitals and in the axillae; local sweating may be due to hysteria (sometimes bromides or hematidrosis); migraine (one side of head); peripheral neuritis or neuralgia (along course of nerve); cervical carries, thoracic aneurysm or tumor pressing on cervical sympathetic (one side of face, neck or chest, with contracted pupil and congested face on same side); rickets (head and neck during sleep); chronic pleurisy (one cheek sometimes); exophthalmic goiter (sweating may be confined to head); Raynaud's disease (affected parts); or paretic dementia. The palm is hot and clammy from excitement, recent exertion, rheumatoid anthritis, etc. Excessive sweating of the hand is sometimes seen in progressive muscular atrophy. By way of treatment Cushny recommends local applications of belladonna ointment, liniment or plaster. Frank uses local applications of a ten to twenty per cent solution of formalin in alcohol, or tannic acid and formalin.

Beverages.—Dilute alcoholic liquors increase the flow of gastric juice and are rapidly absorbed, being burned in the capillaries to the extent of $1\frac{1}{2}$ or 2 ounces of alcohol daily. When used continually they probably combine with the nervous tissue of the brain; they interfere with proper metabolism and predispose to disease.

The alkaloidal beverages, tea, coffee, cocoa, chocolate, kola and mate, are nerve stimulants and are closely related to uric acid. Hence their constant and excessive use is very likely to excite migraine and other uricacidemic conditions. Cocoa is the most nourishing of these drinks, since it contains 50 per cent fat and 12 per cent proteins. Tea and coffee, if used, should be prepared by a few minutes' infusion with nearly boiling water, as prolonged boiling drives off the aromatic oil and causes the water to take up bitter, astringent tannin, a radical foe to eupepsia.

Lemon juice, containing about thirty grains of citric acid per fluid ounce, is of special value as a preventive of scurvy and is also very useful in chronic rheumatism. The prevalent prac- of swilling soda water, phosphates and the like during warm weather, tends to derange digestion through fermentation and to increase heat production by the oxidation of the sugar in these sweet drinks.

Denver and Gross College of Medic

Fourteenth and Arapahoe Streets

Medical Department University of Denver

EDMUND J. A. ROGERS, A.M., M.D.,
Professor of Surgery.

THOMAS H. HAWKINS, A.M., M.D.,
Professor of Gynecology and Abdominal Surgery.

EDMUND C. RIVERS, A.M., M.D.,
Professor of Ophthalmology.

ROBERT LEVY, M.D., Secretary.
Professor of Laryngology, Rhinology and Otology.

HENRY SEWALL, PH.D., M.D.,
Professor of Physiology.

WILLIAM H. DAVIS, M.D.,
Professor of Dermatology and Venereal Diseases.

CHARLES B. LYMAN, M.D.,
Professor of Fractures and Dislocations.

WILLIAM J. ROTHWELL, M.D.,
Professor of Medicine.

JOHN M. FOSTER, M.D.,
Professor of Otology.

CAREY K. FLEMING, M.D.,
Professor of Gynecology and Abdominal Surgery.

FRANCIS H. MCNAUGHT, M.D.,
Professor of Obstetrics.

LEONARD FREEMAN, B.S., A.M., MD.,
Professor of Surgery.

HORACE G. WETHERILL, M.D.,
Professor of Gynecology and Abdominal Surgery.

JOSIAH N. HALL, B.S., M.D.,
Professor of Medicine.

CHARLES A. POWERS, A.M., M.D.,
Professor of Surgery.

CHARLES F. SHOLLENBERGER, M.D.,
Professor of Pediatrics.

HOWELL T. PERSHING, M.Sc., M.D.,
Professor of Nervous and Mental Diseases.

EDWARD C. HILL, M.Sc., M. D.,
Professor of Chemistry and Toxicology.

HERBERT B. WHITNEY, A.B., M.D.,
Professor of Medicine.

HORACE G. HARVEY, A.B., M.D.,
Professor of Fractures and Dislocations.

SHERMAN G. BONNEY, A.M., M.D., Dean,
Professor of Medicine.

MOSES KLEINER, M.D.,
Professor of Therapeutics.

GEORGE B. PACKARD, M.D.,
Professor of Orthopedic Surgery.

T. MITCHELL BURNS, M.D.,
Professor of Obstetrics.

WALTER A. JAYNE, M.D.,
Professor of Gynecology and Abdominal[S

CHARLES B. VAN ZANT, M.D.,
Professor of Physiology.

CARROLL E. EDSON, A.M., M.D.,
Professor of Therapeutics.

MELVILLE BLACK, M.D.,
Professor of Ophthalmology.

JAMES M. BLAINE, M.D.,
Professor of Dermatology and Venereal Di

WILLIAM C. MITCHELL, M.D.,
Professor of Bacteriology.

DAVID H. COOVER, M.D.,
Professor of Ophthalmology.

SAMUEL B. CHILDS, A.M., M.D.,
Professor of Anatomy.

JAMES H. PERSHING, A.B.,
Professor of Medical Jurisprudence.

JOHN A. WILDER, M.D.,
Professor of Pathology.

SAMUEL D. HOPKINS, M.D.,
Professor of Nervous and Mental Diseases.

PHILIP HILLKOWITZ, B.S., M.D.,
Professor of Pathology.

WILLIAM C. BANE, M.D.,
Professor of Ophthalmology and Otology.

Four years' graded course. Sessions of eight months each. 23d Annual Sessions begins September 15, 1903. Matriculation fee, $5.00. Tuition fee, $100.00. Well-equipped laboratories in all departments and excellent clinical advantages in dispensary and hospitals.

The climate of **COLORADO** offers many advantages to students whose health compels them to leave the east

Catalogue on application.

Sherman G. Bonney, A.M., M.D., Dean

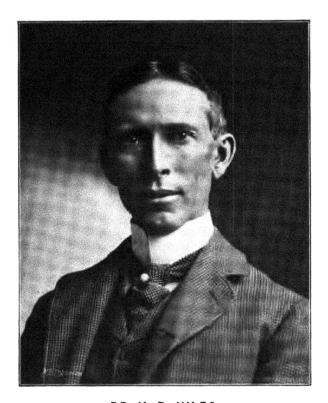

DR. H. D. NILES,

Retiring President of the Rocky Mountain Inter-State
Medical Association.

DENVER MEDICAL TIMES

VOLUME XXIV.   OCTOBER, 1904   NUMBER 4.

PRESIDENTIAL ADDRESS.*

By H. D. NILES,

Salt Lake, Utah.

"WESTWARD THE STAR OF EMPIRE WENDS ITS WAY."

The phenomenal growth and magnificent work accomplished by the American Medical Association during the past decade has taught us many lessons. We have learned something of the advantages of systematic, well organized committee and section work. We have been profoundly impressed with the achievements made possible by a unity of purpose and a combination of forces. We have learned the value of an association journal that at all times and under all circumstances advocates our causes, and that each week brings us into close touch with the best thoughts and work of our professional friends and fellow members. In shaping our conduct we have been taught to look beyond the narrow limits of any written or printed code and find guidance in those generous impulses that spring spontaneously from a spirit of good fellowship, cordiality, and kindly feeling toward each other. We must all acknowledge with gratitude our indebtedness to those who have perfected this superb organization, and I am sure that none who are able to spare the necessary time and money will willingly forego the pleasure and instruction these annual meetings offe,. or for any reason withhold their cordial support from our National Association.

But the American Medical Association is becoming so large that, in spite of the division of labor, it is getting more difficult each year to crowd the necessary work into the few days available, and at the same time give a large number of men an opportunity to bring their best ideas before the association. Moreover, a large proportion of the members are separated by long distances and many dollars from the meeting place each year, and to some it

---

*Read before Rocky Mountain Inter-State Medical Association, September, 1904.

means annually approximately three weeks time, and a consider-able outlay of cash for three days scientific refreshment.

Then too, there are professional interests that belong to cer-tain parts of the United States that cannot well be taken up in a national organization. It has, therefore, come about that in various parts of the country, sectional societies have been formed to meet the special requirements that a national society could not be expected to cover.

In consideration of those men who feel that they cannot reg-ularly attend the meetings of the larger association and who still hold in high regard professional interests and public welfare of their own section, and for the purpose of reducing, improving and systematizing our society work, the American Medical Asso-ciotion has now under consideration a plan for establishing seven or eight large branch associations, each to include a number of states, and all to be governed by constitutions and by-laws furnished by the parent association. In the far west the Rocky Mountain Inter-State Medical Society has, in a large measure, already cov-ered the field, but in view of the facts already stated, and for reasons to be mentioned, the time has come in my judgment, for this association to seriously consider the advisability of including a larger territory and a broader line of work, in harmony with the proposed action of the American Medical Association.

Between the eastern slope of the Rocky Mountains and the Pacific Coast line lies a vast territory that includes thousands of miles of fertile soil, immense tracts of grazing lands, the greatest forests in the world, and mineral riches beyond the estimation of man. The development of the marvelous resources of this vast empire is but just begun, and it requires no prophetic vision for one familiar with the facts and the coexisting conditions to realize that within the next half century this region is certain to be peopled with millions of seekers of fortune, fame, health, and homes, who will expect and deserve from the medical profession every care, attention and protection that our science offers to the most favored of mankind.

Those who have witnessed or learned of the transformation that has been accomplished in the past fifty years, more particu-larly those who have experienced the hardships and trials inci-dental to the practice of medicine and surgery on the frontier and are now able to view the modern hospital structures and conveni-

ences erected, it may be, upon the former site of log cabins—
surely will not doubt any reasonable prediction as to the advancement and growth of our professional work during the next fifty
years.

We of the West need, therefore, not only to be prepared for
our present labors but we must hold ourselves in readiness to
assume the new and greater responsibilities that are certain to be
thrust upon us in the near future. In this region, and at this
time, this work of preparation for present and future duties, if it
is to be most effective means an organization and combination of
our forces, a personal and professional acquaintance with each
other, a unity of purpose associated with deliberate and concerted
action. Moreover we need to be self reliant.

In the past we have intuitively turned our eyes to the east
for instruction and aid, and too often, it may be, we have bowed
to the orders and authority of our eastern brethren in questions
which they could not, from the nature of things, be as well qualified to pass judgment upon, as we. In legislative and sanitary
matters at least we should know our needs and be ready to secure
them ourselves.

Only a few years ago we were without colleges, journals,
hospitals, and laboratories, and with neither inclination or opportunity to carry on original researches ourselves or even impart
such knowledge as we possessed to others, and the western surgeon's preparatory and post-graduate education was made to cost
him more in time, money and effort than now seems necessary or
wise. I mean no disrespect to our eastern brethren nor do I feel
myself lacking in fraternal spirit, when I express the opinion that the
time is not so far distant when we will be able to contribute our
share of thought and knowledge in the advancement of our science,
and that we will have builded colleges, laboratories, hospitals and
established journals worthy of creditable recognition in any part
of the world.

The Pacific Ocean on the west and the plains on the east,
form barriers that prevent our close communication with others,
and we must learn to face and solve the problems that confront us
alone. To meet the conditions and accomplish these objects we
need to form an association in which every state in this section
shall be represented. It has been urged that there are already too
many medical societies. This may be true, but if so, there is all

the more reason for us to be loyal to those who have a right to claim our allegiance.

The most important objects of this branch of the American Medical Association we cannot hope to accomplish in our state, county, national or international associations. For example, we would all welcome a reciprocity clause in our statutes that would permit the licensed practitioner of any of our states to be exempt from examination should he desire to practice his profession in any other state of this section. As a solid body we might reasonably hope to influence legislative action in this and other questions of interest to western men. Is it fair or just we should wait upon the slower action of our eastern friends? Laws and practices regarding sanitation and preventive medicine are easier to rightly formulate and execute in a new country, than to change or improve in an older country.

We need more hospitals and better ones. The management of these institutions should be inspired by a spirit of fairness, that will lead them to extend their peculiar conveniences and educational advantages beyond the favored few on the various staffs, to the general profession of this section so that no regular practitioner of this region shall be deprived of hospital privileges and advantages.

Our colleges need our support, and if we give them our united support as we can, and should, we will transform them into institutions that will deserve and may receive their full share of outside patronage,

We have some excellent journals, perhaps we have too many journals, but certainly none receive sufficient substantial support. A few good journals that would record all our best work and thought would merit and should command the support and cooperation of every well informed medical man in this western country. Personally I believe that one such journal should be under the control or our association. No one who visits regularly the hospitals of this and other countries will question the statement that, as a whole, the work done in our western institutions will conpare, not unfavorably, with that of any part of the world, and this work as well as the ideas of the workers is worthy of record. The papers read in our societies may be lacking in fine spun theories, but as a rule they are the product of earnest, thoughtful, logical men, and I believe our journals should have the privilege of first publishing these papers. If they are willing to represent us, they should have the opportunity to present to the medical world our best endeavors. If they offer us their hearty support we certainly should not withhold from them our unwavering loyalty.

The association of laboratory researches with operating rooms experiences is each year becoming more essential to our progressive advancement, and there is reason, I believe, for us to encourage such scientific work in our hospitals, colleges, and elsewhere, in such a way as so bring our profession generally into close touch with those studies and investigations that now are too often confined to a privileged few. I know of no good reason why, at the present time, our western laboratories should not be so equipped and managed as to supply our broadest requirements.

At this time as in all ages; here, as in all parts of the world, the strongest opposition to scientific progress has come from the victims of a blind, unreasoning faith in the supernatural. The manufacture and sale of nostrums and cure-alls, the practice of all kinds of quackery from osteopathy to Christian Science will continue to menace the lives and health of individuals and communities so long as the ignorant and superstitious indicate their willingness to be victimized. In the interest of humanity it becomes the sacred duty of every true follower of rational medicine to do his full part in stamping out these false teachings, and all such frauds and deceptions as endanger the health and lives of our people. Ridicule will not suffice; logical argument alone will not avail; individual appeals will not succeed. We must combine our forces, and design and carry out broader and more liberal plans than have yet been employed if we are ever to overcome these opponents to progress and prosperity. Public sentiment, at the present time, is not unanimously in sympathy with our purpose, the public press is, for obvious reasons. arrayed against our cause. We need the confidence of the public and the co-operation of the press. We need most of all to realize that the real support of quackery and charlatanism comes from the victims of delusions, who are sincere in their false beliefs, and hence, must be led rather than driven to rationalism. All these thoughts lead up to the conclusion that if we are to eliminate the curse of quackery, the practice of quack methods, and the sale of nostrums and cure-alls, we must systematically plan and carry out our warfare as a united, organized body,

above the suspicion of being influenced by personal or selfish mo-
tives.   The western profession cannot honorably disregard this
duty they owe their people.

Briefly then my plea is for the association of our western
professional men into a strong organization that shall have for its
aim the accomplishment of these and other objects which we may
feel are worthy of our endeavors and which we can never hope to
secure single handed.

The work is before us; the time opportune. Are we of the
Rocky Mountain Inter-State Society ready and willing to join
hands with the profession of our sister states in this cause? This
question I am impressed is the most important that can be pre
sented to this Society now or in the future. I ask you, therefore,
to give it your most thoughtful consideration, weighing with
scrupulous care and exact fairness, advantages and disadvantages,
alone and in discussion. I submit this question to you firm in the
conviction that your combined judgments will surely lead to wise
conclusions on a subject so vitally near the welfare of western
medicine, western institutions and western people.

NORMAL OBSTETRICS.

(CHAPTER SIX.*)

THE OBSTETRIC ANATOMY OF THE FOETUS AT TERM.

By T. MITCHELL BURNS, M.D.

Denver, Colo.

Prof. of Obstetrics, The Denver and Gross College of Medicine.

PART I. THE FOETAL HEAD AND TRUNK.

The Foetal Head.—Its Shape, Size and Divisions.

The shape of the head is ovoidal, the large end being the
occipital.

The head is the largest part of the foetus, (i. e. the long diameter of the head is greater than any diameter of a cross section of
the trunk after a little compression).   Very rarely the compressed
shoulders are larger than the head.

---

*For personal reasons chapters III, IV and V will not be given until later.

The head is divided into the face and the cranium, and the cranium into the vault and base.

The Vault and Base of the Cranium.—The vault is the larger and comprehensible part of the head. The compressibility permits the moulding of the head and the diminution of its diameters during labor. The base is the smaller and non-compressible part of the head. Its lack of compressibility prevents injury to the vital centers. The bones of the vault are the frontal (two halves), parietal and squamous portions of the occipital and temporal bones. (The bones of the base are the rest of the occipital and temporal bones, the sphenoid and ethmoid.)

The Sutures and Fontanelles of the Vault of the Cranium.—The study of these sutures and fontanelles is of great importance, because it is by their situation that the position of the fœtus in the vertex presentation is determined by vaginal examination. An easy method of studying the sutures and fontanelles is to cover the head of the new born baby with a blanket, carefully feel the sutures and fontanelles and then uncover and examine.

The Sutures of the Vault.—The sutures of the vault are membranous spaces composed of periosteum and dura mater uniting the edges of adjacent bones.

The most important sutures are the sagittal, frontal, coronal and lambdoidal.

The sagittal, (inter-parietal), is between the parietal bones, and extends from the anterior to the posterior fontanelle. It is a straight suture.

The frontal, (inter-frontal), is between the two halves of the frontal bone, and extends from the glabella to the anterior fontanelle. It is a straight suture.

The coronal (fronto-parietal), is between the frontal and parietal bones, and extends from the antero-lateral fontanelle of one side to that of the other and passes through the anterior fontanelle. It is a curved suture with its concavity anteriorly, i. e., toward the frontal bone.

Tho lambdoidal, (occipito-parietal), is between the occipital and parietal bones, extends from the postero-lateral fontanelle of one side to that of the other and passes through the posterior fontanelle. It is a suture made up of two straight sutures united at the posterior fontanelle at nearly a right angle, and having the concavity of its angle directed toward the occiput.

The sutures are diagnosed by the following characters:

The sagittal suture is straight and between the anterior and posterior fontanelles.

The frontal is straight, a continuation of the long end of the anterior fontanelle, and ends near the nose.

The coronal is curved; its concavity contains a broad surface, (the frontal surface) and the frontal suture. It passes through the breadth of the anterior fontanelle, and at the anterior fontanelle it forms nearly a right angle with the sagittal and frontal sutures.

The lambdoidal forms nearly a right angle. At the vertex of this angle is the posterior fontanelle. Its concavity contains a narrow surface (the occipital) and no suture, and each half forms an obtuse angle with the sagittal suture.

The Fontanelles of the Vault.—The fontanelles are membranous interspaces at the junction of two or more sutures.

The most important fontanelles are the anterior and the posterior.

The anterior fontanelle, (the large fontanelle or bregma), is formed by the junction of the frontal, sagittal and the two halves of the coronal suture. It is diagnosed by its situation, size and shape (3 S's.) It is situated at the junction of four sutures (the frontal, sagittal and the two halves of coronal). It is generally ten times larger than the posterior fontanelle. Its shape is that of a kite or arrowhead, with its longest end anteriorly continuous with the frontal suture. (Its posterior end is continuous with the sagittal structure. Its lateral ends with halves of the coronal suture.)

The posterior fontanelle (the small fontanelle) is formed by the junction of the sagittal and the two halves of the coronal suture. It is diagnosed by its situation, size and shape (3 S's). It is situated at the junction of three sutures (the sagittal and the two halves of the lambdoidal). Its size is generally one-tenth that of the anterior fontanelle. Its shape is triangular with the apex at the sagittal suture. During labor it is often obliterated by pressure causing the parietal bones to override the occipital, so that in place of a small triangular fontanelle at the junction of these sutures, there is only a triangular depression, of which the floor is formed by the occipital bone and the edges by the overriding parietal bones.

The lateral fontanelles are four in number, one at each anterior and posterior inferior angle of the parietal bones. They are of little obstetric value as they are rarely felt in normal labor. They can be diagnosed, however, by their situation, size and shape, being at the union of three irregular sutures and near the ears, of small size and irregular shape. The ears themselves, which are easily felt, are much more important landmarks in diagnosis. The back of the ear can be diagnosed by its flaring from the head and the finger passing beneath it.

Supplementary fontanelles are sometimes found in the course of the sutures from failure of perfect ossification. They are at the junction of only two sutures, generally near the anterior or posterior fontanelle, of good size and of irregular outline.

The Diameters of the Fœtal Head.—A knowledge of the diameters is necessary for an understanding of the plastic phenomena and mechanism of labor.

The six most important diameters of the head are the occipito-mental, the occipito-frontal, the suboccipito-frontal, the suboccipito-bregmatic, the cervico-bregmatic and the biparietal.

The occipito-mental (O. M.) extends from the tip of the chin to the farthest point on the occiput and measures $5\frac{1}{4}$ inches.

The occipito-frontal (O. F.) extends from the middle of the forehead to the farthest point on the occiput, $4\frac{1}{2}$ inches.

The suboccipito-frontal (S. O. F.) extends from the junction of the occiput with the neck to the farthest point on the frontal bone and is $4\frac{1}{2}$ inches long.

The suboccipito-bregmatic (S. O. B.) begins at the junction of the occiput with the neck and extends to the bregma and its distance is $3\frac{3}{4}$ inches.

The cervico-bregmatic (C. B.) extends from the junction of the head and neck in front to the bregma and is $3\frac{3}{4}$ inches long.

The bi-parietal (B. P.) extends between the eminence on the parietal bones (parietal bosses) and measures $3\frac{3}{4}$ inches.

(Text books vary in the situation of some of these diameters. The author has selected those situations which make the diameters represent the greatest distance between the two named bones or correspond with the name of the diameter.)

The memorizing of these diameters is facilitated by their being written in the order of their situations, the more or less antero-posterior and vertical diameters first (beginning at the top

of the occiput and working down to the neck) and the transverse
last; by their lengths corresponding to the order of their situations;
by the second and third diameters being just $\frac{3}{4}$ of an inch less than
the first, or $4\frac{1}{2}$ inches; the fourth, fifth and sixth being $\frac{3}{4}$ of an
inch less than the second and third, or $3\frac{3}{4}$ inches; and by being
written in outline thus:

O. M. $5\frac{1}{4}$.
O. F. $\left.\right\}$ $4\frac{1}{2}$
S. O. F.

S. O. B.
C. B. $\left.\right\}$ $3\frac{3}{4}$
B. P.

The Circumferences of the Head.—The important circumferences of the head are:

O. M.

O. F.

S. O. F.

S. O. B.

C. B.

Each of these circumferences corresponds in name and relatively in length to the same diameter of the head.

Male and Female Heads.—Male heads are relatively more
ossified and larger than female heads.   Hence still-births are
more frequent and the maternal mortality greater in cases of labor
in which the child is a male.

The Fœtal Trunk; the Diameters.—The transverse diameters of the shoulders and the breech are longer than the antero-
posterior.   It is not necessary to remember the length of the
diameters of the trunk, because they are all more compressible
than the diameters of the head and their longest diameter, the
bis-acromial, 4.7 inches, being compressible one inch, becomes as
small as the smallest diameter of the head.

The important diameters of the trunk are:

Bis-acromial, (B. A.) 4.7 inches.

Dorso-sternal, (D. S.) 3.7 inches.

Bis-trochanteric, (B. T.) 3.5 inches.

Sacro-pubic, (S. P.) 2 inches, increased to 4 inches by including lower extremities.

PART II. THE ATTITUDE, FORM, LIE, PRESENTATION AND POSITION OF THE FOETUS.

The Attitude.—The attitude of the foetus means the relation of the foetal head and extremites to the trunk. The head is bent forward so the chin nearly rests on the chest, the arms are crossed in front of the chest and the legs are flexed in front of the abdomen, or more briefly, the head and extremities are flexed upon the trunk. This attitude allows the foetus to occupy the least possible space and to correspond in shape with the shape of the uterine cavity.

The Form.—The form of the foetus as a whole is ovoidal, the smaller end of the ovoid being the head.

The Lie.—The lie of the foetus is the term used to denote the relation between the long axis of the foetus and the long axis of the uterus. In the first third of pregnancy it is usually transverse, in the latter two-thirds it is generally longitudinal.

The Presentation.—The presentation of the foetus means the part of the foetus which presents at the pelvic inlet or is most dependent in the pelvic cavity.

The Different Presentations.— The different presentations are the vertex, (top of the head presenting), face, breech and left shoulder and by some the brow.

The Vertex Presentation.—The vertex presentation occurs in 90 per cent. of all cases of labor. Its frequency is due to the shape of the foetus, the motion of the uterus and the motion of the foetus, and the center of gravity being in the head end of the foetus.

Change of Presentation.—A change of presentation may occur. The most frequent change is from the breech to the vertex, less frequent from the shoulder to the vertex. (A change from the vertex to the face or shoulder is rare, but most face presentations are the result of change from the vertex to the beginning of labor due to the head impinging on the brim). The rarest change is from the vertex to the breech.

Change of presentation is due to plenty of room, discomfort and firm resistance for the feet. Hence, the feet being against the brim in the breech causes this presentations to change more often than any other. As pregnancy advances changes become less frequent because of less room.

Malpresentations.—Malpresentations are more frequent in premature delivery, because there is more room than at term and because death of the fœtus, a frequent complication of premature delivery, shifts the center of gravity to the breech end.

The Site of the Head in Vertex Presentations at Term.— In the primigravida (one who is pregnant for the first time) at term the head is generally in the pelvic cavity; in the multagravida (one who is pregnant for more than the first time) it is usually at the inlet or in one of the iliac fossae, because of the relaxation of the abdominal walls.

The Position.—The position of the fœtus signifies "the relation of certain fixed points of the presenting parts to certain fixed points of the pelvic inlet." In the vertex presentation the fixed points are the occiput of the presenting part and the four cardinal points of Capuron, the ilio-pectineal eminences and the sacro-iliac joints of the pelvic inlet; i. e., the occiput is in relation with one of the ilio-pectineal eminences or sacro-iliac joints. The cause of the position in all presentations is the long diameter of the presenting part accommodating itself to the nearest long diameter of the inlet, i. e., to one of the oblique diameters.

The Position of the Vertex Presentations.—1. L. O. A. Left Occipito-Anterior. The occiput is to the left and anterior in relation to the left ilio-pectineal eminence, and the long diameter (the sagittal or antero-posterior) of the head is in the first oblique.

The L. O. A. position is called the first position, because it is first in frequency, since it is the easiest position for the fœtus to assume, as it corresponds best with the shape of the uterus, the abdomen and the pelvic inlet, the long diameter of the head being in the longest diameter of the inlet. (The first oblique is the longest diameter of the inlet because the second oblique is shortened by the presence of the rectum).

2. R. O. P. Right Occipito-Posterior. The occiput is to the right and posterior in relation to the right sacro-iliac joint, and the long diameter of the head is in the first oblique. This is called the second position because it is second in frequency. It is second in frequency because, while the diameter is the same, the position is not quite as good as the L. O. A.

3. R. O. A. Right Occipito-Anterior. The occiput is to the right and anterior in relation to the right ilio-pectineal eminence, and the long diameter of the head is in the second oblique. It is not so frequent as the other positions, for while the situation in the uterus may be as good, the diameter of the inlet is smaller.

4. L. O. P. Left Occipito-Posterior. The occiput is to the left and posterior in relation to the left sacro-iliac joint, and the long diameter of the head is in the second oblique. This is by far the least frequent of the positions and most often causes prolonged labor. Just why it is less frequent than the third position is not easy of explanation. The following facts seem to explain the cause: The uterus is generally more on the right side of the abdomen, i. e., to the right of the vertebral column. This leaves the left posterior quadrant of the uterus smaller than any of the others, because of the projection of the vertebral column into it. When the long diameter of the head is in the first oblique the promontory has no effect, and when the long diameter is in the second oblique and the occiput is anterior, i. e., in the R. O. A. position, the promontory does not interfere with the narrow face as it does with the broad occiput in the L. O. P. position.

The Position of the Fœtal Back.—The position of the fœtal back depends somewhat upon the position of the mother. When the mother is in the dorsal decubitus the back of the fœtus, whatever the position of the occiput at the inlet, tends to be toward the back of the mother because the vertebral column tips the fœtus to the side.

The Positions of the Other Presentations.—The position of the other presentations will be described under Abnormal Obstetrics.

THE X-RAY TREATMENT OF URETHRAL CARUNCLE*

By G. H. STOVER, M.D.
Denver, Colo.

The X-ray is now so well established as a remedial measure in a large number of pathological states that one who devotes himself exclusively to this line of work would have too many interesting cases for a single paper if he attempted to go over the work done since your last meeting.

I therefore consider it more suitable, instead of a general paper, to speak of the treatment of a most intractable condition by a new method; I am not aware that any other radiologist has treated urethral caruncle by the x-ray.

*Read before the Rocky Mountain Inter-State Medical Association, September, 1904.

This is a most painful and annoying affliction, and one that seems very apt to return after surgical treatment.

These extremely sensitive tumors, with a bright red surface, just at the meatus urinarius, are easily recognized, and no other similar condition in this region gives rise to so much pain; by this alone they may be differentiated from other affections of this locality, prolapse of the urethra, etc.

The fact that these growths are quite vascular led me to believe that the x-ray, with its well known action in causing an obliterative endarteritis, should be a rational and scientific method . of treatment.

My first case is that of patient No. 122. The tumor first appeared fifteen years ago, and the original growth and two recurrences have been removed by the knife. When this patient consulted me there was a tumor the size of a finger end, very red and tender and inclined to bleed easily, It was so painful that she could not sit in a chair comfortably. Twenty-five x-ray exposures were given, using a tube of medium low vacuum, at a distance of five inches from the growth, the seances lasting ten minutes each. The size of the growth diminished after the fourth or fifth exposure, and the pain became gradually less. When the patient discontinued treatment she had no more discomfort, the surface did not bleed, and it has taken on the appearance of normal mucous membrane; there was still some thickened tissue present.

The other patient was No. 127. The tumor had been removed by the knife some six years previous to her visit to me; it soon recurred and has remained sore ever since, causing a great deal of pain in walking and during urination. Only six exposures were needed; as this sore was quite superficial, a tube of fairly low vacuum was used, at a distance of six inches, with ten minute seances, during a period of about three weeks; after the fourth exposure the patient stated that she had no more pain or soreness.

These results are of course very gratifying, but a considerable time must elapse before I will say that they have been cured.

CHARCOT'S JOINTS.*

By BYRON C. LEAVITT, M.D.

Denver, Colo.

Upon January 28th, 1904, I was consulted by a man, aged forty-two, both of whose ankles were swollen, the right knee being also swollen, and in a condition of knock-knee. Until February 1902 he had never had any trouble with his joints. At that time he retired at night as well as usual, and slept well all night. When he awoke his right knee was as large as his head, but was not painful or sensitive to the touch. About three weeks later swelling appeared suddenly in his right ankle, and four weeks after this in the left ankle. This condition had remained ever since, the size of the swellings considerably diminishing. There had never been any sensitiveness to touch. There had been intermittent painful periods, especially at times of storms or threatening of storm, this being at localized spots, anywhere from the knee to the ankle on the right side, or in the left foot.

The history and general appearance excluded osteo- and rheumatoid arthritis. I learned that the diagnosis of sarcoma had been made over a year before I saw him, and a very competent surgeon had then told him that he would have to have an amputation at once, to save his life. As he had lived this length of time with no great change, it was evident that this disease could be eliminated from the diagnosis.

I took X-ray pictures of the swollen joints, which I have to show. The condition of knock-knee is evident in the right knee; also the proliferated bony tissue, and the loss of the ligamentous tissue in the ankle joints.

This appeared so evidently a case of Charcot's joints that I immediately examined for symptoms of locomotor ataxia, and found Argyll-Robertson pupils, loss of knee-jerk, inability to stand with the eyes closed, a history of shooting pains, and nearly all the typical symptoms of that disease.

The patient remained in about the same condition until July of this year, when he suffered much more severe pain in different parts of the body, lost control of his bladder and bowels, and died the last of that month.

---

*Read before Rocky Mountain Inter-State Medical Association, September, 1904.

The most trouble was with the knee, and a support for this was advised, but the patient kept neglecting to have it attended to. Excision was not advised because of the tendency of the bones not to unite in this disease.

Bradford and Lovett state that in this disease "the cartilage disintegrates, the ends of the bones are exposed and may be rapidly worn away, the synovial membrane and the ligaments thicken and ulcerate. This process may result in spontaneous luxation, in severe cases, synovial effusion may be present, and suppuration may occur. Hypertrophy of the epiphyses may take place as well as the formation of osteophytes, but atrophic changes predominate. The essential character of the affection is the rapid melting away of cartilage and bone.

I have written this paper in the form of a report because I was so much interested in the case, and because it seems to me to be sufficiently typical of Charcot's joints to bring out clearly the landmarks of a disease which is but slightly mentioned in text-books and yet which quite frequently accompanies locomotor ataxia, as well as other diseases of the nervous system.

PERNICIOUS ANEMIA, WITH A REPORT OF CASES.*

By J. N. HALL, M.D.

Denver, Colo.

I have recently had the opportunity of studying eight cases of this disease rather closely and believe the results of this study and of the treatment will be of some interest. I am indebted to my associate, Dr. H. R. McGraw, for much painstaking work in the study of the blood, and to Dr. R. W. Arndt for permission to report two of his cases which I saw with him at the Denver City and County Hospital. Seven of the cases were males between the ages of 30 and 53 and one was a woman of 70. Two were physicians, three were ranchmen, one a laborer, one a smelter-man, while the woman was a housewife.

I shall give a brief synopsis of each, with comments upon it.

Case 1. A physician of 34 years, from an Eastern state. Tuberculosis of the left apex with hemoptysis five years ago. Full recovery. He had previously lost his right forefinger from septic infection. Three years ago he became anemic, and his blood count at that time showed 1,700,000 reds, 2,000 whites, 37% hemoglobin. HCl. was noted as absent at this time.

Without a definite diagnosis he came to New Mexico, and immediately improved, his reds rising to 4,000,000, and his hemoglobin to 70%.

He relapsed and came West again a year ago, with some improvement. He was able to work moderately in the intervals.

Upon examination I found his temperature running to nearly 100° daily. Reds 3,000,000, hemoglobin 55. Nucleated reds present, marked poikilocytosis; no parasites found in stools. No increase of eosinophiles. Liver slightly enlarged. Teeth sound. Marked venous hum in neck. Notable pulsation in vessels of neck. Soft apical murmur transmitted to left. Heart area not increased. No edema. Urine rather dilute, but contained no albumin nor sugar. The nervous system showed nothing abnormal excepting slight numbness of fingers and toes, which had been present for some months and was evidently not the effect of arsenical medication.

---

*Read before the meeting of the Rocky Mountain Inter-State Medical Association, Denver, September 6, 1904.

He was placed in bed upon a light diet. Upon giving small doses of Fowler's solution diarrhoea came on, and he lost nearly a million reds in the next fortnight. Then under the hypodermic use of cacodylate of soda he slowly improved.

Five weeks after I first saw him he had suppuration of the right middle ear. Dr. Levy found the prostration so marked that we resorted to vigorous stimulation, it being necessary to use adrenalin and other drugs to prevent death from collapse. He was unconscious for nearly a week, the pulse being little more than perceptible. The mitral murmur was much more marked.

Four weeks later it became necessary to open the mastoid, to which the ear trouble had extended. The hemoglobin stood at 55 at this time, and the blood was so watery that we feared severe hemorrhage, but operation was imperative. Under chloroform Dr. Black operated as quickly as possible, but the terrible oozing obscured the wound most of the time. Hot water and adrenalin were of much service, and the patient came out of the anaesthetic in better condition than we expected, notwithstanding the loss of much blood.

From this time he improved rapidly, and in four months returned to his practice in practically perfect health, and has remained so for six months. His blood pressure was 165 m m. by Riva-Rocci instrument. Hemoglobin 100, reds 4,290,000. Heart sounds normal. Why the blood pressure remains above normal I am unable to explain.

It is striking in this case to note the previous septic infection of the finger, the pulmonary tuberculosis with recovery, the two relapses, the inability to take arsenic by the mouth, and the rapid recovery when given hypodermically. I do not attribute especial influence to this climate, although one cannot but be impressed with the fact that both of the physicians in this series came from Eastern states and made prompt recovery in Colorado.

Case 2. Ranchman, 30 years of age, referred to me by Dr. Dulin of Las Animas. No previous illness of note excepting typhoid 13 years ago.

For four and a half months he had headache, dyspnoea, palpitation, edema of feet, lemon-yellow color, and feeling of exhaustion. No especial loss of weight. He was extremely apathetic.

Upon examination I found the temperature 100°, pulse about 100, soft and running up quickly upon the least exertion. Palpable venous hum in the neck, audible to second intercostal space. Heart area extends one-half inch to left of left nipple. Soft systolic apical murmur heard also in tricuspid area. Pulmonic second sound accentuated. Liver area nearly doubled in size, lower edge of organ palpable two inches below ribs. Spleen slightly enlarged. Marked edema of feet. Several small retinal hemorrhages, notably two in the upper and inner quadrant of the right eye.

Hemoglobin 30, reds 1,200,000, whites 7,000. Reds extremely pale, varying greatly in size, with marked poikilocytosis; nucleated reds present. Urine moderately increased in amount, sp. gr. 1008, no sugar, no albumin, a few hyaline casts after centrifuging.

Several badly decayed teeth were found. He was placed in bed, with diet gradually increasing as he improved, and Fowler's solu-increased daily until 20 minims after each meal were given. The teeth were attended to promptly.

In four weeks his hemoglobin was 70, reds 3,360,000, almost normal under the microscope. The edema disappeared, liver normal in size. Blood pressure 85 by Gaertner's tonometer. He had lost about 7 pounds from the clearing up of his dropsy.

He went home, continuing his arsenic treatment for two months under Dr. Dulin's care. At the end of this time his hemoglobin was 100, reds 5,600,000, absolutely normal microscopically.

He stopped his medicine for five months, and suffered a relapse, the hemoglobin falling to 50, and the reds to 2,000,000. He was placed upon the cacodylate of soda hypodermically, but did not improve materially. Under Fowler's solution with HCl and bone marrow he gradually improved and three months later he considered himself well.

About July 20th he had an attack of appendicitis, with walling off of an abscess, and was sent to Denver again by Dr. Dulin. Dr. Grant opened and drained this abscess and the patient is now convalescent. Hemoglobin 95%.

In view of the recent theory of the origin of pernicious anemia from chronic poisoning by the colon bacillus the attack of appendicitis is of especial interest. I shall in future look with care for a history of the disease in such cases.

Case 3. Ranchman, 54 years of age, referred to me by Dr. Wm. Greig of Sterling. His mother is said to have died from pernicious anemia. Well marked specific history, several attacks of pneumonia, and two of typhoid.

Patient is very pale, with lemon-yellow color. He has lost 15 pounds in weight. Has moderate edema of feet. Many decayed teeth. Heart little enlarged. An aortic diastolic murmur is heard transmitted to apex and a mitral systolic murmur transmitted to the left. Liver area one-half greater than normal. Spleen and glands negative. Retinae very pale, no hemorrhages, optic disks pale.

Hemoglobin 35%, reds 1,200,000, whites 5,625. Marked poikilocytosis and oligochromemia. No nucleated reds found. Whites normal in appearance and proportions.

Urine 1018; a trace of albumin and a few finely granular casts were present. Total solids for 24 hours, 42 gm.

Test breakfast shows no HCl, no lactic acid, no acidity of any kind.

In 15 weeks under rest and increasing doses of Fowler's solution the patient recovered. Hemoglobin then reached 96%, reds 4,800,000. Soon after this the patient developed well marked scleroderma affecting the neck and trunk especially, for which I referred him to Dr. J. M. Blaine. He improved somewhat under thyroid extract and oily inunctions.

His further course was disturbed by a specific spinal meningomyelitis, somewhat benefited by iodide treatment. He gradually failed and died about 15 months after I first saw him.

Case 4. Ranchman, 54, referred to me by Dr. H. L. Stevens of Laramie, Wyoming, and seen but once.

Was well until 7 months ago. Is now breathless and has lost 20 pounds of flesh. Is very pale, but not yellow.

I found a fairly marked pyorrhoea alveolaris. Moderate edema of feet. Heart negative. Liver considerably enlarged and palpable. Spleen moderately enlarged, glands negative. Retinae normal. Urine 1015, negative. Reds 2,000,000, whites normal, hemoglobin 40. Marked variation in size, color and form of reds. A few nucleated reds were present. Nervous system normal. Under large doses of arsenic the patient made a rapid recovery and remains well.

Case 5. Physician, 51 years of age. Malaria in 1881, but no other serious illness. A slight and transient hemiplegic attack two years ago followed by complete recovery. He states that he has been anemic for two years, and gradually failing. He has lost 23 pounds. He is very pale and sallow. Dyspnoea and palpitation are noticeable. Slight edema of feet. Marked pulsation in vessels of neck. Heart slightly enlarged with soft systolic murmur. Marked hemic hum in neck. Liver a little larger than normal. Spleen negative. One small retinal hemorrhage in each eye. Blood pressure 140 m m. by Riva-Rocci instrument.

Blood examination shows hemoglobin 40%, reds 1,724,800, whites 11,600. Many poikilocytes and nucleated reds. One immense megaloblast seen.

Under rest, liberal diet and arsenic he improved in six weeks up to 90% of hemoglobin and 3,600,000 reds, and has remained in about this condition for about five months. He has resumed practice and considers himself fairly well. A certain tingling and numb feeling in the fingers and toes has caused us to hesitate in pushing the arsenic. I believe these symptoms are due to the disease, but do not dare to disregard them so long as his condition remains so reasonably good.

Case 6. A feeble woman of 70, seen but twice with Dr. H. R. McGraw. She was too feeble to rise from bed. She was very pale with a yellowish shade. Marked pulsation in the vessels of neck. Heart considerably enlarged with loud systolic mitral murmur. Slight edema of feet. Liver, spleen and glands negative. The hemoglobin was 18%, reds 800,000. The usual conditions were found with the microscope. She failed rapidly and died; the whole course of the disease being but three or four months.

Case 7. Smelterman, 53 years of age, seen with Dr. Arndt at the Denver City and County Hospital. Face very pale, with yellowish tinge. Hemic murmur in neck. Heart negative. Liver slightly enlarged. Spleen and glands negative. Hemoglobin very low, reds 2,300,000, whites 12,000; nucleated reds, megaloblasts and poikilocytes abundant.

He appeared at the point of death and died in a few days after admission. The autopsy showed, aside from the usual pigmentation in the liver, small healed tuberculous foci in the lungs, and pyorrhœa alveolaris.

Case 8. Laborer, 34 years old, seen with Dr. Arndt at the Denver City and County Hospital. Has been sick 15 months. Very pale and waxy in color. He has many carious teeth. Heart, liver, spleen and glands negative. Reds 263,000, whites 2,900, hemoglobin 15 per cent. Many nucleated reds, some megaloblasts, marked poikilocytosis. Urine negative.

The patient died one week after admission. Autopsy showed an extremely pale gastric mucous membrane, considerable deposit of reddish pigment in the liver, and much dark staining of the wall of the ileum. Aside from marked pallor there were no findings of especial interest.

Case 9. Attorney, 51 years old. Has had chronic appendicitis for years, and probably gall stones, with two or three attacks of jaundice. Right kidney floats. Marked emaciation. Operation was recommended in June, 1903, but declined.

One year later he returned to town, and I found that a typical pernicious anemia had developed. Lemon yellow color. Extensive edema of feet. Urine clear. Hemoglobin 38 per cent.; reds, 1,600,000, whites normal. Poikilocytosis marked. Nucleated reds present. The liver was moderately increased in size, spleen and glands negative.

Under treatment with arsenic he improved slowly. Subgallate of bismuth was given to prevent the flatulence which was so distressing, and with good effect. Diarrhea compelled a suspension of the Fowler's solution when a dose of 16 minims was reached, but it was soon resumed in smaller dosage.

Sept. 3, 1904, his hemoglobin was 85 per cent., reds 3,724,-800, whites 7,875. A few nucleated reds and poikilocytes were found. His general condition is good. Operation for the gall stones has again been recommended by Dr. Freeman and myself.

The most striking points in the consideration of these cases seem to me to be as follows:

The frequent marked enlargement of the liver. In some instances the diagnosis of cancer was made on this account, the yellow color of the skin passing for jaundice.

The marked pulsation of the vessels of the neck. The peripheral vascular relaxation is very notable in many cases, and this pulsation becomes, in such instances, a prominent feature in the examination.

The frequent presence of serious defects in the teeth, and of pyorrhœa alveolaris. Although we may not credit the theory of intoxication from the swallowing of pus organisms therefrom, we cannot disregard so unhygienic a condition in our treatment.

The frequent absence of HCl from the gastric juice. It would doubtless be found absent or decreased very frequently if we examined for it always. The administration of this acid should be a part of our treatment in all such cases.

The need of rest in the treatment. So long as there is fever I believe the rest is as important as it is in tuberculosis.

The frequent presence of cord symptoms or those of peripheral nervous disease. In no instance here given were the former marked, but in one or two previous cases I found them present, and even simulating locomotor ataxia, as in the case of a physician seen with Dr. S. D. Hopkins, due doubtless to patches of sclerosis in the posterior and lateral columns or to hemorrhagic foci in the substance of the cord. The possibility of confusion between the numbness and tingling of the extremities in this disease and the beginning of an arsenical neuritis must be constantly in mind. With the late Dr. Tyler I saw a fatal arsenical poisoning develop because of neglect of this precaution, the patient continuing the arsenic for weeks after it was ordered stopped by Dr. Tyler.

The frequent relapses are striking, and particularly annoying because of the absence of any known cause. I shall look with particular interest to see if the patient whose appendix was removed relapses. If the colon bacillus intoxication theory proves well founded we may well watch the appendices of our patients with this disease.

The especially pernicious course of this disease is well illustrated by case 6. I have seen several other rapidly fatal cases in old people.

The beneficial effect of the sub-cutaneous use of an arsenical preparation when arsenic cannot be bourne by mouth is to be noted in case 1. Hydrochloric acid, salol and bone marrow seem to be of occasional use, but arsenic is vastly more certain to help the average case.

The commonly noted increase of eosinophilic cells in the blood of those harboring intestinal parasites should make us feel less hesitation in making a diagnosis of pernicious anemia when we find a normal number only.

SYPHILITIC DISEASES OF THE NERVOUS SYSTEM.

In discussing this highly important subject in one of his clinical lectures, Gowers emphasizes the facts that syphilitic disease of the nerve centers affects primarily the adventitious tissue; and that the real nerve elements are involved only secondarily, and the simple inflammatory changes they undergo are not amenable directly to antiluetic remedies. The characteristic specific process is neoplastic, and is characterized pathologically, even to the naked eye, by desseminated caseation. The prognosis depends very largely on the duration of the symptoms before treatment was begun. Thus, if paraplegia from gummatous compression has lasted only a month, recovery will probably be perfect in time; whereas, after a year's duration the return of function may be very slight, and at best will not be great. Tissue elements of recent formation, chiefly cellular, undergo granular disintegration, the results are quickly removed; but the older cells become fibrillar, with progressive contraction, which cicatrization appears to be promoted by treatment. Under treatment with mercury to the physiologic limit, Gowers concludes that the syphilitic disease proper should be removed in six or eight weeks. Mercury also has a beneficial influence on this as on all secondary inflammation. He orders a dram of the ten per cent. oleate to be rubbed into the skin with the same small piece of flannel twice a day for three or four days, and then continued once a day until the end of a week. If the gums then show no sign, resume the two daily rubbings until they do. It is perhaps a little better, because of the counter irritant effect, to make the inunction near the affected part.

After such an energetic course of eight weeks, omit the mercury for two, four or six months, and give the patient three or four weeks treatment with iodide (10 grains three times a day) every four months during the first year after any true specific symptoms, and every six months for the next three or four years. Gowers does not think it wise to give iodide and mercury together in full doses, except for a short time in a very urgent case.

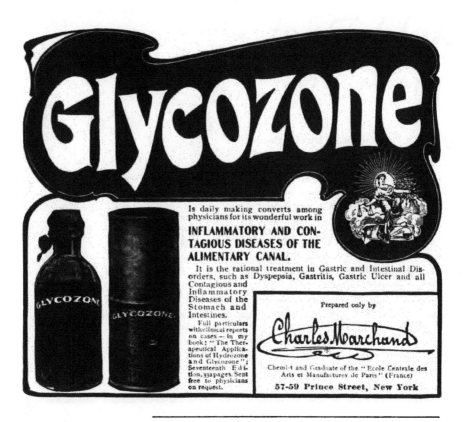

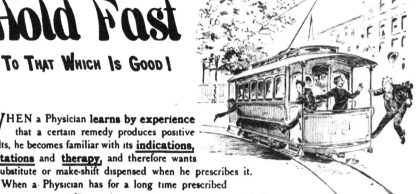

DENVER MEDICAL TIMES

THOMAS H. HAWKINS, A.M., M.D., Editor and Publisher.

COLLABORATORS:

Henry O. Marcy, M.D., Boston.
Thaddeus A. Reamy, M.D., Cincinnati.
Nicholas Senn, M.D., Chicago.
Joseph Price, M.D., Philadelphia.
Franklin H. Martin, M.D., Chicago.
William Oliver Moore, M.D.. New York.
L. S. McMurtry, M.D., Louisville.
Thomas B. Eastman, M.D., Indianapolis, Ind.
G. Law, M.D., Greeley, Colo.

S. H. Pinkerton, M.D., Salt Lake City
Flavel B. Tiffany, M.D., Kansas City.
Erskine M. Bates, M.D;, New York.
E. C. Gehrung, M.D, St. Louis.
Graeme M. Hammond, M.D, New
James A. Lydston, M.D., Chicago.
Leonard Freeman, M.D., Denver.
Carey K. Fleming, M.D., Denver,

Subscriptions, $1.00 per year in advance; Single Copies, 10 cents.

Address all Communications to Denver Medical Times, 1740 Welton Street, Denver, Colo.
We will at all times be glad to give space to well written articles or items of interest to the profession.
[Entered at the Postoffice of Denver, Colorado, as mail matter of the Second Class.]

EDITORIAL DEPARTMENT

THE INFECTIOUS SICK ROOM.

Isolation and disinfection are the sanitary keynotes in preventing the spread of infectious diseases. The sick room should be cleared of all unnecessary furniture and of carpets, curtains and bed-hangings. It is best located at the top of the house, or as far as practicable from the rest of the household. Good light and ventilation destroy and diminish germs. An open fire is convenient to burn infected things and aid ventilation. A sheet saturated with some disinfectant solution may be hung over the door. The acting nurse should keep aloof from the remainder of the household, and sleep in an adjoining room. The attending physician should cover his clothing with a long gown kept just outside the patient's door and sterilized immediately after being used. He should wash his hands with soap and water, followed by mercuric chlorid (1:1000) or other good antiseptic before leaving the sick room. Nurses should keep their hands clean and disinfected, and may also employ some simple antiseptic gargle or spray for the throat and nose. Remnants of food had best be burned and the eating utensils scalded. After an attack of infectious disease, the entire body and the hair must be bathed and washed with hot soapsuds, and the patient dressed in clean clothing from another apartment before leaving the room. The body

of a person dead from an infectious disease is to be enveloped in
sheets saturated with carbolic acid or mercuric chlorid solution.
In cases of dysentery, cholera and plague the anus should be
plugged with a pledget of cotton previously soaked in a strong
antiseptic solution.

Infected matter should be thoroughly disinfected before
throwing into vaults. The disinfection of stools is necessary in
typhoid, dysentery and cholera. One per cent. of active chlorinated lime thoroughly disinfects typhoid and cholera stools in
ten minutes. This germicide is best placed in the vessel before
the excreta, and should be well mixed therewith. Carbolic acid
is uncertain for the destruction of spores, but a 2% solution destroys typhoid and cholera bacilli and gonococci. A 5% solution
is an effective disinfectant for sputum, vomit and feces. A 2%
solution is used as a wash. Carbolized soap solution consists of 3%
soft soap and then 5% of the commercial acid in 100 parts of water. Infected clothing and bedding are soaked in this for 2 or 3
hours, and it is used for scrubbing floors and furniture. Mercuric chlorid solution, 1 :5000-1 :1000, is also employed in washing and scrubbing. A teaspoonful of common salt to the quart
of solution prevents precipitation by albuminous liquids. A 4%
solution of hot washing soda is useful for scrubbing, both as a
detergent and a disinfectant. A 2% solution is used for boiling
cloths, vessels and instruments.

Articles that are safely boiled should be so disinfected, first
soaking stained goods in cold water. Valueless articles are best
promptly burned. Steam apparatus is essential for bulky matters, such as bedding, carpets and clothing. Hot air is inferior
and may scorch and damage many things, but may be employed
carefully for furs, leather, books, etc., and to dry articles moistened by steam.

Previous to fumigation, one should paper over all crevices
and openings, including the fireplace, and keep the room closed
for 24 hours, then ærate thoroughly. Metal surfaces should be
washed over with 2% carbolic acid solution, and such furniture
should be removed from the room if sulphur fumigation is employed. Strip the paper from the walls, or rub over with bread

48 hours old. Whitewash the ceilings and wash the floor with acidulated chlorid 1:1000, or with a 5% solution of carbolic acid.

Formaldehyde destroys highly resistant bacteria and spores, but has little penetrating action. From personal experience, Abbott endorses the use of formalin containing 10% of glycerin, by means of a simple copper retort and a key-hole tube. Five hundred cc. of the mixture is sufficient for 1,000 cubic feet.

The irritating odor is readily removed by exposing ammonia water to the air of the disinfected room. The autoclave is recommended in the U. S. quarantine regulations, for disinfection with formalin (one pound per 1,000 cubic feet) or formochloral, passing the heated gas through the key-hole by means of an escape tube.

Sulphur dioxide, to be reliable, must constitute 4% by volume of the air capacity of the room. Since the gas must unite with water, forming sulphurous acid, in order to exert a germicidal effect, it is well to spray objects with a hand atomizer or generate steam from boiling water along with the evolution of the sulphur vapors. Sulphur fumigation is preferable to formaldehyde in its greater penetration and in the fact that it kills fleas, mosquitoes, bugs and rats. On the other hand, it corrodes metals and bleaches colored fabrics. Sulphur dioxid liquefied by pressure and kept in cans, is very convenient, requiring only to be let out of the container into air previously moistened with steam.

Walls, ceilings and other surfaces may be disinfected by spraying them with a 1:1000 solution of mercuric chlorid or formalin, and rubbing down carefully with bread or damp cheese cloth. It is well, if possible, to repaint and repaper rooms that have been infected. Mere fumigation is by no means sufficient to combat the house infection produced by tuberculosis. The dust-laden walls, hangings, bedding and furniture should all be carefully cleaned at stated intervals, and certainly after the death of the tuberculous occupant. Concerning infected stables and cellars, Abbott recommends to saturate the surfaces thoroughly over night with 5% creolin or sulphocarbolic acid solution, or with a 2% solution of chlorinated lime, and to cleanse them the following morning with a 2% solution of boiling washing soda. Cellars and common stables should be whitewashed.

President Amador of the Republic of Panama has appointed the following officers of the Fourth Pan-American Medical Congress, to be held in Panama the first week in January, 1905:

Dr. Julio Ycaza, President; Dr. Manuel Coroalles, Vice-President; Dr. Jose E. Calvo, Secretary; Dr. Pedro de Obarrio, Treasurer, and Dr. J. W. Ross, Dr. T. Tomaselli, Dr. M. Gasteazoro, Committeemen.

There will be but four sections: Surgery, Medicine, Hygiene and the Specialties, to which the following officers were appointed:

Surgical Section—Major Louis LaGarde, President; Dr. E. B. Harrick, Secretary.

Medical Section—Dr. Moritz Stern, President; Dr. Daniel R. Oduber, Secretary.

Section on Hygiene—Colonel W. C. Gorgas, President; Dr. Henry E. Carter, Secretary.

Section on Specialties—Dr. W. Spratling, President; Dr. Charles A. Cooke, Secretary.

EDITORIAL ITEMS.

Medical Education in Japan. Japan, says the *Medical Fortnightly,* has 31,000 physicians and eight medical schools.

For Syphilitic Allopecia.—Fox directs to apply a five per cent. oleate of mercury ointment.

Tinea Kerion.—The tricophyton fungus disease is treated by Bulkley by epilation and washing with one per cent. bichloride solution.

For Barber's Itch.—J. J. Pringle advises epilation of about a square inch daily, followed by the application of diluted ointment of the red oxide of mercury.

Defluvium Capillitii.—The temporary thinning of the hair after fevers is treated by Fox with a lotion of tincture of cantharides 10, glycerine 2, and cologne water to make 100 parts.

Eczema Capitis.—The "milk crust" of children is treated by Fox by the local use of a mixture of one part of oil of cade to three parts of oil of sweet almond.

Black Urine.—The *Medical Council* states that melanuria is often observed after eating damson plums. When taking ferric chloride or nitric acid, the urine may turn black after it cools.

For Threatened Baldness.—Bartholow recommended the following: ℞ Ext. jaborandi fl. oz. i; tinct. cantharidis dr. iv; linimentum saponis q. s. ad. oz. iv: Rub into scalp once a day.

Cardiac Neuralgia.—In neuralgias of the heart Abbott *(Alkaloidal Clinic)* gives strychnine arsenate in moderate doses in the intervals, continued for months.

For Lupus Vulgaris.—Jackson advises a nutritious diet, cod-liver oil and iodide of iron; also multiple scarification deep enough to penetrate all softened tissues and repeated in five or six days.

Prevention of Baldness.—Brush the hair twice a day with a fairly stiff brush, says Robinson, and tip it every other week. Wash the scalp at intervals with warm rain water and a good simple soap.

Fragilitas Crinium.—Cleavage and friability of hairs is due to local scalp disease (seborrhea), fevers or debility. Jackson directs to cut hairs above cleft and keep scalp in good condition. Shaving may be of service in beard cases.

Fermentation or Aseptic Fever.—Nancrede recommends cold sponging, laxatives and free diuresis induced by the ingestion of large amounts of water by mouth or rectum; also careful regulation of diet.

For Strumous Children.—Shoemaker prescribes the following: ℞ Hydrarg. chlor. corros. gr. 1-48; tinct. gentianæ m. i; syrupi aurantii m. x; aquam q. s.: A teaspoonful four times a day at mealtime.

Meteroism in Pneumonia.—H. Schiller *(American Medicine)* states that meteorism of considerable degree is one of the worst prognostic symptoms in pneumonia. When it is distinct it indicates a severe and often deadly course.

Pseudoleukemia.—The modern and most successful treatment is the use of the x-rays. Arsenic, iron, strychnine, phosphorus and cod-liver oil are of service as adjudvants. The diet should be nourishing and largely of animal origin.

For Chlorosis.—Hershey prescribes fresh pills of ferrous sulphate and potassium carbonate aa. 1½ grains t. i. d. p. c. in occasional cases. Bartholow used the following: ℞ Ferri sulph. exsic. gr. ii; strych. sulph. gr. 1-40: One pill t. i. d.

After-Treatment of Puerperal Fever.—E. P. Davis recommends uid extract of ergot m. xx. and strychnine sulphate gr. 1-60 every six hours night and day. He considers these drugs indispensable.

For Scrofulous Children.—℞ Hydrarg. perchloridi gr. 1-28—1-32; liq. potass. ars. m. i-iv; tinct. ferri. chlor. m, ii-vii; acidi phosphor. dil. m. iv-xv; syr. limonis q. s.: One-fourth to a dram in water after meals.—Goodman.

Referred Pains.—Says the *International Journal of Surgery:* Pains over the iliac crests, the groins, the front of the thighs, the inner aspect of the legs or feet, or the big toe, are often evidences of lumbar caries.

Anchylostomiasis.—Friedrich Schultze recommends the ethereal extract of male fern, 2 to 2½ drams at one dose, preceded and followed in a few hours by castor oil. If this treatment fails, give four or five grams of thymol in a little wine, cognac or beer.

Treatment of Paronychia.—Incision is usually required. In mild cases *(Gould and Pyle's Cyclopedia)* place arm in sling and keep finger constantly wet with boric acid lotion, followed by boric acid ointment. Quinine and other tonics are indicated.

Note Results.—Berberine, says Waugh *(Critic and Guide)* is the direct remedy for dilated stomach. Give, he says, one grain of it daily for a month to women with uterine prolapse, who do not care to continue wearing a pessary, and note results.

Seborrhea Oleosa.—In the ordinary or mixed type Fox tells us to shampoo twice a week in the morning with tincture of green soap, and apply each evening a mixture of 10 parts of oil of sweet almond, 1 part of carbolic acid and 100 parts of alcohol, with enough oil of citronella to perfume.

Treatment of Alopecia Areata.—Nervine tonics, and equal parts of bay rum and tincture of cantharides as a lotion night and morning, are recommended by Fox. He also uses oleate of mercury locally, and if this fails, the strong liquor ammonia or other stimulating wash.

Conglomerate Superficial Perifolliculitis.—This appears as a diffuse, roundish red patch, with pustules or a conglomerate patch of small red papules, at the back of the hand or wrist. Stelwagon instructs to press out secretion, cleanse and apply antiseptic salves or lotions.

Onychomycosis.—Fungous disease of the nails may be due to favus or tinea trichophytica. Mycelia and spores are to be found in the scrapings. Stelwagon directs to keep nails closely cut or pared and apply solution of mercuric chloride (1 to 5 grains per ounce) several times a day, or a dram to the ounce solution of sodium hyposulphite.

Ungual Ulcers.—These may arise from the chloral habit (red spots on back of hand) or from handling irritating drugs. The simultaneous ulceration of a number of nails has been noted in syphilis, syringomyelia and Morvan's and Raynaud's syndromes. A boric acid or other mild ointment is the best local application.

For Hypertrichoses.—To remove unwelcome hairs from the female physiognomy Fox directs to use a galvanic battery of 16 to 20 cells, insert a sharp, small needle to the root of the hair and connect with the negative electrode; after 10 or 20 seconds pull out the dead hair with forceps.

For Dandruff.—Barie directs to rub the hairy scalp every night with a' 1:30 solution of mercuric chloride in alcohol. Bronson prescribes an ointment of ammoniated mercury 20 grains, calomel 40 grains, and petrolatum one ounce: Apply once or twice a day. This, he says, is excellent in simple dandruff, and should be combined with an occasional shampoo.

Premature "Idiopathic" Alopecia.—This form of baldness affects the forehead and vertex. It is often hereditary and is slowly progressive. Stelwagon recommends the following lotion: ℞ Tinct. cantharides dr. iv, tinct. capsici oz. ss., olei ricini dr. ss.; alcohol ad. oz. iv: Rub in thoroughly daily or every second or third day.

Local Anesthesia.—Gant *(New York Medical Journal)* gets good results by injecting sterile water between the layers of skin in the line of injection, then through this line or bleb into the subcutaneous tissues. Internal thrombotic hemorrhoids distended with water are quite insensitive.

Chlorosis of Fecal Intoxication.—Andrew Clarke recommended a combination of one-half grain each of aloin, iron sulphate, ext. belladonna, ext. nux vomica, ipecac, myrrh and soap, giving one pill of this composition an hour before the last meal should bowels not act during the day.

Bleeding Piles.—Boas (quoted in *Medical Standard)* has cured 25 cases of rebellious hemorrhoidal bleeding by the daily injection of 20 cc. of a ten per cent. aqueous solution of calcium chloride just after the morning evacuation of the bowels. The injections should be continued two or three times weekly after the bleeding is arrested. They have no influence on the hemorrhoid nodules.

Dermatitis Papillaris Capilitii.—Keloid acne is characterized by hard, congested papules, changing to uneven tumors, over which the hair is lost or bunched and crusted by the offensive discharge. The usual site is the back of head and neck. In treatment Stelwagon advises stimulating applications, particularly sulphur and ichthyol. Depilation is also of value.

Lupus Erythematosus.—In the early stages Jackson directs to use a lotion of one dram each of zinc sulphate and potassium sulphuret, three drams of alcohol, and rose water to make four ounces. Green soap or its tincture, well rubbed in with flannel, should be used in more chronic cases; also pure carbolic acid or multiform punctures by electrolysis.

Falling of Hair Following Erysipelas.—After cutting the hair short, Shoemaker uses the galvanic alternated with the faradic current every day or two, and singes the hair ends every two or three weeks, if the hair is dry and lustreless and the glands plugged up. He also applies equal parts of oil of ergot and fluid mercury oleate.

Anemia of Acute Nephritis.—Bruce prescribes as follows: ℞ Ferri et ammon. cit. gr. v; potassii cit. gr. xv; ext. scillæ fl. m. i; spt. eth. nit. m. xxx; syr, aurantii m; aq. dest. ad. oz. i: Take t. i. d. after meals. For anemia following acute nephritis he gives: ℞ Tinct. ferri chloridi m. x; tinct. digitalis m. v; spt. juniperis m. x; glycerini m. xxx; aq. dest. ad. oz. i: Take t. i. d. after meals.

After-Treatment of Post-Partum Hemorrhage.—Buchtel uses hypodermoclysis of normal salt solution under the breast in sufficient quantity to replace lost blood, and gives one drop of fluid extract of cereus gradiflora every 15 minutes till the normal color is restored. He orders frequent feeding with freshly prepared bouillons and prescribes strychnine arsenite in small doses during convalescence.

Non-Infectious Puerperal Fever.—Hirst recommends heat to breast; evacuation; castor oil and enema for constipation; When the fever is accompanied by pain or tenderness over the lower abdomen, G. E. Herman directs to apply a linseed poultice mixed with one-fourth its bulk of mustard or sprinkled with oil of turpentine and administer opium.

Puerperal Endometritis and Endocolpitis.—Hirst advises frequent repeated irrigations of the whole genital tract and if accessible touch with silver nitrate solution a dram to the ounce. In all cases G. E. Herman directs to support the patient's strength with easily digested food and alcohol, using quinine for the nervous system and opium for pain. If the temperature is very high, he uses tepid baths, tepid sponging or the wet pack.

Leukemia.—Osler recommends fresh air, good diet and abstention from worry and care. Arsenic in large doses is the best remedy; quinine when malarial history. Now and then inhalations of oxygen are of value in some cases. Thornton gives two or three ounces of bone marrow (taken from bones after boiling) daily, or ten grains of dried red bone marrow three times a day. Hartshorne prescribes dilute nitromuriatic acid, 10 to 20 drops in a wineglassful of water t. i. d.

Treatment of Psoriasis.—Van Harlingen directs to remove scales with a solution of one dram of salicylic acid in four ounces of alcohol, well rubbed in, or with spiritus saponis alkalinus (two parts of green soap in one part of hot alcohol—filter) used as a shampoo. Then rub in well with a soft brush a mixture of one dram of oil of cade to the ounce of oil of almond; or apply an ointment of ammoniated mercury, 20 to 40 grains to the ounce.

Bleeding Stigmata.—Hematidrosis, or ephidrosis cruenta, consists in a bloody secretion from the sweat glands, sometimes preceded by erythema or miliaria and accompanied by malaise and slight fever. The common cause is hysteria. It may also be due to imposture, epilepsy, blood dyscrasiæ, vicarious menstruation or malarial paroxysms. The points of election are on the face, ear, breast, navel, hands and feet.

Pityriasis Rubra Pilaris.—The follicular form of pityriasis appears as brownish or yellow-red pinhead point papules with a horny central spine and fine white scales, forming plaques about the hair follicles. Hardway recommends pilocarpine by the mouth or hypodermically for excessive dryness of the skin; also sodium arseniate internally in increasing doses; soothing pastes and lotions for inflammatory condition; tar and pyrogallic acid in more chronic states; and salicylic acid plaster for thickened patches on the palms and soles.

Simple Pityriasis.—When affecting the scalp, which is nearly normal in appearance, this disease is characterized by diffuse branny dandruff and distressing itching. Jackson directs to rub well into scalp once a day or less often an ointment consisting of 7 drams white wax, 5 ounces liquid petroleum, 2½ ounces rose water ointment, 36 grains of borax and 7 drams of sulphur. Fox rubs in equal parts of rose water ointment and white precipitate ointment.

Seborrhea Sicca.—On the crown of the head Jackson recommends a thin ten per cent. sulphur ointment rubbed into the scalp. or for the oily form a three to ten per cent. resorcin lotion (dilute alcohol with two or three per cent. of castor oil) if sulphur irritates. Apply every day for four days, then wash head; apply every other day again for ten days and wash; gradually lengthen intervals to once a week for at least three months.

For Ringworm of the Scalp.—Crocker directs to shave at least ¾ inch beyond margin of lesion, then paint daily with salicylic acid dr. x in an ounce of collodion for a week, at the end of which time remove crust by prying off and apply for another week, and so on. John Edwin Hayes prescribes one dram of carbolic acid, two drams each of turpentine and tincture of iodine, and three drams of glycerine: Apply twice daily with a camel's hair brush to affected spots.

For Anemia in Children.—J. Lewis Smith prescribed, ℞ Ferri et ammon. acetat., ammon carb. aa gr. i; syrupi, aquæ anisis aa. dr. ss.: A teaspoonful after meals. Garrod gives ferrum reductum 1-12 to ½ grain; infants under a year can easily take two grains t. i. d. If there is constipation, add ½ to 2 grains of powdered licorice root. Sugar of milk is a good vehicle. For the anemia of young girls at puberty Robinson uses Vallet's pil, ferri. carb., one after meals.

Anemia of Children.—Jacobi's method of treatment comprises the following: Outdoor exercise; strychnine or beef with milk (never milk alone); syrup of iodide of iron, ten drops t. i. d. for a child of two years; ferri subcarb. gr. iv—viii, bismuth subcarb. gr. xii-xxiv and sodium bicarb. gr. xvi-xxx for a 2-year-old with gastric irritation; Fowler's solution, one or two drops after meals in chronic cases with torpid stomach; strychnine sulphate a useful adjuvant to arsenic and iron.

Septic Metritis.—A. F. A. King advises thorough antiseptic cleansing of uterine cavity by irrigation and curettage, first cleansing vulva and vagina thoroughly; cold compresses or ice-bags over uterus just above pubes; in diphtheritic cases cauterize diseased patches with silver nitrate or zinc chloride; general treatment by food and stimulants; early hysterectomy when muscular walls infiltrated with pus.

Puerperal Pseudo-Rheumatism.—This joint complication is of gonorrheal origin and the arthritis may last from one to six months uninfluenced by salicylates. In the way of treatment Peroguin advises rest of joint by plaster of paris bandage, with early passive movements in plastic form; puncture and subsequent injections of weak antiseptic solutions for serous and purulent varieties; also local treatment of gonorrhea in the genital tract.

Treatment of Pelvic Peritonitis.—Hirst advises expectant treatment at first—counter-irritation and poultices over lower abdomen, thorough drainage of bowel by strong purgatives, and copious hot vaginal douches. If the symptoms persist much beyond 8 hours in their original intensity, suppuration is probable —the abdomen should be opened and any abscesses evacuated, cleansed, disinfected and drained; distended tubes and ovaries must be removed and hysterectomy may be necessary.

Treatment of General Peritonitis.—Garrigues gives ⅛ to ¼ gr. of morphine every half hour till respiration is reduced to 12 per minute, at which point the breathing is kept for days or weeks if necessary by regulating doses and intervals; if the heart is depressed he adds atropine. He also recommends stimulants and fluid diet and enemas of glycerin or castor oil or turpentine for hympanites. Hirst states that the only possible chance in general diffus suppurative peritonitis is the earliest possible performance of abdominal section, with free irrigation of abdominal cavity.

For Proctitis.—Gant advises removal of source of irritation, and a soothing, easily digested diet. Clear bowels of scybala by injections, Epsom salts, Seidlitz powders and mineral waters. Absolute rest in bed is indicated. In mild cases apply cold to the hips and anus or inject cold water into the rectum. Frequent injections of alum, zinc, silver, lead or sublimate are useful in long standing cases; very hot water for gonorrhœa; lime water or salt water for thread-worms.

Onychia.—Inflammation of the nail bed is usually syphilitic in origin. Syphilitic onychia is best treated *(Gould and Pyle's Cyclopedia)* with black or yellow wash, a weak solution of corrosive sublimate, calomel powder or ointment and internal antisyhpilitic remedies. Non-luetic onychia may be treated with finely powdered lead nitrate, or daily painting with silver nitrate (ten grain per ounce of water). Removal of the nail, cauterization of matrix and dressing with iodoform gauze, are required in malignant cases, along with tonics and nourishing diet.

Eczema of Scalp.—In addition to constitutional treatment, Robinson recommends to wash head well with a shampooing liquid and free from crusts, scabs and secretions. Then cut hair short and apply an ointment of one-half dram each of white precipitate and dilute nitrate of mercury ointments, one dram each of lapis calaminari and palm oil, two drams of oil of bitter almond, and one ounce of vaselin.

Treatment of Favus.—Clip the hair short, says Hardaway. Soak parts in oil, or poultice and then wash with soap and hot water to remove crusts. Then epilate hairs with epilation forceps from a small area each time and apply mercuric chloride, two to four grains to the ounce of alcohol. Prevent dissemination of disease by treating the whole scalp with a saturated solution of boric acid. For epidemic favus painting with tincture of iodine or weak mercuric chloride solution in collodion is usually effective.

Pernicious Anemia.—Osler prescribes Fowler's solution in increasing doses, beginning with 3 minims t. i. d.; increasing to 5 minims at end of first week, to ten minims at end of second, to 15 at end of third week, and if necessary up to 20 or 25 minims. Arsenic is sometimes better borne as arsenious acid in pill form. Rest in bed with massage and a light, nutritious diet in small quantities at fixed intervals, should be enforced. Grawitz gives calomel, salol and other intestinal antiseptics for pernicious anemia with indicanuria.

Treatment of Chlorosis.—Osler relies on iron in the form of Blaud's pill (each containing two grains of sulphate of iron), giving one t. i. d. during first week, two in second, three pills in third week t. i. d. He continues this dose for four or five weeks at least before reducing, and persists in the use of the drug for at least three months, resuming subsequently, in smaller doses if necessary for recurrence. Good, easily digested food is indicated; alkalies to relieve dyspeptic symptoms; and a saline purge each morning if constipation is present.

Dr. Shrady Retires.—After the exceptionally long period of 38 years of continuous editorial management of the *Medical Record,* Dr. Geo. F. Shrady retires to a well-earned rest, with the best wishes of the medical profession of America. Dr. Thomas L. Stedman, for twenty years associate editor of the *Record,* becomes editor-in-chief.

The Los Angeles Journal of Eclectic Medicine.—We are in receipt of the first number of this journal, published under the auspices of the Southern California Eclectic Medical Association, and edited by O. C. Welbourn, M. D. This number has a prepossessing appearance and has for a frontispiece a. photogravure of a cottage covered with roses.

For General Hyperidrosis.—Louis Heitzmann advises iron, strychnine, arsenic, cinchona or mineral acids and a regular mode of living in all cases of long standing. Bromides may have a good effect in nervous individuals. Atropine, 1-120 to 1-50 grain one to three times daily, is a good remedy. A dusting powder of 30 to 50 grains of salicylic acid and one ounce each of zinc oxide and venetian talc, may be dusted on freely every few hours.

Bacteria in the Dead Body.—The common occurrence of streptococci and colon bacilli in the heart's blood, by migration from the lungs or intestines during the agonal or post-mortem period nearly invalidates any diagnostic deductions that might be made from their presence. R. B. H. Gradwohl *(Medical Fortnightly)* points out that the blood of the median basilic vein after death gives negative findings, unless there is a history of general sepsis before death, and in these cases the bacteria from the arm correspond with those at the site of infection.

Removal of Sebaceous Cysts.—If on the face and the orifice is discernible *(American Text-Book of Surgery),* dilate with a small probe and press out contents, repeating procedure from time to time. The best treatment generally is transfixion of the cyst and overlying integument with a curved bistoury, pressing out contents and then grasping edges of cyst wall with two pairs of forceps, twisting and pulling out each half. Careful dissection is required if the wen is too adherent for removal in this way.

Heat as an Analgesic.—Kellogg *(Modern Medicine)* praises the use of the hot sponge where fomentations fail. The sponge is dipped in very hot water, the excess of water squeezed out, and the sponge is gently rubbed over the surface of the painful part. A higher temperature can be employed in this way than in any other. Another very efficacious method is the use of the ordinary incandescent light, wrapped in a piece of flannel and applied to the painful part. The heat of the electric lamp is very penetrating.

"Under the Turquoise Sky."—This is the taking title of a handsome brochure of 78 pages, issued by the Chicago, Rock Island & Pacific railway, and to be had for the asking. It contains much graphic information about Colorado, its scenery, history, cities and resorts, natural resources and industries. It is very handsomely illustrated with many half-tone views, depicting the scenic splendor of this state. Prospective tourists should by all means procure this pamphlet from the general passenger agent of the C. R. I. & P. R. R., Mr. Chas. B. Sloat.

A Method for Preventing the Pain Following Clamp and Cautery Operations for Hemorrhoids.—Howard Lilienthal *(Medical Record,* August 27) prevents edema and consequent pain after the operation by making six or seven radiating incisions through the skin, well into the subcutaneous tissue, by means of scissors. The rather smart bleeding is easily checked by a little pressure and a dry dressing. In six hours a wet dressing may be applied. There is a free flow of serum from these incisions for the next day or two.

Treatment of Intestinal Autointoxication. — Professor Combe, of Lausanne (quoted in *Medical Record),* recommends a farinaceous diet in numerous small meals without drinks; lying down for an hour after meals on back or right side, and getting rid of products of putrefaction in intestines by means of thorough colon irrigation and a disinfectant dose of calomel (5 to 22 grains), given twice at intervals of two hours, and followed by castor oil. This should be repeated in ten days, and afterward at longer intervals.

For Anemia.—Diet and hygiene are of prime importance, says Potter. Nourishing, digestible food should be given in as large quantities as can be assimilated—at first milk, eggs, animal broths—afterward fish, poultry, game, mutton, etc. Moderate daily outdoor exercise is indispensable. Bathing, particularly sea bathing, aids the restoration of breath. Red wines are often useful. When headache is produced by ordinary tonics, Fothergill gives thrice daily an ounce of infusion of quassia containing 5 or 10 grains of potassium bromide and 5 grains of iron and potassium.

Thinning of Hair From Nervous Depression.—Van Harlingen advises regular daily to weekly shampooing of scalp with soap spirit, followed by inunctions with dropper and soft tooth brush of a mixture of 15 grains carbolic acid, 2 drams glycerine and 1 ounce cologne water. Cold water douches, friction, frequent brushing and stimulating washes are also useful. J. J. Pringle states that the galvanic or faradic brush is of service in cases where the neurotic origin is obvious and where anesthesia or other nerve disturbance is present.

Removal of Superfluous Hair.—One of the best depilatories, as suggested by Duhring *(Journal of American Medical Association)*, consists of from two to four drams of barium sulphide, with enough starch and zinc oxide to make an ounce. The sulphide should be mild and freshly made, and kept tightly corked. At the time of the application sufficient water is added to make a paste, which is spread thickly over the part and allowed to remain one or two minutes, then scraped off, and soothing ointment or dusting powder is applied. The application is repeated every week or two, or as soon as the hair has reappeared.

Treatment of Scrofula.—Thompson's may be summarized as follows: Fresh air, warm clothing, baths, nitrogenous food, cod-liver oil, one or two drams an hour after meals—suspend

Editorial Items continued on Page 216

BOOKS.

THE DOCTOR'S RED LAMP.—A Book of Short Stories Concerning the Doctor's Daily Life. Selected by Charles Wells Moulton. The Saalfeld Publishing Co., Chicago, Akron, O., New York.

This is the second volume in the "Doctor's Recreation Series." Many of the stories are by standard authors, some are old favorites, and all relate episodes that will appeal to the practitioner's recollections. They are stories that will interest the doctor, the doctor's wife and children, and likewise the patients in the waiting-room. The book is illustrated with a number of fine art reproductions. The associate editors of this series are Nicholas Senn, Wm. Henry Drummond, John C. Hemmeter, Wm. Warren Potter, Titus Munson Coan, Emory Lanphear, Albert Van Der Veer, Winslow Anderson, W. J. Bell and Henry W. Roby.

TWENTY-SEVENTH ANNUAL REPORT of the Board of Health of the State of New Jersey and Report of the Bureau of Vital Statistics. 1903.

A TEXT-BOOK OF DISEASES OF WOMEN.—By Chas. B. Penrose, M. D., Ph. D., formerly Professor of Gynecology in the University of Pennsylvania; Surgeon to the Gynecean Hospital, Philadelphia. With 225 illustrations. Fifth Edition, Revised. Philadelphia, New York, London: W. B. Saunders & Co. 1904. Price, $3.75 net.

Dr. Penrose's work is worthy of its exceptional popularity. Though not dogmatic, he is clearly certain of his convictions, and in general recommends in each case but one rule of action. The trend of the text throughout is direct and practical. The illustrations are not ornate, but are in keeping with the text, being instructive and readily understood. The present edition contains much new matter, bringing the work right down to date. We consider Penrose particularly suited for the use of medical students.

THE THEORY AND PRACTICE OF INFANT FEEDING.—With notes on Development. By Henry Dwight Chapin, A. M., M. D., Professor of Diseases of Children at the New York Post-Graduate Medical School and Hospital. Second Edition, Revised, With Numerous Illustrations. New York: William Wood & Co. 1904.

This is a good and useful book. The titular subject is considered in four parts: "Underlying Principles of Nutrition," "Raw Food," "Practical Feeding," and "Growth and Development of Infants." The author shows a thorough first-hand knowledge of the subject, which he presents in clear and simple, but forcible language. There is no physician who has to do with babies but would be benefited by a careful perusal of this volume. The text is illustrated with 109 figures, many of which are photogravures.

A TEXT-BOOK OF PATHOLOGY.—By J. McFarland, M. D., Professor of Pathology and Bacteriology in the Medico-Chirurgical Hospital, Philadelphia. Handsome Octavo Volume of 818 Pages, With 350 Illustrations, a Number in Colors. Philadelphia, New York, London: W. B. Saunders & Co. 1904. Cloth, $5.00 Net; Sheep or Half Morocco, $6.00 Net.

The author of this work has taught the subject of pathology for thirteen years, and is the author of a well-known manual on the pathogenic bacteria. The forelying book, like other of his writings, is characterized by clearness and thoroughness. The work is, therefore, especially suited to the needs of students. The text is admirably illustrated with black and white and colored reproductions from the microscope and the clinic. Both general and special pathology are fully covered, and the information given is in accord with the latest researches. To acquire the principles of pathology, on which the scientific practice of medicine is founded, we know of no better work than this of McFarland.

PRACTICAL APPLICATION OF RŒNTGEN RAYS IN THERAPEUTICS AND DIAGNOSIS.—By Wm. A. Pusey, A. M., M. D., Professor of Dermatology in the University of Illinois, and Eugene W. Caldwell, B. S., Director of the Edward N. Gibbs Memorial X-Ray Laboratory of the University and Bellevue Hospital Medical College, New York. The Second Edition Thoroughly Revised and Enlarged. Handsome Octavo Volume of 690 Pages, with 195 Illustrations, Including Four Colored Plates. Philadelphia, New York, London: W. B. Saunders & Co. 1904. Cloth, $5.00 Net; Sheep or Half Morocco, $6.00 Net.

The interest of the medical profession in the subject of this excellent work is shown by the demand for a second edition within a year. The authors have treated their topics in the most practical way, paying almost no attention to points of theoretic controversial interest. The value of the x-ray method in diagnosis is firmly established. The therapeutic uses and limitations are clearly defined in this volume. The most modern technique for examination and treatment is described in explicit detail. Many clinical cases are summarized and very satisfactorily illustrated. Nearly all the voluminous literature of 1903 on the subject of radio-therapy is included in a condensed form in the present volume. Concerning the local and internal therapeutic application of radio-active water, Pusey states that "this idea can only be ranked at present as a bizarre suggestion."

SERUMS, VACCINES AND TOXINES IN TREATMENT AND DIAGNOSIS.—By Wm. Cecil Bosanquet, M. D., Oxon., F. R. C. P., London; Physician to Out-Patients, Victoria Hospital for Children. Chicago: W. T. Keener & Co. 1904. 12mo; Limp Cloth. Price, $2.00.

This is a book that is needed, dealing as it does chiefly with the clinical side of the subject, the importance of which can hardly be overestimated. The author's statements are clear and concise, and are founded in the main on original authorities. If he seems somewhat dogmatic at times in his conclusions as to the value of orotherapy, he is justified in pleading that for practical purposes definite assertions are necessary. It behooves physicians to keep in the current of modern thought, and such a book as this is bound to help them greatly.

CLINICAL UROLOGY.—By Alfred C. Croftan, Professor of Medicine, Chicago Post-Graduate Medical College and Hospital; Physician in Chief to St. Luke's Hospital. Illustrated. New York: Wm. Wood & Co. 1904.

Croftan is always instructive and interesting as a writer. The title of the present volume is well chosen, being chiefly devoted to the pathology of metabolism from the standpoint of urinary analysis. The author himself has done considerable original work, particularly on the purin bodies. The methods he recommends are generally practicable. The text is suitably illustrated with pictures of urinary sediments, etc. Practitioners will find this an excellent work for ready reference as well as for systematic study.

THE STUDENT'S HAND-BOOK OF SURGICAL OPERATIONS.—By Sir Frederick Treves, Bart., K. C. V. O., C. B., LL. D., F. R. C. S., Sergeant Surgeon in Ordinary to H. M. the

King; Surgeon in Ordinary to H. R. H. the Prince of Wales; Consulting Surgeon to the London Hospital. New Edition, Revised by the Author and Jonathan Hutchinson, Jun. F. R. C. S. 12mo; 486 Pages; 121 Illustrations. Price, $2.50. Chicago: W. T. Keener & Co. 1904.

This is a convenient compendium of operative surgery by a thorough master of the subject. The book is abridged from the author's "Manual of Operative Surgery," and is to be commended for its systematic style. The illustrations are excellent. The thin paper and limp cover permit the volume to be carried readily in the pocket.

A Physician's Practical Gynecology.—By W. O. Henry, M. D., Omaha, Neb. Professor of Gynecology in the Creighton Medical College. With Five Full Page Illustrations and 61 Illustrations in the Text. Lincoln, Neb.: The Review Press.

This little volume is designed as a practical guide to medical students and general practitioners. The diagnosis and treatment of the commoner pathologic conditions are succinctly described, much as they would be in a clinical lecture. The author's statements and directions are quite reliable, and can be confidently followed. The book is well printed and handsomely illustrated.

A Hand-Book of Pathological Anatomy and Histology.— With an introductory section on Post-Mortem Examinations and the methods of Preserving and Examining Diseased Tissues. By Francis Delafield, M. D., LL. D., Emeritus Professor of the Practice of Medicine, College of Physicians and Surgeons, Columbia University, New York; and T. Mitchell Prudden, M. D., LL. D., Professor of Pathology and Director of the Department of Pathology, College of Physicians and Surgeons, Columbia University, New York. Seventh Edition. With 13 Full-Page Plates and 545 Illustrations in the Text in Black and Colors. New York: Wm. Wood & Co. 1904.

This elegant volume requires no introduction to our readers, since it has long been the accepted standard in many medical colleges. The present edition has been revised by Prof. Prudden, aided by a number of collaborators, each eminent in a special field. The endeavor has been in the present volume, when it would not conflict with the more practical aims of the work, to consider disease as an adaptive process, and to view pathology as one aspect of the diverse manifestations of life and of energy,

rather than as belonging to a special and exclusively human domain. The more recent phases of pathology, such as immunity
and Ehrlich's side-chain theory, are considered at length. The
rich collection of high grade illustrations are in keeping with the
scientific character of the text. In its latest form this work as
a whole is unexcelled.

LEA'S SERIES OF MEDICAL EPITOMES.—Magee and Johnson's
Epitome of Surgery. A Manual for Students and Practitioners. By M. D'Arcy Magee, A. M., M. D., Demonstrator of Surgery and Lecturer on Minor Surgery; and
Wallace Johnson, Ph. D., M. D., Demonstrator of Pathology and Bacteriology in Georgetown University Medical
School, Washington, D. C. In one 12mo volume of 295
pages, with 129 engravings. Cloth, $1.00, Net. Lea Broth-
ers & Co., Publishers, Philadelphia and New York. 1904.

There is a great deal of information in this compact volume,
which is quite fully illustrated, considering its moderate price.
Leading points are brought to the notice of the student by means
of heavy type. The questions are put at the end of each chapter,
where they belong.

SELECTIONS.

AMENORRHEA.—Celerine and aletris cordial rio, equal parts, teaspoonful every four hours, is a most efficient remedy for amenorrhœa.

COMMENT ON ANTIKAMNIA AND HEROIN TABLETS.—Under the head of "Therapeutics," the *Medical Examiner* contains the following by Walter M. Fleming, A. M., M. D., regarding this valuable combination: "Its effect on the respiratory organs is not at all depressing, but primarily it is stimulating, which is promptly followed by a quietude which is invigorating and bracing, instead of depressing and followed by lassitude. It is not inclined to affect the bowels by producing constipation, which is one of the prominent effects of an opiate, and it is without the unpleasant sequels which characterize the use of morphine. When there is a persistent cough, a constant 'hacking,' a 'tickling' or irritable membrane, accompanied with dyspnœa and a tenacious mucus, the treatment indicated has no superior. In my experience I found one 'Antikamnia & Heroin Tablet' every two or three hours, for an adult, to be the most desirable average dose. For night-coughs, superficial or deep-seated, one tablet on retiring, if allowed to dissolve in the mouth, will relieve promptly, and insure a good night's rest."

AN ACTIVE DEPLETANT FOR PELVIC CONGESTIONS.—The presence of congestion or inflammation, whether acute or chronic, involving the female pelvic cavity, forms grounds for anxiety. Glyco-Thymoline in contact with mucous membrane everywhere produces the following physiological activities in direct proportion to the vascularity of the structure. On the law of exosmosis, which determines the passage of fluids through animal membranes from a rare to a more dense saline medium, this solution through its stimulating and hygroscopic property brings about a rapid depletion, drawing outwardly through the tissues the products of inflammation and materially reducing the danger of septic infection. The following clinical cases bear with interest on the subject: Chas. Le Cates, M. D., Philadelphia, Pa., records: Mrs. A., consulted me in reference to her condition. Made a thorough examination and found uterus much enlarged, very turgid, degeneration of the endometrium, discharge rather profuse. Treatment—Hot vaginal douche, 10 per cent. Glyco-Thymoline. I then irrigated the uterus with pure Glyco-Thymoline and tamponed the vagina with lamb's wool saturated with Glyco-Thymoline. This treatment was given twice and three times a week. Improvement was rapid, congestion was reduced and patient discharged in six weeks.

McKesson & Robbins.—Gentlemen: I think it a duty to express to you my commendation of a dental preparation which you are offering the public under the name of Calox. Theoretically and practically it answers all the requirements of a perfect dentifrice, the first named quality appealing to me at once as sound in precept, the latter confirmed by personal use.

A Calmative and Nerve Tonic.—For nervous irritability, and insomnia accompanying the menopause, Daniel's Conct. Tinct. Passiflora Incarnata should be administered in teaspoonful doses every hour, gradually lengthening the intervals as the nervousness is controlled. Its action is especially gratifying with neurasthenic patients. It relieves neuralgia and gives results where other calmatives are powerless. Several cases recently reported of hysteria and sleeplessness in patients of all ages, due to dissipation, overwork, and other causes, indicate that the practitioners are obtaining splendid cures from Passiflora, and dwell with emphasis on the fact that no bad after-effects are encountered. Passiflora gives quietude and refreshing sleep, and may be employed with assurance in all affections of the nervous system.

Intestinal Parasites With Illustrations.—Battle & Co. will send these illustrations free of charge to physicians upon application.

EDITORIAL ITEMS.— Continued.

once a month for ten days and in very hot weather—a peppermint lozenge takes away bad taste; potassium iodide for glandular hyperplasia, syrup of iodide of iron a useful tonic for young children, m. x-xxx two or three times a day; calcium sulphide; hypophosphites of calcium and sodium with oil when bones or joints implicated; hypophosphites with sodium bicarbonate for glandular enlargement; extirpation of glands if unsightly or painful.

Fruit Tablets for Constipation of Young Children.—The following tablets, says Chapin, are agreeable and efficient. Take four ounces each of raisins, figs and dates and two ounces of ground senna leaves; remove the seeds from the raisins and dates, and finely chop the fruit; then mix on a table, adding the senna to the chopped fruit little by little, putting in sherry enough to make a paste; roll into a mass half an inch thick and cut into half-inch squares; place the tablets between sheets of paraffine paper in a box. One or two of these tablets may be given at night and repeated in the morning if necessary to get the result.

For Cholera Nostras.—Dawson Williams directs to withdraw all solid food and milk, allowing only iced barley water, iced veal broth or chicken broth and iced water. Apply a mustard poultice or hot stupe to the abdomen. If there is much pain, give fifteen minims of laudanum with one dram of compound tincture of camphor or ten grains of bismuth subnitrate. Castor oil is an efficient remedy in the early stage. Check prolonged diarrhœa by astringents. Old, feeble and very young patients often need free stimulation with brandy or champagne.

Surgical Treatment of Tetanus.—In the *Journal of the American Medical Association* of August 13th John B. Murphy reports a case of tetanus in a boy successfully treated by repeated aspiration of the cerebro-spinal fluid and injection of morphine, eucaine and salt solution. About 15 cc. of the cerebro-spinal fluid was withdrawn each time after spinal puncture and 3 or 4 cc. of sterilized physiologic saline solution of morphine (1-75 gr.) and b. (3-50 gr.) injected. He prefers eucaine to cocaine because the former admits of boiling for sterilization and there is less idiosyncrasy to intoxication.

Dextrinized Gruels.—In summer diarrhœa and other forms of putrefactive autointoxication, Chapin directs to use gruels prepared as follows: Beat up one or two heaping tablespoonfuls of barley, wheat or rice flour with enough cold water to make a thin paste; or use two to four heaping tablespoonfuls of rolled oats. Pour on a quart of boiling water and boil for at least fifteen minutes, preferably in a covered double boiler, as the gruel will not then burn. If the mixture is to be dextrinized after it is cooked, place the cooker in cold water, and when the gruel is cool enough to be tasted add one teaspoonful of diastase solution or cereo, and stir. This will thin the gruel. Strain, add salt to taste and cool.

Bromidrosis.—For offensive perspiration on soles or in axillæ, John W. Taylor directs to wash the parts involved twice daily with a solution of five grains of potassium permanganate and ten grains of borax in one-half gallon of water. Unna recommends a 25 to 50 per cent. ointment of formalin in lanolin, applied once or twice daily. Fox employs antiseptic solutions (after washing with alum solution and drying), such as one per cent. potassium permanganate or chloral; allowing to dry spontaneously; boric acid in socks, and dusting powder of five parts of salicylic acid and 45 parts of starch.

A Non-Toxic Preparation of Iodine.—To obviate stomachic disturbances V. H. W. Windgrave (quoted in *Medicine*) uses the following formula: Iodine, 2.5 gm.; tannic acid, 4 gm.; alcohol, 38 cc.; syrup to make 75 cc. The iodine is dissolved in the alcohol; the tannic acid and 30 cc. of syrup are added. The solution is heated to just below the boiling point until it gives no evidence of iodine with the starch reaction. This requires about twenty minutes. It is then cooled and the remainder of the syrup is added with flavorings. Each dram contains two grains of iodine. This combination is especially useful in children with chronic lympadenitis or enlarged tonsils.

Treatment of Sycosis.—Stelwagon says: Remove crusts with warm embrocations. If parts are tender and painful, use bland oils, cold cream, zinc oxide ointment or boric acid lotion, 15 grains per ounce. Most cases demand from the start such astringent stimulating remedies as diachylon ointment (ten to thirty grains of calomel may be added to each ounce), a five to twenty per cent. ointment of oleate of mercury, precipitated sulphur one to three drams to the ounce of benzoated lard, or ten to twenty-five per cent, ichthyol ointment. It is usually necessary to change from one application to another. Shaving is advisable when bearable (taking the place of epilation), to be continued for some months.

Chromidrosis.—In this affection we see localized colored excessive sweating, with micrococcus tetragenus infection (red) or pigmentation. There may be a fine brick-dust deposit on the skin in uricacidemia, a green deposit in copper workers, a blue sediment from indican or ferrous sulphate; pink from potassium iodide; red from leptothrix or bacterium prodigiosum; black or sepia-colored in mental disease. The colored deposit can be removed with chloroform or ether. Aside from this, Heitzmann directs to improve the general condition and remove any underlying cause, especially anemia, chlorosis, hysteria and menstrual and uterine disorders.

Bacteriuria.—Keyes *(New York Medical Journal,* Aug. 27) sums up an article on this subject as follows: Baceriuria is certainly not "a simple urinary infection without parietal lesion." The theory that bacteriuria is but a symptom of catarrh in certain parts of the urinary tract is, on the other hand, fully in accord with the observed facts. Thus bacterinria is a symptom, not a disease. Yet it is the chief, the only striking, feature of certain diseases, notably certain varieties of catarrhal pyelitis. Any of these may become suppurative. It would further appear that cystitis never causes bacteriuria. Prostatitis and spermatocystitis, exceptionally, cause bacteriuria.

Treatment of Rachitis.—Goodhart and Starr advise good fresh air and outdoor exercise; good milk, gravy, custard pudding, broccoli or cauliflower for twelve months and upward—underdone pounded meat with well-cooked cauliflower and gravy when eighteen months or more; reduced amount of milk, or substitution of cream and whey or fresh beef juice, when digestion much disordered; cod-liver oil, twenty drops to one dram t. i. d.; syrup of lactophosphate of calcium and iron in one-half to one dram dose well diluted; a teaspoonful of malt extract twice a

The bone-forming and nerve-strengthening hypophosphites in Scott's Emulsion make it especially useful for young children. Scott's Emulsion contains nothing that children should not have and everything that they should.

SCOTT & BOWNE, Chemists, 409 Pearl St., New York.

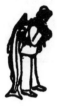

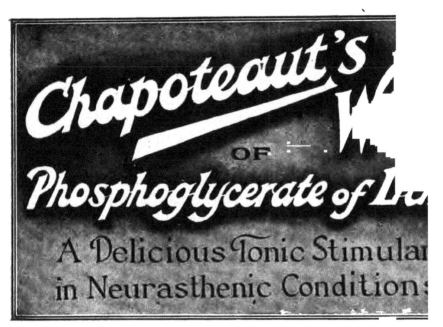

Chapoteaut's

OF

Phosphoglycerate of L

A Delicious Tonic Stimular
in Neurasthenic Condition:

Agents: E. Fouge

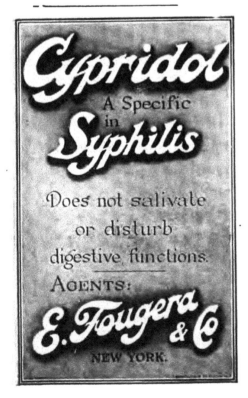

Cypridol

A Specific
in

Syphilis

Does not salivate
or disturb
digestive functions.

AGENTS:

E. Fougera & Co

NEW YORK.

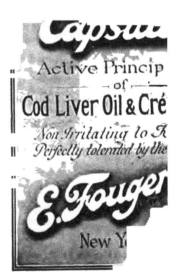

Capsu

Active Princip
of

Cod Liver Oil & Cré

Non Irritating to R
Perfectly tolerated by the

E. Fouger

New Yo

day; orange or lemon juice well sweetened whenever a scorbutic tendency. Treat convulsions, diarrhœa and bronchitis on general principles.

Dermatitis or Eczema Seborrhoicum.—This disease of the scalp appears in sharply limited (red border), somewhat elevated and scaly patches. It shows a watery exudation when scratched, and greasy, yellowish scales or crusts. There is considerable itching. The disease spreads downward from the scalp, and tends to be chronic. By way of treatment Bulkley states that six per cent. of resorcin in zinc ointment or in solution with a little alcohol and glycerine, often clears off a well-defined eruption in a very few days, and is particularly applicable for the scalp. Wet the surface thoroughly morning and night with the solution and a large medicine dropper.

Puerperal Endometritis.—The method of treatment advised by J. Whitridge Williams may be outlined as follows: Remove lochia for cultures, explore interior of uterus with sterile finger, and curet or not according to conditions. Douche with several litres of boiled water or sterilized salt solution and pack with gauze. If infection is streptococcic, desist at once from further local treatment. In putrid endometritis other injections may be used. If infection has extended beyond uterus, local treatment should not be persisted in. Strychnine and large quantities of alcohol should be given by way of general tonic treatment. If fever is high, abate with cold sponging or bathing. If process has extended beyond uterus (paramerritis or pelvic peritonitis), apply hot poultices or fomentations to lower abdomen.

Capillary Leptothrix.—In this condition, due to excessive sweating in the axillæ or groins or on the scrotum, the hairs are rough, with an uneven steamed look, and showing adherent concretions (sometimes red) of micro-organisms. Remove concretions, says Jackson, with soap and water, and prevent return by use of mild antiparasitic lotions and dusting powders, after use of soap and water. In the so-called piedra there are dark, stony, rattling nodules on the hair shafts, from fungi or hair dressing, and likewise removable with hot water. In the probably parasitic trichorrexis nodosa the hair shafts are beaded with oval, light gray, transparent nodules. For this condition Jackson states that continued shaving probably offers the best hopes of any plan.

Baldness Due to Favus.—In this form of alopecia the hair is dry and brittle and cupped with sulphury saucer-like crusts, containing the microscopic fungus. The disease may leave whitish, irregular scars. By way of treatment Stelwagon directs to remove the crusts with oily applications and soap and water, and keep hair closely cut in parts affected; depilation is usually necessary to cure. Apply thoroughly twice daily a parasiticide ointment or lotion, such as mercuric chloride 1 to 4 grains per ounce of alcohol and water, carbolic acid 1 part to 3 or more parts of glycerine, 10 per cent. oleate of mercury, or 2 parts of precipitated sulphur and 1 part each of green soap and oil of cade and 4 parts of lard.

Night Sweats of Phthisis.—Knopf recommends a glass of cold milk with a little cognac before retiring; also to eat something or take an eggnog in the night if feeling faint. Wake up two hours before given hour of perspiration, and take nourishment. Sponge with water and vinegar or lemon juice. Make a compress of several thicknesses of rather coarse linen, folded in the form of a shawl (or, better, three different cloths—a narrow one for each apex and a wider one to wrap around the chest), soak in water at 55° F., wring out and apply over apices and around thorax, cover with thick flannel band, fasten in place and leave on over night, rubbing chest and shoulders dry in the morning. An occasional sweat bath may be used for relatively strong patients who seem to improve under its use.

Treatment of Sapremia.—Playfair directs the practitioner to wash out the uterus carefully for one or two days at least twice daily, with not more than two quarts of 1 :2000 bichloride solution—may be alternated with 1 :50 carbolic acid or with iodine dropped into warm water until it has a pale sherry color. If there is a local slough or necrotic ulcer on vulva or vagina, scrape its surface freely and cover with iodoform. Curette very carefully when retention of a portion of placenta or membranes is suspected or when a highly offensive discharge indicates necrosed decidua—then swab cavity of uterus well with tincture of iodine. When the septic intoxication is due to lesions of the

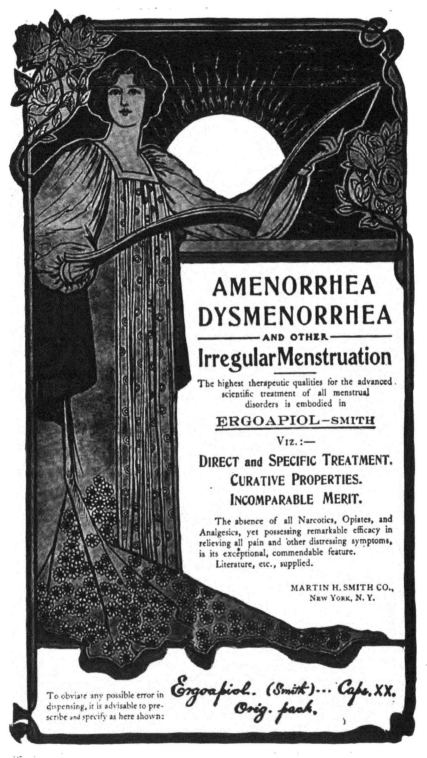

AMENORRHEA
DYSMENORRHEA
—AND OTHER—
Irregular Menstruation

The highest therapeutic qualities for the advanced scientific treatment of all menstrual disorders is embodied in

ERGOAPIOL—SMITH

Viz.:—

DIRECT and SPECIFIC TREATMENT.
CURATIVE PROPERTIES.
INCOMPARABLE MERIT.

The absence of all Narcotics, Opiates, and Analgesics, yet possessing remarkable efficacy in relieving all pain and other distressing symptoms, is its exceptional, commendable feature.
Literature, etc., supplied.

MARTIN H. SMITH CO.,
NEW YORK, N. Y.

To obviate any possible error in dispensing, it is advisable to prescribe and specify as here shown:

Ergoapiol. (Smith)... Caps. XX. Orig. pack.

vulva or vagina, Grandin cauterizes with silver nitrate 60 grs. to the ounce of distilled water, and sprinkles with iodoform, bismuth or aristol.

The Physiologic Action of Digitalis.—Sajous *(Monthly Cyclopedia of Practical Medicine,* August) compares the similar action on the heart and blood pressure of digitalis and suprarenal extract. He shows apparently that the effect of digitalis cannot be a direct one upon the heart, and cites evidence in proof of his assertion that digitalis increases the contractile energy of the heart and raises the general blood pressure by augmenting indirectly (through excitation of the pituitary body) the functional activity of the adrenals and thus raises the proportion of adrenal secretion supplied to the heart. In the light of his views, the so-called cumulative action of digitalis is not due to accumulation of this drug in the organism, but to the excessive stimulation of the vasomotor centers to which its injudicious use gives rise by over-exciting the functional activity of the adrenals. The excessive constriction of the cardiac arteries thus provoked becomes the source of the cardiac arrest.

For Secondary Anemias.—Osler recommends etiologic treatment and plenty of good food and fresh air in traumatic cases and for inanition. Toxic cases (lead and mercury) require elimination of the poison and nutritious diet with full doses of potassium iodide. Ringer advises the use of calcium phosphate in anemia of women from rapid child-bearing or excessive menstruation. Brower uses the chloride of gold and sodium, 1-20 grain t. i. d., increased to 1-10 grain t. i. d. for secondary anemias and chlorosis. Arsenic, iron and red bone marrow are recommended for the anemia of exophthalmic goitre. Calcium lactophosphate was prescribed by Bartholow for the anemia of nursing mothers and for anemia due to suppuration. Thompson uses cod-liver oil with small doses of arsenic in rheumatic anemia. For hydremic anemia Koplik praises the desiccated thyroid extract in combination with iron. T. Henry Jones gives ½ grain of gray powder with 2 grains of saccharated carbonate of iron morning and evening for the anemia of infantile syphilis.

Puerperal Venous Septicopyemia and Septicemia.—Ring's treatment may be summarized as follows: Vaginal antiseptic douches (2% creolin, 5% carbolic acid of 1:3000 bichloride solution; very gentle use of intrauterine antiseptic douche only when uterus is known to contain putrescent matter; avoid curette; iodoform suppositories containing 100 gr. iodoform and 10 gr. each gum arabic, glycerine and starch. In cases of hemorrhage introduce very carefully and gently a tampon of iodoform gauze. Give cardiac stimulants (whisky p. r. n., strychnine, digitalis, strophanthus) and nutritious liquid food (milk, beef tea, beef extract and other meat broths and animal juices every hour or two). Give an early laxative of castor oil or 5 to 10 grs. of calomel with double as much sodium bicarbonate. To reduce temperature give 5 grs. or more of quinine every two hours when temperature is above 101 degrees or phenacetin 5 grs. to a dose, vinegar, bay rum or alcohol. Use morphine to relieve pain —combine with 1-100 gr. atropine if much depression of heart. For metastatic abscesses give tincture of iron m. xx-xxx three or four times a day, and evacuate pus and drain antiseptically if accessible, as in joints.

Rocky Mountain Interstate Medical Association.—At the last meeting this association Doctors Kahn, Hawkins, Jackson, Baldwin and Fleming were appointed to consider the suggestions in President Niles' address and reported back to the association as follows:

"*Resolved,* That a committee of fifteen of re-organization be appointed by the retiring president with power to act, and this committee be empowered to invite the President and Secretary of the State Societies of California, Oregon, Nevada, Washington, Montana, Utah, Idaho, Arizona, Wyoming, Colorado and New Mexico to meet with the next conference at Portland, Oregon. This committee further recommends that the Board of Trustees of the Rocky Mountain Interstate Medical Association consult with the committee on reorganization regarding the time and place of the next meeting."

Report was adopted and President Niles and the retiring president appointed the following committee: S. C. Baldwin, Chairman; E. J. A. Rogers, Thos. H. Hawkins, C. K. Fleming, A. C. Ewing, Hubert Work, Donald Campbell, Leonard Freeman, Edw. Jackson, Sol G. Kahn, I. B. Perkins, J. N. Hall, Geo. P. Johnson, J. H. Bean, H. D. Niles.

LIFE IN KENTUCKY.

Man born in the widls of Kentucky is of feud days and easy virtue. He fisheth, fiddleth, cusseth and fighteth all the days of his life.

When he desireth to raise hell he planteth a neighbor, and lo, he reapeth twenty-fold.

He riseth even from the cradle to seek the scalp of his grand-sire's enemy and bringeth home in his carcass the ammunition of his neighbor's wife's cousin's uncle's father-in-law, who avengeth the deed.

Yes, verily, his life is uncertain and he knoweth not the hour when he may be jerked hence.

He goeth forth on a journey half-shot and cometh back on a shutter, shot.

He riseth in the night to let the cat out and it taketh nine doctors·three days to pick the buckshot from his person.

He goes forth in joy and gladness and cometh back in scraps and fragments.

He calleth his fellow-man a liar and getteth himself filled with scrap iron even to the fourth generation.

He emptieth a demijohn into himself and a shotgun into his enemy, and his enemy's son lieth in wait on election day, and lo, the coroner plougheth up a forty-acre field to bury that man.

Woe, woe is Kentucky, for her eyes are red with bad whisky and her soil is stained with the blood of damijits! Selah.—*Maysville (Ky.) Ledger.*

Denver and Gross College of Medic

Medical Department University of Denver

EDMUND J. A. ROGERS, A.M., M.D.,
Professor of Surgery.

THOMAS H. HAWKINS, A.M., M.D.,
Professor of Gynecology and Abdominal Surgery.

EDMUND C. RIVERS, A.M., M.D.,
Professor of Ophthalmology.

ROBERT LEVY, M.D., Secretary.
Professor of Laryngology, Rhinology and Otology.

HENRY SEWALL, PH.D., M.D.,
Professor of Physiology.

WILLIAM H. DAVIS, M.D.,
Professor of Dermatology and Venereal Diseases.

CHARLES B. LYMAN, M.D.,
Professor of Fractures and Dislocations.

WILLIAM J. ROTHWELL, M.D.,
Professor of Medicine.

JOHN M. FOSTER, M.D.,
Professor of Otology.

CAREY K. FLEMING, M.D.,
Professor of Gynecology and Abdominal Surgery.

FRANCIS H. McNAUGHT, M.D.,
Professor of Obstetrics.

LEONARD FREEMAN, B.S., A.M., MD.,
Professor of Surgery.

HORACE G. WETHERILL, M.D.,
Professor of Gynecology and Abdominal Surgery.

JOSIAH N. HALL, B.S., M.D.,
Professor of Medicine.

CHARLES A. POWERS, A.M., M.D.,
Professor of Surgery.

CHARLES F. SHOLLENBERGER, M.D.,
Professor of Pediatrics.

HOWELL T. PERSHING, M.Sc., M.D.,
Professor of Nervous and Mental Diseases.

EDWARD C. HILL, M.Sc., M. D.,
Professor of Chemistry and Toxicology.

HERBERT B. WHITNEY, A.B., M.D.,
Professor of Medicine.

HORACE G. HARVEY, A.B., M.D.,
Professor of Fractures and Dislocations.

SHERMAN G. BONNEY, A.M., M.D., Dean,
Professor of Medicine.

MOSES KLEINER, M.D.,
Professor of Therapeutics.

GEORGE B. PACKARD, M.D.,
Professor of Orthopedic Surgery.

T. MITCHELL BURNS, M.D.,
Professor of Obstetrics.

WALTER A. JAYNE, M.D.,
Professor of Gynecology and Abdominal S

CHARLES B. VAN ZANT, M.D.,
Professor of Physiology.

CARROLL E. EDSON, A.M., M.D.,
Professor of Therapeutics.

MELVILLE BLACK, M.D.,
Professor of Ophthalmology.

JAMES M. BLAINE, M.D.,
Professor of Dermatology and Venereal D

WILLIAM C. MITCHELL, M.D.,
Professor of Bacteriology.

DAVID H. COOVER, M.D.,
Professor of Ophthalmology.

SAMUEL B. CHILDS, A.M., M.D.,
Professor of Anatomy.

JAMES H. PERSHING, A.B.,
Professor of Medical Jurisprudence.

JOHN A. WILDER, M.D.,
Professor of Pathology.

SAMUEL D. HOPKINS, M.D.,
Professor of Nervous and Mental Diseases.

PHILIP HILLKOWITZ, B.S., M.D.,
Professor of Pathology.

WILLIAM C. BANE, M.D.,
Professor of Ophthalmology and Otology.

Four years' graded course. Sessions of eight months each. 23d Annual Sessions begins September 15, 1903. Matriculation fee, $5.00. Tuition fee, $100.00. Well-equipped laboratories in all departments and excellent clinical advantages in dispensary and hospitals.

The climate of **COLORADO** offers many advantages to students whose health compels them to leave the east

Catalogue on application.

Sherman G. Bonney, A.M., M.D., Dean

DENVER MEDICAL TIMES

| Volume XXIV. | NOVEMBER, 1904 | Number 5. |

ECTOPIC PREGNANCY, WITH REPORT OF A CASE OF REPEATED TUBAL GESTATION.*

By A. W. KERR, M. D.

Member of American Medical Association; member Western Surgical and Gynecological Society; member Rocky Mountain Interstate Medical Society; member Utah State and Salt Lake County Medical Societies; Gynecologist to St. Mark's Hospital.

Salt Lake City, Utah.

Ectopic Pregnancy occurs when for any reason the product of conception is arrested in its progress to its normal habitat, the uterus.

The different forms as usually described include tubal (which may be interstitial, isthmial or ampullal), ovarian and abdominal. Secondary forms include tuba-abdominal, tuba-ovarian and broad ligament pregnancy.

Prior to 1883 ectopic pregnancy was of interest only from a pathological standpoint. Lawson Tait operated the first case about that time, and did much to elucidate the subject. Before 1876 extra-uterine pregnancy was considered very rare, but with the gradual development of abdominal surgery its relative frequency became more recognized. Noble found it in from 3% to 4% of all his laparotomies.

Aetiology: Definite and positive statements concerning the exact cause of this condition are difficult to make. Among the causes usually given are: Congenital deviations from normal type (of Fallopian tubes) *e. g.*, exaggerated convolutions, diverticula and atresias, sagging and attachments by adhesions, resulting in distorting of the tubes; pressure from adjoining organs; thickening of the tubal walls, either congenital or acquired; diminishing peristalsis; desquamative salpingitis or hyperplasia destroying the cilia or causing atresia; growths either in the canal or the walls, and obscure conditions preventing coaptation of the fimbriae with the ovum or ovary. M. Herzog has demonstrated tubal pregnancy occurring in a diverticula of a tube.

*Read before the Rocky Mountain Inter-State Medical Association. Sept., 1904.

Duhrssen believes that occasionally the arrest of the ovum may be due to puerperal atrophy of the tube, impairing its normal peristalsis.

Williams states that in a considerable number of cases he examined, the corpus luteum was situated, not in the ovary corresponding to the pregnant tube, but in the opposite one.

Mandle, Schmidt, Kustner and others elicited a history of gonorrhoeal salpingitis, or inflammatory conditions in over two-thirds of their cases.

Webster is of the opinion that the explanation for the comparative infrequent occurrence of ectopic gestation is that the decidual reaction, which he considers essential to the proper implantation of the fertilized ovum, readily occurs in the uterus, but is usually lacking in the tubes. He maintains that tubal pregnancy can come about only when the tubes are capable of this reaction. He considers such an occurrence probably represents a reversion to an earlier type and may be looked upon as a sign of degeneracy.

The experimental work on lower animals, done by Tainturer, Mandle and Schmidt seems to confirm the Webster theory. An artificial obstruction was produced in the generative tracts of rabbits by applying ligatures to one or both sides, at a certain period of time after copulation. When these were placed about the middle of the cornua, ova were arrested above them and went on to development, but when the uterine ends of the tubes themselves were ligated, extra-uterine pregnancy never occurred, notwithstanding the fact that in rare instances degenerated ova could be demonstrated above the ligatures.

In a control series of experiments in which the uterine end of only one tube was ligated, pregnancy occurred in the non-ligated, but not in the ligated uterine horn, thus showing that the experiments had been performed at the proper time. These observers therefore concluded that something more than mere mechanical obstruction was necessary and believed that a decidual reaction was the essential pre-requisite for the production of tubal pregnancy.

Taylor reported 43 cases of extra-uterine pregnancy in which no history of previous inflammatory disease could be elicited.

Ovarian pregnancy, which is quite rare, only six cases (Williams) being reported in England in the last 100 years, results from the fertilization of the ovum before it escapes from the Graafian follicle.

Pathology: The most common variety of tubal pregnancy is that occurring in the isthmus, or central portion of the tube; while the rarest form is the interstitial, or that variety that occurs in the inner portion of the tube, as it passes through the uterine muscle.

It is said that about one-fourth of the cases of tubal preg-. nancy rupture before the twelfth week, the other three-fourths terminate by tubal-abortion at an early period.

In tubal abortion the connection between the ovum and the tube wall is loosened, the former becoming completely or partially separated from its site of implantation as the result of hemorrhage, due to the sudden opening of the maternal vessels of the growing trophoblast and chorionic villi. The entire extrusion of the ovum through the tubes into the peritoneal cavity constitutes what is designated complete abortion. After this occurs the hemorrhage usually ceases. If the separation of the ovum from the tube is only partial, the ovum remains in situ and the hemorrhage continues. These two varieties are distinguished as complete and incomplete tubal abortions; the latter occurring more frequently than the former—10 to 1—according to Wormser. Kelly illustrates a case in which the ovum was observed in the act of abortion. Williams had two such cases.

When the bleeding is moderate in amount, and the ovum remains in situ, it may become infiltrated with blood and increase considerably in size, being changed into a structure analogous to the fleshy mole observed in uterine abortions. The hemorrhage usually persists as long as the mole remains in the tube and the blood slowly oozes from the fimbriated extremity into the peritoneal cavity, where it may become encapsulated constituting a hematocele. If the fimbriated extremity is occluded the tube may gradually become distended with blood—a hemato-salpinx.

After incomplete tubal abortion small portions of the chorion may remain attached to the tube wall and give rise to a placental tubal polypus, analogous to a uterine polypus, which is found after incomplete uterine abortion.

Abdominal Pregnancy: Most authors, while admitting its theoretical possibility, are extremely sceptical as to its actual occurrence. Vaight, Martin and others have shown that the fertilized ovum may become implanted upon the fimbria ovaria. Such cases closely simulate primary abdominal pregnancy because the surface to which the ovum is primarily attached is so small that as pregnancy advances the edges of the placenta soon extend beyond the primary seat of implantation and become attached to the surrounding organs, thus giving the impression that it was primarily implanted upon the peritoneum. A microscopical examination enables one to differentiate between the two conditions.

The uterus enlarges, but to a less extent than in intra-uterine pregnancy, being up to the fifth month about one-third smaller. Rupture of the tube with death of the ovum checks uterine growth and involution follows. If the ovum continues to live, the uterus continues to enlarge, but to a less degree than before rupture. At full term the uterus of an extra-uterine pregnancy is from four to six inches in depth. The more remote the place of implantation of the ovum from the uterus, the less the increase in size of that organ.

A decidua resembling the decidua vera of normal pregnancy is formed in the uterus and is thrown off, sometimes in one complete cast as debris, about the time of primary tubal rupture, accompanied often by metrorrhagia. The decidua is from one-eighth to one-fourth inches thick, rough upon its uterine and smooth upon its inner surface, and shows no trace of decidua reflexa nor of decidua serotina.

Changes in the Tube and Ovum: The tube enlarges from increased vascularity and hypertrophy of the muscularis. This is followed by free development of connective tissue and often by more or less disappearance of the muscular fibers, particularly after minute rupture, disintegrating them by small extravasations giving rise to inflammatory and cystic changes. Pressure atrophy of the wall may also occur opposite the placental attachment.

When the ovum is retained in the middle or inner portion of the tube closure of the *ostium abdominale* usually occurs about the seventh or eighth week. Complete closure does not occur when the ovum is retained near the outer extremity of the tube, thus favoring tubal abortion.

A decidua is formed in the pregnant tube. It is also occasionally found in the non-pregnant tube. The amount of decidua vera varies in different cases, but it shows the characteristics of the true decidua of the uterine pregnancy, namely a superficial compact and a spongy lower layer.

A tubal mole is due to arrest of development of the ovum, caused by extravasation of blood from the circulation of the embryo into the subchorionic villi; the placenta, as in intra-uterine pregnancy, is made up of loosely held masses of chorionic villi with intervillous spaces.

Termination of Extra-Uterine Pregnancy: Small embryos extruded into the peritoneal cavity become absorbed unless the placenta retains its attachments to the Fallopian tube and still offers conditions suitable for the continuance of the circulation. Sometimes the young foetus is absorbed while still within the tube, leaving an amorphous mass of tissue attached to the umbilical cord. Occasionally the only indication of its previous existence is a portion of the cord in the amniotic cavity. When the foetus has attained a certain size before rupture, it is not absorbed and may terminate in suppuration, mummification or lithopedion or adipocere formation. Suppuration may result in septicaemia or perforation of the adjoining viscera.

Mummification results from the absorption of the amniotic fluid. The soft tissues assume the appearance of parchment paper.

A lithopidion may result from the deposit of lime salts in the foetus. Literature contains reports of more than 30 cases of lithopedions that have remained in the abdomen from 20 to 30 years before their removal at operation or autopsy.

Rarely the foetus is converted into a yellowish greasy mass designated as adipocere. The fatty material is supposed to be due to the action of an ammoniacal soap.

Diseases of the Extra-Uterine Ovum: In cases where an extra-uterine pregnancy goes on uninterrupted beyond the first few months, the ovum is exposed to all the diseases which may occur in the ordinary uterine form. Thus hydatiform mole has been observed by Otto and Wenzel; hydramnios by Teaffel, Webster and others, and malignant tumors of the decidua by Marchand and Ahfeld.

Symptoms: The three principal ideas it is well to emphasize are:

First—History and subjective and objective symptoms of pregnancy.

Second—Sudden, severe cramps in the pelvis, and

Third—A dark bloody uterine discharge.

Ordinarily the patient considers herself pregnant, has the usual subjective symptoms and may suffer from slight pains in the ovarian region (Williams).

The menses were suppressed in 43% of the cases of Martin and others. In many cases the first manifestation of an abnormal pregnancy is the sudden occurrence of intense pain in one or other ovarian region, followed by faintings and collapse. This signifies tubal abortion or rupture.

In cases of tubal abortion the patient usually soon rallies, but if rupture has occurred, the symptoms are more severe—collapse, pallor, and pain in the lower abdomen and sub-normal temperature being present. In cases that become infected, later, with pyogenic bacteria, the temperature may be from 100° F. to 102½ F., but this is not an early symptom. An examination of the blood shows diminution of the red blood corpuscles and of the hemoglobin. Bi-manual, vaginal and rectal examinations frequently reveal the presence of a large fluctuating mass which fills more or less of the pelvic cavity. In case of doubt a vaginal section into the cul-de-sac of Douglas will often reveal the presence of blood.

A secondary abdominal pregnancy may result if the patient survives the rupture of a tubal pregnancy, provided the placenta has not been detached too extensively. In these cases the usual symptoms of pregnancy persist, but the patient feels more pain, due principally to the pulling apart of the adhesions which have formed between the sac and the adjoining abominal organs.

If a secondary abdominal pregnancy or an uninterrupted tubal gestation goes on to full term, false labor sets in associated with distinct pains similar to those in the early stage of normal labor. False labor may last from a few hours to several days and is soon followed by the death of the child.

After the death of the foetus the circulation in the placenta gradually ceases, the amniotic fluid is absorbed and the sac of the foetus retracts and occupies a smaller space than formerly. Then the mass may remain stationary in size for a number of years. The foetus may undergo any of the changes previously mentioned.

Combined and Multiple Pregnancy: Twenty-two out of

500 cases of tubal pregnancy collected by Parry were complicated by a co-existing intra-uterine pregnancy.

Twin and triplet tubal gestations have been reported.

Repeated Tubal Pregnancy: The case I wish to report belongs to this class. Primrose in 1594 (according to Parry) was the first person to describe such a condition. With the increased employment of abdominal surgery, the abnormality has been noticed more frequently. Pestalozza collected 111 cases. The time intervening between the pregnancy varies from a few months to several years. In my case the interval between the two tubal pregnancies was about 19 months.

Diagnosis: An unilateral tubal tumor, found in a patient giving the usual subjective and some of the objective symptoms of pregnancy would indicate an ectopic gestation, especially if the patient has been sterile for a number of years. The tubal tumor is soft and doughy and corresponds roughly in size to the supposed duration of pregnancy. The unruptured pregnant tube may be mistaken for a retroflexed pregnant uterus. A careful, bi-manual, vaginal and rectal examination of the uterus and tubes will usually enable one to differentiate this condition from uterine abortions. The discharge of uterine decidua associated with tubal enlargement gives strong presumptive evidence of tubal pregnancy, but occasionally the uterine decidua has been cast off at an early period and been replaced by normal endometrium by the time the patient is examined. Tubal rupture or abortion may be suspected if the patient complains of pain in the lower abdomen and faintness and shows symptoms of more or less collapse, especially if one can elicit a history pointing to a pregnancy. If rapid recovery from collapse occurs the probabilities are that a tubal abortion has taken place.

The patient may be seen some time after she has recovered from the primary shock, due to abortion or rupture. In such cases vaginal and bi-manual examination will show a mass on one side of the uterus which is usually mistaken for pelvic inflammation. A fluctuating tumor is sometimes felt posterior and lateral to the uterus. Vaginal exploratory incision may be resorted to in case of doubt. This will reveal the presence of a dark, bloody fluid.

After ectopic gestation has reached full term the diagnosis is comparatively easy and is based upon a history of pregnancy followed by false labor pains and a gradual decrease in the size of the abdomen. The uterus is displaced by a large tumor in which the outlines of the child can occasonally be distinguished.

Treatment: As soon as an unruptured tubal pregnancy is diagnosed, a laparatomy for its removal is indicated to avoid the danger to the patient from rupture of the tube and hemorrhage. In 1883 Tait performed the first laparotomy for the purpose of checking hemorrhage from a ruptured tubal pregnancy. Schauta found, after a careful study of literature on the subject, that 123 cases operated upon showed a mortality of 5.7%, while 121 cases treated wit hout surgical intervention presented a mortality of 88.9%

For the majority of cases an abdominal incision is preferable to operating through the vagina, because of the free exposure of the field of operation. The tubal mass is clamped on either side by long forceps. The hemorrhage being thus controlled, the blood is swabbed out, ligatures applied and the mass removed.

If the patient's condition justifies it, and the uterine appendages on the opposite side are diseased, they should be removed. The abdominal cavity may then be carefully flushed out with warm normal salt solution to remove all blood clots. Subcutaneous or intravenous injection of the same solution may be used in desperate cases to prevent shock.

Kelly and others claim good results in the treatment of pelvic hematoma by making an incision through the vaginal fornix, evacuating the blood and diseased tissue and packing with sterile gauze.

In the later months the treatment of ectopic gestation differs according as the foetus is alive or dead. In a secondary abnormal pregnancy the child usually lies in the peritoneal cavity inclosed in a sac made up of foetal membranes and surrounded by adhesions; the placenta being usually within the tube or broadly implanted on the pelvic floor. Prompt laparotomy in these cases to avoid the danger to the mother of sudden severe hemorrhage, is recommended by Williams.

As a rule, in advanced cases, the complete removal of the gestation sac is difficult and can only be done by performing a hysterectomy. When it becomes evident that an attempt to completely remove the placenta would endanger the life of the patient, the sac should be incised, the placenta being avoided and the foetus removed. In a case of this kind which I assisted Fr.

F. Henrotin operate (in the Chicago Policlinic in 1896) after removing the child, which was fully developed, but dead, he sutured the margins of the sac to the abdominal wound and put in a large Mikulicz drain. The patient made a good recovery, although she had to remain in the hospital for about six weeks.

The use of modern aseptic methods of operating has reduced the mortality when the child is still alive from 93% to 31%.

The death of the foetus renders the operation much less dangerous to the mother. Some authorities, therefore, recommend the injection of about ½ gr. of morphine sulphate into the foetal sac which, it is stated, is sufficient to kill the foetus, but does not affect the mother. The operation should be delayed for six or eight weeks after the death of the foetus in order to allow the maternal blood spaces in the placenta to become obliterated, thus facilitating its removal without hemorrhage. In such cases, however, should the patient develop any dangerous symptoms, immediate operation is indicated.

Case of Repeated Tubal Pregnancy: August 19, 1902, I was first called to see patient. The following is briefly the history of the case:

Mrs. C., married, age 32, mother of one child, a boy 12 years of age. No normal pregnancy since. About one month previously was taken with severe pain in lower abdomen. She had been treated medically without any, except temporary, relief. The temperature was at times as high as 102°. A bi-manual pelvic examination showed a mass in the region of the right tube which was quite painful on pressure. I advised operation and patient was sent to the hospital and operated August 21, 1902, by Dr H. D. Niles and myself. The right tube was ruptured and incorporated in an inflammatory mass of exudate. Large blood clots were in the abdominal cavity. The right tube and ovary was removed, normal salt solution was given the patient sub-cutaneously while she was on the operating table. She made a very satisfactory recovery and left the hospital September 6th, two weeks after the operation. Her health was good for over a year and a half. March 22, 1904, I was again called to see her. She complained of pain in the lower part of the abdomen and there was a discharge of blood from the uterus, and she gave rather indefinite symptoms of pregnancy. The pain persisting, I made a pelvic examination March 28, 1904, and a mass was found in region of left tube. Temperature normal or slightly below. Ectopic tubal pregnancy being suspected, I again advised her to go to the hospital and on March 29, 1904, I, assisted by Dr. Jackson, did a second laparotomy on her. I removed the left Fallopian tube, but did not remove the left ovary. The left tube was ruptured about the middle and there was considerable black clotted blood in the peritoneal cavity, which was removed by thoroughly flushing with warm normal salt solution. The patient again made a satisfactory recovery and left the hospital in three weeks.

In conclusion I wish to emphasize the following points:

(1) Take a careful history of all cases.

(2) Do not depend on the patient's statements entirely, but make a thorough pelvic examination.

(3) Operate promptly.

References: Williams' Obstetrics; M. Herzog, F, Henrotin, International Text Book of Surgery; Kelly's Operative Gynecology; Pryor's Gynecology.

VOMITING IN TUBERCULOSIS.

By DANIEL S. NEUMAN, M. D.
Denver.

For the proper rational therapeutics in vomiting of tuberculosis, one must carefully analyze the cause of its production.

Vomiting in itself is only a symptom of some morbid process and should be treated according to the cause.

Taking into consideration the fact that the already lessened vitality of the tubercular patient demands a proper amount of nourishment, which is impossible at the time vomiting occurs, it has to be controlled as soon as possible, as it has a demoralizing effect on a patient, and prevents a good many, from fear of its occurrence, from eating a proper amount of food.

It is my intention carefully to separate the causes of its production and give its differential diagnosis and treatment.

VOMITING IN TUBERCULAR PATIENTS.

	Occurrence	Nausea	Effect on Cough	Character of Vomited Matter
Morning Vomiting	In the morning (mostly before breakfast)	None	Relieved by vomiting	Mucous and gelatinous Matter
Dyspeptic Vomiting	After introduction of food	Precedes vomiting	Has no effect on cough	Undigested food
Nervous Vomiting	Comes at regular periodical intervals	May continue after vomiting occurs	None	No special characteristic.
Vomiting from Stomach Cough	During the eating	None	Stops	Undigested food. (Patient after vomiting enjoys fresh meal)
Vomiting from Constipation	Two or three times a week	Constant and becoming more and more severe till vomiting occurs	Gradually diminishes after vomiting occurs	Foul and toxic
Vomiting from Gastric Ulcer	After solid food has been taken	None	Becomes more marked after vomiting occurs	Gelatinous and from time to time bloody
Vomiting from absence of HCl in Gastric Juice	Fifteen to twenty minutes after food introduced	Constant all the time, not relieved by vomiting. Hiccough often present	Persistent	Absence of HCl in vomited matter
Toxic Vomiting (due to swallowing Sputum)	May occur any time	Precedes vomiting	Relieved by vomiting	Mucous and albuminous
Vomiting from Cough	Follows paroxysm of coughing	None	No effect	Mixed with mucus and sputum

Morning Vomiting.—Due to irritation produced by over-filled bronchial tubes from sputa collected over night. .

Vomiting very seldom occurs 'during the day. This type of vomiting by itself is only physiological, as it tends to empty the respiratory passages and upper part of the alimentary canal.

Treatment: Increase of expectoration during the day must be encouraged. A glass of hot milk in the morning and a cup of weak tea may often facilitate the removal of the source of irritation.

Saline draught, inhalations of Comp. Tr. Benzoin, every morning and evening often beneficial (before. retiring to bed and soon after patient is awake in the morning). (Nothnagel.)

I often obtain good results from the following mixture:

℞ :
Infusi rad. ipecach 50.00
Liquor ammonii anisat 3.00
Aquae 100.00
Syr. althaeae 20.00
Misce. Signa: Tablespoonful in water every three hours.

Vomiting in Hypochlorhydria—Due to insufficient amount of hydrochloric acid in gastric juice.

This type is easily recognized, as vomiting invariably follows after the introduction of food into the stomach.

Marked by profuse anemia; all secretory organs are disturbed.

Sometimes violent hiccoughs precede vomiting.

Fermentation (gas and dry eructations) and constipation are often present. The stools are foul, tongue pale, patient refuses to eat, and the mouth is dry, owing to diminished secretions. To determine the quantity of hydrochloric acid in the stomach, it is best to examine the gastric juice three or four hours after administration of the Leube-Riegel test meal.

Treatment:

℞ :
Acidi hydrochlorici diluti 8.00
Aquae destillatae 160.00
Mucil gummi arab. . . . .
Syr. rubi idaei aa 20.00
Misce. Sig.: Tablespoonful every three hours.
Or

R:

Strychninae sulph. 0.02

Acidi hydrochlorici diluti 14.00

Ext. condurango fl. 42.00

Elix. gentianae 112.00

Misce. Signa: Tablespoonful in water (through glass tube) one-half hour before eating (Hemmeter).

If constipation complicates, I use the following prescription:

R:

Caffeinae citratis 0.30

Acidi hydrochlorici diluti 10.00

Ext. cascarae sagradae aromatici . . 102.00

Misce. Signa: Teaspoonful in water one-half hour before eating.

The tendency of salines is to deplete the circulating blood; hence they are unsuitable in these cases.

Dyspeptic Vomiting.—(Due to catarrhal gastritis). Associated with pain, eructations, anorexia and constant nausea.

Pain, as a rule, is relieved by the act of vomiting and increased by taking food. The tongue is usually furred, and in some cases a red line on the gums occurs.

Absolute aversion to the taking of meals.

The earliest and commonest symptom is loss of appetite.

Vomiting occurs in short time after introduction of food and is preceded by nausea.

Treatment: Out door exercise, hydrotherapy and massage are always of value. We should exclude hot breads, cereal foods, stews, preserved fish, cheese, etc., from the patient's diet (Nothnagel).

If fermentation is present give small doses of resorcin.

R:

Tinct. cardamomi 8.00

Tinct. nucis vomicae 4.00

Acidi hydrochlorici diluti 10.00

Ess. pepsini 60.00

Aquae 38.00

Misce. Signa: Teaspoonful in water three times a day immediately after meals.

Vomiting Caused by Gastric Ulcer.—The early symptoms are somewhat obscure.

Ulceration is almost invariably attended by symptoms of chronic gastric catarrh (hemorrhage may be attributed to tuberculosis itself).

Vomiting (from time to time mixed with blood) occurs every time after solid food has been taken. Food renders pain more severe. Existence of pain on pressure over a limited area.

Treatment: Predigested liquid food. Bismuth subnitrate in doses of at least 1.00 to 1.50.

> B:
> Ext. belladonnae 0.10
> Bismuthi subnitrat 13.00
> Sodii bicarbonatis 5.00
> Misce; ft. pulvis No. 20.

Signa: One powder before and one after meals (six powders a day).

Or we may give nitrate of silver pills 0.02, one pill before meals.

Toxic Vomiting.—Due to overloading the stomach with sputa containing tubercular bacilli (mostly occurs in children).

Vomiting may occur any time. Most prominent symptoms are distended stomach and formation of the gases from decomposition.

Character of vomited matter: Profuse and gelatinous.

Treatment: The stomach should be washed two or three times a week, and antiseptic antiferments should be used. The patient should be strongly warned against swallowing the sputum.

> B:
> Acidi carbolici 0.50
> Tincturae iodi 1.00
> Aquae cinnamoni 59.00
> Misce. Signa: Teaspoonful in water every three or

four hours.

Salol in large doses is sometimes very beneficial.

Vomiting Due to Constipation.—Due to diet, prolonged mental worry, insufficient amount of liquids introduced into the system, or drugs.

Symptoms: Coated tongue, bad taste in the mouth, vertigo, despondency and irregular pulse, due to auto-intoxication from ptomains.

Treatment: Instruct patient to go to the closet at a certain hour every day. Free drinking of water.

Diet should contain considerable amount of fresh or cooked fruits.

Massage applied along the line of the colon. Electricity (Nothnagel).

Daily administration of a large quantity of cod liver oil (Thornton).

Leube recommends

B:
Pulv. rad. rhei. 20.00
Sodii sulphat 10.00
Sodii carbonat . . . .
Sodii bicarbonat aa 50.00
M. Signa: At bed time one-eighth to one teaspoonful in glass of warm water, as may be necessary.

Nervous Vomiting.—Is due to hysteria and neurasthenia.

Through the vomiting centre, transferred to the vagus, phrenic or intercostales. It comes on at more or less regular periodical intervals, without nausea and without reference to the character of the food. Attacks of vomiting are usually accompanied by migraine.

Treatment:

B:
Potassii bromidi 16.00
Aquae 120.00
M. Signa: Teaspoonful every three or four hours.

The following prescription I have found almost specific:

B:
Tinct. belladonnae 1.00
Aquae laurocerasi 5.00
M. Signa: Five drops, three times a day, in water.

In some cases strychnine or liquor potassi arsenitis is of service.

In obstinate cases the following prescription is of great service:

R:
Morphinae hydrochloratis 0.20
Cocainae hydrochloratis 0.30
Tincturae belladonnae 5.00
Aquae amygdalae amarae 25.00
M. Signa: Ten to fifteen drops every hour (Ewald).

Vomiting from cough may be subdivided as follows:
From stomach cough.
From nasopharingeal cough.
From laryngeal cough.

Vomiting due to the stomach cough is noticed in a good many cases. Its physiological basis is somewhat obscure, but usually due to some factor, as the gastritis, etc. Cough, anorexia and vomiting in these cases go hand in hand.

Treatment:

R:
Ext. valerian 1.00
Ext. belladonnae 0.10
Pulvis zingiberis . . . .
Ext. gentianae aa 1,00
M, ft. pill No. 20.
Signa: One pill in the morning and one at bed time.

Vomiting from laryngeal cough may be due to laryngeal tuberculosis, ulcerations, tuberculous tumors, lupoid, etc.

Treatment: Local, according to the cause of its production.

Catarrh of the nosopharynx often gives rise to cough which terminates in vomiting, A local examination is necessary for its determination and treatment.

Nothnagel recommends

R:
Iodi pur. . . . . 0.10 to 0.30
Potass. iodid . , ... 1.00 to 3.00
Glycerin . . , ... 10.00
Mix and apply to nasopharynx every one or two days.

To diminish the sensitiveness of larynx use internally acidum hydrocyanicum dilutum in small doses (one to two drops every three or four hours).
Or

℞:
Ext. hyoscyami fl 1.00
Aquae amygdalae amarae 20.00
Misce. Sig.: Ten drops in water every three or four hours.

Vomiting in phthisis is also often due to the abdominal compression from coughing, and it is easy to diagnose by the irregular movements of the diaphragm; in fact it resembles the vomiting during an attack of whooping cough (E. Thornton).

Reflex vomiting from enlargement of bronchial vessels, is due to great amount of fluid in the circulation, usually increased after introduction of food. It is best treated by free administration of salines (E. Thornton).

NORMAL OBSTETRICS.
(CHAPTER SEVEN.)

THE DURATION OF PREGNANCY AND THE PREDICTION OF THE DATE OF LABOR, AND THE PERIOD OF PREGNANCY.

By T. MITCHELL BURNS, M.D.

Denver, Colo.

Prof. of Obstetrics, The Denver and Gross College of Medicine.

THE DURATION OF PREGNANCY.

Knowledge.—A knowledge of the duration of pregnancy is important, because by knowing it the date of labor may be estimated. It is important medico-legally, because upon its knowledge may depend the moral reputation of the patient and the legitimacy and hereditary rights ot the infant.

Average Duration.—The average duration of pregnancy is 280 days reckoning from the first day of the last menstrual period. The exact duration of pregnancy, i. e., the time from conception to labor, is not known, because the date of conception is unknown. (Conception may occur from one to thirty days after intercourse.)

Extremes in Duration.—The extremes of the duration of pregnancy are 7, 12 and possibly 15 months. Lusk says that

pregnancies lasting over 285 days are very rare, but the American
Text Book and other works consider pregnancies of ten, eleven
and twelve months as fairly common, because of the positive variations in the duration in the lower animals. The average duration of gestation in the cow is 285 days, and the extremes are
183 and 356 days.

Prolonged Pregnancy.—Prolonged pregnancy is the term
given to pregnancy of unusual length. Pregnancy is apparently
prolonged by conception occurring just before the first menstrual suppression. This brings the actual date of labor about
three weeks later than the reckoned time. Another cause of apparent prolonged pregnancy is conception following menstrual
suppression from some other cause. Pregnancy is really prolonged
at times from lack of uterine irritability, and possibly some fœtuses
requiring more than the average time to mature, as is the case with
some plants.

Precocious Pregnancy.—Precocious pregnancy is the term
applied to pregnancy of short duration. Pregnancy of short duration may be due to increased uterine irritability or unusually
rapid development of the fœtus. Exertion, fatigue, indigestion,
and mechanical irritation tend to hasten the onset of labor, i. e., to
shorten the pregnancy. First pregnancies are generally of normal
duration or less, i. e., they tend to shorter duration than subsequent
pregnancies.

Medico-legal Duration of Pregnancy.—In American and
English Courts, the physician decides as to the legitimacy of cases
which represent the extremes, but in most other countries the extreme duration of pregnancy which is recognized is stated in the
statutes.

In Prussia the legal extreme is 302 days since the death of
the husband or the last possible intercourse. This is more than
in any other country.

THE PREDICTION OF THE DATE OF LABOR AND THE PERIOD OF
PREGNANCY.

Several methods are used to predict the date of labor.
1st. The Menstrual Method.
As the duration of pregnancy is generally ten lunar
months, or 280 days from the first day of the last menstrual period,

it is customary to count nine calendar months forward or three calendar months backward from the first day of the last menstrual period and then add seven days to obtain the date of labor.

An error from one to three weeks is not rare, because of the variations in the duration of pregnancy and the differences between the time of conception and the last menstrual period.

When conception occurs just before the time for the menstrual period, frequently the period is only partially suppressed. Because of this clinicians are careful to ask the character of the last period.

The menstrual method is the method used as a rule. The following methods are of value only in special cases or after considerable experience.

2nd. The Intercourse Method. By counting 280 days from the date of the supposed fruitful intercourse the date of labor is obtained. This method is of value when there has only been one intercourse or when means have been used to prevent conception at other times.

3rd. The Quickening Method. Adding 22 weeks to the date of quickening is supposed to give the date of labor.

This method is of little value except when conception occurs during lactation or when the menses continue after conception, as quickening varies at least a month in the time of its appearance.

4th. The Height of the Fundus Method. Before the fourth month (calendar) the fundus is generally in the pelvis. At the end of the fourth month (rarely at the end of the second or third month) the fundus is at the brim, at the end of the fifth month half way between the brim and the navel, at the end of the sixth month at the navel, at the end of the seventh month half way between the navel and the sternum, at the end of the eighth month nearly to the sternum, in the last three weeks a little lower than at the end of the eighth month (due to the sinking of the uterus).

In this method the patient is examined in the dorsal relaxed position (i. e., on her back with the limbs flexed), and the height of the fundus is marked by pressing the ulnar side of the hand into the abdomen just above the fundus.

This method is of considerable value, as after a little experience it will rarely result in a wrong prediction.

The height of the fundus of course depends upon the size of

the uterus (due to the size of the fœtus and the amount of liquor amnii), but a full bladder or rectum may raise the fundus in the early months if not noted, and cause an error.

5th. The Size of the Fœtus Method. When in doubt by the other methods this method is of great value in the latter part of the pregnancy after experience, as by it one can say positively that according to the size of the fœtus the date of labor should be so many months later.

The Period of Pregnancy. The period of pregnancy is determined by counting the number of months since the first day of the last menstrual period, since the day of the supposed fruitful intercourse, or since the date of quickening and by noting the height of the fundus and the size of the fœtus.

SHOCK, GENERAL NERVOUS AND SURGICAL.*

By GEORGE C. STEMEN, A. M., M. D.

Denver, Colo.

In presenting this paper before this Society, I shall offer no apology, as its importance is always its excuse. Shock has been, and is today, a great source of worry to the surgeon and, I may add, to the general practitioner as well. There are several forms of shock, which require great care on the part of the surgeon to properly control, but I shall speak of but two forms in this paper, general nervous shock and surgical shock. We must admit that this subject, like many others, has not received that close attention during the past that its importance demands, and but little literature has been added since the writings of Jordan, Pirogoff, Savory and others. The clinical observations and the experimental work, so far, afford but slight satisfactory proof of the nature and etiology of shock, and it therefore remains for some member of the profession of the clinical field to prove by investigation its etiology, and to formulate such therapeutic or prophylactic measures as will insure a greater degree of certainty in the treatment of this condition. Pirogoff describes shock as "trau-

*Read before Rocky Mountain Inter-State Medical Association, September, 1904.

matic torpor or wound stupor." Savory says that it is a "paralyzing influence on the action of the heart, due to sudden and severe injury to the nerves." Fischer believes "it to be a weakness of the heart's action, caused by a reflex vasomotor paralysis." Blum says "that it is an arrest of the heart's action, due to reflex irritation of the pneumogastric nerve." Groeningen believes "that the spinal cord is the part of the central nervous system principally involved." Lyden is of the opinion that "the brain does not participate in the shock." Many other writers believe it to be a paresis of the heart, and of the peripheral parts of the circulation, which accounts, to a large degree, for the coldness and pallor, which are invariably present, and to the weakened condition of the brain, which are due to the sluggish flow of the blood within the brain, as a result of the paresis of the heart, and its lowered action, due to the vaso-motor reflexes. From the opinions of the able writers just quoted, as to the etiology of shock, it is evident, to my mind, that this very important subject needs the attention of our profession to prove, by future study and investigation and experimental research, which, if any, of the theories now advanced should be accepted as truths, and if not, to prove what shock really is. It is evident, however, that all the organs of the body are actuated by, and regulated through, the influence of the great nerve centers, and any impression made upon these nerve centers, either by accidental or intentional means, causes, by reflex action, a degree of functional disorder which is characterized by a general depression of the powers of life, known to the profession as shock. All know that when the functions of the various organs are harmoniously and regularly performed health prevails, but when they are disturbed by injury, the conditions of health are changed to that of disease, however sudden the changes may be. If the injury be of such a nature as to produce a marked derangement in the functions of the local nerves, the reflex action may so depress the powers of life as to result in what is termed collapse or shock. If this condition immediately follows the injury it is designated as primary shock, but when it comes after the lapse of several hours or several days, as it is claimed by some writers that it may do, then it is known as insidious, or so-called secondary shock. This division may appear to be arbitary, as it is frequently extremely difficult to make a clear distinction between the primary and secondary symptoms.

In both conditions, however, there is the common feature of depression, the degree of which depends upon the severity of the injury. It is generally conceded that the unusual mortality following severe injuries is out of all proportion to the extent of the injury sustained. This condition, I believe, is due to the mental excitement or fright attending the accident. Therefore the mental condition of the patient should be carefully considered. Most surgeons aim to give sufficient importance to the psychical influences in considering the etiology of shock. In my opinion mental impressions and fright are the chief elements to be considered in connection with the cause of the degree of shock so often following severe injuries.

Men employed in hazardous occupations, as on our railroads, in shops, mines, and in the army, and in time of war, are constantly being brought face to face with the fact that, from the nature of their calling, they are liable at any moment to severe bodily injury. The intensity of the shock is greater in men injured in the employments above enumerated, than usually attends accidents received by a person knocked down and run over in the street or accidentally shot, and the cause I believe is this, that, on the one hand there is a constant element of fear and alarm, while on the other hand this element of fear is entirely absent.

To what degree fright may contribute to the condition called shock, may be illustrated by a few cases coming under my observation. Some years ago I was called to see a young man who had fallen from the top of a box car while the train was running at about ten miles per hour. There was found a simple fracture of the left leg and a slight scalp wound. No other injury could be found, yet in two hours he died of shock. Post mortem examination failed to reveal any cause of death, and I believe in this case death would have occurred from shock had there been no bodily injury. The terror induced by the contemplation of the consequences of the fall, was sufficient, in his case, to produce a state of mental depression from which it was impossible to recover. Some time after the case reported above, a man 37 years old, a laborer, in good health, was standing upon the railroad track waiting for an incoming freight train to pass. An outgoing passenger train struck him, crushing both legs, throwing him under the wheels of the freight train, crushing both arms. He was removed to a hospital and the ordinary cardiac stimulants administered. There was no pronounced shock, yet I did not think it possible that the man could survive more than a few hours. He was made as comfortable as possible, but on the following morning, fourteen hours after the receipt of the injury, there was still no evidence of shock and a quadruple amputation was made. The operation did not entail any perceptible shock, and the patient lived for nine days, dying of sepsis. I would not have it understood that I have drawn my conclusions from the cases just reported, for I could cite a number all tending in the same direction. In fact, all my experience as a surgeon leads to the conviction that when a wound is inflicted without warning, the attending shock is of little consequence. To further illustrate this point, there are numerous cases reported when insane persons have, by their own act, received serious injuries without the condition of shock being manifest. From the report of the above cases and the personal observations of many able surgeons, it is believed that mental depression, the sequence of the terror caused by the accident, is one of the principal elements entering into the production of shock. Agnew said: "The intensity of shock depends on a variety of conditions." Enumerating these conditions under the head of constitutional peculiarities, mental and physical, he says: "A timid or cowardly person exposed to some sudden accident will, even though the bodily injury be slight, suffer a more serious prostration than one who is fearless and indifferent to danger." Cases are reported on good authority of persons who, upon entering the operating room for operation have fainted and died. A case was mentioned recently of a strong, vigorous man who had been suffering some days from an abscess of the finger caused by a splinter of wood. An incision was made to give vent to the pus, when the patient raised himself from the bed, fell back and expired. Such results can only be explained on the theory of some individual peculiarity or idiosyncrasy of organization. On the other hand we find a class of cases of persons of a cold, phlegmatic temperament, with strong nerves and firm, defiant muscles, who endure all forms of injury and mutilation without an expression of pain or any depression of the vital forces, and so it is, that in some cases there may be a crushed leg or arm with but a slight depression of the general vitality. There can be no question that many cases of instantaneous death are the immediate result of a general shock, without any serious lesion of any organ of the body. I may further say that I never witnessed an extreme degree of shock occurring in a person who has been injured while in a state of intoxication. Time will not permit a too lengthy discussion of the after, prolonged or so-called secondary symptoms of shock. Suffice it to say that they are varied and many. They may simply be the continuation of the primary symptoms or they may be entirely different in every respect. A considerable length of time may pass between the primary and the so-called secondary or insidious forms. Is there such a condition as secondary or delayed shock? McLeod affirms that he has seen several cases of delayed shock. The elder Hamilton says he never met with such a condition unless there was a rupture of some large blood vessel accompanying the accident. Very few, if any, surgeons would be willing to admit today that they have ever seen a case of secondary shock. The symptoms which were the cause of leading our surgeons of a quarter of a century ago to describe secondary shock, were not the result of the immediate effect of the injury or operation, but came from some complications, such as acute sepsis, internal hemorrhage, etc. There must, however, be some prolonging of certain symptoms of shock, for numerous cases are reported in which a chain of symptoms are traceable to an injury received some time in the past. It may be weeks, and in some cases, months, and even years, before these prolonged or, it may be delayed, symptoms present themselves as formidable foes in the treatment of certain cases. They may at the onset be slight and very liable to be overlooked by the surgeon, and the patient may pass from his hands into those of some specialist, especially on diseases of the nervous system. Chief among the after, or delayed effects of shock are sleeplessness, disturbance of the circulation, headache, nervousness, disorders of secretion, photophobia and abnormal size of the pupil, loss of memory, menorrhagia and other menstrual disturbances of the genito-urinary system, especially as regards sexual matters, disturbance of digestion, impaired assimilation, neurasthenia, hysteria, etc. These various conditions may be real and in many cases are. The majority of such cases, however, after the development of some of the conditions above enumerated, are no longer the legitimate property of the surgeon, but are, or at least should be, the property of the specialists. What has been said of general nervous shock may, to a very large degree, be said also of surgical shock, yet in surgical shock we not only have the conditions as mentioned in nervous shock, but in many instances of accident we have the additional burden of hemorrhage to contend with, which adds very greatly to the already present disturbing elements of shock. The etiology of surgical shock, barring hemorrhage, is about the same as the etiology of nervous shock and, therefore, can only be explained by assuming a permanent or temporary paralysis of a reflex origin. Experimental research has given us much valuable information as regards the etiology of shock, but much more work in the same direction is badly needed before we will be able to present, with any degree of certainty, an etiology proven by facts. The experiments recorded by Goltz, Crile, Regner, Richet, Gutschs, Boice, Belzold, Beyer, Weir Mitchell, Morehouse and Keen, are of great value, and I believe that the continuation of experimental research will soon reveal to the medical profession some startling truths in regard to the etiology of shock. Senn says: "The danger of shock from operations has been greatly diminished by the use of anesthetics." Yet we have reason to believe that many of the deaths which have occurred on the table since anesthetics have been almost universally employed, and which have been attributed to their use, have resulted from shock. Time will not permit going into the pathology, symptomatology, diagnosis and prognosis of shock now. The preventive treatment has received during the past few years considerable attention and is worthy of careful consideration. Dudley P. Allen has demonstrated by his experiments the value and great importance of prophylactic measures with a view to diminishing or preventing shock, following operations. I believe that the consensus of opinion among all surgeons is that the treatment of shock is purely symptomatic. Without going into detail in regard to the treatment so far as the diffusible and cardiac stimulants are concerned, I dare to say that they all have their place as valuable therapeutic agents in the treatment of this condition. Rectal enemata of hot normal salt solution and subcutaneous and intravenous infusion of the same solution, have been tried and found valuable. It has been my habit for the past few years, when through with a serious abdominal operation, when there have been extensive adhesions and a considerable handling of the viscera has been necessary, to fill the abdomen with hot normal salt solution or hot water, from 6 to 10 degrees warmer than the body temperature, and close tne abdomen, leaving the fluid to be absorbed. The most beneficial results have followed this procedure. Acting upon this knowledge, some eighteen months ago I thought that severe and dangerous shock might be more rapidly overcome by intra-abdominal injections of hot salt solution or hot water, believing that shock may be due to paresis of the abdominal viscera. I have employed this procedure in five cases of severe shock during the past eighteen months with the most gratifying results. I may say, however, that I did not follow this procedure to the exclusion of any other therapeutical measure, for in all cases, except one, treated in this manner, I also used strychnine and spartein as an adjunct to the intra-abdominal injection. The surgical procedure necessary is no more difficult or dangerous than the intravenous or hypodermo-clysis method. The heat applied directly to the abdominal viscera has caused marked reaction in a few moments in all cases. The number of cases in-which I have employed this method are insufficient to base results upon, and I only mentioned it now in hopes that some surgeon who may have a severe case of shock may also use this method, thereby demonstrating its value as a therapeutical agent in this serious condition.

DISCUSSION OF DR. STEMEN's PAPER.

DR. COFFEY: I have been very much interested, indeed, to hear this very excellent paper by the doctor. He believes that one of the principal elements in shock is the mental impression. I think that is proven in a great many ways. For instance, it is a common thing for the patient's friends, even at the sight of the operation, to faint. Another thing is in the case of vaccination; the sight of the operation will often cause fainting on the part of the person undergoing the operation, and the very dread of it, as we know, has much to do with it.

Shock from hemorrhage, I believe, has been greatly overestimated. A shock from hemorrhage, even if it is so great that you can not detect the pulse, is not so serious as other kinds of shock.

I believe, however, that the prime factor in the cause of shock is the method of giving the anesthetic. I heard Dr. Mayo remark the other day that he believed that the cause for the present craze for local anesthetic is that, as a rule, there are so many incompetent and incapable men who give the anesthetic.

For the past three years we have not had a regular anesthetist who has not given a thousand anesthetics before he has come to us. Our present anesthetist has been giving anesthetics for us a little over two years, and during that time has given a little over thirteen hundred anesthetics, and during that time we have not had a case of shock which we could say was due to his work. We have not, during this time, been called upon to use artificial means of respiration. During this time we have probably had a hundred cases where we just called in a man to give the anesthetic, and in at least ten per cent of these cases the patients "have not taken the anesthetic well," and we have began to use artificial means of respiration. For instance, I had one begin artificial respiration very soon before the operation began. I examined the pulse myself before the patient was under the anesthetic. The man administering the anesthetic says to me: "Doctor, do you think the man is all right; he is not breathing; he is not taking it properly." So he kept on with his artificial respiration. Pretty soon the patient broke out into a hearty laugh, showing he was not in a state of anesthesia at all, and that the doctor knew nothing as to where his patient was.

I believe the time is coming when anesthesia will become a specialty. I think there is no field in the domain of surgery, outside of the operation itself, so important as anesthesia. I believe you can get along with almost any kind of an assistant, but you must have a man at the head of the table with ideas of his own.

The anesthetist, if he knows his business, can tell you when you are overdoing, and he knows exactly where his patient is all the time, and in that way is able to guard you against those dangers, by leaving a part of the operation for another time.

The second most important cause of shock, I believe, is the exposure of the peritoneal surface of the intestines. Therefore, the most important part of the abdominal operation, as far as the shock is concerned, is the thorough walling off of the peritoneal surfaces, so that it is entirely unexposed to the air, before the operation is begun. I think that is something which has been frequently mentioned, but sufficient stress has not been laid upon it.

I am very much pleased with the Doctor's paper, and feel that I have learned from it.

Treatment of Suppurative Parametritis. In the very early stages, says Etheridge, keep patient in bed under influence of opiates, with local application of ice-bags. Maintain general health with alcoholics, quinine and strychnine. If suppuration seems to be inevitable, replace cold with hot applications and pouches. As soon as focus of pus can be discovered, open and drain. It is usually best to locate pus with exploring syringe and open along needle with thermocautery or sharp-pointed scissors, taking care to avoid any pulsating vessels, and withdrawing scissors open. Explore pus cavity and, if it communicates with other cavities, enlarge openings between them sufficiently to secure free drainage. Irrigate abscess frequently with an antiseptic solution and maintain free drainage until cavity closes throughout. If there is much new tissue formation after the abscess is closed, use pelvic massage, hot douches and iodine locally.

Simple Chronic Rhinitis. Nasal catarrh, so common in this western country, depends largely on deformities of the nasal septum and other parts of the nose. Sudden atmospheric changes, hygienic errors, anemia and scrofula predispose. The chief symptoms are mouth-breathing from nasal stenosis (especially at night, disturbing sleep), hawking and coughing (mostly mornings), sometimes with retching and vomiting; impaired hearing and tinnitus aurium, asthenopia, and chronic headache, worse in the morning. Inspection shows bony deformities, particularly septal deflections and spurs; nasal mucous membrane bright-red-gray and swollen (swelling does not all disappear with cocaine), with rounded and somewhat irregular surfaces, coated with limited amount of grayish, translucent mucus; white "grubworm" swelling at back end of lower turbinates; thick, tenacious plugs of mucus in nasopharynx; follicles and glands of lower pharynx enlarged.

The Influence of Weather Changes. Bartley and Chapman record some experiments on pigeons (*Brooklyn Medical Journal*), which seem to show that the unrest manifested by birds before a storm is due to a rise in body temperature. They have noted a similar rise in human beings. This atmospheric effect seems to take place through the sympathetic nervous system; hence it is more marked in hysterical individuals and convalescents.

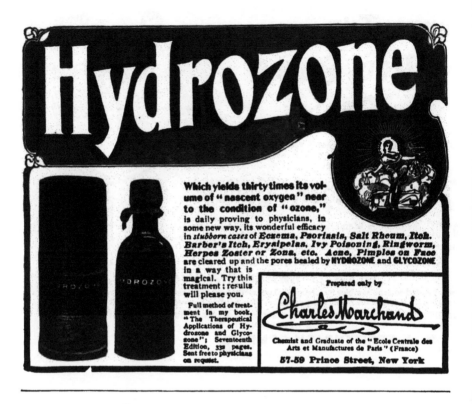
—15—

DENVER MEDICAL TIMES

THOMAS H. HAWKINS, A.M., M.D., Editor and Publisher.

COLLABORATORS:

Henry O. Marcy, M D., Boston.
Thaddeus A. Reamy, M.D., Cincinnati.
Nicholas Senn, M.D., Chicago.
Joseph Price, M.D., Philadelphia.
Franklin H. Martin, M.D., Chicago.
William Oliver Moore, M.D.. New York.
L. S. McMurtry, M.D., Louisville.
Thomas B. Eastman, M.D., Indianapolis,Ind.
G. Law, M.D., Greeley, Colo.

S. H. Pinkerton, M.D., Salt Lake City
Flavel B. Tiffany, M.D., Kansas City.
Erskine M. Bates, M.D:. New York.
E. C. Gehrung, M.D, St. Louis.
Graeme M. Hammond, M.D, New York.
James A. Lydston, M.D., Chicago.
Leonard Freeman, M.D., Denver.
Carey K. Fleming, M.D., Denver, Colo.

Subscriptions, $1.00 per year in advance; Single Copies, 10 cents.

Address all Communications to Denver Medical Times, 1740 Welton Street, Denver, Colo.
We will at all times be glad to give space to well written articles or items of interest to the
profession.
[Entered at the Postoffice of Denver, Colorado, as mail matter of the Second Class.]

EDITORIAL DEPARTMENT

FOOD ADULTERATIONS AND SOPHISTICATIONS.

There are three kinds of adulterations; addition of harmless substances, addition of injurious matters, and abstraction of some valuable constituent from food. Adulteration is generally more fraudulent than harmful. Sophistication interferes with the digestibility and proper balance of food materials.

Most states have laws prohibiting adulteration in general or special forms of it, and most large cities have some special regulations in this regard. According to H. W. Wiley, of the National Department of Agriculture, probably less than five per cent of articles of food are adulterated. The latest report of Edward N. Eaton, State Analysist of Illinois, shows that of 712 food products analyzed, 412 were adulterated or illegally labeled.

The following numbers represent the specimens examined and those found fraudulent: Baking powder, 44-44; butter, 49-36; catsup, 47-45; lemon extracts, 34-27; vanilla extracts, 26-20; olive oil, 25-13; vinegar, 360-192.

Desiccation and sterilization or pasteurization are the only proper methods of preserving perishable foods, but in practice chemical preservatives are very frequently added to "embalmed" flesh, fruits and vegetables. The most common of these preservatives are borax, boric acid, benzoic acid, salicylic acid, sodium chlorid, sulphite and silicofluorid; potassum nitrate and fluorid;

sulphurous acid, formaldehyd, abrastol and saccharin. They all retard the normal process of digestion. According to Vaughan, however, dusting the surfaces of hams and bacon, which are to be transported long distances, with borax or boric acid, not exceeding 1.5 per cent by weight, is effective in preventing meat becoming slimy, and is not objectionable from a sanitary standpoint.

Coal-tar anilin dyes are used largely for coloring milk, butter, oleomargarin, jams and jellies, preserves, confectionery, sausages, etc. Tea may be faced with lead salts or Prussian blue. Sugar is treated with ultramarine to give a bluish-white color. The green color of pickles is heightened with chlorophyl, sometimes fixed by means of copper sulphate.

Spices are generally sophisticated with starches, sawdust, ground shells, and fruit stones, dirt, charcoal, hulls and cheaper spices. Artificial nutmegs are easily broken into a powder when treated with boiling water. Confectionery is made largely of glucose, which is further adulterated with talc, terra alba, baryta and fusel oil. Ground coffee is nearly always mixed with chicory, and tea leaves often with other leaves. "Lie tea" is an imitation made with dust and tea sweepings, starch and gums.

Flour is sometimes adulterated with corn meal. The contained water in flour should not exceed 15 per cent. Alum is normally present in flour and bread to the extent of 6 to 10 grains in a 4-pound loaf. The addition of alum makes the loaf whiter and more hygroscopic and also prevents souring. Gluten meals generally contain starch. Lard and cottonseed oil are sometimes added to skimmed milk cheese as a "filling."

Fruit syrups aften contain no fruit whatever, but are made of anilin colors and flavors. Artificial honey consists of glucose, cane sugar, molasses and syrups, with dead bees introduced for effect. Maple sugar is commonly sophisticated with cane sugar, and maple syrup with glucose, cheap cane syrups and the juice of hickory bark. Dark molasses is bleached with sodium sulphite and zinc dust, the latter being removed with oxalic acid. Jams and jellies often contain glucose, gelatin, cheaper fruits, cores, parings and seeds. Preserves are made for sale with pumpkins, turnips, glucose, cheap fruits, vegetable seeds and refuse products. Milk is improved in appearance with caramel, annatto, aniline dyes and gelatin or chalk. Ice cream is sometimes made to deceive by means of poisonous dyes and flavors. Raspberry sauce is sometimes created wholly from gelatin. Vanilla extract is commonly adulterated with tonka; also with vanillin and artificial colors and flavors. Vinegar is sophisticated with glucose and mineral acids; wines, with sulphur and plaster of Paris. Cheap wines are made largely from other fruits than the grape. Champagne has been concocted entirely from gooseberries and water. Gin is often made from a mixture of water, sugar, cinnamon, alum, capsicum, cream of tartar and a little alcohol. Hanson states that fusel oil with other adulterations will make a very fair whiskey for five cents a gallon. Acids are often added to liquors to imitate the acid reaction of mellow age. Fruits and "cider" usually consists of a weak solution of cider vinegar, flavored with rose water and sparingly sweetened.

Oleomargarine is as nutritious as butter, but hardly so digestible. Lard is much adulterated with cottonseed oil, or beef stearin and excess of water. "Compound lard" may be made of maize, sesame and peanut oils. Olive oil, "imported" or otherwise, generally comes from the cottonseed.

"No man is so poor but that he should be supplied with honest food." Deleterious preparations ought to be strictly prohibited by law. Adulterations and sophistications not manifestly injurious should be plainly labeled according to law, so that any who prefer them on account of the price can have them. Interstate traffic in these goods should be regulated by national laws, and the manufacture and sale of them within the state by state boards of health.

EARLY STAGE OF HYPERTROPHIC RHINITIS.

The mucous membrane is very spongy and bright pinkish in color. Probe pitting last but a moment. Cocaine causes marked contraction. Coakley recommends a cleansing spray of six grain of sodium bicarbonate and three grains chloride to the ounce of water. If the patient must go out of doors at once, follow cleansing with an oily spray of forty grains of menthol, fifteen grains of camphor, thirty m. of encalyptol, fifteen m. of oil of pinus pumilio and benzoinol to make two ounces. When these sprays do not completely relieve swelling, use light linear cauterization along middle of inferior turbinate with galvanocautery (cherry red heat or trichloracetic or chromic acid crystals—first cocainizing and wiping dry area to be cauterized and neutralizing excess of acid (if this is used) with sodium bicarbonate solution on a pledget of cotton.   If by chance the septum has also been cauterized prevent synechiae by keeping a pledget of cotton between parts, and renewing it daily after spraying nose with salt and soda solution.   Fowler's solution internally, five to ten drops t. i. d., is a useful remedy·

LATER STAGE OF HYPERTROPHIC RHINITIS.

The mucous membrane has become a rather pale pink and firmer.   Probe pitting lasts several seconds or minutes.   There is only partial contraction from a cocaine spray.   Coakley directs to cauterize with the galvanocautery down to the bone at one sitting, or by repeated applications of chromic or trichloracetic acid in the same line.   Remove prominent projecting parts with a cold wire snare, checking hemorrhage with very hot normal saline solution or hydrogen peroxide, or by plugging nostril with a long strip of inch-wide sterile gauze.   Syringe the nasal cavity gently with a normal salt solution.

THE LYING-IN ROOM.

This apartment should be the sunniest and best ventilated in the house.   It should have no connection with the sewer, and ought not to be too near the water closet.

A rectal injection of soap-suds and water and a full bath should be given at the onset of labor, followed by the donning of clean clothing throughout.   Thorough scrubbing of the genital region with antiseptic soap solution and hot water is now in order. During labor pledgets of absorbent cotton, soaked for half an hour in 1:1000 mercuric chlorid, should be used to wipe away from before backward any feces that may emerge from the anus.

If leucorrhea or blenorrhea is present, the vagina should be thoroughly scrubbed in the early stage of labor with tincture of green soap, hot water and pledgets of cotton, and then be douched with 1:2000 mercuric chlorid solution, using finally a little clear water.   All water employed for douches and for washing the external parts ought to have been boiled.   Hirst reports three cases of tetanus contracted from intrauterine douches of unboiled water containing two per cent of creolin.

The position and presentation of the fetus can generally be determined by abdominal palpation, and vaginal examinations should be restricted as much as possible, since there is always some degree of danger from sepsis in this procedure. The accoucheur should cut his finger nails short and clean them scrupulously. The hands and arms should be scrubbed for ten minutes, as Furbringer recommends, with a nail brush, hot water and tincture of green soap, scrubbed again with alcohol and then immersed for at least two minutes in 1:1000 mercuric chlorid solution. The finger is now anointed with five per cent carbolized vaselin and inserted directly into the vagina, while the other hand lifts up the upper buttock as the woman lies on her side. A basin of antiseptic solution shauld be kept by the bed for frequent immersion of the hands.

Forceps and other metallic implements used about the person of the woman in childbed, should be boiled in water containing a handful of baking soda for at least five minutes. The few instruments that would be injured by boiling may be sterilized for at least a half hour with a 1:1000 solution of mercuric chlorid in boiled water, or in a two per cent solution of carbolic acid The labor must be so conducted as to avert, if possible, injuries to the maternal tissues, such as perineal tears or excessive bruising by long continued pressure. In the third stage and the early puerperium great care should be taken to secure complete evacuation of the uterine cavity, and to keep the womb thoroughly contracted, thus avoiding sapremia and the absorption of germ products into the uterine sinuses and blood channels.

Post-partum hemorrhages are generally due to uterine inertia, from local or general exhaustion. Occasionally they depend on retention of secundines, and exceptionally on lacerations. To prevent this alarming accident, Davis insists on sufficient nourishment; also chloral hydrate in ten-grain doses every three hours, or in a larger dose per rectum, and ammonium bromid, twenty grains, or trional, ten grains, in broth or soup with whiskey and hot water. Labor ought not to be allowed to drag on too long without assistance. The placenta should never be delivered in the absence of pains. The hand is simply kept above the womb till the latter empties itself and suddenly rises a couple of inches, when the placenta may be pressed out of the vagina, using the uterus as a piston. When there is a history of former hemorrhages, the pregnant woman should exercise and keep the skin and bowels active. The fetus should be delivered slowly and the membranes punctured when the os is nearly dilated. Calcium chlorid, ten grains t. i. d., for two weeks before delivery, is recommended by some writers.

During the lochial period the parous woman should wear constantly an antiseptic vulvar pad of salicylated cotton wrapped in iodoform or carbolized gauze. These pads, kept in place with perineal napkins pinned in front and behind to the abdominal band, should be burned as soon as soiled and be replaced with new ones. Whenever they are changed the blood and clots should be removed from the vulva into a bed-pan, by washing with a stream of boiled water.

Post-partum vaginal douches are not usually needed in private practice, unless sapremia is developing, but a hot antiseptic douche, just after the third stage of labor, acts favorably in soothing pain and encouraging uterine retraction. The use of frequent small doses of quinin or ergotin after labor, by promoting uterine contraction serves to close the doors, namely, the veins, lymphatics and Fallopian tubes, against infection. The physician himself ought to be as scrupulously clean about his obstetric patients as if he were performing a major surgical operation. If a general practitioner is treating infectious patients at the time he is called to attend a woman in labor, he should take a full bath and make a complete change of clothing.

A special obstetric bag containing instruments, ergot, quinin, carbolic acid, carbolized vaselin, iodoform gauze, green soap alcohol, mercuric chlorid, a new nail brush, rubber bed-pan and a long linen gown, is very convenient and servicable. The gown should be put on before making an examination of the patient.

The obstetric nurse must observe the same cleanly precautions as the obstetrician regarding her hands and clothing. She should take a full bath, scrub her hair and scalp thoroughly with soap and water, then rinse with a 1:1000 solution of mercuric chlorid. Her nails ought never to be in mourning, lest her patient's family also need to don the habiliments of woe. The cardinal principles of the puerperium are to keep the mother clean and the baby warm.

EDITORIAL ITEMS.

Ointment for Coryza. After cleansing, Gygaz directs to apply a solution of 12¼ grains of chloral in four drams of castor oil.

A Spray for Coryza. Gleason recommends a solution of 10 grains of menthol or camphor to the ounce of fluid albolene.

Stagnin. This is an extract from horse-spleen, used to increase the coagulability of the blood in cases of menorrhagia.

Rheumasan. This is a combination of salicylic acid and superfatted soap, used locally in rheumatic complaints.

Women in Medical Societies. Dr. Lucy Waite (*Medical Age*), reports 4376 women as listed in the medical societies of this country.

Bile Beans. These consist (*Alkaloidal Clinic*) of cascara, rhubarb, licorice and oil of peppermint, coated with gelatin.

For Debility with Dropsy. Hare gives fluid extract of chimaphila in the dose of ½ to 1 dram.

Dyspeptic Anorexia. Debove and Remand give sodium arsenite 1-64 to 1-32 grains in water two or three times a day.

For Febrile Thirst. Allay thirst with ice-cold water containing 1:1000 hydrochloric acid.

Anorexia Nervosa. The Weir-Mitchell rest treatment is best for adults. Gymnastics and hydrotherapy are useful in hysterical children.

Rheumatic Pneumonias. Bruce gives 16 grains of salicin and 30 minims of fluid extract of licorice in an ounce of water every six hours.

Alcoholic Pneumonia. Mays recommends tincture of capsicum, ½ to 1 dram every two or three hours for nervous depression, etc.

Actinomycosis. Wm. Ewart recommends potassium iodide and eucalyptus or, better, operative measures.

Acute Miliary Tuberculosis. Loomis employed morphine in small doses—1-20 grains hypodermically every six or eight hours.

Phthisical Lobular Pneumonia. A. Jacobi gives from the outset two drops of fluid extract of digitalis every four hours.

Hydatids of Lung. Powell advises thoracentesis and removal of cysts when adhesions are present, as shown by pains and pleurisy.

To Abort a Cold. Potter gives 7½ grains of sodium salicylate in one half dram each of syrup of orange and aromatic spirit of ammonia every four hours.

Inhalation for Coryza. Wunshee directs to inhale from the hand four or five drops of a ten per cent solution of menthol in chloroform.

A Snuff for Coryza. Levy has employed a mixture of six grains of cocaine hydrochlorate and one dram each of powdered extract of suprarenal capsule and powered acacia.

Antiquity of Syphilis. Adachi (quoted in *Progressive Medicine*) has found characteristic lesions in bones in a shell-fish heap dating from the stone age in Japan and at least thousands of years old.

Fatal Rhus Poisoning. The *Alkaloidal Clinic* states that a man aged 42 died at a Chicago hospital of ivy poison after two months' suffering.

Consolidation of Southern Medicine and Gaillard's Medical Journal. These two excellent medical publications are now one, the first amalgamated number appearing in October.

Race Suicide from the Gynecologic Standpoint. Grandin (*Medical News*) asserts that nearly 45 per cent of sterile marriages are the direct result of gonorrhea.

Japanese Surgery. It is estimated (*Detroit Medical Journal*) that three per cent will cover all the deaths of wounded who have returned to Japan after having been treated in the field.

Bad Taste in Mouth. Ringer recommends podophyllin or mercury for a cankery taste in the morning. If these fail, use a mouth-wash of potassium permanganate.

For Foul Breath. W. H. Weaver directs to clean the tongue diligently every morning with a tongue-scraper, using afterward a disinfectant mouth-wash on the tongue and teeth.

Anorexia of Debility. Hare prescribes: ℞ Acidi arseniosi gr. 1-40; ext. nucis vom. gr. 1-5; quin. sulph. gr. i: One pill t. i. d., after meals.

Pica of Pregnancy. Jewett states that all efforts at controlling the abnormal cravings of these patients is usually futile. The most that can be done is to keep them from harmful things.

Atony of Stomach from Debility of Alcoholism. Hare recommends tincture of capsicum, five to ten drops every four or five hours; or oleoresin of capsicum in pill form in the dose of ½ to 1 grain.

For Bulimia. Beale recommends dilute hydrocyanic acid three to five drops, and sodium carbonate, fifteen to twenty grains, in an ounce of water one-half hour before meals.

Appetite in Old Age. To increase it Charcot and Loomis recommend aromatic bitter infusions (quassia, columbo, gentian) combined with strychnine, quinine and iron.

For the Cough of Old Age. Waring prescribes as follows: ℞ Ammonii chloridi gr. v.; ext. glycyrhizae gr. v.; spt. eth. sulph. co. m. x.; aquam q. s. A teaspoonful every two or three hours.

Active Congestion of the Lungs. Bartholow prescribed two parts of tincture of aconite root with three parts of tincture of opium, giving thirteen drops at once, followed by five drops every hour or two.

Hypostatic Pneumonia. ℞ Camphorae gr. i.: ether q. s. ad ft. pulv.; ammonii chloridi, pulv. ipec. co. aa. gr. ii. A powder every hour or two till relieved.—Shoemaker.

Acute Catarrhal Pneumonia. Shoemaker prescribes: ℞ ammon. chlor. gr. xv.; potassii iodidi gr. ii.; tinct. ipecac. m. iv.; mist. glycyrrhizae comp. q. s. A tablespoonful every four hours.

Broncho-Pneumonia. Solis-Cohen gives amyl nitrite m. iii. in one-half dram each of alcohol and glycerin; ammonium carbonate, gr. v. *pro dosi;* strychnine sulphate gr. 1-24 t. i. d.; quinine gr. v., morning and evening.

Ether Pneumonia. Try to prevent this complication, says Anders, by thorough cleansing of the mouth and naso-pharynx, followed by the topical use of an efficient antiseptic solution.

Vulvar Lymphangitis. When not deep-seated, says King, this condition may be benefitted by the constant application of compresses wet with lead and opium wash.

Chronic Bronchitis with Emphysema. Fothergill gives five grains of ammonium carbonate in one-half dram of tincture of squill, and one dram of infusion of serpentaria, three times a day.

Morning Cough of Phthisis. Knopf directs to relieve these attacks with a glass of hot water and some lemon juice, with but little or no sugar—or give five to ten drops of ammoniated spirit of anise.

Constitutional Treatment of Coryza. Shoemaker says: Encourage emunctories; then within forty-two hours get charged with quinine and calcium sulphide, after first reducing fever with aconite, gelsemium or veratrum; alkaline expectorants if needed, followed by acids and antiseptics.

Etiology of Acroparesthesia. This symptom, says Dejerine and Egger (*Progressive Medicine*) is caused by an irritative lesion of the posterior roots in their intramedullary portion, and there is much resemblance between these disturbances of sensation and those of tabes.

Tinnitus Aurium. Bryant (*Laryngoscope*) recommends in chronic cases massage behind the angle of the jaw applied with finger or vibrator. He likewise advises sleeping with the head high and stopping mouth-breathing, if present; also counter-irritation.

A Curious Effect of Antipyrin. Two cases have been reported (*New York Medical Journal, July 16*) of black spots confined to the penis, occurring after the ingestion of antipyrin. These spots disappeared spontaneously but slowly.

Alcohol Depression and Longing for Drink Following Debauches. Zedekoner uses a mixture of two drams chlorated water, 5¼ ounces decoction of althea and two drams of cane sugar: A tablespoonful every two or three hours.

Alcohol Habit. C. Carter has employed with success hypodermic injections three or four times a day of small doses (less than 1-100 gr.) of atropine. It produces, he says, a great distaste for alcoholic liquors in from one to five days.

Editorial Items continued on Page 272

BOOKS.

A TEXT BOOK OF MATERIA MEDICA: Including Laboratory Exercises and Histologic and Chemic Examinations of Drugs.—For Pharmaceutic and Medical Schools, and for Home Study. By Robert A. Hatcher, Ph. G., M. D., Instructor in Pharmacology in Cornell University Medical School of New York City; and Torald Sollmann, M.D., Assistant Professor in Pharmacology and Materia Medica in the Medical Department of the Western University of Cleveland. 12mo volume of about 400 pages, illustrated. Philadelphia, New York, London: W. B. Saunders & Co., 1904. Flexible leather, $2.00 net.

We have gone through this book with exceptional interest and profit. It seems to us to teach the subject of materia medica in the right way, that is, by actual macroscopic, microscopic and chemical study of official and unofficial drugs. The arrangement of the text conduces to its ready comprehension. The recognition of adulteration is given much attention. The book should prove a first-class vade mecum for both students of medicine and of pharmacy.

A HAND-BOOK OF SURGERY.— For Students and Practitioners. By Frederic R. Griffith, M.D., Surgeon to the Bellevue Dispensary, New York City; Assistant Surgeon at the New York Policlinic School and Hospital. 12mo volume of 570 pages, containing 417 illustrations. Philadelphia, New York, London : W. B. Saunders & Co., 1904. Flexible leather, $2.00 net.

Dr. Griffith's work is an example of multum in parvo. By systematic condensation he has managed to convey in this small volume all the essentials of surgery, including the specialties, medicolegal examinations and microscopic technique. Special attention is given to minor surgery and bandaging. The underlying principles of surgery are clearly outlined. The text is fully illustrated with well selected figures. We think this work will be appreciated and largely utilized by students and recent postgraduates.

HOW TO COOK FOR THE SICK AND CONVALESCENT.—Arranged for the Physician, Trained Nurse and Home Use. By Helena V. Sachse. Second edition, revised and enlarged. Philadelphia: J. B. Lippincott Company, 1904.

As a general thing, proper food is far more important than

medicine in aiding nature to throw off disease. The forelying volume contains a great number of recipes of food formulas which appear to be accurate and carefully written with due regard to the demands of good health. There is a complete index affixed to the text, and a very convenient preliminary classification of recipes. We think the book can be profitably recommended by physicians to nurses and mothers.

PROGRESSIVE MEDICINE.—A quarterly Digest of Advances, Discoveries and Improvements in the Medical and Surgical Sciences. Edited by Hobart Amory Hare, M.D., and H. R. M. Landis, M.D. Volume III, Sept. 1904. Lea Bros. & Co., Philadelphia and New York.

The largest section of the present volume is a review of progress in diseases of the thorax and its viscera, including the heart, lungs and bloodvessels, by Wm. Ewart. This resume is very instructive and should be especially helpful to general practitioners. The section on dermatology and syphilis, by Wm. S. Gottheil, contains, with much other matter, an interesting illustrated summary of some cases of feigned eruption. There is an excellent section on diseases of the nervous system, by Wm. G. Spiller; and on obstetrics, by Richard C. Norris.

REFRACTION AND HOW TO REFRACT.— Including sections on optics, retinoscopy, the fitting of spectacles and eye-glasses, etc. By James Thorington, A.M., M.D., Professor of Diseases of the Eye in the Philadelphia Polyclinic and College for Graduates in Medicine. Third Edition. Two hundred and fifteen illustrations, thirteen of which are colored. Price, $1.50. Philadelphia: P. Blakiston's Son & Co., 1012 Walnut St., 1904.

Dr. Thorington's manual is deserving of its considerable popularity. The text is systematic and inductive, necessarily somewhat dogmatic and above all clear and concise. The great number of diagrams and other illustrations are of great service in lightening the labors of the student and practitioner, to whom this book can be safely recommended.

TEXT-BOOK OF NERVOUS DISEASES AND PSYCHIATRY.— For the use of students and practitioners of medicine. By Charles L. Dana, A.M., M.D., Professor of Nervous Diseases and of Mental Diseases in Cornell University Medical College; Visiting Physician to Bellevue Hospital; Neurologist to the Montefiore Hospital. Sixth Revised and Enlarged Edition. Illustrated by Two Hundred and Forty-Four Engravings and

Three Plates in Black and Colors. New York: Wm. Wood & Co., 1904.

This work has the advantage over some of the older books on neurology in being based as far as recent advances permit, on neuroanatomy, pathology and bacteriology. The author has gone into each subject thoroughly, collating the actual professional experience of himself and others in the endeavor to present each topic as a complete whole. His classification of mental diseases differs somewhat from other authorities, his tendency being to limit the major psychoses in favor of the minor mental derangements. His literary style is lucid and entertaining. The comprehensive nature of the work renders it a satisfactory neurologic guide to practitioners, and the needs of students are given special consideration. The illustrations are mostly clinical and pathological in character.

LECTURES TO GENERAL PRACTITIONERS ON THE DISEASES OF THE STOMACH AND INTESTINES.—With an account of their relations to other diseases and of the most recent methods applicable to the diagnosis and treatment of them in general; also "The Gastro-Intestinal Clinic," in which all such diseases are separately considered. By Boardman Reed, M.D., Professor of Diseases of the Gastro-Intestinal Tract, Hygiene and Climatology in the Department of Medicine of Temple College, Philadelphia; Attending Physician to the Samaritan Hospital. Octavo; 1021 pages. Illustrated. Price $5.00. New York: E. B. Treat & Co., 241–243 W. 23rd St., 1904.

This substantial volume, built up in part from lectures to the author's students, is a practically complete exposition of diseases of the alimentary tract. The text is arranged in eighty-two lectures, comprised in four parts, namely, Anatomic, Physiologic, Clinical and Diagnostic Data; Methods of the Examination; Methods of Treatment; and the Gastro-Intestinal Clinic, under which separate diseases, symptoms and syndromes are considered. The diagnostic and therapeutic methods described by the author are of the modern type, and are such as American patients will tolerate. He does not narrow his observations to the gut and the stomach, but for example, regards uranalysis indispensable in gastro-intestinal affections, and devotes three chapters to the relations here concerned. Diet and mechanical measures are given more attention than in most other works of the kind. We commend this volume to our readers for its intrinsic merits and practical usefulness.

KIRKES' HAND-BOOK OF PHYSIOLOGY.— Revised by Frederick C. Busch, B.S., M.D., Professor of Physiology, Medical Department University of Buffalo. Fifth American Revision. With Five Hundred and Thirty-five Illustrations, including many in Colors. New York: Wm. Wood & Co., 1904.

This work has been a long time before the medical profession, and is equally a favorite with students and teachers. Its great popularity has led to frequent careful revisions and the addition of many more and better illustrations. The present edition has all the sterling features with which we are familiar, and such new ones as the the most recent progress in physiologic science has brought forth. In no particular that we can notice is the work defective, and we trust it will continue to hold a position in the van of medical text-books.

NAGEL'S EPITOME OF NERVOUS AND MENTAL DISEASES.—A manual for Students and Physicians. By Joseph Darwin Nagel, M.D., Consulting Physician to the French Hospital, New York. In one 12mo volume of 276 pages, with 46 illustrations. Cloth $1.00, net. Lea Brothers & Co., Publishers, Philadelphia and New York, 1904.

In this neat and compact volume the author has arranged the essentials of nervous and mental diseases in a convenient form for students' use. The information given on each subject is brief but precise. Each of the eleven chapters is followed by a list of review questions. Forty-six figures illustrate the verbal text.

DISEASES OF THE NOSE, THROAT AND EAR and their Accessory Cavities. By Seth Scott Bishop, M.D., D.C.L., LL.D., Author of "The Ear and Its Diseases"; Honorary President of the Faculty and Professor of Diseases of the Nose, Throat and Ear in the Illinois Medical College; Professor in the Chicago Post-graduate Medical School and Hospital; Surgeon to the Post-graduate Hospital and to the Illinois Hospital; Consulting Surgeon to the Mary Thompson Hospital, to the Illinois Masonic Orphans' Home, and the Silver Cross Hospital of Joliet, etc. Third Edition. Thoroughly Revised, Rearranged and Enlarged. Illustrated with 94 Colored Lithographs and 230 Additional Illustrations. 564 Pages, Royal Octavo. Price, Extra Cloth, $4.00 net; Sheep or Half-russia, $5.00 net. F. A. Davis Company, Publishers, 1914–16 Cherry St., Philadelphia.

We are quite familiar with this work, and almost never fail to find what is sought when we consult it. For the general practitioner the book meets every practical requirement. The author's descriptions are clear and precise; his directions for treatment are explicit and may be relied upon for a successful issue in curable cases. A praiseworthy feature of the text is the consideration given to his fellow specialists in America. We note, for instance, several references to the work of Drs. Robt. Levy and Melville Black, of this city. The present edition has been carefully revised, with such alterations and additions as were needed to make it represent the most recent advances. The exceptional array of beautiful colored plates and other illustrations merits special mention.

SAUNDERS' QUESTION COMPENDS.—Essentials of Medical Chemistry. Sixth Edition. Thoroughly Revised. Essentials of Chemistry, Organic and Inorganic. Containing also questions of Medical Physics, Chemical Philosophy, Medical Processes, Toxicology, etc. By Lawrence Wolff, M.D., formerly demonstrator of Chemistry at the Jefferson Medical College, Philadelphia. Sixth Edition. Thoroughly Revised. By A. Ferree Witmer. Ph.G., formerly Assistant Demonstrator in Physiology at the University of Pennsylvania. 12mo volume of 225 pages, fully illustrated. Philadelphia, New York, London: W. B. Saunders & Co., 1904. Cloth, $1 net.

The fact that this little work has reached the sixth edition is proof of the demand for such compendiums. In the present revision Dr. Witmer makes mention of the more recent discoveries in physical chemistry and organotherapy. The text is arranged catechismically.

A TEXT-BOOK OF CLINICAL DIAGNOSIS.—By Laboratory Methods. For the use of Students, Practitioners, and Laboratory Workers. By L. Napoleon Boston, A.M., M.D., Associate in Medicine and Director of the Clinical Laboratories of the Medico-Chirurgical College, Philadelphia; formerly Bacteriologist at the Philadelphia Hospital and at the Ayer Clinical Laboratory of the Pennsylvania Hospital. Octavo volume of 547 pages, with 320 illustrations, many of them in colors. Philadelphia, New York, London: W. B. Saunders & Co., 1904. Cloth, $4.00 net; Sheep or Half Morocco, $5.00 net.

This, the latest work on clinical diagnosis, is up to date in every particular. The work is a practical storehouse of latter-day chemic and microscopic methods of distinguishing disease. The author has devised quite a number of original tests, which will appeal to the busy physician because of their convenience and simplicity. Among the newer subjects fully considered are serum diagnosis, cyto-diagnosis, purin estimation, Bence-Jones albuminuria and inoscopy. The text is profusely illustrated. The beautiful colored plates on the blood and urine are exceptionally good.

SELECTIONS.

Causerie Therapeutique, Cacodylic Medication with Women.—One of the most interesting points in the communication of Prof. Gautier to the Academy of Medicine, was that which proved the close relation existing between the presence of arsenic in the organism, and the menstrual function. Indeed, while noticing that under the influence of cacodylate of soda the hair of women was becoming more abundant—which is a direct consequence of the exciting action of arsenic on the epidermic appendixes—he noticed also less irregularities in the menstrual periods. A point that very well confirms the fact that the menstrual blood always contains arsenic (o milligr 28), while the common blood does not contain any. This role of arsenic in the capital manifestation of woman life was well set forth by M. Gautier in the following lines:

"Thus arsenic and iodine are normally eliminated each month with the menses, and this flow has for its origin and purpose a sort of depletion of the vital portions of the economy which are rich in phosphorus, and more especially of those which are elaborated by the thyroid. After having been elaborated in the thyroid, the particular nucleo-proteids formed in that gland are at all times carried away in the lymphatics and deposited in the blood, to perform there the part of excitants of vitality, and of cell reproduction. These thyrodian proteids nourish the skin and its appendices, which are always arsenical. But each month their surplus passes out with the menses, except in cases of pregnancy, when the globulines and the thyrodian nucleo-proteids are utilized by the body of the new being, which needs phosphorus, iodine, and arsenic of such exceedingly plastic form."

Will F. Shultz, M. D., has used sanmetto quite extensively as a genito-urinary tonic in chronic atonic conditions of the genito-urinary organs resulting from chronic specific urethritis, and has met with most excellent results.

Covington, Ky.

A Corrector of Iodism.—Dr. W. H. Morse reports (*Southern Clinic for May*) success in the use of bromidia, which he says has aroved corrigental of iodia. Discussing his results he says: Vomiting is so frequent and troublesome a symptom, in many diseases beside irritation and inflammation of the stomach, as to demand much practical attention from the physician. So, although the causes are so various, and although we are actually treating a symptom, for this symptom bromidia is remarkably effectual. We have all employed the remedy for colic and hysteria, two disorders where nausea and vomiting are as pronounced as they are persistent, and almost the first evidence of relief is shown by the disappearance of these disagreeable symptoms. It is quite as efficacious for the nausea and vomiting from ulcer or cancer of the stomach. There is nothing that will more quickly check the vomiting, and the hypnotic effect is quite in order.

KENNEDY'S EXTRACT OF PINUS CANADENSIS is a valuable agent in chronic diseases of the mucous membranes, and admirable for the removal of morbid discharges of every kind.

HAGEE'S CORDIAL OF COD LIVER OIL COMPOUND is one of the most popular cod liver oil preparations on the market. All the nutritive properties of the oil are retained and the disgusting and nauseating elements are eliminated. Combined with hypophosphites of lime and soda it offers to the profession a reconstructive of great value.—*St. Louis Medical Review.*

PAIN.—Lord Lytton said: "There is purpose in pain." How true is the fact, especially from a diagnostic point in diseases of women. Dysmenorrhea, that distressing manifestation of uterine obstruction most frequently caused by congestion, is only one of the many instances. To equalize pelvic circulation and remove uterine engorgement is the object to be attained and is best accomplished by administering Hayden's Viburnum Compound.

Dr. James Charles Copeland says, in his "Medical Treatise' in the chapter on Menstrual Life of Women: "For dysmenorrhea characterized by sharp, colicky pains, there is nothing better than Hayden's Viburnum Compound."

RESPIRATORY TRACT: AFFECTIONS, SYMPTOMS AND TREATMENT.—By Dr. Arthur B. Smith, Springfield, Ohio. The average physician is frequently vexed in finding a condition which resists his best efforts to bring about a cure. This holds good in almost every disease at some time or other, but particularly in affections of the respiratory tract, where there may be a great variety of symptoms in several cases of the same disease.

Almost every physician has some favorite prescription for coughs, bronchitis, laryngitis, etc., which he uses until suddenly it seems to lose its efficacy—why no one knows. Then another remedy takes its place until it, too, fails to give the desired result. It is rarely that one finds a cough remedy which will be consistently good in the majority of cases. Theoretically there appears to be a well-founded objection to the use of cough syrups in general, but nevertheless there are times when nothing else gives satisfaction; therefore, the physician pins his faith to that remedy from which he and his patients derive the most good. It is not always easy to find such a remedy, but when it is once found, it is equally difficult to dispense with, and often the physician is almost compelled to resort to a routine treatment

Some time ago my attention was called to a preparation composed of a solution of heroin in glycerine, combined with expectorants, called Glyco-Heroin (Smith). It possesses many advantages not shown by any other preparation I have used, and has none of their disagreeable features.

In citing some of the cases treated with this remedy I shall not go into a minute description of any case, but briefly state the conditions which existed and the results obtained, which were uniformly good:

Case 1. S. B., aged 16. Caught a severe cold while traveling. This developed into an unusually severe attack of bronchitis with mucous rales, pain, cough and some slight fever. Prescribed Glyco-Heroin (Smith), one teaspoonful every two hours, decreased to every three hours. After a few doses were taken there was a decided improvement, the respirations were slower and deeper, the expectoration freer and the temperature normal. In a few days the patient was practically well and able to return to school. No medicine except Glyco-Heroin (Smith) was given and the results from its use were excellent.

Case 2. W. L., aged 31. Acute bronchitis. Painful cough, with difficult expectoration, particularly when in a reclining posture. Glyco-Heroin (Smith) in teaspoonful doses every three hours gave speedy relief and a cure was effected in a few days.

Case 3. S. W., aged 60. Chronic bronchitis. Had coughed for years, with expectoration of a thick, yellow, purulent and very offensive matter. Had lost flesh gradually until about twenty pounds below usual weight. No appetite, very constipated, pains all over chest, night sweats and insomnia. Patient on the verge of nervous prostration and greatly weakened. She was given bromides, a tonic, and Glyco-Heroin (Smith), the latter in the usual dose at intervals of two hours. The first few doses were not well borne, as they seemed to cause some nausea, but by giving a smaller dose and then gradually increasing it, tolerance was soon obtained, and the results were remarkable. The cough and expectoration greatly decreased, the appetite improved and the patient became much better in every way. The treatment was continued as before, except that the Glyco-Heroin (Smith) was given every three hours. In three weeks the patient was eating almost everything she pleased, and sleeping well. The night sweats had stopped, together with the cough, and, as the patient expressed it, she "felt like another woman." At present she is in perfect health and needs no medicine except an occasional laxative.

Case 4. B. E., aged 26. Severe bronchitis accompanying an attack of influenza. Various remedies were tried in this case, with negative results, until Glyco-Heroin (Smith) was given in teaspoonful doses every three hours. In a short time decided relief was obtained and the cough stopped permanently.

Case 5. W. H., aged 5. Whooping cough. Spasmodic paroxysms of coughing, sometimes being so severe as to cause vomiting. Tenacious mucus was present, requiring great expulsive effort to loosen it. There was little fever, but the patient was much prostrated and weakened by the cough. Glyco-Heroin (Smith) was given in 10 drop doses every two hours with good results.

EDITORIAL ITEMS.— Continued.

Successful Treatment of Inoperable Cancer. The editor of the *Medical Record* (*Oct. 6*) calls attention to three cases of inoperable cancer (thorax, tongue, neck) treatment respectively and successfully with the X–rays, and hypodermic injections of one per cent soap solution and of twenty per cent solution of Chian turpentine in sterilized olive oil every other day. The practical moral, he says, would seem to be that cases so hopeless in their natural evolution should not be abandoned without a rational experimentation along some one of these lines.

Thirst of Intestinal Troubles. In acute intestinal catarrh W. W. Johnston gives cracked ice, carbonic acid water, and barley, or rice-water in moderation. In cholera morbus he uses cracked ice sparingly at first, more freely later.

Removal. Dr. Geo. F. Butler has severed his connection with the Alma Springs Sanitarium, at Alma, Michigan, where for nearly five years he has been Medical Superintendent, and has returned to Chicago, where he will henceforth limit his practice strictly to internal medicine.

Anorexia of Early Suberculosis. Penzoldt recommends basic orexin powder, five to eight grains daily at 10 a. m. If the remedy fails after a trial of five to ten days, suspend for a week and then give a second course.

Passive Pulmonary Congestion. An important preventive measure is to change the patient's posture from time to time. By way of treatment Shoemaker prescribes a pill every three or four hours, containing $\frac{1}{3}$ gr. ergotin, $\frac{1}{4}$ gr. ext. digitals, and 2 grs. of Dover's powder.

For Acute Salpingitis. Skene recommends rest and anodynes for relief of pain; counter-irritation and attention to bowels, and iodine and mercury locally when acute symptoms subside; layarosalpingotomy and removal of tube when pyosalpinx or hydrosalpinx is present.

Late Stage of Phthisis. Castel administers Hoffmann's anodyne and fluid extract of opium in syrup of lettuce. In the hopeless stage Hare advises a resort to normal liquid or fluid extract of cannabis indica.

For Pneumonic Cough. A favorite prescription consists of two minims each of dilute hydrocyanic acid and chloroform, and 14 minims each of tinct. hyoscyamus, syrup of tolu, camphor water and mucilage of acacia: A teaspoonful every half hour or hour.

Diphtheritic Vulvitis. Thoroughly cleanse parts with concentrated solution of salicyic acid, a five per cent solution of thymol, or with lime water; or dust with iodoform, boric acid or potassium chlorate.—Winckel-Parvin.

Gangrene of Vulva or Vagina. The *American Text-Book of Gynecology* directs to excise parts if recognized early enough and obliterate resulting wound with sutures; or disinfect with a strong antiseptic solution.

Emphysema. Grindelia, says Waring, is of great service for the dyspnea and cough. For accompanying bronchitis Taylor employs expectorants, such as ammonium carbonate, (5 to 7 grains) wine of ipecac and tincture or infusion of senega; also mustard plasters or linseed poultices.

Pulmonary Gangrene. Knopf directs to treat vigorously with tonics (digitalis, caffeine, alcohol); employ pneumotomy and drainage if circumscribed. Wm. Ewart also advises surgical operation if tne lesion is limited and the patient has good vitality.

Treatment of Pulmonary Abscess. Powell says: Endeavor to keep abscess cavity as empty and disinfected as possible. Help expectoration by change of posture. Employ disinfectant inhalations and keep up patient's strength. Surgical intervention may be necessary.

Treatment of Chronic Rhinitis. Gleason directs to cleanse with an alkaline solution, then apply on cotton a mixture o ten grains of iodine and thirty grains of potassum iodide with an ounce of glycerine, following this application with a spray of abolene or liquid vaseline. Tonics are always in order.

Serous Diarrhea. In the serous form of diarrhea. after the bowels have been cleared of all irritating matter, the following (*Clinical Review*)is a serviceable mixture: ℞ Bismuthi subnit. gr. xx; tinct. kino m. xxx; tinct. zingiberis m. x; tinct. cardamomi comp. ad ℥ii.: Repeat in from two to four hours.

Fetor of Breath from Gastric Fermentation. Thornton recommends sodium hyposulphite, a teaspoonful in water after meals and ten grs. of charcoal every three hours. Correct achlorhydria, if present, by giving pepsin, dilute hydrochloric acid and strychnine sulphate after meals.

Chronic Alcoholism. Gowers recommends bitter tonics; tincture of capsicum, 10 mimins before meals, or when craving comes on; cocaine hydrochlorate, 1–10 to ¼ gr. after food, combined with ⅛ minim of alcoholic solution of nitroglycerin, 4 minims of liquor strychninae, and some liquid preparation of pepsin.

Craving for Alcohol. A. L. Loomis has prescribed: ℞ Tinct. capsici m. i; tinct. nucis vom. m. iv; tinct. cinchonae co. q. s: A teaspoonful every two or three hours. Hare writes for: Tinct. capsici m. v; tinct. opii deod. m. viii; spt. ether nit. m. xv; spt. lavand. co. q. s.: A desertspoonful every four or five hours.

Phthisical Loss of Appetite. Debove directs to take beef and remove all the fat and tendons. Hash rather coarsely, spread on plates and dry in the oven at 194° F. When it is dried hard, grind in a mortar and strain through a fine silk sieve. Tubefeed as bonillon, to which may be added the whites and yolks of two eggs previously beaten.

Thirst of Diabetes. Phosphoric acid, says Butler, diminishes thirst and lessens the quantity of urine. Pilocarpine nitrate, 1-24 gr. in diluted spirit, say be placed on the tongue four times a day. Duchenne recommends potassium phosphate, two parts in 75 of water—a dram of the solution twice or thrice daily in wine or hop tea.

Diet in Pneumonia. Powell advises to use milk (may be diluted with effervescent water or flavored with tea or coffee), cream, strong beef tea, mutton or chicken broth, with perhaps some farinaccous thickenings. Food and stimulants should be given in reasonable quantities at intervals of about two hours.

Chronic Interstitial Pneumonia. N. S. Davis, Jr., advises cure of the primary affection; good hygiene, especially fresh air; pulmonary gymnastics—bend body to unaffected side and back; and residence at high altitudes. Ringer recommends inhalations of iodine night and morning.

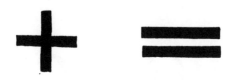

Distilled Water + Salicylic Acid + Soda + Pancreatin + Pure Lofoten Cod-Liver Oil = Hydroleine.

Note the simplicity of the above formula. It contains just enough soda to produce the slightly alkaline medium necessary for the fat-splitting action of pancreatin. A trace of salicylic acid keeps the whole combination sweet and stable.

No attempt has been made to medicate Hydroleine. It's simply absolutely pure Cod-Liver Oil rendered thoroughly digestible by Nature's method of emulsifying fats. That's why Hydroleine is absorbed and assimilated when the plain oils and the ordinary, mechanically-prepared emulsions are ineffective. Sold by all druggists. Write for literature.

THE CHARLES N. CRITTENTON CO., Sole Agents,
115-117 FULTON STREET, NEW YORK

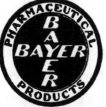
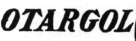
—17—

Pneumonic Phthisis. When pneumonia passes into pulmonary tuberculosis Hughes prescribed: ℞ Ammonii carb. gr. x; ammonii iodidi gr. v—x; aquae chloroform ℨii; syr. pruni virg. ℨi.: Take every five hours diluted. Alternate with the following: ℞ Sig. potass. arsenit. m. v; massae ferri carb. gr. v; vini xerici ℨi; aquam ad. ℨss.

Cytodiagnosis in Nervous Disease. Niedner and Mamlock (quoted in *Medical News*) have examined the centrifugated sediment in a number of nervous diseases and find hyperlymphocytosis (more than five lymphocytes in a microscopic field under a magnifying power of 400 to 500) as a characteristic feature of syphilitic and parasyphilitic affections of the central nervous system.

Dysmenorrhea of Anteflexion. J. W. Long directs to operate two weeks before expected flow—dilate, irrigate, curette, pack, and remove gauze in six days; amputate the cervix if it is greatly hypertrophied. Coitus is in order before and after the flow. In the menopausal anteflexion of old maids dilation of the cervix and a gauze drain are all that are usually needed.

Gonorrheal Metritis. Garrigues advises washing out the uterus at least once a day with mercuric chloride (1:3000) or zinc chloride (1:100) through a glass tube. Paint interior of uterus all over twice a week with twenty per cent zinc chloride solution or 1:12 silver nitrate. Pack the womb once or twice with iodoform gauze, and finally leave a strip well dusted with iodoform in the uterine cavity.

New York Skin and Cancer Hospital. The governor of the New York Skin and Cancer Hospital announces that Dr. L. D. Bulkley will give a sixth series of Clinical Lectures on Diseases of the Skin, in the Out-Patient Hall of the hospital on Wednesday afternoons, commencing Nov. 2nd, 1904, at 4:15 o'clock. The course will be free to the medical profession.

Influenzal Coryza. Bishop directs to put to bed and relax the bowels if necessary, and use antipyretics for high fever. He also recommends coryza tablets, each containing 1–12 grain of morphine, 1–600 grain of atropine and 1–6 grain of caffeine, for pain and nasal obstruction. Spray throat, he says, three or four times a day with three per cent solution of camphor-menthol in lavolin or benzoinol.

Curtain-Like Inferior Turbinate. Such a formation touches
the floor of the nose and retains mucus between the pendulous
border and the outer wall of the nose. Relief, says Coakley, is
secured by removing the lower portion of the inferior turbinate
by means of a cold snare with a horizontal loop.

Hyperemesis Gravidarum. Norris (*Progressive Medicine*)
has frequently observed the good result of intestinal lavage for various manifestations of the toxemia of pregnancy, and it has come
to be a routine practice with him to employ this measure in all
cases of excessive vomiting. For the cases associated with hysteria isolation and intestinal lavage have been almost uniformly
successful.

For Nausea. Beale advises the use of dilute hydrocyanic
acid, one to five minims, with sodium bicarbonate before eating;
aqua ammonia, 6 or 5 drops in water, and counter irritation.
Ingraham recommends a two per cent solution of cocaine, applied
well up in the nasal cavities. In men addicted to excessive smok-
ing, Hare employs the compound spirit of ether in capsules or
ice-cold water—dose one or two drams.

After Fevers. In convalescence from prolonged fevers Hare
prescribes: ℞ Acidi nitrohydrochlor. diluti m. i—iiv; tinct. nucis
vom. m. ii; tinct. cardamomi comp. m. xxx; tinct. gent. comp. q.
s.: A teaspoonful in water after meals. Following malarial
fevers he considers quassia particularly useful, in the dose of
one-half to one dram of the tincture.

Convalescence. Butler advises the use of simple bitters one-
half to one hour before meals, changing from one to another every
week or two. They are best given in liquid form. Following
acute diseases Hare has found freshly prepared nitromuriatic acid
generally preferable. He gives purgative doses for gastrointestinal
torpor, shown by thick yellow coating of tongue.

Night Cough of Phthisis. Burney Yeo has recommended
croton-chloral in moderate and quickly repeated doses until tolera-
tion is discovered. Shoemaker prescribes ℞ Codeinae gr. $\frac{1}{8}$; tinct.
belladonnae m. iiss; syr. pruni. virg. q. s: A teaspoonful when
cough annoys. Ringer gives a teaspoonful of glycerine in lemon
juice at night.

Senile Pneumonia. Leonard D. White commends strychnine as the most important drug. He also advises the use of the

Scott's Emulsion is a scientific pharmaceutical preparation, the medicinal ingredients of which are pure cod liver oil, with hypophosphites of lime and soda and glycerine. In this preparation the oil has been artificially digested by mechanical processes, thus preparing it for immediate absorption into the circulating fluid and supplying what deficient digestive ferments fail to supply. The utility of this expedient in the dietetic management of many morbid states has received the approval of high authority.

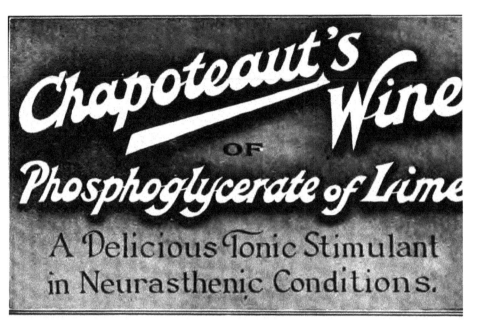

A Delicious Tonic Stimulant in Neurasthenic Conditions.

Agents: E. Fougera & Co., 26-30 N. William St., N. Y.

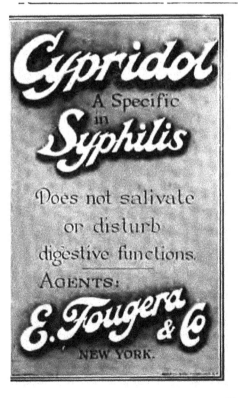

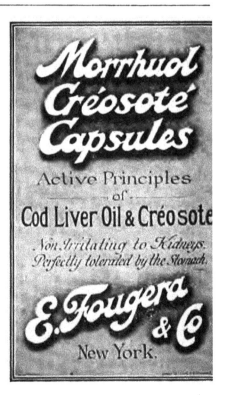

hot pack or infusion of digitalis, if kidneys do not functionate; caffeine for cardiac complications; whiskey or brandy in small doses frequently repeated; liquid nourishment; an enema daily, if needed, of oil and suds; room well ventilated and not above 60°F.

Pelvic Cellulitis. Hirst states that this affection will yield in the majority of cases to rest in bed, counter-irritation and poultices over lower abdomen and hot vaginal douches. If these fail, abdominal section should be made, and if inflammation is confined strictly to the pelvic connective tissue, close abdominal wound; if infected area has suppurated, open by incision above Poupart's ligament or through the vaginal vault.

Mississippi Valley Medical Association. The officers elected at the 30th Annual Meeting of the Mississippi Valley Medical Association, held at Cincinnati, O., Sept. 11–13, are as follows:

President, Bransford Lewis, M.D., St. Louis; First Vice-President, Frank Parsons Norbury, M.D., Jacksonville, Ill.; Second Vice-President, J. H. Carstens, M.D., Detroit, Mich.; Secretary, Henry Enos Tuley, M.D., Louisville, Ky.; Assistant Secretary, John F. Barnhill, M.D., Indianapolis, Ind.; Treasurer, S. C. Stanton, M.D., Chicago, Ill. Next place of meeting Indianapolis, Ind., October, 1905. Henry Enos Tuley, Secretary.

Distressing Cough with Tenacious Expectoration. Knopf prescribes ℞ Codeinae gr. ⅛—1-6 (or heroin, gr. 1–16), acidi sulph. dil. m. ii; glycerini, aquae l, aurocerasi aa. m. x; syrupiprun. virg. m. xx; syr. tolu. q. s: A teaspoonful whenever cough becomes distressing—not more than six doses as a rule in 24 hours. For this same annoying cough Murrell prescribes: ℞ Codeinae gr. ⅛; acidi hydrochlor, dil. m. i; spt. chloroformi m. iii; syrupi limonis m. iii; aquam q. s.: A teaspoonful as occasion demands.

Diphtheritic Metritis. If the cervix is attacked, says Garrigues paint the inner surface once thoroughly with a 50 per cent solution of zinc chloride. Wash out the uterus with carbolized water once a day. Introduce an iodoform pencil (5 drams iodoform, ½ dram starch, ½ dram of glycerin, 1 dram acacia) to fundus and leave to melt. Give quinine, stimulants and ferric chloride internally. If the disease is true diphtheria, antitoxin is, of course, the first thing to use. Sustain vital powers with alcohol, strychnine, digitalis and frequent forced feeding.

Treatment of Pulmonary Edema. Osler directs to treat primary condition, use active catharsis in acute cases, and free venesection if cyanosis. For heart disease, prompt treatment is needed, says Taylor, with the usual cardiac tonics, diuretics and purgatives; for Bright's disease, diaphoretics and purgatives or vapor baths; in elderly people with failing heart, cardiac and general tonics. Ammonium carbonte is particularly valuable. For local edema from loss of tone after inflammation, iron, mineral acids and sometimes small doses of digitalis are recommended by Powell.

Treatment of Hyperesthesia Gastrica. For underlying anemia a good remedy is iron (chloride in egg water) with full doses of arsenic on a full stomach, along with vegetable bitters. Locally Ewald employs morphine with one-tenth as much atropine sulphate in bitter almond water; also cocaine hydrochlorate, gr. 5-6 to ½. He treats the hysterical form as follows: ℞ Morphi hydrochlor. two parts, cocaine hydrochlor, 3 to 5 parts, tinct. belladonnae 50 to 100 parts; bitter almond water 250 parts: Take 10 to 15 drops every hour. Or give chloral in three to five per cent solution, sometimes with cocaine every one-half to two hours; or bromides up 30 or 45 grs. two or three times a day.

Tuberculac Cough. Shoemaker prescribes: ℞ Creasoti m. i-iii; tinct. gent. comp. m. xxx; spt. frumenti ad. ʒii: Take four times daily. Tyson has the chest painted twice a day with a mixture of one dram of croton oil, two drams of tincture of iodine and five drams of ether. Coghill advises the use of the respirator with three parts of guaiacol to one part of chloroform, and Murrell employs inhalations once or twice daily of compressed air made to bubble through six per cent solution of formaldehyde. Mays prescribes: ℞ Tinct. capsici m. ii-xv; ext. euphorb. pilulif. fl., tinct. benzoini co. aa. m. x; chloroformi m. i-ii: Take four times daily.

Treatment of Acute Metritis. Garrigues recommends rest in bed; an ice-bag or ice-water coil over the symphysis (warm poultice or hot-water bag if due to menstrual suppression from cold); vaginal douches of plain warm water (100°—105° F.) t. i. d. or oftener; a luke-warm sitz bath once or twice a day, or a general warm bath every other day if necessary movements do not hurt patient; five grains of quinine every four hours. Keep the bow-

The Family Laxa= tive

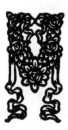

California Fig Syrup Company

San Francisco,
California.

Louisville, Ky.
New York, N. Y.

The ideal, safe, family laxative, known as "Syrup of Figs," is a product of the California Fig Syrup Co., and derives its laxative principles from senna, made pleasant to the taste and more acceptable to the stomach by being combined with pleasant aromatic syrups and the juice of figs. It is recommended by many of the most eminent physicians, and used by millions of families with entire satisfaction. It has gained its great reputation with the medical profession by reason of the acknowledged skill and care exercised by the California Fig Syrup Co. in securing the laxative principles of the senna by an original method of its own, and presenting them in the best and most convenient form. The California Fig Syrup Co. has special facilities for commanding the choicest qualities of Alexandria senna, and its chemists devote their entire attention to the manufacture of the one product. The name "Syrup of Figs" means to the medical profession "the family laxative, manufactured by the California Fig Syrup Co." and the name of the company is a guarantee of the excellence of its product. Informed of the above facts, the careful physician will know how to prevent the dispensing of worthless imitations when he recommends or prescribes the original and genuine "Syrup of Figs." It is well known to physicians that "Syrup of Figs" is a simple, safe and reliable laxative, which does not irritate or debilitate the organs on which it acts, and, being pleasant to the taste, it is especially adapted to ladies and children, although generally applicable in all cases. Special investigation of the profession invited.

"Syrup of Figs" is never sold in bulk. It retails at fifty cents per bottle, and the name "Syrup of Figs," as well as the name of the California Fig Syrup Co., is printed on the wrappers and labels of every bottle.

The advent of the season in which

COUGH,
BRONCHITIS,
WHOOPING COUGH,
ASTHMA, ETC.

Impose a tax upon the resources of every physician renders it opportune to re-invite attention to the fact that the remedy which invariably effects the immediate relief of these disturbances, the remedy which unbiased observers assert affords the most rational means of treatment, the remedy which bears with distinction the most exacting comparisons, the remedy which occupies the most exalted position in the esteem of discriminating therapeutists is

GLYCO-HEROIN (Smith)

GLYCO-HEROIN (Smith) is conspicuously valuable in the treatment of Pneumonia, Phthisis, and Chronic Affections of the Lungs, for the reason that it is more prompt and decided in effect than either codeine or morphine, and its prolonged use neither leaves undesirable after effects nor begets the drug habit. It acts as a reparative in an unsurpassable manner.

> DOSE.—The adult dose is one teaspoonful, repeated every two hours, or at longer intervals as the case may require.
> To children of ten or more years, give from a quarter to a half teaspoonful.
> To children of three or more years, give five to ten drops.

MARTIN H. SMITH CO.,

PROPRIETORS.

SAMPLES SUPPLIED

CARRIAGE PAID, UPON REQUEST   NEW YORK, N. Y,

—22—

els open. When the most acute symptoms have subsided, exchange ice-bag for Priessnitz's compress, paint tincture of iodine on the abdomen and roof of vagina, and introduce a glycerin tampon into the vagina.

Hypertrophy of Posterior End of Inferior Turbinate. Posterior rhinoscopy reveals a large, rounded mass with pale, uneven, smooth, reddish mulberry-like surface at the posterior end of the inferior turbinate. Coakley advises removal of the swelling with cold snare, or better with galvanocautery snare at red heat. Control hemorrhage with hot water or hydrogen peroxide or Bernay's sponge or packing with gauze, or by applying from behind on a cotton-wound nasopharyngzal applicator a thick, syrupy solution of tannic acid in water. These measures failing, plug posterior nares with absorbant cotton with the acid of a gum elastic catheter and a strong, small piece of twine a yard long—never leaving plug in situation more than 24 hours.

Pleural Exudates and Transudates. From an accurate laboratory study of 36 specimens, Herbert S. Carter (*Medical News, Oct. 1*) concludes that the diagnosis of tuberculous pleurisy may be based on the high specific gravity of exudate (1:012-1.024; average 1.018); and a large amount of fibrin and albumin, with accompanying lymphocytosis. There is usually at the outset a considerable rise of temperature, which may average 103.-4°. A diagnosis of post-pneumonic serous effusion lies in its high specific gravity (averaging 1.0165), large fibrin and albumin content, and polymorphonuclear lencocytosis (average 71.7 per cent.) The temperature is usually much lower than in the tuberculous cases, unless complicating an active pneumonia, averaging at outset about 101°. Both pleural transudates and tuberculous pleurisies show a lymphocytosis, but the latter has a high fibrin and albumin content, the former a small amount of these.

Blood Pressure from the Therapeutic Aspect. Comparing the value of drugs in this regard, S. B. Briggs (quoted in *Progressive Medicine*), stated that the use of capsicum causes a rise of equal height and duration as that from whiskey, but without the subsequent fall produced in the case of whiskey by depression of the vosomator centers. Strychnine and digitalin, given subcutaneously, raise the pressure less quickly but for a longer time (one to three hours)—longer after strychnine than after digitalin.

Their combination is therefore a most valuable agent in shock and
in toxic states. Subcutaneous injections of normal saline solution
are not found to be true cardiovascular stimulants any more than
alcohol, and their uses must be explained from some other point
of view.

Goutiness. Oliver's experiments (quoted in *Progressive
Medicine*) confirm the view that goutiness is primarily due to a
retention of waste products dependent upon a disturbance of
lymph-capillary intermediary circulation, their removal being prevented either by excessive capillary blood pressure, or by a diminution of that pressure such as to reduce the fluid exchange between blood and tissue.

Brandycardia. Ewart (*Progressive Medicine*) sums up
his rational views as follows: There is first the great distinction
between the physiologic and the pathologic slowness of the heart.
Thd first group contains not only the congenital or inherited variety, but that also which may occur in pregnancy. Slow action is
part of the order of things in certain individuals, and is not to be
acquired. The pathologic or original slowness is in its etiology
most various, but occurs under two distinct types, the paroxysmal
and the continuous or chronic; the latter, being associated with
vascular disease, is less common and more unfavorable. The paroxysmal variety has different degrees of gravity. An important
groupe is that regarded by Satterthwaite as connected with gastro-
intestinal irritations, and reminds us of the similar etiology of
some paroxysmal tachycardias. Another strong analogy is brought
out by the results of treatment. Remedies addressed to the abnormal rhythm are not only useless as correctives, but apt to do harm.
It is the *causa causans* that we should endeavor to treat. The
pathologic slowness of heart is, I believe, to be regarded as an
evidence of weakness rather than of strength, both in the chronic
variety and in the paroxysmal, and the foundation for all treatment in both forms seem to be rest rather than stimulation. As
insisted by Satterthwaite, alcoholic over-stimulation is the worst
form of accelerator treatment in these cases.

A CASE OF AESTIVO-AUTUMNAL MALARIA.*

BY D. MACDOUGALL KING, M.B.,

Denver, Colorado,

The infrequency with which malaria is met in Colorado and the comparatively great frequency with which typhoid is met, ought, I think, to make a case of malaria, of decidedly typhoidal appearance, one of more than ordinary interest to our Society.

The case I am about to report is that of a young man, 30 years of age, who came to Colorado some three months ago. Previous to coming here he had lived all his life on a farm in southern Missouri. For the last seven years, at irregular intervals, especially in the summer, he has experienced attacks of pain of a dull character across the abdomen, accompanied with fever, frequently followed by sweats, but never preceded by a chill. For the last two or three years these attacks have become much more severe, and the intervals are always accompanied with lassitude, stiffness, and sometimes aching pains. There is nothing in the family history particularly interesting, save that Mr. F. had two brothers similarly affected. The one came to Colorado and recovered, while the other remains at home in misery. Three years ago the patient is said to have had typhoid fever, and several months ago, upon consulting three specialists in St. Louis, he was informed by them that his stomach was "full of ulcers."

I was first called to see the patient on September 5th, 1904. At that time his temperature was 103 degrees and he complained of an intense headache and of feeling sore all over. He wore a listless typhoidal expression. The skin was considerably jaundiced, and the lips and mucous membranes were rather pale. His tongue was furred and breath fetid, abdomen distended and very tender, and the bowels constipated. The spleen was much enlarged, extending upward to the lower border of the fifth rib and downward to two inches below the costal margin in the anterior

---

*Read before the City and County of Denver Medical Society.

axillary line. The liver, probably as a result of the upward pressure of the distended gut, was slightly displaced in an upward
direction, reaching, in the mammary line, to the lower border of
the fourth rib. The pulse was running at 120 and dicrotic in
character, and along the left margin of the sternum could be
heard a soft systolic murmur of probably hæmic origin.

The diagnosis appeared to rest chiefly between typhoid and
malaria, with a possibility of both conditions existing in the form
of the so-called malario-typhoid. One might also have included
the possibility of a septic condition of the liver. The only way,
to my mind, to be positive about the diagnosis, was to have a careful blood examination. Accordingly, after having the patient removed to St. Luke's Hospital, I sent a blood specimen to Dr.
Mitchell to be examined for the Widal reaction, and called in Dr.
Arneill to examine for plasmodia. Dr. Mitchell reported the
Widal reaction to be negative, but, much to my delight, Dr. Arneill very quickly and successfully demonstrated plasmodia of the
variety known as the "crescent" of Laveran, which is diagnostic of
malaria of the æstivo-autumnal form. According to Osler's description, the crescents are developed within the red blood corpus-
cle, the margin of which may usually be seen on the concave surface of the crescent. The border is very sharply defined, the protoplasm uniform, homogeneous with coarse pigment granules, often
in the form of rods, which are collected about the center. These
features may readily be observed in the specimens which Dr. Arneill has kindly prepared for exhibition.

The further examination of the blood revealed 70 per cent of
hemoglobin and an absence of any leukocytosis, thereby lessening the possibility of a septic condition of the liver which might
have existed.

From the fact that a blood examination had never before been
made, and the extreme importance of such an examination in
making a correct diagnosis, one might readily ask the question:
Was the attack which occurred two years ago and was diagnosed
as typhoid fever, really a case of typhoid or malaria fever? The
patient reports that, during the attack, he was badly jaundiced,
he perspired very profusely on numerous occasions, and the attack,
lasting between three and four weeks, came to a sudden termination. Without the microscope on that occasion, I feel confident
in saying that an intelligent diagnosis was an utter impossibility.

The treatment was not begun until the plasmodia had been demonstrated, as the administration of quinine causes a disappearance of the plasmodia from the peripheral circulation. As soon as the diagnosis was assured, the system was put under the influence of quinine as quickly as possible. This was accomplished according to Osler's method, viz: By giving calomèl, grains three, in half grain doses, and administering, hypodermically, thirty grains of the bisulphate of quinine with five grains tartaric acid. As this caused considerable local irritation, a pledget soaked in a ten per cent solution of cocaine, was placed on the site of injection for three minutes before administration. The injection was administered two hours before the rise in temperature was expected, there being no chill. Between the attacks, which were of an atypical singly tertian variety, an attempt was made at administration of quinine by rectal suppositories, but the patient was unable to retain them. The stomach being in an irritable condition, the hypodermic was used entirely. In addition to the quinine, between attacks there were used, three times a day, three minims of liquor arsenicalis, directly after nourishment, twenty minims dil. muriatic acid, one-half hour after nourishment, and a quarter grain of podophyllin, one-half hour after nourishment.

The results were most encouraging. Three days after the first administration of quinine the temperature dropped permanently to normal. The patient was then placed on Gudes' peptomangan and left the hospital a week later. As the stomach had greatly improved he was able, after going home, to take, per os, three grains of quinine five times a day. This he continued for four days and as, at that time, the stomach showed signs of returning irritability, the quinine was dropped except for one day in each week.

TYPHOID FEVER. *

By A. C. EWING, M.D.,

Salt Lake City, Utah.

There has been so much written about typhoid fever, its etiology, pathology, general characteristics, treatment, etc., and by
men renowned as investigators in medical science, that it would
seem presumptuous in me to make an effort to add anything prac
tical to the management or treatment of a disease that has baffled
the skill of the profession from the days of Hippocrates to the
present time. Yet, however old a disease may be, the fact that it
is still the subject of much discussion makes it ever new to all
busy investigators after truth. Though its etiology is well understood, its pathological lesions familiar to all, there are many
things about typhoid fever that are still obscure; for aside from
the Brand method of cold water bathing, but little real advancement has been made as to the *cure* since the days of our fore-
fathers. It seems that certain glands (possibly all) have what
might be called a "selective function," that is, each variety of
gland selects, or takes up from the blood certain poisons or germs.
For example: The parotid gland selects a certain unknown poison or germ and as a result we have parotitis, or mumps. The
spleen seems to select the malarial germ, the lungs the pneumococcus. The liver acts as a crucible to germ life, besides having
the power to arrange from the blood chemical material to make
bile, and the stomach, pepsin and hydrochloric acid. "May not
the office of the glands of Peyer be to select from the contents of
the bowel the bacillus of Eberth, thereby setting up an inflammation of these glands as in a case of specific parotitis, and where
the selective office of the spleen renders it a victim of hypertrophy and abscess?"

There is no doubt that the primary cause of typhoid is the
bacillus discovered by Eberth in 1880, and upon entering the alimentary canal finds lodgement (whether selected or not) in Peyer's
patches. First, a hyperplasia is produced, then an inflammation,
followed (unless a resolution takes place—which is doubted by
many) by partial or complete strangulation of the blood supply,
resulting in ulceration, necrosis, and general systemic infection.

*Read before the Rocky Mountain Inter-State Medical Association, Sept., 1904.

The germ is carried by so many different ways, that makes it sometimes difficult to trace the real source of infection. That it gains access to the human body through the medium of water, milk or food, is not questioned, through the water that is used in drinking or cooking, and when traceable to milk, the bacilli are usually introduced in the water with which the milk is diluted or through the water used in washing the milk cans and bottles. Other common ways of infection are by the hands that have been contaminated by the dejections, as well as the conveyance of the germs to our food through the medium of the common house fly. So as it has often been demonstrated that typhoid fever is an index of the purity of the water and milk supply of a city, we cannot be too diligent in our inspection of the milk furnished the people, and the protection of our drinking water from sewage pollution.

Most clinicians ascribe the severity of an attack to the degree of infection. Mild cases, the so-called paratyphoid, is thus accounted for rather than the stronger resistance some have over others in throwing off the disease. Others have thought or have advanced the idea that dilution of the poison by the spring rains is why attacks are milder at this time of the year than in the fall when drouths have concentrated the poison. Vaughan has made some interesting investigations as regards what he calls "atypical forms" of Eberth's bacilli, differing from the standard forms sufficiently to be classed as "varieties." This fact may account for the decidedly atypical types all of us occasionally encounter.

McClintock claimed that immunity is observed in those having had one attack, and attributed the immunity to the presence in the blood of certain enzymes, which, when brought in contact with the bacilli of typhoid digest, or cause the bacilli to be dissolved. One attack does give a certain immunity, but according to my observation, it is not longer than from four to six years. I have taken advantage of this supposed immunity and have injected the serum from convalescents into the subcutaneous tissue of those sick with typhoid, but with indifferent success. The theory, I think, is a good one, but the method was abandoned, owing to the difficulty of procuring the serum. Inoculation for immunity has been tried, Billings having reported success with the inoculation of some 2,000 soldiers during the Cuban war. From other and later reports however, the procedure offers but little hope of complete immunization. It is well to note, that with a thorough knowledge of the cause, together with the means of disposal of the dejecta, the morbidity has been greatly reduced and the mortality lowered.

As to the diagnosis: Its objective and subjective symptoms are well defined, as a rule, and with the characteristic rise and fall of temperature, together with the aid of Widal's blood and the diazo reaction tests, none of us need experience but little difficulty in differentiating typhoid from a few other diseases whose symptomatology bears a likeness that is striking, and at times, confusing. The leucocyte count is a great help when one is in doubt as to differential diagnosis between typhoid, meningitis, and appendicitis; the two latter showing marked leucocytosis. In this disease there is a "constant stream of pathogenic germs aside from the bacilli of Eberth, infecting the intestinal tract." To prevent the invasion into the blood and the tissues of the toxic elements resulting from these germs, there must be present the destructive fluids and the resisting powers of the intestinal cells. The intestinal wall is usually sufficient in holding back the damaging bacilli and their toxins so long as ulceration does not occur, but so soon as necrosis of Peyer's patches takes place, toxæmia supervenes— the toxins taking a short and easy route into the blood and general system along with the chyle. Once these toxic elements enter the circulation, we get all the characteristic phenomena peculiar to this disease, and so long as the morbific agents remain active, so long will the disease continue.

Nature is constantly striving at elimination, throwing off the poison by the bowels, kidneys, skin and even the lungs; hence our treatment should be directed largely along this line—that of elimination. That there is elimination by the lungs is evidenced by the "typhoid odour" always present and so marked at times that one can almost make a diagnosis by the breath alone. It is probable this may account also for the so-called typhoid cough. We know but few infectious diseases in which we are able to meet the causal indications. Malaria we can control by quinine, syphilis by mercury and potassium iodide, acute rheumatism by sodium salicylate, and diphtheria by antitoxin—and we might add the thyroid extract in the treatment of myxædema, and the encouraging specific treatment in tetanus and yellow fever. After looking over the achievements of the past, can we be satisfied with the progress thus far made in the use of specific medication? The usual typhoid treatment with most physicians, of the present day, is to depend almost wholly upon the vis medicatrix naturæ—to treat symptoms as they arise and make but little effort (if any) to remove the underlying cause. "Excuse for this kind of treatment is rational only when the cause is unknown, or if known, it is irremediable. Another excuse might be, that when we know the cause to be transient, and of such a nature, that it may be with safety left to itself." When such conditions as these exist, if we but regulate the various functions of the body and gird them up as nearly as possible to a normal physiological condition, is about all one need do. But in the disease under consideration, we know the primary cause and can unerringly interpret the origin of the multiplicity of its symptoms. One should not lose sight of nor undervalue the forensic strength that is laid up in the storehouse of nature, but I am confident that we have drugs at our command, the proper administration of which, if they do not destroy will at least inhibit the growth and virulence of these enfeebling devitalizing germs, and thus relieve nature before she has exhausted the supply from which she manufactures the arms necessary for her defense. · We wish to oppose one of the old-time notions in regard to typhoid, and still exists in the minds of many able physicians, and that is, that it is a let-it-run-its course disease. In other words, that it is a disease of a self-limiting character; that we should simply watch a patient as he passes "successively through the infection, ulceration, intoxication, wasting, lowered vitality and dissolution and make no effort to treat the disease per se." Toxins already absorbed into the blood are speedily gotten rid of, if the focus of infection is discovered and can be reached. It is the continuous *fresh* supply of toxins that does the mischief. The object then aimed at in the treatment is to turn our batteries on the micro-organisms at the point where the defense is weakest and if we are not able to kill, we can at least inhibit their activity and thereby reduce the production of their poisonous excreta.

This is an era of antisepsis, and so far as my limited experience goes, intestinal antisepsis is the sheet-anchor in the treatment of this formidable disease. Antisepsis may be accomplished by certain drugs acting upon the germs and the diseased glands and follicles as local antiseptics, and by the well-known power of a number of systemic antiseptics (such as calomel, podophyllin, &c.)

in stimulating glandular secretion.   All admit that bile is an intestinal antiseptic, and in cases where this secretion is interfered
with we lose one of nature's greatest means of bowel disinfection.
It is claimed that the bacilli have been found in the gall bladder,
but if so I venture to say they were as dead as door nails.   So,
with small, repeated doses of calomel we favor not only the reduction of intestinal toxicity by greater fæcal evacuations, but also
the increased flow of antiseptic bile, thereby lessening the chances
of further infection.   Peristaltic action, not too active, is helpful
in this disease, by preventing the stagnation of poisonous matter
in the intestines—a circumstance most favorable for auto-intoxication—especially when daily colonic flushing, which I always use,
is barren of results.   I am not in the habit of stopping a diarrhœa, it being mostly due to fermentative changes going on in the
bowels, and should therefore rather be encouraged than otherwise.
There is a vast difference, be it remembered, between a germicide
and an antiseptic; the former destroys the germ, while the latter
inhibits its growth and multiplication.   It requires 1 to 1,000
mercuric chloride to destroy the anthrax spores, but only 1 to
300,000 strength will prevent their development.

Doctor M. M. Felt, President of the Concord, New Hamp-
shire Medical Association, in an address before that body in July
last, in speaking of intestinal antisepsis says: "In my opinion
much of the beneficial effect of the internal administration of calomel is due to its antiseptic and disinfectant or germicidal influence on the ptomains and toxins in the alimentary canal."

In fact, Bouchard, and many others, long ago, verified the
utility and practicability of intestinal antiseptics; and yet, on the
other hand, very many able physicians contend that they are useless, the great difficulty being, they claim, to get the antiseptic
unchanged to the source of infection.   Some of the radical opponents of intestinal antiseptics, in order to gain a point, are now
claiming that the intestinal lesions are, instead of being primary,
the result of metastases.

That the disease originates in the infection of Peyer's patches,
there is no doubt.   One can readily understand why antiseptics
per se would be of no use in a disease like tuberculosis—you cannot get the medicine in contact with the germs; but in typhoid it
is different, as we here have an avenue to the seat of the disease
practically open.   My mode of treatment of typhoid is to some

extent original, in so far as I know, in the administration of intes-testinal antiseptics. Taking advantage of a well-known fact that an oil is not absorbed from the stomach, but is passed through the pylorus into the duodenum in its original state and is taken up by the lacteals and used in the economy only after its thorough emulsification, I administer the antiseptics, composed usually of resorcin, and boric acid, incorporated in pure olive oil. Owing to the fact that there is a scarcity of bile and pancreatic juice, a swift and thorough emulsion of the oil does not take place, thus favoring the results ought to be accomplished. The infinitesimal mouths of the lacteals being unable to take up the but partially emulsified globules, the oil is allowed to pass on slowly through the intestinal labyrinth, giving out its germicidal properties all along the way. Thus, by repeated doses the intestinal canal is kept more or less completely under the influence of an efficient germicide or antiseptic—the bacilli and other germs being either destroyed or driven to corner; helpless, and unable to perform their deadly excretory function. This, with the graduated cold bath, and strychnia, when needed, constitute the treatment I have adopted the past two years with signal success. Resorcin is not only an ideal antiseptic (equal to that of boric acid) but possesses besides both antifermentative and antipyretic properties. Strych-nia in its action approaches that of electricity. It is a direct ton-ifier of the nervous system and indirectly of muscular fiber, there-by equalizing blood distribution and relieving an over-worked heart. I usually give 5 grs. of resorcin and 10 grs. of boric acid incorporated in ʒii of oil every three or four hours. I am now using the resorcin and boric acid in tablet form coated with salol. If a little saccharine and oil of peppermint are added, the mixture is not unpleasant to take; and besides, the oil is a decided nutriment to the patient. Dr. Gilman Thomson, in a paper entitled: "Modern Treatment of Typhoid Fever," read recently before the New York Medical Association avers that the "apparent" good accomplished by intestinal antiseptics is due to intestinal antifermentatives. Then he goes on and says: "Persistant tympanites, with a rigid, distended and tender abdomen is a condition more to be dreaded than any symptom, not even excepting intestinal hemorrhage."

As to the "why," the advocates of intestinal antiseptics do not wish to keep up a controversy, so the treatment is beneficial to the patient. One cares not whether the administration of a drug acts as an antiseptic or as an antifermentative, so long as one gets good results. The most radical opponents to the treatment will certainly admit that it is decidedly more rational to administer the intestinal antiseptic (or intestinal antifermentative if you please) *before* the abdomen becomes "tender" and "rigid"—before the "serious distention" of the bowel occurs,—thereby lessening to a marked degree the stretching of the eroding ulcers—thus avoiding the consequent danger of an extreme perforation. (I will say here in way of parenthesis, that when the symptoms point to an extreme and unmistakable perforation, no valuable time should be lost with opium, adrenalin, etc. The case then resolves itself into a surgical one, and the treatment which has been encouragingly successful, is the opening of the abdomen immediately, and closing the rent). The graduated bath is preferable in the majority of cases; the Brand, or very cold one, being used only in cases where the stimulant effect of the cold plunge on the psychical centers is urgently demanded. The bath, when the antiseptic treatment is used, from the start, is not needed so much for its antipyretic action, but more for its effect in the elimination of toxine through the kidneys and skin. Examination after the bath shows the toxicity of the urine has increased to six times that of the normal. (Billings.) Give plenty of sterilized water, but *do not over-feed*. Unlike ordinary cases of temporary indigestion, where one or more of the digestive secretions may be deficient or at fault, we are here confronted with a condition in which not only are the *essential* glands temporarily disabled, refusing to secrete their respective ferments, but where almost the entire alimentary tract is involved. Over-feeding in a dilemma like this will only result in putrefactive changes, with accompanying distention and elevation of temperature. Sterilized milk is generally the best diet, with the addition to it of a little lime water, and given in moderate quantities. When this disagrees, and it will with some, resort may be had to the peptonoids, and egg albumen, followed by diluted hydrochloric acid to favor its digestion.

Typhoid fever, as well as the entire range of infectious and contagious diseases, invites us to patient, pains-taking investigation, and if the "bacteriologist and the clinician would join hands in a quest for antagonists to disease, specific medication would perhaps add many new triumphs to match the sombre achievements of pathology and the brilliant successes of surgery!"

DISCUSSION OF DR. EWING'S PAPER.

Dr. Wiest. I am hardly prepared, Mr. Chairman, to open the discussion of this paper on "Typhoid Fever." I have listened to it with a great deal of pleasure and profit. The treatment which Dr. Ewing suggests is one which is quite new to me, and seems to be very rational; and that is to get the intestinal antiseptics to the seat of the trouble in a medium which is not greatly interfered with before it gets to the diseased portion.

I would like to remark upon his suggestion, which is, of course, old, and yet never so old but what it is of service to us; not to over-feed the patients. I believe that in typhoid fever pretty near a starvation diet is quite the thing, just so you do not deplete your patients' strength to too great a degree. There is more danger from over-feeding than from a very, very light diet, because you can combat a weakness caused from lack of food later on after you have the disease under control.

Dr. Munro. I think, as Dr. Ewing has pointed out, it is emphatically necessary to get at these cases of perforation early with surgical treatment. Osler, I believe it was, urged some years ago that the surgeon and the physician should watch typhoid cases together. I do not believe that there is any one group of symptoms that always points to a definite perforation; or to the time when perforation has taken place; but if the physician is willing to let the surgeon visit his cases with him, that is, of course, the cases where there is at least suspicion of any abdominal infection, I think we can lower the mortality.

There is no question but that in these cases, if they are operated upon in the very early stages, before a general peritonitis has taken place, a large proportion can be saved; at least after an individual perforation. They may die later of secondary perforations, or of the typhoid infection, but I believe a large majority can be saved if they can be operated upon promptly. During a number of years we have watched a good many cases of typhoid at the city hospital in Boston, and it seems to me that in going over them year after year, those patients whom the physician allowed us to follow along conjointly, were the ones that gave us the best results. Moreover, I think it is only fair to say that the surgeon's definition of spasm is different from that of the physician, and that the surgeon who is dealing with intra-abdominal

infections will detect a spasm a little more quickly than a physician, and it is most important that this detection should be made
early in the history of these cases.

NORMAL OBSTETRICS.

(CHAPTER EIGHT.)

THE MATERNAL CHANGES DURING PREGNANCY.

By T. MITCHELL BURNS, M.D.,

Denver, Colorado.

Professor of Obstetrics, The Denver and Gross College of Medicine.

THE IMPORTANCE OF STUDYING THE MATERNAL CHANGES.

The study of maternal changes is of importance because it
is essential to the study of the diagnosis, hygiene and pathology
of pregnancy.

The Different Maternal Changes.—The maternal changes
include changes in the nutrition and body weight, the form, pose,
nervous system, face, thyroid gland, breasts, thorax, respiration,
heart, blood, abdominal walls, digestive system, liver, spleen, lymphatics, bowels, bladder, urine, pelvic bones and ligaments, the
vulva, vagina, uterus, tubes and ovaries, ovulation, menstruation
and changes in other organs and functions. (The preceding order, that is, first, the more general symptoms, then the more local
changes arranged according to their situation from the head downward, is used to aid the memory.)

The Cause of the Maternal Changes.—These changes are
due to the presence of the growing ovum in the uterus modifying
the nervous system so that it produces qualitative and quantitative changes in the blood.

The Nutrition and Body Weight.—The nutrition and body
weight during the first three months are diminished from lack of
food due to the nausea and vomiting, increased work and to the
nervous condition, but there are many exceptions to this rule
where there is an increase of weight from the beginning. After
the third month, or at least after quickening, the weight increases
from return of the appetite and increasing digestion. Many pri-

migravidæ feel in better health all through the nine months than they ever have before. This is due to the normal condition of the uterus, which is rarely as perfect in a multigravida, as the phenomena of labor have left their markings. Loss of weight may occur in the last two months from conditions unfavorable to nutrition, as death of the fetus and its retention in utero, recurring nausea and vomiting, albuminuria and other toxemias. The average increase in weight at term is about 1-10.

The Form.—The form becomes stout. The parts that especially enlarge are the abdomen, hips, buttocks and breasts.

The Pose.—The pose is marked; the shoulders are thrown back, and there is a carefulness of step.

The Nervous System.—The nervous system is usually affected. Nervousness is frequently present. The mental condition sometimes undergoes a complete change. Cheerful women become ill-tempered, and ill-tempered cheerful.

Fear is often present and as a result the patient expects that she or her baby is going to die or that the baby will be marked. Meddlesome neighbors are the most frequent cause of excessive fear. They talk of all the frightful cases that have ever happened in their imagination, and exaggerate any real cases about which they have heard.

In the early months the mental condition is generally depressed; rarely the melancholia ends in mania. The memory is weakened, especially in those who bear children in close succession.

Neuralgia and pruritus from increased sensibility, often occur. Numbness from impaired circulation is generally present at some time during pregnancy, and occurs especially in the limbs. Dizziness is another nervous symptom.

The Face.—The face becomes changed in complexion and expression and is pigmented. In the early months the expression is often anxious and the complexion anemic; later the complexion is generally plethoric.

Pigmentation of the face, or "the mask of pregnancy" is most marked upon the forehead and is of a dirty brownish color or rarely nearly black. As a rule it disappears after labor or at least after lactation, but sometimes it remains permanently. It is closely allied to the skin disease called chloasma, or "liver spots," and probably is due to the condition of the liver, as the liver changes of pregnancy and chloasma are relieved by phosphate of soda.

The Thyroid Gland.—The thyroid gland enlarges. Lusk says, that where goitre is endemic or when there is a predisposition to enlargement of the gland pregnancy may cause temporary or permanent goitre.

The Breast Changes.—The mammary glands undergo changes both primary and secondary. The primary changes: These changes occur between the second and third month and are increased sensitiveness and tingling, especially of the nipples, enlargement of the primary areolæ, nipples, veins, and whole breast and increased pigmentation of the primary areolæ and nipples. The increased sensitiveness and tingling is due to congestion. The primary areola, or colored area around the nipple, increases in size to 1 or $1\frac{1}{2}$ inches and becomes edematous. The veins appear in blue streaks.

The breasts enlarge from increase of glandular, connective and adipose tissue. The glandular tissue gives the knotty feeling to the breasts.

The pigmentation of the primary areolæ and nipples is rose or brown, according as the complexion is light or dark.

The secondary changes: These changes occur between the 5th and 6th month and consist of the appearance of the secondary areola, the colostrum, the glands of Montgomery and striæ.

The secondary areola appears around the primary and resembles dusty blotting paper upon which drops of water have been sprinkled. It is due to growth of non-pigmented sebaceous follicles.

Colostrum, the milk-like fluid of the breasts, is generally present in the last three months and may be present as early as the third month.

The glands of Montgomery are 10 or 12 enlarged sebaceous follicles or rudimentary mammary glands, which appear in the areola. The striæ (striæ gravidarum, lineæ albicantes or cicatrices of pregnancy) are reddish or glistening streaks, (white if old), which appear on the skin of the breasts and are due to the stretching of the skin from the increase of tissue beneath it. (Striæ occur on the breasts and other parts of the body of the non-pregnant from the same cause. They are often seen at puberty, in obese women, and pathologic distension.)

Postfebrile atrophy also causes this striation, especially after typhoid and scarlet fever. (It may be idiopathic.)

The Thorax.—The thorax is increased in breadth, but diminished in depth, and generally towards the end of pregnancy the vital capacity of the lungs is some diminished by the high position of the fundus.

Respiration.—In primigravidæ the respiration becomes more oppressed than in multigravidæ because of the higher position of the fundus. Near the term this oppression lessens more in primigravidæ because the uterus sinks more than in multigravidæ. (The amount of carbon consumed is increased and the amount of carbonic acid exhaled is augmented.)

The Heart Changes.—The heart changes consist usually of an eccentric hypertrophy of the left ventricle to compensate for the increased amount of work the heart has to do. When this hypertrophy does not occur, there is an increase in the frequency of the heart beat to take its place. With the hypertrophy the pulse is usually below 70, without it the pulse is often 100 to 120. This hypertrophy disappears after labor or lactation. A rapid pulse is sometimes due to the unstable condition of the nervous system. The pulse often has the same frequency whether the woman is lying, sitting or standing. This is due to the hypertrophy of the heart.

The Blood.—The blood is increased in amount. In the first half of pregnancy it is generally hydremic, because of the drain on the system made by the growing fetus, the increased tissue waste and the inability to take and assimulate food. The leucocytes are increased in number.

In the second half of pregnancy there is as a rule not only an increase above the average of the total number of red blood corpuscles but also of the hemoglobin. The fibrin diminishes up to the sixth month, but after the sixth month increases and at term is two-fifths more than normal. This explains why blood clots more readily in labor at term than in a miscarriage.

The Abdominal (Wall) Changes.—The abdominal (wall) changes consist of alterations in the size and shape of the abdomen, the thickness of the wall, the condition of the navel, the appearance of striæ, pigmentation and costal pain and the separation of the recti muscles.

The size of the abdomen increases progressively after the 4th month and sometimes after the 2nd month.

The shape changes. At about the 2nd month the depression normal above the iliac crests lessens, and flattening of the lower abdomen somtimes occurs from sinking of the uterus. Later the shape changes markedly by the antero-posterior diameter increasing more rapidly than the transverse.

The thickness of the wall is lessened from stretching, but in the well-nourished there is a compensatory thickening from a deposit of fat.

The navel at the 5th month begins to diminish in depth, at the 7th month it is level with the skin and subsequently protrudes.

Striæ occur on the lower abdomen and also on the nates and thighs in the latter half of pregnancy.

Pigmentation of a dirty brownish color occurs on the linea alba from the pubes to the navel, and often encircles the navel and extends upward to the sternum.

Costal pain, i. e., a painful sensation at the costal insertions of the abdominal muscles, is not rare. It is due to the distention of the abdomen causing pulling on the insertion of the abdominal muscles, or is referred from uterine congestion. It occurs especially in multigravidæ because the existing relaxation of the abdominal muscles allows the abdominal contents to sag against the abdominal wall and to pull on its muscles, and because of the relative frequency of uterine congestion in multigravidæ. It occurs more often on the right side because the uterus, being inclined to the right, causes more sagging on the right side.

Separation (diastasis) of the recti muscles generally occurs. It is due to the stretching of the abdomen from the increased intra-abdominal pressure and to the standing posture. (Pathologically it is due to short vertical abdominal diameter and contracted pelvis; the latter prevents the entrance of the fetus into the pelvis.) Diastasis is best noticed after labor, as then the whole width of the hand can be passed in between the two recti muscles above the fundus. It generally disappears two or three weeks after labor. If permanent, it causes constipation and necessitates the use of the forceps in future labors.

The Digestive Apparatus.—Nausea and vomiting, or "morning sickness," generally begins soon after the suppression of the menses and continues up to quickening or until the system gets used to the uterine irritation which causes it. (Quickening probably acts by creating new thoughts, thoughts of the future baby rather than of self). This sickness usually occurs in the morning upon rising. In the latter part of pregnancy it may occur from pressure of the fundus upon the stomach or pathologically from blood or kidney disorder.

The appetite is frequently capricious, and "longings" or desire for peculiar articles of food occur.

The Liver, Spleen and Lymphatics.—The liver, spleen and lymphatics are enlarged. (Fatty infiltration of the liver is said to occur beginning around the portal vein and consisting of spots varying in size from that of a pin head to a millet seed).

The Bowels.—The bowels as a rule are constipated but diarrhea may occur, especially at the time for a menstrual period.

The Bladder.—The bladder changes its location with the changes in the position of the uterus, i. e., as the uterus sinks it becomes lower, as the uterus grows it rises into the abdomen. This is due to the close proximity and attachment of the bladder to the uterus.

Vesical irritation is present at the beginning of pregnancy and frequently continues until term. This irritation is due to the same cause as the changes in the position of the bladder, and also probably to the close relation of the uterine and vesical nerve supply.

The Urine.—The urine is increased in quantity. The total solids are diminished, except the chlorides and urea. Albuminuria to the amount of 6 per cent is said to exist in 10 per cent. of all pregnant women near term, and most of these cases are considered to be physiologic, but it is best to regard all cases of albuminuria as pathologic. The worst cases of eclampsia may previously show only a small percentage of albumin. Physiologic glycosuria is generally present in the latter months of pregnancy.

Kiestein is a peculiar floculent precipitate found on the surface of the urine of pregnant women after it has been standing covered. It is also found on the urine of anemic non-pregnant women and some men, being merely a scum of "triple" phosphates.

The Pelvic Bones.—The pelvic bone changes are slight. (Osteophytes, or bone-like deposits on the inner surface of the pelvis and skull are sometimes present, but may also be found in men.)

The Pelvic Ligaments.—The pelvic ligaments become infiltrated with serum and allow the pelvic joints to give a little, but the majority of authorities believe that this is not sufficient to be of any real value in labor.

The Vulva.—The vulva increases in color, size, secretion and temperature. The color of the vulva becomes bluish or pinkish. The labia gap.

Crosswise or oblique "pinkish streaks on a livid background" run outward from the front part of the vaginal orifice, especially near the urinary meatus.

The blood of the vulva gives the characteristic blood changes more often than the blood from other parts of the body not connected with the genitals.

The Vagina.—The vagina increases in color, size, secretion and temperature as does the vulva. The change in color is especially marked on the lower anterior vaginal wall. The length of the vagina is considerably increased. The papillae in the vagina increases in size and feel like granules. The vaginal secretion is so augmented at the beginning of pregnancy and near term as to constitute a leucorrhea.

The Uterus.—The uterine changes consist of a change in the structures, size and growth, shape (dimensions), situation, weight, capacity, attitude, relations, pressure, properties and the special changes in the cervix (viz., size and growth, softening; mucous plug, shortening and stretching of anterior lip).

The structures of the uterus (muscular fibres, connective tissue, blood vessels, lymphatics and nerves) all increase in size and number (hypertrophy and hyperplasia).

The mucous membrane thickens to form the maternal part of the placenta and the deciduae.

The cervical ganglia increase three times in size.

The size and growth of the uterus increase from the beginning of pregnancy. The site of this increase is mainly the fundus and body.

Stretching of the uterine wall occurs in the latter months, from the uterus not growing as rapidly as the ovum.

The thickness of the uterine wall at the middle of pregnancy is over half an inch ($\frac{5}{8}$) and at term less than half an inch (3-16).

The presence of the ovum in the uterus is not essential to the growth of the uterus, as the uterus grows in extra-uterine pregnancy as much as the nutrition is increased.

The normal anteflexion is increased some by the posterior wall of the fundus and body growing a little faster than the anterior.

The shape of the exterior of the uterus in the first three months is pyriform, in the middle three months more spherical, and during the last three months more ovoidal or balloon-like. These changes in the shape are due to the fact that at first the ovum is growing only in the upper segment, later growing relatively more rapidly in the lower segment than in the upper.

The shape of the cavity of the body, as soon as the ovum fills it, becomes ovoidal and so continues until term. The larger end of this ovoid is at the fundus.

Asymmetry of the body externally and internally occurs often at first from the ovum growing in one part of the cavity. This causes a bulging of a portion or a half of the external surface. Sometimes a well marked external longitudinal furrow exists between the bulging part and the rest of the uterus.

The dimensions of the uterus each month can be remembered by the following rules: The length at the end of the first and second months is three inches. (The anterio-posterior and transverse diameters of the uterus are the ones which are mainly increased in the early months). After the second month the length equals in inches one and one-half times the number of months, e.g., at six months nine inches. The width, (of the body) equals in inches a little more than the number of months, e.g., five months five inches plus. The thickness (body) is in inches a little less than the number of months, e.g., four months four inches minus.

The situation of the uterus is estimated, as is the size, by the height of the fundus.

The height of the fundus each month is given in chapter seven: "The Duration of Pregnancy and the Prediction of the Period of Pregnancy and the Date of Labor."

Sinking of the uterus and fetus, i.e., a slight lowering, occurs from one day to three weeks before labor and is especially marked in primigravidae. In primigravidae the cervix descends from its high position at the brim nearly to the pelvic floor, and the fetus descends a little in the uterus. The sinking of the uterus is due to the resistance of the abdominal muscles, or better, to the constantly increasing intra-abdominal pressure. A proof of this is the fact that in multigravidae when the muscles are relaxed it does not occur. The cause of the fetus descending in the uterus is the increasing irritation which forces the upper segment to retract and enlarge the lower segment. Sinking of the uterus sometimes occurs in the first months of pregnancy from the increased weight of the uterus.

The weight of the uterus increases so that at term it is two pounds. The virgin womb weighs one ounce.

The capacity of the uterus at term is about 500 times that of the virgin uterus which is estimated at one drachm (3.55 c.c.).

The attitude of the uterus during pregnancy is one of ante-flexion, dextroflexion and dextro-torsion. Its ante-flexion is due to an increase of the non-pregnant ante-flexion, from the increased weight of the upper part of the uterus and the extra growth of the posterior wall of the uterus. Its dextro-flexion (right lateral obliquity) is due to the presence of the rectum on the left side, the spine in the median line and the dextro-torsion. The dextro-torsion (left lateral rotation) is due to the embryonic development of the uterus.

The relations of the uterus at term are as follows: The anterior surface, lower fourth, the bladder; the anterior surface, upper three-fourths, the abdominal wall, but in the dorsal decubitus often the small intestines and omentum; the fundus, the transverse colon and stomach; the lateral wall, the ovary, tube, broad ligament and colon; the posterior surface, the rectum, promontory and small intestines.

The pressure of the contents of the gravid uterus is not directly upon the surrounding structures, except that the lower end of the fetus may in the last few weeks press on the pelvic inlet. In other words, the intra-abdominal pressure simply increases at all points equally as pregnancy advances.

The Properties of the Uterus.--The properties of the uterus during pregnancy are those of the non-pregnant uterus enhanced. They are growth, contractility, elasticity (expansibility and retractibility), softening, sensibility and irritability.

Growth has been described.

Contractility is due to the uterine muscular fibres alternately shortening and lengthening. It constitutes the intermittent contractions of the uterus, which are always present in the pregnant and non-pregnant state. These contractions are not painful during pregnancy or in the non-pregnant unless they are increased by irritation. During labor they become painful ("labor pains") from the exaggerated irritation causing increased frequency and severity. In multiparae for 2 to 4 days after labor they often cause "pains" ("after pains") from some residual irritation, particularly from imperfect retraction of the uterus or the retention of clots. (Any foreign body in the uterus of sufficient size will cause painful uterine contractions.) The contractions during pregnancy occur every 30 to 5 minutes and last about one minute.

Expansibility is that property of the uterus which allows it to expand during pregnancy and to conform to the shape of the contents.

Retractility is that property of the uterus by which after expansion it returns to the size of its contents. This causes the walls of the uterus to increase in thickness. Retractility aids involution and prevents hemorrhage.

Expansibility and retractility constitute elasticity. (Many obstetricians use the term elasticity for expansibility, and consider retractility as distinct from elasticity. This is erroneous. While retractility of the uterus is not just the same as that of a piece of rubber, the law by which it acts is the same).

Softening of the uterus begins with pregnancy and varies in different parts of the uterus. The softening of the cervix will be described under, "Changes in the Cervix." The uterine body softens unequally; the lower segment, between the 6th week and the 3rd month is especially soft, from the ovum occupying only the upper segment (Before the 6th week the softening is not very marked, and after the 3rd month part of the ovum occupies the lower segment). Sometimes near term, if the uterus is much stretched, the lower segment becomes tense instead of soft. The upper segment becomes more elastic and softer as pregnancy advances but because of its thickness and elasticity, it rarely feels as soft as the lower segment, and it is alternately hard and soft from the presence or absence of the uterine contractions. The two halves of the upper segment in the first two or three months are often unequal in consistence, on account of the ovum occupying more of one-half. This causes the unoccupied half to feel relatively softer.

Uterine sensibility and irritability are more or less increased, but the amount varies greatly in different patients.

The Changes in the Cervix.—The changes in the cervix are an increase in the size and growth, softening, the formation of a plug of mucus in the canal, rounding of the external os, erosion of the vaginal surface, apparent shortening of the whole cervix, and stretching of the anterior lip.

The cervix grows up to the 4th month, but the main cause of its enlargement is hyperemia.

Softening of the cervix begins at the external os, and is much more rapid in multigravidae because of the previous softening. Softening of the cervix is normally always present. (In pathologic cases, as hypertrophic elongation or induration, which are very rare, it is generally absent).

Softening of the cervix during the premonitory stage of labor will be described under chapter twelve, "The Physiology and Mechanism of Labor."

The cervical canal is filled with a plug of mucus.

The external os becomes more round. In primigravidae it changes from a transverse slit to a circular opening.

Erosions of the vaginal surface of the cervix, it is said, can generally be felt in the latter months of pregnancy.

Apparent shortening of the cervix occurs from the edema increasing its width and allowing the examining finger to sink into it, also from the uterus rising into the abdomen, and in primigravidae near term by the head stretching the anterior lip of the cervix.

Stretching of the anterior lip of the cervix before labor occurs in primigravidae because the head descends a little into the cervix one day to three weeks before labor and in descending (the internal os being posterior to the center of the head) presses mainly upon the anterior lip and thins it.

The posterior lip and posterior wall of the canal remain of the usual thickness, and if the head is pushed up the anterior lip returns to its former length, showing that there is no real shortening of the cervix. In multigravidae the thinning of the anterior lip does not generally occur, because as a rule the head rests in one of the iliac fossae. (All this in reference to stretching of the anterior lip will be found under chapter twelve, "The Physiology and Mechanism of Labor").

Real shortening, or effacement and dilation of the cervix, are no longer supposed to take place normally before labor. The author has seen in some cases of "false labor pains," and cases without any pain, more or less real shortening or effacement and from one to three fingers dilation of the cervix in the premonitory stage of labor, and noted that these did subsequently only partially disappear, but it is a question whether these should be classed as normal as they were really due to the beginning of a premature labor. Formerly real shortening and dilation were thought to occur at the seventh month and many theories of explanation were offered. Of these Bandl's is the most important, because of the facts it contains.

Bandl's theory: In the last two months of pregnancy the upper half of the cervical canal dilates from above downwards, becomes the future lower uterine segment which subsequently never disappears and what is called the internal os is not the real internal os, but is simply the lower limit of the dilation at the time of the examination. This theory is based on the following facts: During pregnancy the body of the uterus becomes divided into an upper and lower segment separated by a slightly thickened band, called the retraction ring, or ring of Bandl. Before pregnancy, i.e., in the virgin eturus, the peritoneum is closely attached to the uterine walls as low down as opposite the internal os. Near term and after labor, instead of being attached as low as, what is at this time called, the internal os, it is attached only as low as Bandl's ring. In the nulliparous uterust he cervix and the body are of about equal length (the body being a little shorter) but in the multiparous uterus the body is nearly two-thirds of the whole length of the uterus.

The author has seen the lower segment in many miscarriages as well developed as in the uterus at term, and does not believe that dilation occurs before labor, but that the lower segment is always present and pregnancy causes it to stretch and grow, and that the portion of the external surface which was nearly opposite the close attachment of the peritoneum is carried upward by its growth. (The following case seen by the author, seems to favor Bandl's theory, but must be only an unusual retraction of the lower segment: In introducing his hand to remove an adherent placenta after a forceps delivery, he found the cervix funnel-shaped from relaxation, the small end of the funnel being at the internal os.   Above the internal os could be felt a retracted thick-walled lower segment with a cylindrical canal, just large enough to admit two fingers and about as long as the canal of the cervix. This thick lower segment was pushed into the cervix by an assistant, and then felt like something entirely distinct from the cervix, because of its comparative hardness).

The Changes in the Ovaries Tubes and Uterine Appendages. —The ovaries, tubes and uterine appendages increase in size during pregnancy.   The ovaries, tubes and broad ligaments lie parallel with and close to the sides of the uterus.   The ovaries are at the junction of the upper and middle third of the uterus, and can be felt through the abdominal wall midway on a line between the navel and the anterior superior spine of the ilium.

The round ligaments increase greatly in size, and at the end of gestation feel like a whip cord extending from the side of the uterus to the inguinal canal.

Menstrual Suppression.—Menstrual suppression has been discussed under the physiology of the reproductive organs.   It depends on the excess of nutrition, of blood (congestion), being taken up daily to supply the ovum and the mother's body with the hypernutriment necessary for the continuance of pregnancy.

Ovular Suppression.—Ovulation is probably stopped, but on this point, however, there are no data of any great value.

Other Changes.—The other changes are rare or of little importance.

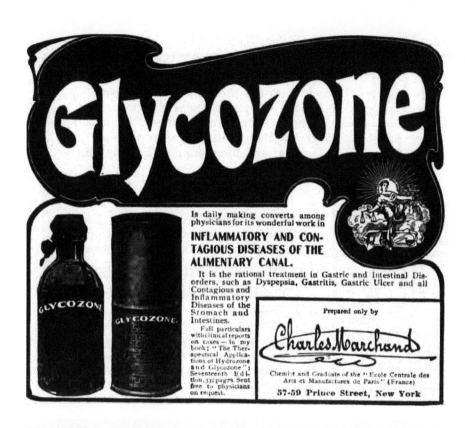

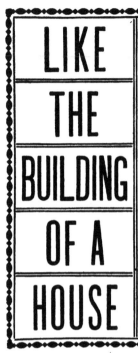

DENVER MEDICAL TIMES

THOMAS H. HAWKINS, A.M., M.D., EDITOR AND PUBLISHER.

COLLABORATORS:

Henry O. Marcy, M.D., Boston.
Thaddeus A. Reamy, M.D., Cincinnati.
Nicholas Senn, M.D., Chicago.
Joseph Price, M.D., Philadelphia.
Franklin H. Martin, M.D., Chicago.
William Oliver Moore, M.D., New York.
L. S. McMurtry, M.D., Louisville.
Thomas B. Eastman, M.D., Indianapolis, Ind.
G. Law, M.D., Greeley, Colo.

S. H. Pinkerton, M.D., Salt Lake City.
Flavel B. Tiffany, M.D., Kansas City.
Erskine M. Bates, M.D., New York.
E. C. Gehrung, M.D., St. Louis.
Graeme M. Hammond, M.D, New York.
James A. Lydston, M.D., Chicago.
Leonard Freeman, M.D., Denver.
Carey K. Fleming, M.D., Denver, Colo.

Subscriptions, $1.00 per year in advance; Single Copies, 10 cents.

Address all Communications to Denver Medical Times, 1740 Welton Street, Denver, Colo.
We will at all times be glad to give space to well written articles or items of interest to the profession.
[Entered at the Postoffice of Denver, Colorado, as mail matter of the Second Class.]

EDITORIAL DEPARTMENT

CARDIOVASCULAR WEAKNESS OF FEVERS.

Stengel concludes that the pathology of this condition is connected largely with vasomotor depression, as the older writers held, and less with mechanical factors in the heart and vessels. In the management of heart weakness during infectious diseases, he employs strychnine with alcohol (not to exceed six or eight ounces of good whiskey or brandy in 24 hours).

When the circulation requires additional support, particularly when nervous symptoms are prominent, he has found camphorated oil (one grain of camphor in fifteen minims of sterile olive oil) by hypodermic injection most valuable. He frequently gives a grain or two of camphor in this way every second or third hour for several days in succession. He has come to use adrenalin solution in these cases (30 minims in a half pint or pint of normal salt solution subcutaneously or intravenously) only when an acute emergency, such as collapse from hemorrhage or perforation in typhoid fever, has been the indication for prompt support. Digitalis and strophanthus are far less satisfactory in the relief of the cardiac weakness of fever than in the treatment of valvular disease. The cold bath and its substitutes act chiefly as therapeutic agents in reducing the tendency to excessive weakness and in mitigating the nervous symptoms of fever. Generally speaking, the principal indications for cardiac stimulation in infectious diseases are alterations in the apex beat (more diffuse and wavy) the change in the character of the first heart sound (more valvular; sometimes blowing at base) and the depression of the systolic pressure at the wrist. Time and care alone can effect a complete restitution of the heart muscle and other tissues. For this reason, it is best, whenever possible, to forbid an individual just recovering from an infectious disease from resuming his occupation for a considerable period of time. When, despite our efforts, myocardial weakness is developing during convalescence, thermal baths, massage, and the use of arsenic, strychnine and phosphorus are advantageous.

AIR.

The atmosphere is a boundless source of life and a medium of death. Fresh air and plenty of it is absolutely essential to the maintenance of health. Historic examples of the effects of insufficient air are the "Black Hole" of Calcutta, in which 123 out of 146 British prisoners perished in a single night; and the 300 captured Germans, who after the battle of Austerlitz were crowded into a small prison with the result that 140 of them died that day and night. It is said that 61 societies in the boroughs of Bronx and Manhattan are interested in fresh air and summer outings for the poor.

Vitiation of the air is noticed by the sense of smell when the carbon dioxid from respiration reaches .6 pro mille, and this limit should never be exceeded. To meet such sanitary requirements an adult individual at rest should be supplied with 3000 cubic feet of fresh air per hour. The air in a living room can hardly be changed throughout with comfort more than three times in an hour; hence each adult person ought to have at least 1000 cubic feet of room space. Account must also be taken of the products of combustion, a 16-candle power kerosene light giving off five times, and the same intensity of burning gas three times, as much carbon dioxid in an hour as is exhaled in the same time by a man.

The most dangerous vitiation of the respired air, except specific germs, is from the decomposition of organic matter, namely: ammonia, amins, sulphur compounds, ptomains and leucomains.

Chronic poisoning by these and by excess of carbon dioxid, through deficient ventilation, is marked by morning drowsiness and headache, nausea, malnutrition, anemia and debility. Subjects of this common form of poisoning are particularly susceptible to infection. The long continued inhalation of drain and sewer air produces gradual loss of health, anemia, fever, lassitude, headache, sore throat, vomiting and diarrhea. Acute mephitic poisoning from open, foul drains and cesspools is marked by sudden, severe vomiting and purging, headache, prostration and sometimes partial asphyxia.

Up till 1846 the mortality of the British army, crowded in ill-ventilated barracks, was 11.9 per thousand. As more space was allowed to each man, this mortality fell to 2.3 per thousand in 1870, and still lower since that time. The relative death rate from consumption in prison is said to have been formerly about four times that among the free population.

The regular practice of deep and full respiration in the erect posture is a highly important factor in the prevention of pulmonary disease. The chest may be further strengthened by daily ablutions with cold salt water or the shower bath, always taking care on drying to rub with the towel until reaction takes place.

SUNSHINE.

Photographic comparisons prove that the light on a bright day is 18,000 times stronger at the seashore, and 5,000 times as strong on the sunny side of a street as in the ordinary shaded and curtained rooms of a city home.

Sunlight is as essential to human beings as it is to plants. Both grow pale and weakly for want of it The chlorophyl of grass and leaves and the hemoglobin of the blood are increased by exposure to the sun's rays.

Sunlight is actively germicidal. According to Rosenau, objects infected with the bacillus pestis may be sufficiently disinfected on the surface by exposing them all day to a bright sun, providing the temperature is above 30°. Tubercle bacilli are destroyed by direct sunshine in three or four hours. The virus of smallpox is quite resistant to the solar rays.

REST.

Every living thing needs periodic rest. The healthy human infant should sleep twenty out of twenty-four hours. The adult in his prime requires at least seven hours of slumber. Old people are normally light and short sleepers.

When a person cannot sleep well, the cause of the insomnia should be sought out very carefully. Hypnotic drugs ought hardly ever to be resorted to, and then only temporarily. Regular hours, a light evening meal and relaxation of mind and body favor sound and normal sleep.

Sufficient waking rest and harmless recreation prolong life and render it better and happier. Physicians particularly need vacation, to prevent nervous breakdown. They frequently and advantageously combine science and pleasure by attending medical conventions in other cities.

Rest is especially indicated to prevent dangerous complications in typhoid fever, and as prophylaxis against threatening tuberculosis. It is indeed nature's sovereign method of cure.

Pyrosis of Pregnancy.— James H. Etheridge gives sodium bicarbonate or calcined magnesia after meals, or effervescing alkaline mineral waters with meals; also half-dram doses of aromatic spirit of ammonia. It is important to regulate the bowels.

Podophyllin in Helminthiasis.—Neumann (quoted in *Practical Medicine Series*) reports experiences and experiments which show that podophyllin has a specific action on intestinal epithelium, which interferes with the ankylostoma clinging to it. The parasite is thus easily dislodged by male fern after administration of podophyllin.

Gastric Ulcer.—Van Valzah and Nisbet advise restriction to a milk diet for a time. If the hyperchlorhydria is reflex, keep stomach empty for 24 hours. If due to associated hypersthenic gastritis, give alkalies (sodium bicarbonate with magnesia or chalk) in large doses at end of each feeding. Silver nitrate, $\frac{1}{4}$ to $\frac{1}{2}$ grain in water every morning twenty minutes before first feeding, is also very useful in hypersthenic cases.

EDITORIAL ITEMS.

Fourth Pan-American Medical Congress. Dr. Rudolph Matas, of New Orleans, Secretary of Section of General Surgery for the United States, informs us that an arrangement with the United Fruit Company has been perfected by which a steamer of this line will leave New Orleans for Colon on *Wednesday, December, 28th, 1904, at 10 a. m.* (instead of Friday, December, 30th, at 11 a. m. as previously announced) which will reach Colon (Panama) on *Monday, January, 2nd, 1905*, the opening day of the Congress.

In view of the facilities offered to reach Panama via New Orleans it is expected that many will choose this route, and those who intend to do so will please forward their names to Dr. R. Matas, Secretary of Section of General Surgery, No. 2255 St. Charles Avenue, New Orleans, La., not later than *December 22nd, 1904.*

Narkotil. Methyl-ethylene bichloride is a new general an-esthetic.

Pyrolin. This disinfectant consists essentially of magnesium acetate.

Novozon. This is a mixture of magnesium peroxide and carbonate.

Menopausal Flatulence. For this symptom Ringer states that eucalyptol is the remedy.

Vitalin. This is the name given to a disinfectant mixture of resin oil and resin soap.

Flatulence of Pregnancy. Ringer employs sodium sulpho-carbolate, five to fifteen grains after meals.

Intestinal Dyspepsia with Flatulence. Potter states that in these cases salophen is used with decided benefit.

For Acid Dyspepsia. Ringer directs to drink a tumbler of hot water two or three times a day midway between meals.

For Gastrosuccorrhœa. W. H. Allchin (*International Clinics*) has found distinct benefit from atropine or belladonna.

Stomach Flatulence and Acidity. Ringer gives one or two

drams of glycerin several times a day in tea, coffee, or water with food.

Normalin. This is a mixture of hemoglobin and serumal-buminate of arsenic.

Somnoform. This is an anesthetic compound of ethyl and methyl chlorides and ethyl bromide.

Rhomnol. This is a nucleinic acid of French manufacture, obtained from the thymus gland of the calf.

Lofotol. Cod-liver oil is rendered "tasteless" by impregnation with carbon dioxide.

Isopral. Trichloriso-propyl alcohol is a new hypnotic, similar in effect to chloral hydrate.

Lactoserum. This is sterilized milk serum impregnated with carbon dioxide.

Gerdal. This nutrient is a combination of beef juice, albumen and sugar.

Haloform. This is a menthol and formaldehyde preparation, used in coryza.

Anthrasol. This is a purified mixture of coal tar and juniper tar, used in skin diseases.

Exudol. This ointment consists of ichthyol, green soap and various analgesies.

Gonosan. This is a combination of santal oil and the resin of kavakava, used, of course, in gonorrhea.

Hetraline. Dioxybenzene-hexamethylene tetramine is a new candidate for favor in gonorrhea and cystitis.

For Spasm of Pylorus. For immediate relief Hoffmann's anodyne is usually most efficient.

Excessive Cough Following Influenza. Hare recommends oil of sandalwood in doses of five to twenty drops in capsules.

Microsol. This is a disinfectant mixture of copper sulphate and sulphocarbolate, sulphuric acid and water.

Enterin. This new intestinal antiseptic and astringent is a combination of heramethylenetetramine (urotropin) with proteid.

Iodozol. These antiseptic preparations are compounds of sodium, potassium and zinc with diiodophenolsulphonic acid.

Fetid Bronchitis. Taylor recommends inhalations of carbolic acid, turpentine, thymol, eucalyptol and tincture of iodine.

Liniment for Chest. E. Grady recommends fifteen drops of oil of mustard, a dram each of oils of sassafras and cedar, and four ounces of alcohol.

Ozogen. This is a trade name for a three per cent solution of hydrogen peroxide.

For Fermentive Dyspepsia. Hydrogen peroxide, oxygenated water, terebene and creasote are favorably mentioned.

Styptol. Cotarnine phthalate is a uterine hemostatic in the dose of three-fourths grain three to five times a day.

Gastric Indigestion. Beale administers liquor potassae m. xx., or liquor ammoniae m.v., in water before or after meals.

Ronozol Salts. These are antiseptic compounds of sodium-potassium, zinc, and mercury with diiodoparaphenolsulphonic acid.

Pyran.—Pyran, or pyrenol, is an antineuralgic and antirheumatic compound of benzoic and salicylic acids with thymol.

Salocreol. This is combination of salicylic acid and beech-tar-creosote phenols is used by inunction in rheumatic affections.

Diomorphin. This is an aqueous solution of dionin and morphine, suggested as a succedaneun for the latter drug.

Mirmol. Mirmol is a mixture of carbolic acid and formaldehyde, used externally in cancerous and other ulcers.

Vaporin. Naphthene eucalyptol camphor is a new remedy for whooping cough, used by evaporation from hot water.

Nervous Flatulence. Shoemaker prescribes: ℞ Spt. etheris comp. m. xxx; tinct. capsici m. ii; spt; ammon. arom. m. xi; aq. sod. menth. q. s.: A teaspoonful every few minutes till relieved.

Urethritis Petrificans. Calcareous deposits in the urethral wall are generally the results of devitalization from long-contiued gonorrhea.

Menorrhagia at Puberty. Davenport states the drug of most value in the profuse flowing of young girls is iron. The general health must also be improved.

Flatulence of Emptiness. When due to poorness of the

mother's milk, Goodhart and Starr advise feeding the infant during the day and putting to breast only night and morning.

Chronic Gastritis.   Forbid tea, pastry and coarse vegetables, says Osler.   Give bismuth and sodium carbonate, thymol, creosote, carbolic acid.

Tannochrom.   This tannin-chromium-resorcin compound is used as an antiseptic injection in gonorrhea, in the strength of $\frac{1}{4}$ to $\frac{1}{8}$ of one per cent.

Blenorrhol.   This prophylactic of blenorrhea neonatorum is a ten per cent protargol-gelatin, kept for convenience and cleanliness in tubes.

Lactagol.   This is a preparation from cotton-seeds, used to promote the secretion of milk, the idea being derived from the oil cake employed in dairies.

Empyroform.   This is a condensation product of birch-tar and formaldehyde.   It is used in solution with chloroform or in ointments for chronic skin diseases.

For Gastric Fermentation.   Shoemaker prescribes: ℞ Acidi carbol. m. 1–5; syr. acaciae et. aq. cinnamomi aa. q. s.:   A teaspoonful before meals.

Chronic Bronchitis.   A. Goldhammer recommends guaiacol in the dose of five drops t.i.d., increased to fifteen drops, best given in milk or capsules.

Phthisical Bronchorrhea.   Knopf advises the daily intratracheal injection of a mixture of one part each of guaiacol and menthol in six parts of olive oil.

Gastric Hyperacidity.   Potter recommends tincture of nux vomica m. v-x. and dilute nutric acid m. xv. at one dose for pyrosis of atonic dyspepsia.

Cirrhotic Bronchitis.   The treatment, says Fothergill, is the same as for tuberculosis, which it resembles.   Strychnine and fatty foods are especially useful.

For Degenerative Bronchitis.   Fothergill recommends tonics, stimulants, expectorants, carminatives; very low dietary; mental and bodily quiet and good care.

Acute Bronchitis.   Biddle prescribes: ℞ Acidi hydrocyan. dil. m. i; syrupi ipecac m. iv; morp. sulph. gr. $\frac{1}{8}$; syrupum pruni virg. q.s.:   A teaspoonful every three hours.

Acute Bronchitis. Whittaker gives 1–32 to ½ grain of apomorphine hydrochlorate and ½ to 1 drop of dilute hydrochloric acid in syrup and water every two hours.

Acute Primary Bronchitis. Da Costa used opii camph., syrupi acaciae aa. m. x; liq. potas. cit. q. s.: A tablespoonful three times a day in early stage.

For Pyrosis. Ringer recommends hydrochloric acid in small doses shortly before meals for acid pyrosis—after meals when pyrosis alkaline.

For Nocturnal Cramps in the Muscles of the Legs. H. S. Noble (*Practical Medicine Series*) mentions an evening dose of hyoscine as a cure for this annoying complaint.

For Dyspeptic Flatulence. Murrell praises oil of cajeput, a few drops on sugar as needed. Wormley uses cold compresses over the abdomen through the night.

Influenzal Cough with Copious Expectoration. Lyon gives each day three to five pills, each containing four grains of terpene hydrate and sufficient glycerine and simple syrup.

Cough of Typhoid Fever. Alonzo Clark gives from a dram to an ounce of guaiac mixture with six to ten drops of tincture of tolu, repeating the dose every two to four hours.

Antithyroidin. This is the name given to the serum from the blood of sheep deprived of the thyroid gland. It is used in the dose of five grammes for exophthalmic goiter.

Camphossit. This is a condensation product of camphor and salicylic acid, used in the dose of eight grains as an antipyretic and antiseptic in diarrhea and typhoid fever.

Nervol. This combination of sodium-vanadium citrochloride and lithium bromide is recommended as a sedative in hysteria. The dose is a teaspoonful four or five times daily.

Obtundo. This local dental anesthetic is composed of cocaine, chloretone, menthol, nitroglycerine, thymol, and the oils of cloves, wintergreen and eucalyptus.

Senile Atonic Flatulence. Hare prescribes: ℞ Tinct. belladonnae m. v; tinct. physostigm. m. iiss; spt. camphorae q. s.: A
teaspoonful two hours after meals, or whenever needed.

Rum Stomach with Flatulence. Take before meals, says A.
L. Loomis, five to fifteen drops of tincture of nux vomica and one
dram each of compound tincture of gentian and columbo.

For Flatulent Dyspepsia. Shoemaker prescribes: ℞ Bismuthi subnit. pulv. aromat. aa. gr. xx: Take before meals. Castor oil is very useful in pronounced intestinal tympany.

Flatulence of Old Age. Charcot and Loomis recommend a
dry diet; avoidance of potatoes; taking spices and alkalies; cajeput oil, creosote, charcoal, ammonia and compound spirit of ether.

Chronic Gastric Catarrh. Prohibit fats, sugar, starches and
beer, says Flint's Encyclopedia. Alkalies are administered with
benefit. Nux vomica will relieve the majority of cases.

Acute Bronchitis in Feeble Patients. Garrod prescribes: ℞
Bromoformi m. viiss; codeinae phos, gr. i; syr. scillae comp. m.
x; syr. lactucariae q. s.: A dessertspoonful every two hours.

Bronchitis of Children. As an inhalant for the cough, E.
Grady uses a dram of compound tincture of benzoin, five grains
of menthol and ten drops of ether in a pint of boiling water.

Chronic Bronchitis with Chronic Gastric Catarrh. Hughes
prescribes: ℞ Ammonii chloridi gr. xi; tinct. nucis vom. m.
viiss.; infusum gent. co. q. s.: A dessertspoonful in water before meals.

Bronchitis of Old People. Maragliano administers cachets
four or five times daily of five grains of benzoic acid and 2½
grains of tannin. The same combination is useful in bronchorrhea.

Bronchitis of Babies. N. Weist has prescribed as follows:
℞ Ammon. muriat. gr. 1–5; syrupi scillae co. m. iv; tinct. aconiti
m. 1–5; syrupum simp. q. s.: A half teaspoonful every three
hours.

Influenzal Bronchitis. Potter gives five to ten drops every
two hours of a mixture of two parts of fluid extract ipecac, four
parts deodorized tincture of opium and one part of tincture of
aconite.

Disposition to Accumulation of Flatus in Bowels. Wood employs a wineglassful t.i.d. of an. infusion made with one-half ounce each of columbo and ginger, one dram of senna and a pint of boiling water.

Resorcin in Eczema. The use of this drug as an anodyne in acute eczema is highly lauded by F. C. Clark (*Practical Medicine Series*). It may be applied in four per cent solution or ointment.

Vegetable Bitters. W. H. Allchin (*International Clinics*) states that gentian is more suitable when the tongue is red and irritable with prominent papillae. Calumba is to be preferred when the tongue is pale.

The Urine in Rheumatoid Arthritis. Goldthwait and Painter (*Johns Hopkins Hospital Bulletin*) have shown that there is a reversal of the normal calcium-magnesium ratio, twice as much calcium being excreted as ingested.

Gastric Cancer. Van Valzah and Nisbet advise thorough lavage one hour before breakfast, leaving in the stomach not more than a pint of water at a time. Follow lavage in one-half hour with hydrochloric acid tonic. Exclude sweets from diet.

Purpura Angioneurotica. This chronic disorder (*Practical Medicine Series*) shows relapses of cutaneous hemorrhages, gastric crises, hyperesthesia, angioneurotic edema, and a condition of the blood resembling pernicious anemia.

Irritative Dyspepsia. Isambard Owen gives one grain of carbolic acid or creosote or one-half grain of thymol in a pill twice a day, or one dram of sulphurous acid in three ounces of water once or twice daily, or an enema of milk of asafetida.

Gastric Dilatation. Einhorn recommends resorcin in the dose of three to five grains with twenty grains of bismuth subnitrate in a watery mixture. Baudoin gives ammonium fluoride 1–24 grain, increased to $\frac{1}{4}$ grain, t.i.d. in water.

Fluorescent Therapy. H. von Tappeiner (quoted in *Practical Medicine Series*) has got good results by painting superficial skin lesions with a five per cent solution of eosin and then exposing to sunlight.

Editorial Items continued on Page 330

BOOKS,

IN THE YEAR 1800.—Being the Relation of Sundry Events Occurring in the Life of Doctor Jonathan Brush, during that year, by Samuel Walter Kelley, M.D., 1904. The Saalfield Publishing Co., Chicago, Akron, O., New York.

This is lhe third volume of the "Doctor's Recreation Series" and is so far the best of the series. The narrative, told in the first person, depicts life as it was a century ago in Maine, New York City and Philadelphia. The plot of the story is well laid and will hold the reader's interest up to the very satisfactory ending. The characters, except the eccentric villain, are such as one likes to meet in literature or life. The medical and surgical methods of that day are, we opine, truthfully portrayed, without detracting from the story itself; and the same may be said of the considerable philosophy that pervades the pages of this book.

A TEXT-BOOK OF HISTOLOGY.—By Frederick R. Bailey, A.M., M.D., Adjunct Professor of Normal Histology, College of Physicians and Surgeons—Medical Department, Columbia University, New York City. Profusely illustrated. New York: William Wood & Co., 1904.

We have nothing but praise for this handsome and well-written volume, which is equally of service in the laboratory and for class-room work. The first part of the text, on histologic technic, comprises all the essentials of the subject. The second and third parts, on the cell and tissues, offer a clear and concise exposition of basic facts and principles. In the main, or fourth part, concerning the organs, space commensurate to its importance is devoted to the nervous system, and the newer methods of neurologic staining are elsewhere fully described. The text is adorned and elucidated with 286 well chosen figures.

BLOOD-PRESSURE AS AFFECTING HEART, BRAIN, KIDNEYS AND GENERAL CIRCULATION.—A practical consideration of theory and treatment. By Louis Faugeres Bishop, A.M., M.D., Physician to the Lincoln Hospital, New York. Price, $1.00. New York; E. B. Treat & Co., 241–243 West 23rd St., 1904.

We have read through this little volume with much interest and some profit. The author takes ground properly, we think, against the merely mechanical conception of the circulation, and shows from the clinical point of view the relations between the heart and the vasomotor system. He gives not a little good advice on the use of thenitrites, digitalis and other cardiovascular remedies.

THE SURGICAL TREATMENT OF BRIGHT'S DISEASE.—By George M. Edebohls, A.M., M.D., LL.D., Professor of the Diseases of Women in the New York Post Graduate Medical School and Hospital; Consulting Surgeon to St. Francis' Hospital, New York; Consulting Gynecologist to St. John's Riverside Hospital, Yonkers, N. Y., and to the Nyack Hospital, Nyack, N. Y. Frank F. Lisieck, Publisher, 9 to 15 Murray St., New York, 1904.

Dr. Edebohls has achieved considerable success in popularizing his method of treating chronic Bright's disease by stripping the kidney of its capsule. The forelying volume comprises, to the extent of two-fifths, his contributions to medical periodicals on this subject, dating from the first formal proposition in the *Medical Record* of May, 1901. The major portion of the text is entirely new matter, and consists largely of a discussion of his results, along with many tables. Seventy-two cases are recorded, ranging in age from 4½ to 67 years. and the average probable duration of the disease prior to operation was 3 years and 8 months. Eleven years and eight months had elapsed since the first operation, and eight months since the last operation performed upon these seventy-two patients—up to the end of the year 1903. Of these patients, seven died within two weeks following operation, twenty-two died at a more remote period, three disappeared from observation, and forty are known to be living, twenty being improved and seventeen cured.

INTERNATIONAL CLINICS.—A quarterly of illustrated clinical lectures and especially prepared original articles on treatment, medicine, surgery, neurology, pediatrics, obstetrics, gynecology, orthopedics, pathology, dermatology, otology, rhinology, laryngology, hygiene and other topics of interest to students and practitioners. By leading members of the medical profession throughout the world. Edited by A. O. J. Kelly,

A.M., M.D., Philadelphia. Price, cloth $2.00 net. Volume III., fourteenth series, 1904. Philadelphia. J. B. Lippincott Co., 1904.

The special feature of the present volume is the symposium on syphilis in which the following medical men take part: Campbell Williams, A.M., Ohmann-Dumesnil, G. Carriere, G. Milian, Wm. G. Spiller, A. Chaufford, Dr. Gourand, J. W. Ballantyne, Alfred Fournier, Thos. R. Neilson, Wm. S. Gotthiel. This section is well illustrated. Among the fifteen other special articles and clinical lectures, "Observations on Indigestion," by W. H. Allchin; "Lumbar Puncture" by Purves Stewart; and "Hemorrhage at and After the Menopause," by Cuthbert Lockyer, are particularly good.

PRACTICAL DIETETICS WITH REFERENCE TO DIET AND DISEASE.—
By Alida Frances Pattee, graduate Boston Normal School of Household Arts; Instructor in Dietetics. Bellevue Training School for Nurses, Bellevue Hospital, New York City. Second edition, revised and enlarged, twelve mo. cloth, 311 pages. Price by mail, $1.10. Published by the author, 52 West 39th St., New York City.

As instructor in dietetics at various hospitals, Miss Pattee felt the need of a simple and concise manual for nurses, as a classroom text-book and for the graduate nurse as a reference book. This neat and attractive little volume is the outcome of her need, the author having utilized the literary contributions of a number of leading physicians of New York, Philadelphia and Boston. The recipes are of great variety, are clearly written and conveniently arranged. The book should prove invaluable to nurses.

THE PRACTICAL MEDICINE SERIES OF YEAR BOOKS.—Volume IX.
Physiology, pathology, bacteriology, anatomy, dictionary. August, 1904. Price of this volume, $2.00; of series of ten volumes, $5.50. Chicago. The Year Book Publishers, 40 Dearborn Street.

Prof. W. A, Evans contributes to this volume a brief summary on anatomy and an extended and valuable resume of pathology. Prof. Adolph Gehrmann brings out clearly the latest theories and findings in physiology and bacteriology. The "Dictionary of New Words" occupies about thirty pages of the text and will be found convenient for ready reference.

THE PRACTICAL MEDICINE SERIES OF YEAR BOOKS.—Volume VIII.
July, 1904. Price of this volume, $1.00. Chicago. The Year Book Publishers, 40 Dearborn Street.

This volume comprises an excellent outline of the year's progress in materia medica and therapeutics, including physical measures, by George F. Butler and George S. Browning; a summary of preventive medicine, by Henry B. Favill; a review of climatology, by Norman Bridge; notes on suggestive therapeutics, by Daniel R. Brower; and a digest of forensic medicine, by Harold N. Moyer.

THE PRACTICAL MEDICINE SERIES OF YEAR BOOKS.—Volume X. Skin and venereal diseases; nervous and mental diseases. Edited by Wm. L. Baum, M.D., and Hugh T. Patrick, M.D., September, 1904. Price, $1.00; series of ten volumes, $5.50. Chicago. The Year Book Publishers, 40 Dearborn Street.

The increasing interest which dermatologists are taking in constitutional relations is well shown in the part of the present volume devoted to skin diseases. The division on nervous and mental diseases, by Patrick and Mix, is a clear and careful resume of a great mass of somewhat technical literature. There are twenty-seven photographic figures in the text.

A COMPEND OF MEDICAL LATIN.—Designed expressly for elementary training of medical students. By W. T. St. Clair, A.M., professor of the Latin language and literature in the Male High School, of Louisville, Ky. Second edition, revised. Price, $1.00. Philadelphia. P. Blakiston's Son & Co., 1012 Walnut St., 1904.

For medical students whose knowledge of Latin is nil or nearly so, this little volume will be a welcome aid. The didactic method employed is clear and systematic. The vocabulary presented is strictly medical.

THE PHYSICIAN'S VISITING LIST FOR 1905.–Price, $1.00 and upward. Philadelphia. P. Blakiston's Son & Co., 1012 Walnut St.

This is the fifty-fourth successive (and successful) year publication of what was at first called Lindsay & Blakiston's visiting list. It is in many ways a model record volume, and is extremely convenient for carriage. The dose table in the present

edition has been revised in accordance with the new U. S. Pharmacopeia of 1900.

THE MEDICAL NEWS VISITING LIST FOR 1905—Price $1.25; thumb-
letter index, 25 cents extra. Philadelphia and New York.
Lea Bros. Co.

This handsome and durable pocket volume, now in the nineteenth year of issue, has much to recommend it aside from the
adaptability to practical use of the classified ruled records. The
numerous tables on poisons and antidotes, dosage, eruptive fevers,
therapeutic reminders, etc., are of great service for ready reference.
It is published in four styles to meet the requirements of every
practitioner.

HARE'S PRACTICAL THERAPEUTICS—A text-book of practical therapeutics; with especial reference to the application of remedial
measures to disease and their employment upon a rational
basis. By Hobart Amory Hare, M.D., professor of therapeutics and materia medica in the Jefferson Medical College
of Philadelphia. With special chapters by Drs. G. E. De-
Schweinitz, Edward Martin and Barton C. Hirst. New (10th)
edition, much enlarged, thoroughly revised and largely rewritten. Octavo, 908 ages, with 113 engravings and 4 full-
page colored plates. Cloth, $4.00, net; leather, $5.00, net;
half morocco, $5.00, net. Lea Brothers & Co., Philadelphia
and New York, 1904.

This work has gone through ten editions and about thirty
printings in a little more than a decade. The type for the present edition has been entirely reset. The book has been considerably enlarged without increase of price. In addition to the first
three parts on general therapeutic considerations, drugs, other
remedial measures and feeding the sick, the extensive part on
treatment of diseases is virtually a practice of medicine. The author may not be always scientifically exact in his statements, but
he is always practical and progressive, and the continued popularity of his writings attests their merits. The considerable number
of illustrations in the text is a praiseworthy feature.

THE MEDICAL RECORD VISITING LIST OR PHYSICIANS' DIARY FOR
1905.—New revised edition, New York. Wm. Wood & Co.,
Medical Publishers.

This wallet volume occupies the least space of any complete
visiting list that we have seen. Besides the usual ruled blanks for
general and special purposes, there is considerable ready-at-hand

emergency information, such as maximum dosage, poisoning and other emergencies, and a unique obstetric calendar.

GENERAL CATALOGUE OF MEDICAL BOOKS.—P. Blakiston's Son & Co., Philadelphia. Price, 25 cents.

This little leather brochure contains a complete list of the modern publications of all medical publishers with prices arranged alphabetically and in classes.

ESSENTIALS OF BACTERIOLOGY.—Fifth edition, thoroughly revised. By M. V. Ball, M.D., formerly resident physician at the German Hospital, Philadelphia. Fifth edition thoroughly revised. By Karl M. Vogel, M.D., assistant pathologist at the College of Physicians and Surgeons (Columbia University), New York City. 12mo volume of 343 pages, with 96 illustrations, some in colors, and six plates. Philadelphia, New York, London. W. B. Saunders & Co., 1904. Cloth, $1.00 net.

The present edition includes all the recent advances in immunity, yellow fever, dysentery, tuberculosis and other infectious diseases. Use of instruments and methods, pathogenic and non-pathogenic bacteria are discussed concisely but fully. The chief characteristics of the principal bacteria are compared in columns. One is struck with the number and quality of illustrations, considering the low price of the book.

ESSENTIALS OF ANATOMY.—Seventh edition, thoroughly revised, including the anatomy of the viscera. By Charles B. Nancrede, M.D., professor of Surgery and clinical surgery in the University of Michigan, Ann Arbor. Seventh edition, thoroughly revised. 12mo volume of 419 pages, fully illustrated, Philadelphia, New York, London. W. B. Saunders & Co., 1904. Cloth, $1.00 net.

This compact little work, now in the seventh edition, has been carefully revised. The section on the nervous system has been completely rewritten in conformity with the latest researches. The illustrations are excellent for a volume of this kind. The book will doubtless continue to be a *sine qua non*, with a host of medical students.

ESSENTIALS OF MATERIA MEDICA AND PRESCRIPTION WRITING.—Sixth edition, thoroughly revised. By Henry Morris, M.D., College of Physicians, Philadelphia. Sixth edition thoroughly revised. By W. A. Bastedo, M.D., tutor of materia medica and pharmacology at the Columbia University (College of Physicians and Surgeons), New York City. 12mo volume of 295 pages, Philadelphia, New York, London. W. B. Saunders & Co.,1904.   Cloth, $1.00 net.

Dr. Bastedo, in making this revision of Dr. Morris's "Essentials of Materia Medica," has brought the text fully up to date in all particulars, incorporating articles on the new synthetics and other remedies.   The work is clearly written, and appears to be accurate in statement.   It truly contains the essentials of the subject.

ESSENTIALS OF NERVOUS DISEASES AND INSANITY.—Fourth edition, thoroughly revised; their symptoms and treatment.   By John C. Shaw, M.D., late clinical professor of diseases of the mind and nervous system, Long Island College Hospital Medical School.   Fourth edition thoroughly revised.   By Smith Ely Jelliffe, Ph.G., M.D., clinical assistant, Columbia University, department of neurology; visiting neurologist, City Hospital, New York.   12mo volume of 196 pages, fully illustrated. Philadelphia, New York, London.   W. B. Saunders & Co., 1904.   Cloth, $1.00 net.

Even nervous diseases progress as to our knowledge of their nature and therapy.   The present edition of this compendium has been entirely recast by Dr. Jelliffe, so as to bring the order of arrangement in accord with the present status of these important subjects, and to set forth the natural relations of affiliated nervous disorders.   In the section on mental diseases, the general views of such leading psycholologists as Ziehen, Weygandt, Kaepelin, Berkeley and Peterson have been carefully weighed and propounded. Without loss of vital facts, the work has been simplified as much as possible to meet the difficulties of students.

SELECTIONS.

The Correction of Abormal Conditions of the Blood Relative to Surgical Operations.*—By S. C. Emley, A.B., M.D., of Wichita, Kan., late Pathologist Augustana Hospital, Chicago, Ill. Frequently the surgeon is called upon to operate on patients who, when they first present themselves, are in no condition to stand an operation on account of deficient quantity of blood or the poorness of its quality. On the other hand, it is desirable that the patient regain his normal condition as soon as possible after operation, whether the abnormal condition of blood is due to the operation or not.

The ideal remedy is that which will restore the normal condition of the blood in the shortest time with the least disturbance to the rest of the body, the digestive system particularly. Less necessary are palatability and cost of the remedy. To determine which of several preparations best fulfilled the above conditions was the purpose of this investigation.

All of the preparations used being recognized as good, Dr. A. J. Ochsner gave me permission to prescribe them as I saw fit to certain of his patients in Augustana Hospital. Only those cases were selected whose appearance indicated the need of a hematinic. As often as possible similar cases were paired off, one patient being given one preparation and the other patient another, and the results compared. The cases were paired according to pathological conditions, age, sex, general condition and the condition of the blood as to hemoglobin and erythrocytes at the beginning of treatment. The preparations used were malt with iron and manganese; malt with iron, quinine and strychnine; Blaud's pills, and the preparation known as pepto-mangan (Gude).

After watching the effect of the medication on the patients, and observing the records, it is seen that Blaud's pills acted quickly, but constipated; the malt combinations caused nausea in a few patients, and the malt, manganese and iron combinations caused constipation in nearly all. The pepto-mangan, given in milk, was agreeable to take, and in no case did it cause nausea or constipation. While in two cases the Blaud's pills acted more

* Reprinted from Medical News, September 2d, 1904.

quickly than pepto-mangan in two similar cases; on the whole, the latter gave better and quicker results than any of the others, and at the same time caused no digestive disturbances in any of the cases.

Although the investigation was undertaken for the purpose of finding the best hematinic for surgical cases, it was tried in one case of chlorosis and in several obscure medical cases.

The following table shows the results obtained in all those cases where Gude's preparation was given. One to four drachms were given in milk in each case three times a day. The hemoglobin was estimated with Von Fleischel's hemometer, and the erythrocyte count made with the Thoma-Zeiss apparatus. The first blood count was made previous to operation in all surgical cases, and the last a short time before the patient's discharge from the hospital. The second count was never made immediately after the operation because of the temporary derangement due to the anesthetic and the loss of blood.

In the nineteen cases tabulated there is an average increase of 800,000 erythrocytes and of 14.5 per cent. hemoglobin. This improvement was during forty days on an average. The usual time a patient stays in the hospital is twenty-one days when the case is of ordinary severity from a surgical standpoint. Such cases were placed on tonic treatment and showed rapid improvement, but of such cases only one (Case 16) is noted because it might be urged they would improve equally fast with or without a tonic.

It is seen from the following table that even in the cachexia of carcinoma there is a temporary improvement, which shows that in the use of this tonic we are dealing with a powerful hematinic. In Case 17 there was no improvement, the patient dying shortly after the last count. At the autopsy I found a pyogenic abscess in the liver as large as an orange and about 200 c.c. of pus below the right kidney, which explained the retrogression. In all of the other operated cases the improvement was steady and marked, especially in uterine diseases accompanied by loss of blood. In the case of chlorosis (Number 9) the improvement was remarkable, the patient being discharged cured in a little over a month, at which time all the symptoms had disappeared.

Name	Age	Diagnosis	Date	Erythrocytes per 1 c.m.m.	Per cent. of Hemoglobin
1. G. N.[1]....	53	Carcinoma of stomach	9 /29 /03	2,920,000	33
			10 /12 /03	3,400,000	43
			10 /25 /03	3,260,000	42
			11 / 8 /04	2,520,000	36
2. Mr. L.[1]...	49	Carcinoma of stomach	10 /29 /03	2,665,000	27
			11 /23 /03	2,900,000	28
			12 / 5 /03	2,540,000	27
			12 /19 /03	2,300,000	26
3. Miss J....	17	Acute menorrhagia	12 / 4 /03	2,310,000	36
			12 /20 /03	3,565,000	44
			12 /27 /03	4,160,000	49
4. Mrs. E. K,	33	Menorrhagia.........	12 / 7 /03	4,340,000	44
			1 /10 /04	3,565,000	64
			1 /18 /04	5,100,0L0	82
5. Mr. S.....	23	Neurasthenia (?).....	12 /16 /03	4,060,000	60
			1 / 7 /04	4,260,000	65
			1 /14 /04	4,560,000	75
6. Mr. K....	35	Tuberculosis of mesenteric glands	11 /15 /03	3,825,000	62
			12 /10 /03	4,826,000	63
			1 / 4 /04	4,716,000	66
7. Mrs. F....	23	Pelvic abscess........	10 /25 /03	4,060,000	60
			11 /23 /03	5,100,000	69
			12 /11 /03	4,975,000	78
8. Mrs. A....	34	Pelvic abscess........	12 /10 /03	3,195,000	53
			14 /29 /03	4,293,000	58
			1 /11 /04	4,560,000	78
0. Miss A. J.	16	Chlorosis............	10 /25 /03	3,010,000	45
			11 /12 /03	4,950,000	65
			11 /28 /03	5,676,000	80
10. Mrs. H,...	40	Myoma of uterus....	7 /15 /03	2,100,000	42
			8 /17 /03	3,900,000	55
			9 /15 /03	4,500,000	80
11. Johnny L.	13	Tuberculosis of hip..	12 / 1 /03	2,680,000	45
			12 /29 /03	3,600,000	55
			1 /20 /04	4,100,000	62
12. Mr. E. P..	21	Tuberculosis of ankle	10 /29 /03	4,310,000	66
			11 /10 /03	4,850,000	71
			1 /23 /04	5,166,000	75
13. Johnny F.	9	Extensive burn and infection of surface	11 / 9 /03	3,580,000	50
			11 /25 /03	3,900,000	56
			1 /23 /04	4,362,000	68
14. Miss E. B.	17	Perforative appendicitis	11 /25 /03	3,600,000	55
			12 /26 /03	4,000,000	65
			1 /22 /04	4,250,000	69
15. N. N......	29	Suppurative appendicitis	12 /20 /03	4,200,000	60
			1 / 2 /04	4,400,000	66
			1 /20 /04	5,120,000	75
16. Mr. B.....	28	Chronic appendicitis	1 / 2 /04	3,565,000	62
			1 /10 /04	4,320,000	70
			1 /23 /04	4,800,000	78
17. Mr. S.....	37	Gangrenous appendicitis	10 /10 /03	3,300,000	45
			10 /27 /03	3,350,000	45
			11 /27 /03	3,010,000	40
18. Mis W. J..	29	Empyema...........	11 /20 /03	2,740,000	44
			12 /20 /03	3,070,000	52
			1 /22 /04	3,820,000	60
19. Mr. F.....	44	Cholelithiasis Chronic appendicitis	11 /23 /03	3,560,000	57
			12 / 4 /03	4,100,t 00	68
			1 /12 /04	4,640,000	78

[1] Incurable.

THE THERAPEUTIC VALUE OF PEPTO-MANGAN (GUDE).—By Dr. Vehmeyer, Haren, Germany. I was led to resort to Pepto-Mangan (Gude), and my observations extend now over a large field, comprising patients of various ages and conditions of life, so that I am able to formulate a reliable opinion of this preparation in the following conclusions :

1. Pepto-Mangan (Gude) is incontestably a blood-forming preparation, and in this respect is fully equal to every other preparation.

2. Its use. is therefore recommended in all those diseases in which, through an increase of . blood and improvement of its quality, a cure or a beneficial influence upon the organism is to be expected; as for instance, in chlorosis, anæmia, leukæmia, in chronic diseases of the respiratory organs, in many digestive disorders, especially after diarrhœas, and in convalescence from various diseases, especially in weak and anæmic women after childbirth.

3. Owing to its great palatability and tolerance this preparation does not require any correctives, and is adapted especially in obstinate and protracted diseases, in nervous, neurasthenic, and all other persons who are unable to take other iron preparations even for a short time. In people who require iron and are afflicted with nervous dyspepsia Pepto-Mangan (Gude) is not only by far the best ferruginous preparation, but at the same time a stomachic which has a most favorable influence upon the secretory functions of the stomach.

4. Its blood-forming and in general curative properties depend both upon the direct introduction of iron and upon its power of stimulating the appetite and digestion. Owing to its fortunate composition this preparation deserves a general symptomatic employment.

5. Unpleasant by-effects are excluded.

Pepto-Mangan (Gude) therefore constitutes a valuable addition to our list of remedies. I prefer this preparation, which has never left me in the lurch, to all similar products, and am persuaded that within its field of indications it will prove of equal service to others. As regards the dose, it is advisable in general to follow the printed directions, although in individual cases it may be exceeded without the least untoward effects; for it is one of the prominent advantages of the preparation, that while exhibiting in full its curative effect, it never satiates or becomes repugnant, but permits of administration many months, and that it is equally well tolerated by children and adults of both sexes without exciting the least aversion.

SIR WILLIAM ROBERTS ON DIGESTION.—Sir William Roberts, of London, the great authority on digestion, says : " The digestive change undergone by fatty matter in the small intestines consists mainly in its reduction into a state of emulsion or division into infinitely minute particles. In addition to this purely physical change, a small portion undergoes a chemical change whereby the glycerine and fatty acids are dissociated. The main or principal change is undoubtedly an emulsifying process, and nearly all the fat taken up by the lacteals is simply in a state of emulsion."

This eminent authority is confirmed in the foregoing view by various experiments by which it has been ascertained that fat foods pass from the lacteals into the circulation by way of the thoraic duct in the form of an emulsion.

Emulsified cod liver oil as contained in Scott's Emulsion appears in a form so closely resembling the product of natural digestion—as it occurs within the body—that it may well be administered as an artificially digested fat food of the very highest type, in combination with the other ingredients mentioned—glycerine being an emollient of inestimable value. Scott's Emulsion offers to the physician a valuable, exquisite and rare accession to his prescription list.

EVERY PHYSICIAN KNOWS.—In the *North American Practitioner*, under the head of " Intestinal Antisepsis," reported by Dr. Pettingill of New York City, we find some excellent experiences, from which the following is selected :

" Every physician knows too well the advantages to be derived from the use of antikamnia in very many diseases, but a number of them are still lacking a knowledge of the fact that antikamnia in combination with various remedies, has a peculiarly happy effect; particularly is this the case when combined with salol. Salol is a most valuable remedy in many affections; and its usefulness seems to be enhanced by combining it with antikamnia. The rheumatoid conditions so often seen in various manifestations are wonderfully relieved by the use of this combination. After fevers, inflammations, etc., there frequently re-

main various painful and annoying conditions which may continue
namely : the severe headaches which occur after meningitis, a
'stitch in the side' following pleurisy, the precordial pain of pericarditis and the painful stiffness of the joints which remain after
a rheumatic attack—all these conditions are relieved by this
combination called 'Antikamnia and Salol Tablets,' containing
2½ grs. each of antikamnia and salol, and the dose of which is one
or two every two or three hours. They are also recommended
highly in the treatment of cases of both acute and chronic cystitis.
The pain and burning is relieved to a marked degree. Salol
makes the urine acid and clears it up. This remedy is a reliable
one in the treatment of diarrhœa, enterocolitis, dysentery, etc.
In dysentery, where there are bloody, slimy discharges, with
tormina and tenesmus, a good dose of sulphate of magnesia, followed by two antikamnia and salol tablets every three hours, will
give results that are gratifying."

SURGEONS AT PAN-AMERICAN CONGRESS.—Dr. Rudolph Matas,
Secretary of Section of General Surgery for the United States, asks
those who wish to contribute papers to send titles to him at
No. 2255 St. Charles Ave., New Orleans. He also announces
that the United Fruit Company's agents are offering, as a special
inducement to American "Congresistas," a reduction of the regular
fare for the round trip from New Orleans to the Isthmus to
$50 ; that is, $25 each way. The steamers leave New Orleans
each Friday; the last steamer to leave New Orleans in time for the
opening of the Congress will sail on December 30th, 1904, at
11 a.m. It takes about four and one-half days to reach Colon and
seven days on the return trip, on account of a stopover at Port
Limon, where ample opportunity is given to tourists to visit San
Jose, the beautiful capital of Costa Rica—"the Paris of central
America "—where the most picturesque tropical scenery can be
seen at this season under the most favorable conditions.

REAPING PTOMAINES.—A great many people seems to think
that it matters little what kind of material goes into the building
of the human structure !

They feed on thorns and expect to pick roses !

Later, they find they have sown indigestion and are reaping
ptomaines.

It's a wonderful laboratory, this human body. But it can't
prevent the formation of deadly poisons within its very being.

Indeed, the alimentary tract may be regarded as one great laboratory for the manufacture of dangerous substances. "Biliousness" is a forcible illustration of the formation and absorption of poisons, due largely to an excessive proteid diet. The nervous symptoms of the dyspeptic are often but the physiological demonstrations of putrefactive alkaloids.

Appreciating the importance of the command, "Keep the Bowels open," particularly in the colds, so easily taken at this time of the year, coryza, influenza and allied conditions, Dr. L. P. Hammond, of Rome, Ga., recommends "Laxative Antikamnia and Quinine Tablets," the laxative dose of which is two tablets, every two or three hours, as indicated. When a cathartic is desired, administer the tablets as directed and follow with a saline draught the next morning, before breakfast. This will hasten peristaltic action and assist in removing, at once, the accumulated fecal matter.

THERE IS NO SUBSTITUTE FOR SANMETTO IN ACUTE OR CHRONIC PROSTATITIS, CYSTITIS AND NEPHRITIS.—I have prescribed Sanmetto quite extensively in the last ten or twelve years, and I must say I like the remedy very much in all forms of genito-urinary troubles. I can find no substitute for Sanmetto in either acute or chronic prostatitis, cystitis and nephritis. I am not in the habit of giving testimony to proprietary remedies, but I must confess my faith in Sanmetto, and shall continue to prescribe it as long as it gives results.   J. C. DREHER, M.D.

Plainwell, Mich.

THL LOCAL TREATMENT OP ERYSIPELAS WITH ACETOZONE.— I had an ugly case of facial erysipelas in a woman of about thirty-eight years. I used as a local application, to begin with, a saturated solution of boric acid, and depended largely upon tincture ferric chloride as an internal remedy. I got the attack under control and supposed I would have no further trouble, but all at once the disease began to spread over the scalp. The usual remedies did no good. I thought that if Acetozone was the germ destroyer it was represented to be, it should be of use to me. So I made a solution of fifteen grains to two pints of water and used it freely on the scalp. I obtained results at once, and in twenty-four hours the disease had abated.   J. KNOWLES, M.D.

Logan, Iowa.

EDITORIAL ITEMS.— Continued.

Influenzal Cough. Daniel E. Hughes prescribed: ℞ Ammonii chloridi gr. x; tinct. hyoscyami m. xv; syr. ipecac m. v; spt. frumenti dr. ss; aq. chloroformi dr. iss: Take every three or four hours, diluted.

A Simple Cough Mixture. Mays prescribes: ℞ Tinct. benzoini comp. m. viii; ext. euphorbiae pil. fl. m. viii; tinct. capsici m. vi; syr. senegae m. xv; syr. acidi. hydriod. q.s.: A teaspoonful in water every three or four hours.

Mitral Bronchitis. Fothergill advises absolute rest in bed; sedatives watchfully for cough; a resort to digitalis only when acute stage has passed. Mitral lesions are often a result of acute bronchitis, particularly in old people.

Acute Bronchial Cough. A favorite prescription with N. S. Davis is the following: ℞ Morph. sulph. gr. $\frac{1}{8}$; antim. et. potass. tart. gr. 1–12; ammonii chloridi gr. x; syr. glycyrrhiza q, s.: A teaspoonful every three or four hours.

The American Journal of Urology. This new special journal enters the field under the editorial charge of Henry G. Spooner, assisted by a corps of distinguished collaborators. It is published at $3.00 a year by the Grafton Press, 70 Fifth Avenue, New York.

Gastrosuccorrhea. Van Valzah and Nisbet recommend confinement to bed in a darkened room; draughts of hot water; caffeine early to abort; Winternitz compress; thorough stomach washing, followed by doses of calomel and morphine and atropine hypodermically.

The Blood in Rheumatism. Goldthwait and Painter have found high hemoglobin and erythrocyte count and no leucocytosis in rheumatoid arthritis, as contrasted with low hemoglobin, leucocytosis and slight anemia in acute rheumatism and other infectious arthrites.

Bronchitis Depending on a Cardiac Lesion. Mays prescribes: ℞ Strychninae sulph. gr. 1–32; quin. sulph., acetanilidi, caffeinae citrat. aa. gr. $1\frac{1}{4}$; ferri. sulph. gr. $\frac{1}{2}$; pulv. digitalis gr. $\frac{1}{8}$; acidi arseniosi gr. 1–128: One capsule four times a day.

Infantile Flatulence. Goodhart and Starr advise the use of anise or caraway water, a tablespoonful sweetened with a little powdered white sugar in each bottle of food after feeding; to dilute the milk add lime water, baking soda, barley water or gelatin; empty bowels with castor oil and keep baby warm.

Habitual Regurgitation. Van Valzah and Nisbet recommend hygienic and physical measures for the nervous system; intragastric faralization or cervicogastric galvanization; and soothing, easily evacuated, minutely divided food. They consider strychnine more trustworthy than bromides.

Chronic Bronchitis with Gouty or Rheumatic Element and Tough, Scanty Expectoration. A favorite prescription of Mays is as follows: ℞ Sodii salic. gr. iv; potassii acetat. gr. ii; potassii carb. gr. i; vinicolch. rad. m. v; aquam gaultheriae q. s: A teaspoonful four times a day.

Gouty Bronchitis. Bruce advises a smart mercurial and saline purge, low diet, removal of stimulants and employment of an alkaline iodide mixture at short intervals. Shoemaker prescribes: ℞ Liq. potassii m. ss; syr. senegae m. xx; mist. glycyrmizae co. q. s: A dessertspoonful in a wineglassful of water every three hours.

Gouty Bronchitis. Apply sinapisms, says Ferrand, here and there on the chest. Give each morning a wafer containing $1\frac{1}{4}$ grains of powdered squill and $4\frac{1}{2}$ grains of powdered phellandra. Order with each meal seltzer water containing $7\frac{1}{2}$ grains of lithium carbonate. Keep the bowels open with small doses of calomel.

Bacteria of Normal Urethra. Pfeffer (quoted in *American Journal of Urology*) made cultures from the secretions of twenty-four male urethras, that had never had any venereal disease. Thirteen different species of bacteria were isolated, the principal being the pseudo-diphtheria bacillus and the streptobacillus urethrae.

Chronic Bronchitis. Arthur T. Davis has employed wine of ipecac diluted with three parts of water, administered as a spray with steam atomizer or hand-ball-spray apparatus—one to four drams to be inhaled at each sitting once daily, the patient breathing deeply and closing his nostrils with his fingers.

Low Blood Pressure Secondary to High Arterial Tension. In these serious and intractable cases Bishop has found a single large dose of digitalis (fluid extract in capsule) at bed time, often better than divided doses. A nutritious diet (milk often badly borne) and warm saline baths are in order.

Fermentive Dyspepsia. B. W. Richardson prescribes: ℞ Olei creasoti puri m. i; spt. tenuoris m. c; ammon. benzoat. gr. x; glycerini puri m. xxx; infusum caryophylli q. s: A table-spoonful in four ounces of water between meals, two or three times a day. If acidity is considerable, add potassa to each dose, or give as needed.

Piroplasma Hominis. This is the name that has been given to the intracorpuscular parasite causing Rocky Mountain spotted fever (*Practical Medicine Series*). It is a refractile, non-pigmented, ovoid body found near the edge of the red cells and showing ameboid movements. It is probably transmitted to man by a species of tick.

Inward Spasms. These are characterized by considerable flatulence and distension, often limited to or more marked in one part of the abdomen, especially the left side under ribs, accompanied by severe pain, which is temporarily relieved by eructations. By way of treatment Ringer recommends sodium sulpho-carbolate gr. xv., or carbolic acid m. i-ii. immediately before or after food.

Bronchitis of Cardiac Diseases. Ferrand enforces rest in bed at the outset and a strict milk diet. He gives sodium sulphate or scammony (gr. 7½) for obstinate constipation. He also prescribes the following: ℞ Ext. digitalis gr. 1–50; ext. conii gr. 1–30; pulv. ipecac gr. 1–20; oxymel scillae m. xii; mucil. acaciae q. s: A teaspoonful every three hours.

Winter Cough. Ringer gives 2-grain tar pills every three hours. Crook employs three parts of terebene and one part of oil of eucalyptus, giving ten to fifteen drops of the mixture on sugar every hour. T. E. Taylor has used apomorphine, gr. 1–15 every four or five hours; also a spray of wine of ipecac, with an equal volume of water several times a day.

The Clinical Thermometer. Judson Daland (*Medico-Chirurgical Journal*) states that Galileo invented the thermometer about three centuries ago. To Wunderlich, who in 1871 published his sixteen years' study of medical thermometry, we owe the introduction of the clinical thermometer into practical medicine. In the Philadelphia Hospital the use of this instrument began in 1875.

It's Worth Remembering

that fats are always demanded in the treatment of phthisis and other wasting diseases because they check the destructive metabolism of proteids.

Some fats, of course, are better proteid-sparers than others; the most effective are those that are easily digested and oxidized.

Hydroleine contains a notably large per cent. of the most digestible form of the most digestible and oxidizable food-fat known—pure Lofoten Cod-Liver Oil. That's why Hydroleine produces immediate and positive results in wasting diseases. Write for literature.

Sold by all druggists.

THE CHARLES N. CRITTENTON CO.

Sole Agents,

115-117 FULTON STREET, NEW YORK.

TANNIGEN

The Intestinal Astringent.

LACTO-SOMATOSI

The Food and Restorative   **in Diarrheal Diseases.**

ROTARGOL

The Non-Irritating Substitute for Nitrate of Silver.

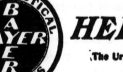

HELMITO

The Urinary Antiseptic and Analgesic.

Internally.

SPIRIN

BEST ANTI-RHEUMATICS.

amples Suppl.
by
FARBENFABRIK
of

To Initiate Diuresis.

THEOCI

THE POWERFUL DIURETI

SOTAN

Externally.

AGURIN

To Maintain Diuresis.

—17—

Senile Endometritis. The chief symptom is a purulent and often offensive discharge, which by retention may give rise to pyometra. This form of disease, says Davenport, is best treated by painting the cavity with pigmentum iodi (one dram each of iodine, potassium iodide and glycerine, with enough water to make four drams) and draining. Curettage does no good.

Cypress Oil for Whooping Cough. It has been noted by Bravo and others (*Practical Medicine Series*) that a few drops of cypress oil poured on the clothes and pillows of children with pertussis gives remarkable results in controlling the paroxysms. O. Soltmann has used ten to fifteen grammes of a one to five alcoholic solution of the oil in this way four times a day. Linen is stained by the oil.

Bronchitis of Infants. E. P. Davis recommends the turpentine chest pack—long layer of turpentine stupe more than sufficient to go around body, and over this flannel another dry one—renew when inner cloth is made dry by heat of body. He gives small doses of paregoric or syrup of lettuce for the cough, or if harsh, two grains of ammonium chloride with syrup of licorice and water for an 8-months child.

Memorrhagia of Endometritis. Hydrastis canadensis, says Davenport (*International Clinics*) seems to be of the greatest value in the menorrhagia due to endometritis. It should be given as the fluid extract in the dose of one-half to one teaspoonful in water after meals and at bedtime, increasing if the flow is profuse. It will have a more satisfactory effect if its use is kept up during the interval between the periods of flowing.

Indicanuria Complicating Typhoid Fever. Judson Daland (*American Medicine*, Oct. 29) has for some years made it a routine practice to examine every forty-eight hours, for indican in the urine of typhoid patients. When found in excess he pays special attention to the mouth and teeth, tonsils, pharynx, nose and accessory cavities. He gives calomel in small doses, followed by sodium phosphate, and if necessary, uses colon irrigation with one or two quarts of warm normal salt solution.

Appendicitis and Meat Diet. H. Speier (*Wisconsin Medical Recorder*) reviews a recent study presented by Lucas-Championniere to the Academy of Medicine, at Paris. This showed

It needs but little physiological knowledge to see how, in case of diabetes mellitus for example, in which disease cod liver oil is the "sheet-anchor," the use of substitutes for cod liver oil would be attended with disagreeable results. Cod liver oil possesses all the good qualities that the proposed substitutes lack, and none of their defects. The highest grade of pure cod liver oil is admirably combined with hypophosphites of lime and soda and glycerine in Scott's Emulsion.

PASSIFLORA

The Commoner Pathogenic Bacteria that Invade the Eye·
Among these micro-organisms, Wood and Woodruff mention the
staphylococcus pyogenes aureus as the chief cause of all forms of
irritation in the conjuctival sac. The streptococcus pyogenes is
present in most purulent inflammations of the conjunctiva, especially in discharge from the lachrymal sac, and is also found in
many forms of corneal ulcer. The gonococcus is the special bacterium of adult gonorrheal conjunctivitis, and, in most cases, of
ophthalmia neonatorum, particularly in that form of it that shows
itself on or before the fourth day after birth, The pneumococcus
is the germ found in a highly contagious form of conjunctivitis,
in serpiginous ulcer of the cornea, and in panophthalmitis. The
small Koch-Weeks bacillus is characteristic of that acute form of
contagious conjunctivitis, commonly known as " pink-eye." The
paired and chained diplobacillus of Morax and Axenfeld is found
in a well defined form of subacute conjunctivitis, accompanied by
slight discharge, which usually runs a course of several weeks'
duration.

that in every section of France the frequency of appendicitis increased in direct ratio with the consumption of meat. In schools, prisons, asylums and convents, where the diet is nearly or entirely vegetarian the disease is very rare. It has not yet appeared among the vegetarian natives of Porto Rico.

Flatulence of Hysterical and Hypochondriacal Subjects. The tincture or fluid extract of valerian is often given in the dose of one-half to two drams. Bartholow has recommended a tablespoonful every hour or two of a mixture of three parts of camphor water and one part of compound tincture of lavender. Shoemaker prescribes: ℞ Tinct. asafetidae m. xx-xxx; tinct. cardamoni m. xv-xxx; spt. ammon. arom. m. ii-iv; aq. menth. pip. m. xxx-lx. Take in water every two or three hours.

Gastric Myasthenia. Van Valzah and Nesbit recommend a mixed diet, small in bulk, finely divided and rather dry, with very little fruit and vegetables. They use abdominal massage, electricity, hydrotherapy (intragastric spray and Scottish douche) and open-air exercise in moderation. Strychnine is the most useful drug; hydrastinine, quinine, ergot and very small doses of ipecac are also beneficial. Use laxatives as little as possible.

Obscure Symptoms of Circulatory Disorder. Among these symptoms L. F. Bishop mentions puffing and blowing sounds in the head; simulation of slight attacks of paralysis, or "clumsiness" of a leg or an arm; slight loss of power of speech, attacks of sciatica, neuritis, and other pains in various parts of the body; congested liver, with marked stomach disorder, or persistent congestion of the lungs and pleural transudation; mental defects and rarely general convulsions; paresthesia and cramps in muscles of extremities. A few doses of nitroglycerine have stopped all complaint of cold extremities in any patients of this type.

Castor Oil for Burns. C. MacLellan (*Practical Medicine Series*) washes the burned surface as well as can be done, then pours the oil freely over the parts, and distributes it evenly with a fine varnish brush. Pieces of plain or medicated gauze, cut in the desired shape and previously soaked in the oil, are applied over the wound and brushed to smoothness. More oil may now be brushed in to thoroughly saturate the gauze, which is then deeply covered with cotton wool. The wool is frequently removed and the oil reapplied upon the gauze covering the wound.

Treatment of Diabetic Coma. Heinrich Stern (*Medical Standard*) states that he has found precipitated calcium carbonate the most valuable drug for this condition. If the patient is still conscious, the medicine is given by the mouth, thirty grains every two hours; a saline cathartic is given every morning, and entero-clysis with large amounts of sodium chloride solution should be performed at least once a day. In case deep coma has set in, the calcium carbonate should be administered by the rectum, in doses of forty-five to sixty grains every four hours suspended in $\frac{1}{2}$ to two pints of hot water by the addition of 25 per cent. its weight of acacia, and preceded on each occasion by salt enteroclysis.

Dysmenorrhea. Davenport states (*International Clinics*) that the most common cause of dysmenorrhea is anteflexion, par-ticularly in connection with lack of development, conical cervix, narrowing of canal at internal os, and abnormal sensibility at point of flexion. The pain in these cases usually begins a few hours after the flow, increasing rapidly, and usually becoming less or disappearing after 24 hours. It is often paroxysmal, usually most in front, and sometimes accompanied by nausea and vomit-ing. The one satisfactory mode of treatment for this form of dysmenorrhea is dilatation under ether, the effect of which may be made more permanent by the insertion of a plug to be worn for some weeks.

Acute Rhinitis. The symptoms include chilly sensations, lassitude, slight fever and muscular pain; stuffy feeling in frontal region, often with headache, neuralgia of antrum and lachryma-tion; dry burning or pricking at root of nose, followed in a few hours by free discharge; anosmia, partial aguesia; and ringing in ears or temporary deafness. The signs are a mucous membrane bluish-red, dry, glazed and swollen (swelling disappears under cocaine in first stage), bathed in profuse watery serum in second stage; secretion scanty, thick, viscid and bright yellow in third stage; posterior nares more or less blocked by swelling of mem-brane; lower pharynx often dry and glazed from mouth-breathing; nursing of infants interfered with to a greater or less degree.

Emphysematons Bronchitis. Ferrand recommends small doses of tartar emetic during attacks, repeated to nausea each morning for three consecutive days and continued for two or three weeks. Rub thorax repeatedly with a mixture of camphorated

The amily axative

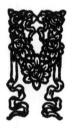

alifornia ig Syrup ompany

an Francisco,
California.

Louisville, Ky.
New York, N. Y.

The ideal, safe, family laxative, known as "Syrup of Figs," is a product of the California Fig Syrup Co., and derives its laxative principles from senna, made pleasant to the taste and more acceptable to the stomach by being combined with pleasant aromatic syrups and the juice of figs. It is recommended by many of the most eminent physicians, and used by millions of families with entire satisfaction. It has gained its great reputation with the medical profession by reason of the acknowledged skill and care exercised by the California Fig Syrup Co. in securing the laxative principles of the senna by an original method of its own, and presenting them in the best and most convenient form. The California Fig Syrup Co. has special facilities for commanding the choicest qualities of Alexandria senna, and its chemists devote their entire attention to the manufacture of the one product. The name "Syrup of Figs" means to the medical profession "the family laxative, manufactured by the California Fig Syrup Co." and the name of the company is a guarantee of the excellence of its product. Informed of the above facts, the careful physician will know how to prevent the dispensing of worthless imitations when he recommends or prescribes the original and genuine "Syrup of Figs." It is well known to physicians that "Syrup of Figs" is a simple, safe and reliable laxative, which does not irritate or debilitate the organs on which it acts, and, being pleasant to the taste, it is especially adapted to ladies and children, although generally applicable in all cases. Special investigation of the profession invited.

"Syrup of Figs" is never sold in bulk. It retails at fifty cents per bottle, and the name "Syrup of Figs," as well as the name of the California Fig Syrup Co., is printed on the wrappers and labels of every bottle.

The advent of the season in which

COUGH,
BRONCHITIS,
WHOOPING COUGH,
ASTHMA, Etc.

Impose a tax upon the resources of every physician renders it opportune to re-invite attention to the fact that the remedy which invariably effects the immediate relief of these disturbances, the remedy which unbiased observers assert affords the most rational means of treatment, the remedy which bears with distinction the most exacting comparisons, the remedy which occupies the most exalted position in the esteem of discriminating therapeutists is

GLYCO-HEROIN (Smith)

GLYCO-HEROIN (Smith) is conspicuously valuable in the treatment of Pneumonia, Phthisis, and Chronic Affections of the Lungs, for the reason that it is more prompt and decided in effect than either codeine or morphine, and its prolonged use neither leaves undesirable after effects nor begets the drug habit. It acts as a reparative in an unsurpassable manner.

DOSE.—The adult dose is one teaspoonful, repeated every two hours, or at longer intervals as the case may require.
To children of ten or more years, give from a quarter to a half teaspoonful.
To children of three or more years, give five to ten drops.

MARTIN H. SMITH CO.,
PROPRIETORS.

SAMPLES SUPPLIED
CARRIAGE PAID, UPON REQUEST   NEW YORK, N. Y,

—21—

ammonia liniment and spirit of turpentine, or else with croton oil. Use saline or drastic cathartics when called for. The diet should consist of fruits, vegetables, milk, eggs, and white meats. Vichy water is a useful sedative to counteract the local irritant effects of antimonials on the digestive tract. In the intervals give each morning for five days in a week 1–65 grains of arsenate of antimony, and each night order a pill composed of 1½ grain each of datura and powdered phellandra. Use sulphur fumigations each morning. Keep bowels free.

How to Live Long. H. Weber (*Practical Medicine Series*) sums up his advice on this question as follows: Moderation in eating, drinking and physical indulgence. Pure air, out of the house and within. The keeping of every organ of the body, as far as possible, in constant working order. Regular exercise every day in all weathers; supplemented in many cases by breathing movements, and by walking and climbing tours. Going to bed early and rising early, and restricting the hours of sleep to six or seven. Daily baths or ablutions according to individual conditions, cold or warm, or warm followed by cold. Regular work and mental occupation. Cultivation of placidity, cheerfulness and hopefulness of mind. Employment of the great powers of the mind in controlling the passions and nervous fear. Strengthening the will in carrying out whatever is useful and in checking the craving for stimulants, anodynes and other injurious agencies.

Treatment of Acute Vaginitis. Davis advises to use four times a day half-gallon vaginal douches of 1:5000 mercurio chloride at 100°F. Apply to lesions, on absorbent cotton, hydrogen peroxide, followed by boric acid or iodoform as a dusting powder. Unload bowels with calomel and soda, followed by a saline or an enema. Use turpentine stupes for pain. Bushong gives thorough and frequent vaginal douches in the dorsal position—one-half gallon or more at 110–111°F. every two or three hours, containing bichloride of mercury (1:10,000 to 1:2,000) or common salt (tablespoonful or more to the gallon of water). When the painful stage has been allayed with douches, make a thorough application of silver nitrate (one dram to the ounce of water) to the whole of involved area, on a small ball of cotton with forceps and speculum.

Pelvic Hematocele. This very dangerous and often deceptive condition is treated by Byford as follows: Rest in bed; ice-water bag over pubes for 24 hours; cold drinks and stimulants in case of syncope; afterward rest in bed for two or three weeks. Apply tincture of iodine over the lower abdomen twice a day and employ saline laxatives and a light diet. When suppuration ensues, puncture mass antiseptically per vaginam with aspirating needle or small trocar as far back and as near median line as it can be reached, carefully avoiding pulsating vessels, and evacuating pus as in pelvic abscess. Abdominal section is indicated when intervention is necessary during first few days, or when the mass is inaccessible by the vaginal route. A firm, non-suppurative mass, after two weeks or more, should be evacuated per vaginam.

Absorbent Paper in Practical Hematology. Tallquist (*Medical News*, Oct. 22) calls attention to the fact that in using white absorbent paper in connection with his color scale, if around the colored spot made by the drop of blood there extends a moist ring (best seen by transmitted light) the number of red blood corpuscles is reduced to one-half or less of normal.

Medication during Cardiac Compensation. The occasional use, says Bishop, during the stage of compensation, of the iodide of sodium as a means of preventing degeneration of the hyper-atrophied heart, is a useful procedure even when no other drug therapy seems advisable. He gives two to fifteen drops of a saturated solution in a half glass of water after meals.

Diseases of the Skin connected with Errors of Metabolism. Bulkley (*Medical Record*, Nov. 26) says at the close of his carefully prepared article: Metabolic errors are exhibited in the excreta from the lungs, skin, intestines and kidneys; and of these the urine best affords a satisfactory indication, as it represents nearly one-half of the total excreta, and practically all of the nitrogenous and soluble mineral substances, together with about one-half of the water expelled from the system. Complete and minute urinary analysis is a very great aid in discovering metabolic errors and in establishing proper therapeutic measures for the cure of many diseases of the skin.

DENVER MEDICAL TIMES

Volume XXIV.   JANUARY, 1905   Number 7

SURGICAL TREATMENT OF DISPLACEMENTS OF
THE UTERUS.*

By R. C. COFFEY, M.D.,

Portland, Oregon.

Practically all text books on diseases of women in giving the supports of the uterus classify the ligaments under the heads of true and false. Under the head of true ligaments are given round, utero-sacral, and utero-pelvic ligaments. The false ligaments are broad, utero-vesical, and utero-rectal. Anatomists and histologists as well as authorities on diseases of women say that the true ligaments are composed largely of muscular fibres with a little elastic and fibrous tissue; that these ligaments are in reality but prolongations of the muscular walls of the uterus; that the false ligaments are simply peritoneal folds which enclose the vessels and other structures going to the uterus, but are said to play no important part in supporting the uterus.

It is claimed by most authorities that the round ligaments are the chief agents in holding the uterus forward. Some modern authorities, however, claim that the utero-sacral ligaments play a still more important part by holding the cervix back toward the sacrum, and other authorities have claimed that intra-abdominal pressure is the chief agent in the support of the uterus. Still other authorities claim that what is ordinarily known as the pelvic floor is the chief support of the uterus. The principal surgical operations for the relief of the displacements have, therefore, been directed to the following lines: first, to make solid the pelvic floor; second, the shortening of the so-called true ligaments, especially the round ligaments; third, the formation of a new ligament by stitching the peritoneal surface of the uterus to the peritoneum of the abdomen, with the idea of forming an entirely new ligament for the support of the uterus.

I think it will generally be admitted that no operation so far devised has given general satisfaction. I shall not attempt to give

---

* Read before the Rocky Mountain Inter-State Medical Association, September, 1904.

the various flaws in each operation, as those who have operated
extensively have no doubt observed the failures of all methods.
The advocates of one method have generally condemned the other

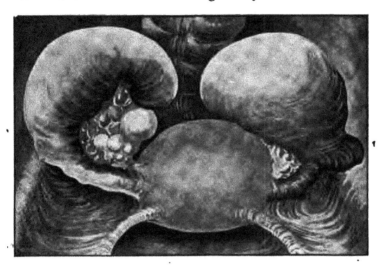

Fig. 1—Ideal case of Pyo-salpinx with accompanying cystic ovary, after
adhesions have been broken up.

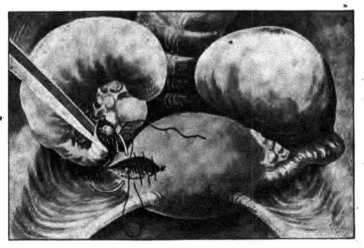

Fig. 2.—Excision of the tube from the cornus of the uterus. Closing the
incision immediately after with catgut.

methods.   The consequence is that many operations for the shortening of the so-called true ligaments are being devised.   And yet

no operation has stood the test of time like one that depends upon a single, frail, peritoneal attachment for its support,—namely: ventro-suspension or ventro-fixation.   The partial failure of these various operations naturally suggests the question, "Are we wrok-

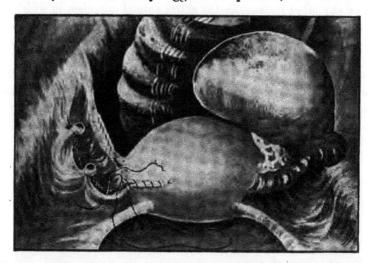

Fig. 3.—Cystic portion of ovary and tube have been removed. Ovary has been sutured with fine catgut. Meso-salpinx has been drawn over to the side of the uterus, turning in the stumps and forming shelter for ovary.

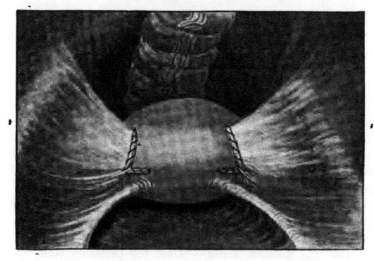

Fig. 4.—The broad ligament has been drawn over and stitched to the side of the uterus, leaving the ovary underneath.

ing upon the right anatomical principles?" If the anatomist and histologist are correct as to the formation of the so-called true ligaments in stating that they are mainly muscular prolongations of the uterus, are we not justified in asking the question, "Is there any other instance in the entire animal organism in which a muscle is used for the support of any organ or tissue?" Second, "Is it not a fact that all muscular fibers when subjected to a constant strain like what would be required to support an organ, inevitably become paralyzed or filled with an inflammatory exudate which becomes organized and thus destroys the ordinary utility of the muscular fibers?" Third, "Is it not conceded by all anatomists

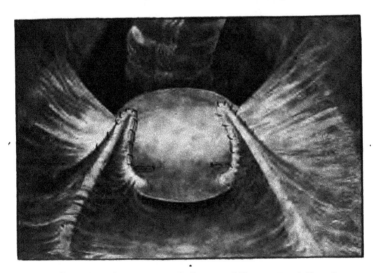

Fig. 5.—Posterior advancement of the round ligaments of the uterus.

and physiologists that the function of a muscular fiber is to contract and thereby produce motion, and has any other use been discovered for a muscular fiber?" I think not. Therefore, are we not justified in questioning, or at best modifying our idea of the functions ordinarily attributed to the so-called true ligaments of the uterus? Shall we not, therefore, look for a somewhat different use for these so-called true ligaments in which they would perform their normal function of contraction and producing motion, and for continuous support and suspension of the uterus?

Then the question arises,—"Does the perineum form the chief support of the uterus?" Most certainly the experience of almost every one will call forth many cases with the perineal support completely destroyed, and yet the uterus and other organs are in their normal position. Then, is it intra-abdominal pressure? Let us look to the other organs in the abdominal cavity. Has not every operator noticed that many times the abdominal cavity, no matter how lax its muscular walls, contains organs all in an absolutely normal position? In these cases there may be absolutely no intra-abdominal pressure, the organs all lying limp when

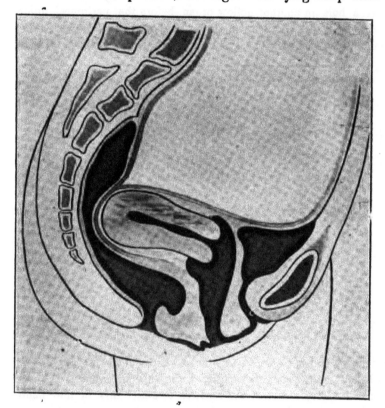

Fig. I.—Section through body showing retroverted uterus.
(Copy from Dudley.)

the abdomen is opened. What supports them? Deaver in his incomparable work on anatomy gives as the entire support of the liver, which is the uppermost and heaviest organ in the abdominal cavity, peritoneal folds; and who has not in the cadaver found that the ligaments of the liver will hold many times the weight of this organ, which of itself is several times heavier than all the generative organs? The spleen is held in place by peritoneum. The stomach and all the intestines are held in place by peritoneum. The kidneys are held in place by simply being behind the peritoneum. Moreover, the best operation which has been given us for the support of the uterus depends entirely upon the attachment of the uterus to the loose peritoneum of the anterior abdominal wall. Adhesion of an abdominal organ covered with peritoneum to another peritoneal surface when firmly organized will tear a hole in another hollow organ before the peritoneal union will separate, as shown by stitching two intestines together. The omentum attached to the abdominal wall becomes very much

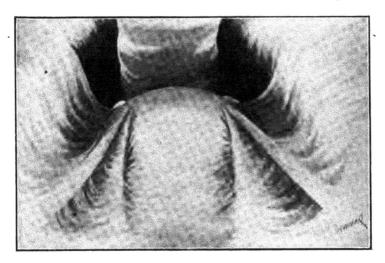

Fig. II.—Retroverted uterus shown from abdominal incision. The ovaries and tubes are beneath and behind the uterus in the cul-de-sac.

thickened and is so firmly adherent to a peritoneal surface that it will hold many times the weight of the lighter organs in the abdominal cavity. I have had occasion to notice this in the "hammock" operation for gastroptosis.

Who has ever known the parietal peritoneum to be found out of contact with the abdominal wall? Is it not a fact that the loose peritoneum of the abdominal wall, even though it may be drawn inches away from the wall and attached to another organ will generally pull the organ to it and retract to its normal attachment? Therefore, considering this fact that peritoneum clings to the abdominal wall under all circumstances, and considering the fact that all of the organs in the abdominal cavity are held by peritoneum, why should we attempt to make an exception in the case of the uterus, especially when we consider the fact that the uterus has running into its sides larger folds of peritoneum and more advantageously placed from a mechanical standpoint than any other organ in the abdominal cavity?

In considering the anatomy of the peritoneum of the pelvic

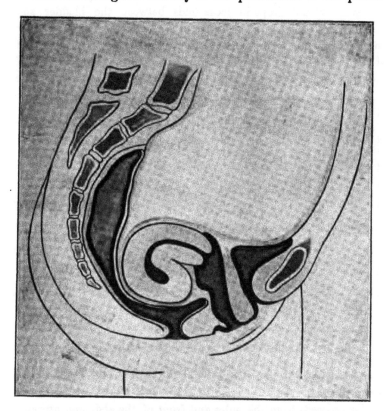

Fig. III.—Section through body showing retroflexed uterus (Copy from Dudley.)

portion of the abdominal cavity, we find that it comes down on the sides of the pelvis from above and is attached firmly in a vertical direction in the long axis of the uterus to the postero-lateral border. It comes in from the sides of the pelvis, covering over the tubes and round ligaments like a blanket, and attaches near the fundus. A portion of that coming from below is attached to the antero-lateral border of the uterus in a vertical direction, in the same manner as that coming from above is attached to the postero-lateral border. That portion of the peritoneum of the uterus dips far down forming what is called Douglas' cul-de-sac, which lies in loose folds capable of expanding and stretching many times its normal length. Coming up from below anterior to the uterus, the peritoneum is spread loosely over the bladder like a cover and drops in loose folds between the bladder and uterus forming the vesico-uterine fold. The loose folds before and back of the uterus are ample to give room for the expansion of the rising of the uterus during pregnancy. That portion of the peritoneum which is attached to the postero-lateral border

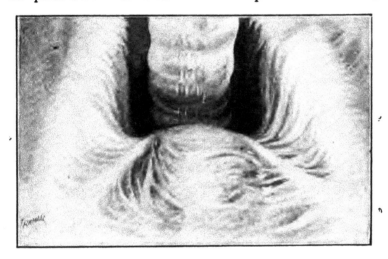

Fig. IV.—Retroflexed uterus shown from abdominal incision.

proceeds from the sides and front of the pelvic cavity downward, forward and inward. That portion attached to the antero-lateral border proceeds from the sides and front of the abdomen upward, forward and inward forming almost a triangle, the apex of which is from one to two inches wide and is attached to the sides of the uterus, while the base of the triangle comes from the sides of the pelvis over a surface of six to ten inches. The roof of the triangle comes from the sides and front of the pelvis to the internal opening of the inguinal canal and proceeds almost directly toward the center and is attached to the fundus of the uterus, forming a tent loosely attached over the round ligament and adnexa of the uterus. The triangular portion of the peritoneum is commonly known as the broad ligament. That portion of the broad ligament coming from either side of the rectum and attaching into the posterior surface of the uterus is commonly known as the utero-rectal ligament. That portion of the peritoneum proceeding from either side of the bladder to the antero-lateral surface is known as the utero-vesical ligament. That portion of the pelvic

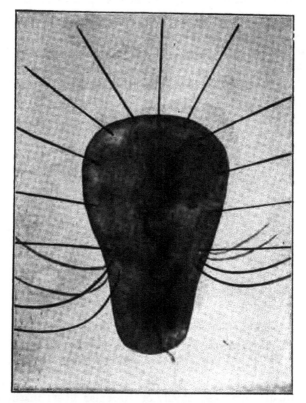

Fig. V.—Side view of the uterus showing attachment of broad ligament. Straight lines indicate points of peritoneum where some tension is made, curved lines peritoneum in fold.

peritoneum lying between the rectum and uterus, behind and between the uterus and bladder in front, lies in loose folds in contradistinction to all that portion of peritoneum which goes to form the broad ligaments, which is normally found in a more or less tense condition. Thus it will be seen that the uterus is slung in a swing composed of the lower portion of the parietal peritoneum, which is arranged in the same manner as the ropes sustain the huge masts of a ship.

The round ligaments come over, not from the front as the text books have led us to believe, but almost directly parallel to the transverse diameter of the uterus, and lie loosely under the peritoneum ready to serve their normal function of moving the uterus and either lifting the uterus upwards to its place in case of a traumatism and possibly lifting the uterus under other conditions, as sexual intercourse, etc.

The utero-pelvic ligaments are muscles, probably ready to move the cervix to its normal position when displacement has occurred or to pull the uterus down under other circumstances.

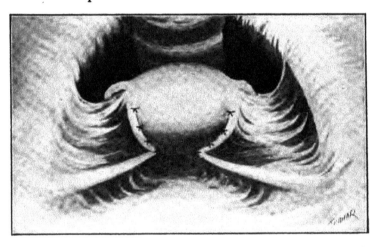

Fig. VI.—Round ligaments have been drawn to the antero-lateral border of the uterus and stitched with thirty-day catgut.

Therefore, inasmuch as the so-called true ligaments of the uterus are admittedly composed chiefly of muscular fiber; inasmuch as the only known function of a muscular fiber is to contract and produce motion; inasmuch as it is contrary to the nature of a fiber to be able to resist a constant strain, no matter how small for a considerable length of time, as is the case of the suspension of any organ; inasmuch as all operations, thus far known, to shorten these muscular ligaments alone without shortening their perito- neal covering have proven successful only in recent and unmarked cases; inasmuch as we find a use for these so-called ligaments in a sphere exactly suited to their normal action, are we not justified in trying to assign them to their normal labor? Second,—Assuming it is not probable that the muscular ligaments of the uterus play any particular part in the constant holding up of the uterus, and inasmuch as we find that laceration of the pelvic floor plays only a small part in the displacements of the uterus; inasmuch as the intra-abdominal pressure seems to influence very little the position of the uterus; inasmuch as every other organ in the abdominal cavity is held in place by the peritoneum; inasmuch as peritoneal surface always clings to the parietas tending to draw any organ to it; inasmuch as the best operation yet devised for retain-

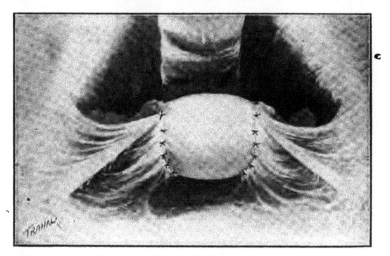

Fig. VIII.—Second loop of round ligament has been brought to normal origin and stitched.

ing the uterus in place is due to a simple adhesion to the peritoneum; inasmuch as peritoneum coming in toward the uterus is arranged in the most advantageous mechanical manner possible for the purpose of suspending the uterus in a movable position, are we not justified in believing that the chief suspensory support of the uterus is its peritoneum? And this being the case, are the operations which are commonly described in text books resting upon an absolutely correct anatomical and mechanical basis?

After the shortening of the muscular ligaments of the uterus a few times with no great success, and having done the suspension operation more than two hundred times with a limited amount of success, some cases having been entirely relieved of symptoms, others having been greatly benefitted, and still a larger number having been slightly benefitted, and a few having been made no more comfortable, I have gradually during the past three years developed an operation, step by step, which has for its chief point the taking up of the slack of various portions of the broad ligaments with intra-abdominal shortening of the round ligament. I shall endeavor to show you by a set of drawings something which I believe has not been published so far, with the statement that while sufficient time to judge of its merits has not elapsed, all doctors who have witnessed the result of this operation will

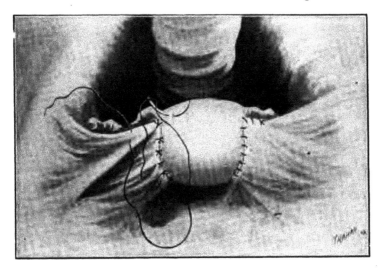

Fig. IX.—Peritoneum of broad ligament being stitched to front of uterus covering in interrupted stitches.

agree with me in saying that the results are more rapid and satisfactory, that the patient is in a better condition after this operation than after those that have commonly been done. I, therefore, submit it to you for criticism.

A little more than three years ago, in finishing up the operation for removal of pus tubes, I began to systematically turn the stumps into the cul-de-sac and suture the peritoneum of the broad ligament to the side and top of the uterus, with the primary idea of protecting any remaining ovarian tissue and the stump from giving rise to adhesions. After watching this result I noticed that the uterus was very satisfactorily held in position by this operation. A little later I began to pick up the round ligament with the broad ligament and advance it posteriorly in those cases where a tendency to retroversion existed. After a few operations had been done, we applied the term "posterior advancement of the round and broad ligament." This gave such perfect satisfaction that I began to study anatomy with the idea of developing an operation along similar lines which could be applied in ordinary cases of retro-displacements in which the tubes and a portion of the ovaries remained.

We made a very careful study of the peritoneum in all these cases and very soon began to do an anterior advancement of the

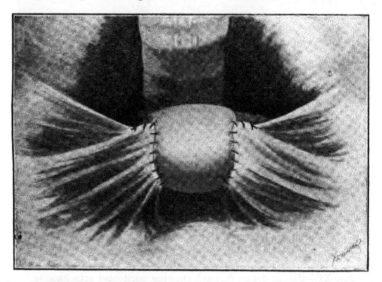

Fig. X.—Completed operation for advancement of round and broad ligament·

round and internal advancement of the broad ligament. About a year and a half ago, we began to construct the drawing, Fig. I, as we were unable to find any drawing in the literature which showed a view of a retroverted uterus from the abdominal wound. After beginning this picture, have each time the abdomen has been opened in these cases carefully packed away the intestines and observed the uterus as it rested in the retroposition. The picture here shown will represent almost the ideal case of retroversion taken from an average of more than fifty cases observed. Fig. II. shows a complete retroflexion. The anterior surface of the uterus, pointing directly upward in number

one, is in number two turned directly backwards resting against
the rectum. In both cases the peritoneum is found in a relaxed
condition. In picture number two, the round ligaments are so
small as to be of practically no value. In both cases it will generally be found that both tubes and ovaries are lying back and
beneath the uterus, which accounts for the disease of these organs
which generally accompanies retro-displacement. It is, therefore,
almost always necessary to eneucleate a number of small cysts and
thus greatly reduce the size of the ovary as a preliminary step of
the operation.

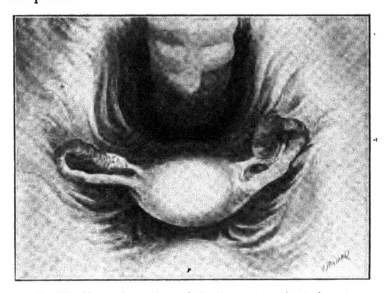

Fig. XI.—Uterus drawn forward showing peritoneal attachments
on back side.

Picture No. 3 shows the peritoneum back of the uterus in a
relaxed condition. The operation I wish to describe then begins:
First—By lifting the uterus up to its normal position, and doing
the necessary operative work upon the ovaries; Second—Seize
the round ligament with its surrounding peritoneum about one
and one-half inches from its origin and stitch it by four or five
interrupted sutures of number three formalin or chromicized catgut to the side and front of the uterus about the insertion of the
broad ligament; Third—Seize the round ligament about an inch
and one-half from the lower suture placed in the first row and

bring this knuckle back to the origin of the round ligament and fasten with interrupted sutures as before. You will notice that each time the round ligament is brought to the side of the uterus, a double layer of peritoneum is also brought down, which in reality is a plication of the broad ligament. At this stage I have been in the habit in certain cases of shortening the ligaments back of the uterus, or rather I may say of plicating the peritoneum back of the uterus. This is done by pulling the uterus well forward either with a vulsellum or simply by the hand of the assistant. A suture is passed through a fold of peritoneum over what is sometimes called the sacro-uterine ligament, and is then passed

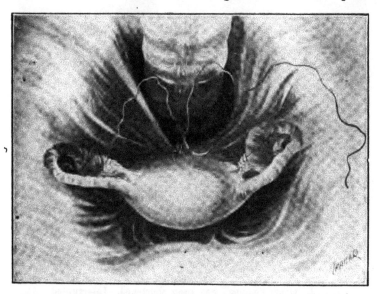

Fig. XII.—One stitch being taken to shorten fold of broad ligament covering sacro-uterine. Corresponding stitch tied on the other side.

through the peritoneum where it is normally attached to the posterior surface of the uterus as shown in figure eight. You will note that a single stitch has been placed on the right side and tied, which leaves a space between this newly formed ligament and the broad ligament. This newly formed ligament is then stitched by four or five interrupted sutures on each side to the posterior surface of the uterus opposite the internal os and to the adjacent broad ligament, thus closing the opening made. The result is shown in figure nine. It will be seen that the ovary practically rests upon a little shelf and the lower end of the uterus is held hack by it. Figure five represents the second plication of the ligaments.

Figure six represents the third step in the front part of the operation,—the covering of all the heavier interrupted sutures by bringing the peritoneum of the broad ligament over them with a continuous suture of number one formalin cumol catgut. I have lately been returning with my continuous suture after reaching the lower interrupted stitch and ending up a little exterior to the cornus of the uterus.

Figure seven shows the completed operation. If the ovarian

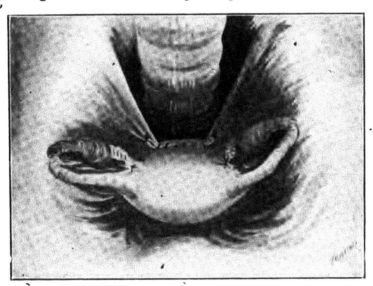

Fig. XIII.—Posterior ligaments shortened. Cystic ovaries have been repaired. Ovary ligament has been shortened. Interrupted
stitches should be used.

ligament allows the ovary to hang too low, a single stitch holds it in good position. The same may be done with the tube, the ope-rator judging of the amount of stitching necessary in each indi-vidual case. Frequently the appendix will be found in the pelvis, and in these cases should always be removed. Less frequently the cecum is found in the cul-de-sac and should be held in place by plicating the mesoappendix and mesoceum.

While I have not done a sufficient number of these opera-tions, and those done have not been of sufficient length of time to call this report statistics, I have done sixty or more by the operation here described, and including those cases in which the first operation described or posterior advancement had been performed, my cases would run to the neighborhood of one hundred. I shall not pretend to give statistics, however, while the operation is so new, but will say that so far the results have been so satisfactory as to leave very little to be desired as far as the comfort of the patient is concerned. I have enquired very carefully after all cases and have frequently written to the doctors for whom I have operated, and they are all of the opinion that the results are far superior as far as the comfort of the patient is concerned to any of the operations they have seen before. No case has relapsed, and no case has required a secondary opening of the abdomen; no case has been pregnant so far, and this to my mind is the unsettled question in the matter. I have examined quite a large per cent of these cases some time after operation, and find the uterus in its normal position and movable.

I have several times left the repair of the cervix and perineum until after this operation has been done for two or three months. I find that the cervix can easily be operated upon three months after these ligaments have been plicated. Theoretically if the muscular ligaments play an important part in the movements of the uterus they would be to a certain extent crippled by this operation, and the ideal operation from a theoretical standpoint would be some extra-peritoneal shortening of the round ligament by some method similar to that described some time ago by Noble of Atlanta, combined with plication of the peritoneum as shown in the last step of the operation here described. Clinically and practically, however, I would not feel like changing unless some unforeseen trouble develops in the future.

This operation here described will never take the place now occupied by the operation of ventro-suspension. I mean by this that it is not an operation which every tyro will use as an introduction in making his debut into abdominal surgery, as a certain amount of familiarity with the pelvis is required to perform this operation with any degree of success. I believe that even experienced abdominal surgeons will do the operation better after they have done it a few times than they will at first. It is like most other operations in that its success will depend very largely upon the ability of the surgeon to adapt his work to the conditions present.

In conclusion, I will say that there has been no sudden and decided discoveries in connection with this work, but the operation as described here has been gradually developed by careful observation for a period of a little more than three years. My views of the subject are entirely different now from what they were during the first part of my study on this subject. The hope of the operation as described here is based on the following principles:

First—The so-called true ligaments of the uterus are chiefly muscular prolongations of that organ.

Second—The only known function of a muscular fiber is to contract and produce motion.

Third—A muscular fiber will under no circumstances stand a constant strain, as is necessary in the supporting of any organ.

Fourth—The uterus is a movable organ and therefore needs an agent to produce this motion. This function is supplied by the muscular ligaments, thus giving them the important function of motor or accessory ligaments of the uterus with the power to restore it under ordinary circumstances when its equilibrium has been disturbed, and possibly to move it under other circumstances.

Fifth—The uterus has by far the greatest peritoneal support of all the other organs of the abdominal cavity, as is shown by the very firm attachment of the broad ligament on the antero- and postero-lateral borders of the uterus.

Sixth—The peritoneum is apparently the universal ligament of all the organs in the abdominal cavity.

I shall not insist that any one adopt the operation here described, but simply throw out these suggestions to be used as food for thought in the development of this subject, as we know that this subject is far from settled at the present time. But I believe that the question of this as well as all other abdominal ptoses will be settled by a method which shall depend upon one idea, namely: *"That the peritoneum with its re-duplications is the universal and chief sustaining ligament of the organs of the abdominal cavity."*

DISCUSSION.

DR. FLEMING. I have listened with considerable interest to Dr. Coffey, and I want to congratulate him upon his operation.

I cannot agree with him, however, in some of his remarks regarding the supports of the uterus. We know that the uterus s a perfectly movable organ, and even in some cases where we have lacerations of the perineum we have no prolapse, and yet we can draw the uterus down regardless of the peritoneum. We can push it up and push it sideways, so to my mind the peritoneum does not in any way support the uterus. I believe that an intact perineum is a very important factor, but the retentive power of the abdomen is the most important. That has been described by Penrose in his most excellent book, and I think he agrees that this retentive power is a very important factor in maintaining the uterus in its normal position.

I think a great many cases of relapse, following suspension operations on the uterus, are due to the fact that the retentive power of the abdomen has not been restored. This, as we all know, is a very difficult matter to do, once the abdominal walls are relaxed.

I think some of our treatment should be directed towards the restoration of this power. It is easy to hold the uterus in position temporarily, but which is the best operation remains to be seen.

We find in suspension, (I think Kelly mentions it) that in the course of a year or two there is a new ligament two or three inches long developed at the attached place, which has been formed by the force which produced the original displacement. This force, I believe, is the lack of retentive power of the abdomen.

Dr. Jayne. This subject is one of great importance, and I have been exceedingly interested and greatly instructed by Dr. Coffey's paper.

I cannot quite agree with him, however, in his conclusions that the false attachment of the peritoneum is the proper method of holding up the uterus. As Dr. Fleming has very well said, this subject is still not fully developed. We are learning every day and by just such suggestions as Dr. Coffey has made. It is only by time and experience with various operations that we will find who is right.

It occurs to me that we are gradually arriving at some definite ideas, and for myself I can say that my ideas are formulated to the extent that I feel the most successful operations for the permanent retention of the uterus are those which depend upon the normal tissues, which, I believe, normally act, not necessarily as supports to the uterus, but as guy ropes.

As to the structures retaining the uterus in its normal position, I do not know that that is a question for discussion at the present time, but I do believe that in the round ligament we have an efficient means of retaining the uterus in its normal position without interfering with the physiological changes incident to pregnancy. It also has the advantage that it undergoes the same physiological changes of involution during the puerperium as other pelvic organs, and we find it efficient after labor. For uncomplicated cases of displacements backward, I believe we have in the Alexander an operation answering all the requirements, with few relapses even after gestation and delivery.

The best operation at present for cases requiring section undoubtedly is the Kelly operation of ventro-suspension of the uterus, but we find that reports show it occasionally interferes with the normal development of pregnancy, and it is followed by other complications in certain cases. It is for this intra-abdominal class of cases especially that a better operation is desired. It would seem to me that efforts directed to the same efficient use of the round ligaments in intra-abdominal operations as is now done in the Alexander would offer a better hope of a solution of the problem than the complicated peritoneal adhesions Dr. Coffey creates by his operation, which he says has not been subjected to the test of a subsequent pregnancy.

Dr. Grant. It seems to me that the only two operations which have permanent features are ventro-suspension and the Alexander, with such modifications as each operator may apply for himself.

The Alexander, as it is well known, is not a suitable operation when the uterus is fixed by adhesions and is not always proper in an enlarged fundus. In all operations we find it necessary to correct general constitutional conditions in order to make the operations permanent.

It is well known that Kelly fixed the posterior surface of the uterus to the abdominal peritoneum, and that is the operation that has given most trouble in labor; but most operators, I believe, now discard that method and fix the anterior wall of the uterus to the abdomen; then we do not have so much trouble and most of the patients go to a normal pregnancy and a normal labor.

Dr. Niles. It has been my lot, and no doubt it has been yours, to read many papers on the displacement of the uterus, but

I am sure that we all feel we have yet to find that which is ideal. I do not feel at this time justified in occupying the time of this Association in a discussion of this particular method, but I do want to say that to my mind this paper, more than I have ever read, more than any I have listened to, presents conclusions that seem reasonable and logical. Whether or not, after more careful study, I should be prepared to accept *in toto*, or in part, the con- clusions advanced in this paper, I do not know, but at this mo- ment I am thoroughly impressed with their reasonableness.

When compared with the Alexander operation, we have a choice between a ligament attached on either side, a single liga- ment, and on the other hand this operation is a general support that extends from the fundus along the side of the uterus down to the uterine fold, and making a uniform support, as this opera- tion affords. I think it has a distinct, absolute, marked advan- tage in that particular respect when compared with ventro-sus- pension.

I have opened quite a number of abdomens where ventro- suspension has been done, and if it is one, two or three years after- wards, the bands that Dr. Kelly has described, which you have all seen, are of a length to be of absolutely no use.

Within the last two months I operated on a case where ven- tro-suspension had been done within a year, perhaps nine months. The three bands were of sufficient strength, but were lax, at least three inches long; were absolutely of no account as a support to the uterus, with the possible danger at all times of obstructing the bowels. At this moment I believe that Dr. Coffey's principle is better than ony one that we have. I believe it is based on good logic. Whether this particular operation is the best way to accom- plish this object or not it is, of course, early to say.

I want to thank the writer of this paper, and again repeat, as far as I am concerned, that I have never met with a method that seemed on its face so logical and reasonable.

DR. BALDWIN. In the start I will say that I know nothing about these cases. I do not know what those ligaments are only from what I can remember from the time when I was a student.

But there were two or three points that impressed themselves upon me, if I caught them right, and I think they are worthy of notice. One is in reference to muscular contraction. In the first place, my opinion is that it is not from non-use that a muscle becomes paralyzed. You may put up a muscle or a limb in a fixed position almost indefinitely without destroying the use of the muscle. The reason that we get paralysis of the muscles in these cases is because of the stretched condition. You put a muscle in extreme extension and keep it there an indefinite length of time and you get paralysis. You then overcome that extension, and without doing anything to the muscle, you will get more or less life later on.

So much for that: Now, Dr. Coffey has spoken of these ligaments. A ligament, according to the anatomical definition, is non-elastic fibrous tissue, and therefore, a ligament should not stretch, but as I have remarked in talking on another subject, whether they stretch or not they become elongated. After they have become elongated, in a great many cases they are useless.

Well now, this operation appeals to me in this way; just so far as the ligaments are concerned, because so far as the uterus, and all that is concerned, I do not know anything about it. But as I understand it, it brings this peritoneum up and in that way supports the uterus. That allows the ligament to become relaxed, I should judge, the same as when you drop a piece of string on the floor. Now when these ligaments are in that relaxed condition, and the weight that has been dragging on them and lengthaning them has been taken off, they will regain their normal condition. A ligament will shorten up the same as it lengthens, if the pressure or the tension on it is removed, and it would seem to me that in this operation, Dr. Coffey would allow the tension there to shorten up, and in that way the ligaments will grow normal of themselves.

DR. COFFEY. I will state in the beginning that I am fully aware of the fact that the idea here advanced is against the principles ordinarily advocated. For that reason I would not insist that any one try the method shown. I simply state what has been my own experience, and it is of little importance as to wnether this particular operation is to be done or not. The method is simply an incident to the principle that "the peritoneum is the universal support of all the abdominal organs."

Now the doctor who first spoke took exception on the ground that the uterus can be pulled down, and therefore, if the broad ligament were the ligament how would it stretch? The fact is we all know, as we stated before, that the peritonum necessarily must stretch. If the peritoneum is an inch or two inches away from the peritoneal wall the tendency is to contract or pull back to that.

Now as to the Kelly operation. I believe this is the best operation which we have had. The Alexander operation has not proven successful, I think, for the very reason that, as many of our authorities claim, the malposition of the uterus produces cystic disease of the ovaries which requires special treatment.

As to the peritoneum, I know it is the general belief that the peritoneum plays practically no part in the support of the abdominal organs. I wish to ask this question, and ask anyone to to answer it: If the peritoneum does not support it, what does support it, are we to spin some fine spun theory that it is intra-abdominal pressure, or some kind of spiritual force that holds up these organs? If the peritoneum does not, then there is nothing that can, because there are no other ligaments in the abdomen other than the peritoneal ligaments; these so-called muscular ligaments.

Relative to this intra-abdominal pressure, if we open the abdomen of certain patients, unless there is a drainage that would create air pressure or intra-abdominal pressure, the bowels are relaxed and they may pick up in a relaxed state, showing that there is absolutely no tension inside, yet all these organs are absolutely in place. Therefore, what can we say of intra-abdominal pressure? When it is not present, as in this case, and these organs do not prolapse, what are we going to hold these organs up with, if not with the peritoneum? The uterus, as we say here, has very much greater peritoneal attachments than any other organ in the abdominal cavity. The uterus is held just as the mast of a ship is supported by attachments in the nature of guy ropes.

Now in conclusion, I will say I do not know whether this operation is the thing or not. It is as satisfactory as far as I have tried it during the last two years and a half, and I would not use any of the old methods at all after using this one.

I want to urge this idea once more, because it is all the idea in the paper: "That the peritoneum, with its re-duplications, is the universal sustaining ligament of all the organs in the abdominal cavity." Now I make this statement with the understanding and knowledge that it is not in entire accord with the generally accepted theory, but as those who oppose the theory are unable to present any other tangible one, I do not feel like giving this up until they do. This operation is simply an incident in the other work we are doing along this line. If it proves as well in future results as it has clinically so far, I believe that some method of this kind will be of benefit in bringing the treatment of uterine displacements to a most satisfactory result.

NORMAL OBSTETRICS.

(CHAPTER NINE.)

THE DIAGNOSIS OF PREGNANCY.

By T. MITCHELL BURNS, M.D.,

Denver, Colorado.

Professor of Obstetrics, The Denver and Gross College of Medicine.

Importance—The diagnosis of pregnancy has always been important, but it is much more so now because of the frequency of abdominal sections. Many a normal pregnant abdomen has been opened in the last few years. A more careful study of the symptoms and signs of pregnancy, especially by abdominal surgeons, would prevent much chagrin, many unnecessary operations and at times death.

While the majority of pregnant abdomens are opened through carelessness, there are cases so complicated that a positive diagnosis is impossible without an exploratory incision, but in such cases the patient should be fully informed in regard to the necessity for the operation and the possibility of pregnancy being present. Nothing does more harm to the medical profession than mistakes like these, which often show up so lively in a few months.

The diagnosis of pregnancy is important in some medico-legal cases, for upon the diagnosis may depend the reputation and even the life of the patient. If a woman condemned to death is found to be pregnant the sentence will be suspended.

The importance of differentiating normal and abnormal pregnancy is shown by the frequency of ectopic pregnancy and the value of early operative interference in such cases.

The Difficulty of Diagnosis in Early Pregnancy.—The diagnosis of early pregnancy is difficult because, 1st, the symptoms in the first two months do not generally warrant a positive diagnosis; 2nd, many of the symptoms may be absent and the patient be pregnant; 3rd, many conditions other than pregnancy cause enlargement of the uterus and abdomen; 4th, many conditions causing enlargement, may coexist with pregnancy; 5th, all the signs and symptoms of pregnancy may be apparently obtained and the patient not be pregnant; and 6th, some patients try to make the examiner think they are pregnant or are not pregnant when the opposite is true. This they do either intentionally or unconsciously.

The Duties of the Examiner.—The duties of the examiner are to take a careful history, to make a thorough examination, to examine not only the pelvic and abdominal contents, but to examine the vulva, vagina, abdomen and breast, and to percuss and auscultate the abdomen, to call in a consultant when in doubt, and not to be afraid to wait if the signs do not warrant a positive diagnosis.

The Method of Study.—To facilitate the study of the symptoms of pregnancy the author believes that it is best to divide them into subjective and objective, to outline and classify them according to their time of appearance and situation, to give their relative diagnostic value and then to fully consider each symptom separately.

The Subjective Symptoms of Pregnancy.—The subjective symptoms, those obtained by the patient, are (1) nervousness, (2) salivation (ptyalism), (3) breast irritation (fullness, tingling and increased sensitiveness,) (4) nausea, vomiting and "longings," (5) frequent micturition, (6) leucorrhoea, (7) menstrual suppression, (8) quickening and (9) special symptoms. Some give other subjective symptoms but the eight here mentioned are the usual ones.

The Objective Symptoms of Pregnancy.—The objective symptoms are those ascertained by the examiner by means of inspection, palpation, auscultation, percussion and mensuration. All the symptoms given in the outlines which follow are considered objective except those which are given in the preceding list as subjective. (It should be remembered that any objective symptom may also be subjective and that most of the symptoms classed as subjective may be objective, but some sensations, as tingling, are purely subjective).

An Outline of the Symptoms of Pregnancy According to their Time of Appearance and Situation.—

First Month:—

1. Nausea and vomiting. ⎫
2. Frequent micturition. ⎬ (Subjective symptoms).
3. Menstrual suppression. ⎭

Second Month, (end of):—

4. The other subjective symptoms except quickening.

Nervousness, salivation, breast irritation, leucorrhoea and special symptoms.

5. General pose.

Shoulders thrown back, carefulness of step.

6. Breast—Primary changes.

Enlargement of primary areola, nipple, veins and whole breast.

Increased pigmentation of primary areola and nipple—brown.

7. Abdominal size and shape.

Flattening from sinking of uterus, or enlargement from rising of uterus.

8. Vulvo-vaginal discoloration, secretion and blood changes.

Blueness, especially on lower anterior vaginal wall.

Increased secretion.

Leucocytosis and increase of resistant cells.

9. Uterine consistence, shape and size.

Cervix—Softening beginning at external os. Some enlargement and apparent shortening from oedema. External os round.

Lower Segment—Softening and compressibility (Hegar's sign).

Upper Segment (body)—Consistency—Alternating from soft and elastic to hard. Shape—Spherical, from increase in antero-posterior diameter; often bulging of one side of body and a longitudinal furrow. Size—Increased.

10. Kyestein.

11. Pulse.—Same in all positions.

Fourth Month (end of):—

11. Quickening (Subjective symptom).

13. Face.—Anemic, peaked and pigmented; expression changed.

14. Abdominal size, shape, pigmentation and striæ.

Shape—Increase in anterio-posterior diameter without corresponding increase transversely.

Pigmentation—Brownish along linea alba.

Striæ—Along groins, reddish if fresh, white if due to previous pregnancy.

15. Vulvo-vaginal discoloration, increased size, secretion and temperature.

16. Uterine fundus, contractions and bruit.

Fundus above brim (sometime at end of second month).

Contractions, intermittent and painless.

Bruit—Uterine, funic and cardiac.

17. Ballottement.

18. Fetal shock.

Fifth Month (end of):—

19. Breast—Secondary changes.

Secondary areola. Colostrum (sometimes end of third month). Glands of Montgomery. Striæ.

20. Navel bulging.

21. Fetal movement (active) by palpation.

22. Fetal parts by palpation.

23. Fetal heart sounds.

The Diagnostic Value of the Symptoms of Pregnancy.— The symptoms of the first two months warrant a probable diagnosis, those of the fourth month an almost certain diagnosis and those of the fifth month a certain diagnosis.

The main symptoms of early pregnancy are: First month— Nausea and vomiting, frequent micturition and menstrual suppression. Second month—Vulvo-vaginal discoloration and blood changes, uterine softening, shape and size (3s). In the diagnosis of early pregnancy special subjective symptoms which the patient has had in previous pregnancies have been of considerable value in the writer's experience.

The main signs of advanced pregnancy are: Fourth month —Quickening, abdominal shape and pigmentation, uterine fundus, contractions and bruit, and ballottement. Fifth month—Breast— secondary changes, navel bulging, fetal movements (by palpation), and fetal heart sounds.

The so-called four certain signs of pregnancy are ballottement, fetal movements by palpation, fetal parts by palpation and the fetal heart sounds (3F's).

The only legal certain sign, is the fetal heart sound.

THE SYMPTOMS OF PREGNANCY CONSIDERED SEPARATELY.

1st. Nausea and Vomiting or Morning Sickness. This is diagnosed by the presence of other symptoms of pregnancy, as menstrual suppression, and vesical irritation, by beginning in the early morning and lessening as the day advances, by the patient feeling nearly well each time after vomiting, (this is not always true in severe cases), and by absence of any primary disease of the stomach. It may appear before or after menstrual suppression. Some women do not have nausea and vomiting during pregnancy. "Longings," or desires for peculiar articles of food, when present, somewhat increase the diagnostic value of nausea and vomiting. Nausea and vomiting and "longings," like many of the other symptoms of pregnancy, may occur in other conditions than pregnancy. Menstrual suppression from any cause tends to cause nausea at times.

2nd. Frequent Micturition (vesical irritation). This condition by itself is of little value, but it enhances the value of menstrual suppression and nausea and vomiting, because it is generally present in pregnancy.

3rd. Menstrual Suppression. This symptom is of great value if the patient has previously always been regular, and especially so if accompanied by morning sickness and vesical irritation. The following points previously mentioned under the physiology of menstruation should be remembered: (1) Absence of menstruation may be due to any acute or chronic disease, particularly "catching cold," to emotion resulting from exposure in the unmarried or newly married. (2) Suppression due to emotion or "catching cold" generally only lasts one or two months. (3) Amenorrhea from causes other than pregnancy does not always prevent conception, as impregnation has occurred before puberty, after the menopause and during lactation and disease when menstruation was absent.

4th. The Other Subjective Symptoms Except Quickening. These are of little importance, but taken together with other symptoms may at times help to differentiate in doubtful cases. These are, as previously mentioned, nervousness, ptyalism, breast irritation (feeling of fullness, of tingling and increased sensitiveness), leucorrhoea and special symptoms. In the ptyalism of pregnancy there is not the fetid odor as in mercurial poisoning, and as a rule the gums are not tender or spongy. These symptoms are of little importance because they occur at puberty, at the beginning of a menstrual period and when menstruation is absent from other causes than pregnancy. Special symptoms which a patient has had in previous pregnancies seem to be an exception, as they have been of considerable value in the author's practice.

5th. The General Pose and Form. The shoulders are thrown back, there is a carefulness of step and an increase of flesh (especially in the outer parts of the groins and over the crest of the ilia. See "Abdominal Shape").

6th. Breast—Primary Changes. These are given under "The Maternal Changes" and are of little value, as many conditions other than pregnancy cause them.

7th. Abdominal Size and Shape. There is a flattening from sinking of the uterus, an enlargement from rising of the uterus and increase of flesh, or no change. The most frequent early noticeable change in the abdomen from increase of flesh is seen in the outer third of the groins above the crests of the ilia.

8th. Vulvo-vaginal Discoloration, Secretion and Blood Changes. There is increased secretion from the vulva and vagina, and blueness appears on the vulva and in the vagina, especially on the lower anterior vaginal wall. Some consider this discoloration a positive sign of pregnancy, but increased congestion from other causes often produces a similar blueness. In the majority of cases if the blood of the vulva (and of the finger) be stained by Gram's iodin-potassium iodid solution, two and one-half or five to one, more red corpuscles will take the deep stain than in normal blood. Leucocytosis is generally present.

9th. Uterine Softening, Shape and Size. The softening, shape and size of the uterus in early pregnancy are all important signs of pregnancy.

Cervical softening: This begins at the external os, is an especially important sign of early pregnancy and is almost always present in some degree. No other condition causes the same amount of softening as pregnancy.

The cervix becomes enlarged and apparently shortened from oedema, and the external os becomes more round, but these changes are not of much value.

Softening and compressibility of the lower uterine segment

(Hegar's sign): This is best detected by bimanual touch. If the uterus is anteflexed, the vaginal fingers are placed in front of the cervix and the external fingers on the abdomen behind the fundus. If the fundus is hard to reach, the vaginal fingers are placed behind the cervix and the abdominal fingers in front of the uterine body. The lower segment is felt soft, compressible and pulsating between two larger objects, the relatively hard cervix and the uterine body, which is hard and resisting during contractions and soft during relaxation. The lower segment when examined at the right time, between the sixth week and the third month, is often so soft that the fingers feel as if they met, and some have compared this thinness to that of a sheet of paper. This sign is due to the ovum, in the first three months, only occupying the upper uterine segment. This softening is not usually sufficiently developed before the sixth week to be felt. It is not always discernible, but it is not simulated to any great extent by any morbid condition and is therefore of great value when definitely found. The consistency of the upper segment alternates from soft and elastic to hard from the absence or presence of the uterine contractions; being soft and elastic between contractions and hard during.

The shape of the upper segment: The spherical shape of the upper segment is due to the ovum growing in its centre. If the ovum grows more in one half of the uterus than it does in the other half—a frequent occurrence—the side containing most of the ovum will be more bulging and it may be separated from the other side by a longitudinal furrow. The bulging side will be dense and the empty side soft and compressible (called by most writers elastic).

10. Kyestein. (See chapter eight, "The Maternal Changes").

11. The Pulse. (See chapter eight, "The Maternal Changes").

12. Quickening. Quickening is the sensation produced in the mother by the first preceptible fetal movement. "Life" is the sensation produced any time by the fetal movement. Patients are asked when they felt "life" first or quickened. The sensation of life is at first like a slight flutter or throb, later like a definite tap or kick. The time of quickening is generally four and a half months. The extremes are three and six months. The early extreme depends upon previous experience (multigravity), the sensitiveness of the patient, the proximity of the uterine to the ab-

dominal wall and the position of the fetus. (The last two depend upon the fact that only parietal peritoneum is sensitive, and that nerves of involuntary muscular tissue do not transmit impressions which becomes conscious unless the irritation is quite severe. Hence if during the motion of the fetus it does not press against the abdominal wall, parietal peritoneum or voluntary muscular tissue, no sensation is usually conveyed). Quickening does not correspond with the first fetal movements. The latter are present at about the tenth week. The site of the sensation is near the site of the motion or at a point some distance from it, e.g., in one of the groins above the pubic symphysis or in some other part of the abdomen; at times about, or above and to one side of the navel, even though the fundus is just a little above the brim. This is due to the sensation being referred. (Burns). The value of quickening alone is slight, as it is often simulated by gas in the intestines and contractions of the abdominal muscles in hysterical women, and especially in such women at the menopause.

13. The Face. (See chapter eight, "The Maternal Changes"). The anemic expression of early pregnancy is quite characteristic, and many of the laity have diagnosed pregnancy by this sign alone.

14. The Abdominal Shape, Pigmentation and Striæ. (See chapter eight, "The Maternal Changes"). The abdominal shape is considered pathognomonic by some.

15. Vulvo-vaginal Discoloration, Size, Secretion and Temperature. (See chapter eight, "The Maternal Changes").

16. The Uterine Fundus, Contractions and Bruit. The uterine fundus: This is felt above the pubes at the fourth month, as a rule, but in some cases it is felt at the second month. (It may be apparently felt above the pubes without being above the plane of the brim, because the brim of the pelvis posteriorly is three and one-half inches higher than in front). (For the height of the fundus each month see chapter seven).

The uterine contractions, (Braxton Hick's sign): (See chapter eight). These are obtained in the early months of pregnancy by placing the patient in the obstetric position (the dorsal relaxed position, with the patient crosswise of the bed, and her feet on chairs), then lifting the uterus up with two fingers of one hand in the vagina and gently grasping the fundus through the abdomen with the other hand for 5 to 20 minutes. In the latter half of pregnancy they are obtained by gently placing the hand on the abdomen in contact with the fundus. The hand is placed gently so as not to excite contractions of the abdominal muscles. Often the contractions can be seen by inspection when the uterus is close to the abdominal wall. They cause a change in the respiratory wave of the abdomen. The usual time of obtaining these contractions is after the fourth month, because before this the fundus cannot be definitely felt through the abdominal wall. Their diagnostic value is considerable, because no other condition produces. as marked contractions as pregnancy. Contractions can be felt in a uterus enlarged from any cause, but enlargement due to soft uterine fibroid (myomata) is the only one to approach the softness of pregnancy.

The uterine murmur, bruit or souffle: This is the sound produced in the uterine arterial branches as their capacity becomes greater than that of their main trunk. It resembles the bruit of an aneurism and is synchonous with the maternal pulse. It is best heard over the sides of the uterus as the uterine arteries are here situated, and especially on the left side as this side of the uterus is more anterior. This bruit occurs in enlargement of the uterus from any cause and in a few ovarian tumors. Its diagnostic value is slight except to show that there is an enlargement of the uterus or possibly of an ovary.

The uterine thrill: This is the sensation conveyed by touch and can be obtained by bimanual examination if the fingers are brought in contact with one of the uterine arteries.

The funic and cardiac bruit: The funic murmur or bruit is produced in the cord from compression and therefore may indicate fetal danger. It is of little diagnostic value, as when it can be obtained the heart sound can be heard. The cardiac bruit is supposed to be due to the same cause and has the same diagnostic value. Both are rare.

. 17. Ballottement. Ballottement (or repercussion) is the feeling of passive fetal movement by the obstetrician, or the sensation experienced by the examiner when the fetus is given a sudden motion. It results from the displacement of a solid body in a liquid. It is obtained by two methods. In the bimanual method the vaginal finger is placed in front of the cervix and the abdominal hand grasps the fundus gently, then a sudden upward movement is given by the vaginal finger with the result that the fetal mass is propelled upward, where it often strikes the abdominal hand and subsequently falls to strike the vaginal finger. In the abdominal method the patient is placed lengthwise of the bed and near its edge either on her back or side. Facing the patient's feet, the examiner places one hand on one side of the lower abdomen and one on the other side, and then gives a quick motion with the lower of the two hands. The lower abdomen is used because ballottement is most easily obtained by moving the fetal head. After feeling in the lower abdomen, the examiner may face the patient's face and place the hands in the same manner on the upper abdomen. It is often well before beginning ballottement to examine for a hard object like the head, and if one is found to practice ballottement at its site. The bimanual method is of special value because it can be obtained first. The abdominal method is the better method for differentiating abdominal tumors.

Ballottement may not be obtainable when the fetus is abnormally large or very small, when there is an excessive or deficient amount of liquor amnii, placenta previa, twins, or after the head is engaged. But according to the author's experience, it can nearly always be obtained in all these conditions by one of the two methods, e.g., after engagement of the head it cannot be obtained per abdomen, but it can easily be obtained per vaginam. Its diagnostic value is great, for it is a certain sign of pregnancy, when elicited by an expert, as no other condition gives the definite sensation of a solid body moving freely in a liquid. (Ballottement is slightly simulated by mutilocular cysts of the ovary, small ovarian cysts with a long pedicle, an anteflexed non-pregnant uterus, a pregnant uterus floating in ascitic fluid, floating kidney, and a calculus resting in the *bas fond* of the bladder). Its value is lessened by the fact that at the time it becomes definite other more important signs, as active fetal movements and the fetal heart sound can be obtained.

18. Fetal Shock. In fetal shock or the sound of the fetal movements there is heard a sudden tap followed by a quick bruit As this sign can be obtained by experts before the heart beat and because it addresses both the sense of touch and of hearing, it is considered of more value, at times, than the fetal heart sounds To the general practitioner it is of little value.

19. Breast—Secondary Changes. (See chapter eight). The secondary areola is a positive sign of pregnancy in those who have

never born children, as no other condition produces this change. The presence of colostrum in the breasts of women who have not born children, is considered almost a positive sign of pregnancy, as those cases where milk is found in the breast of men and girls are very rare. Sudden premature suppression of the milk in nursing women is rather positive evidence of pregnancy if no other cause seems probable.

20. Bulging Navel. This is rarely produced by any other condition than pregnancy.

21. Active Fetal Movements Felt by Palpation. This practically positive sign of pregnancy is obtained by laying the hands gently upon the abdomen. If this method does not elicit active fetal movements they may be excited by pressure of the finger tips as in playing the piano, by using the two hands as in attempting to detect fluctuation, (dipping the fingers in cold water and then applying them to the abdomen), or by touching the site of a localized pain, which may be due to the pressure of an extremity.

22. Fetal Parts Recognized by Palpation. Two methods are employed in the recognition of the fetal parts by touch, the vaginal and abdominal. In the bimanual method the finger is placed in front of the cervix against the lower uterine segment, which is pushed downward and forward by the abdominal hand on the back of the fundus. In the abdominal method the finger tips are pressed inward in different parts of the uterus, and at times the fingers of one hand are pressed toward those of the other hand so as to include more or less of the supposed fetus between the two hands and to lift it up. This sign is one of the so-called certain signs, and is very reliable, but certain growths might be mistaken for a part of the fetus, especially if they were in ascitic fluid. While the parts are not recognized per abdomen until the end of the fifth month, the head may be felt sometimes per vaginam at the end of the fourth month.

23. The Fetal Heart Sound. The character of the fetal heart sound is like that of a new-born baby's heart, and resembles the tick-tack of a watch under a pillow. The frequency of the beat varies considerably; the average frequency is 134, the extremes, 120 and 160. The frequency is increased by any exertion on the part of the mother or fetus, (pressure of the stethoscope or the uterine contractions causing motion of the fetus, increase of maternal pulse, maternal or fetal fever), and ergot. (Ergot in-

creases uterine contraction, and a large dose may first increase the pulse and then diminish it by the tetanic spasm induced). Chloroform diminishes the frequency and force according to the amount used. At the beginning of a uterine contraction the heart beat increases in frequency; at the acme, slows or stops; after the acme suddenly increases, then gradually returns to the normal. (A heart beat below 100 or above 180 indicates that the fetus is in danger and that labor should be ended as soon as consistent with existing conditions). The diagnosis of sex may often (?) be made by the frequency of the pulse. A pulse below 134 indicates a male, because the larger the heart the slower the pulse, but a large female would have a large heart and a slow pulse. A pulse above 134 indicates a female, but a small male would have a small heart, and a fast pulse. The slower the frequency the greater the chances of a boy, and the higher the frequency the greater the chances of a girl. The area of maximum intensity for the fetal heart sound is from three to five inches in diameter, but the fetal heart sound may be heard all over the abdomen. The area of intensity in early pregnancy is over the fundus, in later pregnancy over the part of the uterus where the fetal trunk comes in closest relation with the abdominal wall, i.e., over the fetal back near the heart, except in the face presentation when the front of the chest is anterior, then the fetal heart sound is heard through the front of the body. The fetal heart sound is the most positive sign of pregnancy and of the life of the fetus. The fetal heart sound is simulated by the maternal pulse, but the maternal pulse is nearly always much slower. In these cases where the maternal pulse is fast, the beat of the fetal heart and that of the maternal pulse will seldom be synchronous. The fetal heart sound may be obscured by anything which may come in between the fetal heart and the examining ear, (e.g., thick abdominal wall, large amount of liquor amnii, the dorsum of the fetus being posteriorly, the acme of uterine contraction, the placenta, flatus in the intestines, and abnormally by ascites and other conditions). The absence of the fetal heart sound is not a positive sign that the fetus is dead, as this absence may be due to the presence of some condition which may prevent the heart sound being heard at all during pregnancy.

THE DIFFERENTIAL DIAGNOSIS OF PREGNANCY.

While it is possible to always differentiate pregnancy from any of the diseases which simulate it by the four so-called positive signs of pregnancy, it is necessary to consider the symptoms of certain diseases, because frequently the case has not advanced far enough for the positive signs of pregnancy to be present or to be excluded. Exclusion is a good procedure in the differential diagnosis of pregnancy. Of the following, which may be mistaken for pregnancy, the first five not only cause enlargement of the abdomen, like all the others, but also produce more or less enlargement of the uterus:

Subinvolution.—History of labor followed by prolonged lochia or irregular and excessive menses; uterus large, but does not increase in size, is tender and not elastic; pain in the back and groins; purulent leucorrhoea, often streaked with blood. Subinvolution and pregnancy may both be present. Time is the great element in the diagnosis. Hence it is best to wait a month or so before making a positive diagnosis.

Uterine Fibroids.—Uterus slightly enlarged and the tumor a small lump, or uterus with the tumor may fill the whole abdomen; uterus hard and nodular, at least in places; menses irregular and profuse, growth very slow, intermittent contractions rare; (uterine bruit, dullness on percussion).

Uterine Soft Myomata and Hydatids.—Uterine wall varies in softness and thickness; menses irregular or suppressed; fluctuation; weak uterine contractions in the healthy part of the uterine wall; (uterine bruit and dullness on percussion); periodic discharge of water pathognomomic of hydatids; growth rapid.

Hematometra.—(Accumulation of menstrual fluid in uterus). Very rare; atresia of genital canal; periodic increase in size at time for menstrual period associated with pain; uterus hard and resisting; duration longer than pregnancy.

Physometra.—(Gaseous distension due to decomposition of retained secretions or fragments of ovum) very rare; acquired atresia or stenosis, if latter gas escapes from time to time; tympanites; uterus small; growth slow.

Hydrometra.—(Fluid in uterus due to atresia) very rare; generally after the menopause; uterus small and growth slow.

(All the above conditions cause more or less enlargement of the uterus).

Ovarian Tumors.—Begin on one side; growth slow (exceptionally, faster than pregnancy); tumor soft and more or less on one side; health impaired and ovarian facies; fluctuation more or less general; uterus below tumor and displaced; sometimes amenorrhoea from anemia or internal hemorrhage; absence of intermittent contractions of great value; may have to wait for diagnosis. Ovarian tumor and pregnancy may co-exist, then two tumors and all the signs of pregnancy.

Ascites.—Navel always depressed; middle of the abdomen flat, flanks bulging; no definite tumor; fluctuation general; percussion clear in median line; dull in flanks, but changes with position. Cardiac, hepatic or renal disease is present.

Fat in the Belly Wall.—Fat may be included between the hands and generally lifted up; abdomen is pendulous; usually between forty and fifty years of age.

Pseudocyesis.—(False pregnancy, phantom tumors). Most common near the menopause, also in young hysterical women; many of the subjective signs of pregnancy and sometimes false labor; milk in the breast and enlargement of the abdomen. Enlargement due to fat, gas or contraction of muscles; last two disappear under chloroform—uterus normal size and all other objective signs absent.

Distended Bladder.—(Cause, e.g., incarcerated pregnant uterus or pelvic tumor). Short duration; much discomfort and restlessness; dribling of urine; well marked abdominal fluctuating tumor disappearing on use of catheter.

Fecal Accumulation.—History; tenderness and fullness over distended bowel; tumor may equal six months pregnancy; salines and enemata cause tumor to disappear.

Floating Kidney.—Tumor can be pushed under ribs.

Chronic Peritonitis.—Rarely resembles enlarged uterus.

Malformation of the Uterus.—Diagnosis easy unless complicated by pregnancy; with pregnancy may cause diagnosis of uterine tumor.

Conditions Complicating the Diagnosis of Pregnancy.—Pregnancy may be complicated by extra-uterine implantation, twins, polyhydramnios, death of the fetus, disease of the decidua and other conditions which may greatly interfere with a positive diagnosis. These conditions will be considered under "Abnormal Obstetrics."

Time.—Time in all cases is of great value, unless serious symptoms arise, then an immediate exploratory operation for diagnostic purposes is justifiable.

Exploratory Operations.—Before operating on any case the existence of pregnancy must be excluded if possible. If this cannot be done, the patient or her friend should be so informed, and reasons why the operation is necessary even though pregnancy exists should be given. After such an explanation, even though pregnancy existed, the operation should only reflect the carefulness of the operator and the conscientiousness of his work.

The Exclusion of Pregnancy.—To exclude pregnancy the uterus must be found of normal size. The size of uteri vary so that it is almost impossible to say that a patient is not a month or so pregnant. Advanced pregnancy may be positively excluded by the small size of the uterus or the absence of fetal heart sounds, fetal movements and parts by palpation, ballottement and uterine contractions.

The Diagnosis of Life in the Fetus.—In the early months the life of the fetus is diagnosed by the normal growth of the uterus and the absence of abnormal symptoms indicating death of the fetus. (See "Diseases of Pregnancy").

In the latter half of pregnancy the life of the fetus is diagnosed by the presence of the fetal heart sounds and fetal movements felt by palpation. Absence of either or both of these signs does not prove death of the fetus, but the disappearance of the fetal heart sounds after they have been definitely heard at a previous examanation is suspicious of death of the fetus. (This will be taken up under "Diseases of Pregnancy").

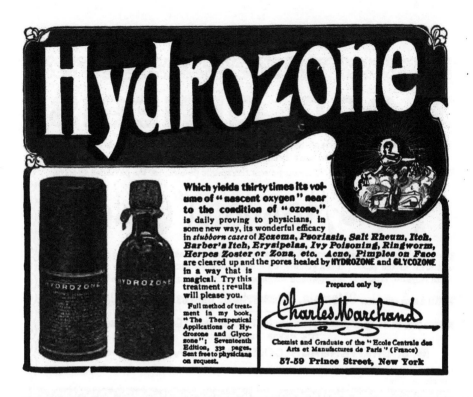

DENVER MEDICAL TIMES

THOMAS H. HAWKINS, A.M., M.D., EDITOR AND PUBLISHER.

COLLABORATORS:

Henry O. Marcy, M.D., Boston.
Thaddeus A. Reamy, M.D., Cincinnati.
Nicholas Senn, M.D., Chicago.
Joseph Price, M.D., Philadelphia.
Franklin H. Martin, M.D., Chicago.
William Oliver Moore, M.D., New York.
L. S. McMurtry, M.D., Louisville.
Thomas B. Eastman, M.D., Indianapolis, Ind.
G. Law, M.D., Greeley, Colo.

S. H. Pinkerton, M.D., Salt Lake City.
Flavel B. Tiffany, M.D., Kansas City.
Erskine M. Bates, M.D;. New York.
E. C. Gehrung, M.D, St. Louis.
Graeme M. Hammond, M.D, New York.
James A. Lydston, M.D., Chicago.
Leonard Freeman, M.D., Denver.
Carey K. Fleming, M.D., Denver, Colo.

Subscriptions, $1.00 per year in advance; Single Copies, 10 cents.

Address all Communications to Denver Medical Times, 1740 Welton Street, Denver, Colo.
We will at all times be glad to give space to well written articles or items of interest to the profession.
[Entered at the Postoffice of Denver, Colorado, as mail matter of the Second Class.]

EDITORIAL DEPARTMENT

ATROPHIC RHINITIS.

The causes of ozena are purulent rhinitis and other chronic infections, and it is the final stage of hypertrophic rhinitis. Characteristic symptoms are crust formation occluding nares, especially in mornings, with distressing fetor; occasional epistaxis from picking nose; sense of irritation in nasopharynx; laryngitis and bronchitis from dryness of air and inspissated mucus; constant "hawking and hemming"; impaired vocal functions, often hoarseness; hearing usually impaired. Each nasal cavity is more or less filled, especially in front with grayish-greenish-yellow musty fetid crusts covering light yellow mucopus. The mucous membrane is somewhat bloodless and attenuated; the bones themselves are shrunken and atrophied in the later stages. The pharyngeal mucous membrane appears dry and glazed like parchment, with a plug of thick mucus in the vault. By way of treatment, Stein recommends the local application of trichloracetic acid (0.5 to 10 per cent) as specifically curative, changing the atrophic to the hypertrophic form. Thornton directs to apply a 25 per cent aqueous solution of ichthyol to the nasal mucous membrane, after cleansing with a 2 per cent solution of the same. Hamm, after cleansing the nose, insufflates with a powder blower a mixture of equal parts of citric acid and sugar of milk. After thorough cleansing with warm Dobell

solution, Levy inserts tampons of dry cotton (Gottstein), allowing them to remain one hour. Kyle's method of treatment may
be summarized as follows: Remove any obstructions; persistent
and thorough cleansing with a douche of very hot water containing eight grains of borax to the ounce, followed by use of equal
parts of hydrogen peroxide, aqueous extract of hamamelis and
cinnamon water; clear nostrils by blowing nose, and use in each
nostril a warm douche, fifteen grains each of borax, sodium bicarbonate, sodium chlorate and potassium bicarbonate with three
minims of carbolic acid in two ounces of water; then drop in four
to six drops of refined carbon oil containing one grain of iodine
to the ounce; if discharge is purulent, after cleansing apply three
per cent zinc chloride; stimulate with 1:5000 formaldehyde solution.

PURULENT RHINITIS.

This form of nasal catarrh usually depends on neglected colds
in the head, sometimes on the presence of foreign bodies, rarely on
Bright's disease (may portend uremia). Sneezing is often a
prominent symptom when exacerbations from taking cold. Chilli-
ness and fever (may be hectic) are sometimes present. The chief
sign of the disease is a bright yellow, or greenish yellow semi-
fluid mucopurulent discharge from both nostrils (usually from
only one when due to a foreign body) obstructing the passages
more or less. The mucous membrane is slightly reddened and
swollen. For the chronic form of the disease, Kyle directs to
cleanse with hydrogen peroxide, followed by a spray or swab every
three or four hours with the following solution: Borax, sodium
bircarbonate aa. gr. x; listerine dr. ii; cinnamon water dr. iv;
aquam ad oz. i. After cleansing, dry with cotton pledgets and
apply an astringent, such as zinc sulphocarbolate, twenty grains to
the ounce of water, or 50 per cent ichthyol. Potassium permanganate, five grains per ounce is useful to control odor. The double
sulphide of arsenic, 1–24 to 1–16 grain t. i. d., may be given after
meals if there is glandular involvement.

SYSTEM REMEDIES IN TUBERCULOSIS.

Cod-liver oil is a preparation that has held its own in tuberculosis since its introduction in 1824. It is more a food than a
medicine. Its value depends chiefly on ready digestibility and

easy oxidation. It is most useful, along with ferrous iodide, in children of the strumous type, and is contra-indicated in the final stages of tuberculosis.

The pure oil is preferable to emulsions. A tablespoonful or more should be taken two hours after meals. The nauseous taste is disguised by floating on strong coffee, orange or lemon juice, ginger bitters, malt extract, ale, beer or weak brandy and soda, or by taking a pinch of salt before and after each dose. Eructations may be prevented by chewing a peppermint lozenge after taking the oil. In rare cases it is well to give the oil by the rectum.

Beechwood creosote is another good remedy, and has had a modern revival. It has no direct effect upon the tubercular process, but does good in many cases, particularly when there is mixed infection, by improving appetite and digestion, checking bowel fermentation, relieving constipation, and sterilizing to some degree the tubercular products in the lung. Creosote is taken best two hours after meals in warm milk or hot water flavored with an essential oil, or in sherry or bitters. Another good way is for the patient to fill capsules with the pure liquid by means of a dropper, taking the medicine in this manner after drinking a glass or two of milk. The dose of creosote may be increased rapidly from one or two minims t. i. d., up to ten or even forty minims, and then be diminished. The drug is contraindicted if the appetite is not enhanced or if the gastrointestinal symptoms grow worse. Guaiacol carbonate and thiocol are derivatives of creosote, to which they are preferred on account of taste. Guaiacol is well administered by external application, but large doses are depressing. Ichthyol is less irritating than creosote to the stomach.

Arsenic is an efficient stimulant of cell growth. It is best given in the form of Fowler's solution, m. ii-iii t. i. d , well diluted, and may be combined with tincture of iron, though chemically incompatible. Jacobi prescribes two minims of liquor arsenicalis daily, in three doses largely diluted after meals, to a child a few years old. Symptoms of over-dosage are prevented by small doses of opiates. The non-poisonous arsenical derivatives, cacodylic acid and its salts, particularly sodium and iron cacodylate, have come into prominence of late years as general roborants in pulmonary tuberculosis. The hypodermic dose of the sodium salt is five to ten cgm. daily.

Cinnamic acid is a comparatively new remedy that stimulates

leucocytosis, and hence phagocytosis, walling in tubercles and favoring encapsulation. Sodium cinnamate occurs as white crystals freely soluble in water. The dose of this drug is $\frac{1}{2}$ to two grains, t. i. d., in pills, or with olive oil in capsules, 1–64 to $\frac{1}{4}$ grain once daily subcutaneously or intravenously. An aqueous five per cent solution is convenient for the hypodermic injection into the gluteal region.

The dose should be reduced if headache, oppression or chilly sensations arise. Oil of cloves, five minims and upward, in capsule after each meal, is of special service, when digestive disturbances are present.

Iron is obviously indicated in anemic cases, and is best given in small doses after each meal—five grains of Bland's pills, three grains of reduced iron, or ten minims of tincture of ferric chloride in glycerin and water. The citrate of iron and quinine, three to five grains in solution, is well adapted for children, as is also the syrup of iodide of iron in five minim doses.

Strychnine is a remedy that appeals with special force to those clinicians who regard the neurologic element as of paramount importance in pulmonary tuberculosis. An excellent tonic pill is one which contains 1–60 grain strychnine, 1–20 grain arsenous acid, and two grains of ferrous carbonate. In no other malady is it more important to keep up the cardiac strength.

Iodine preparations are most useful in the early stages of chronic tuberculosis, particularly in scrofulous subjects and in advanced cases when there is but slight tendency to softening and cavity formation.

The question of the administration of alcoholics in pulmonary tuberculosis is a subject of dispute by good authorities. The recent experiments of Atwater have proved beyond doubt that alcohol has potential value as a fuel food. On the other hand, if liquors are used with indiscretion a chronic alcoholic gastritis may be set up, rendering the patient's general condition much worse, to say nothing of the possible danger of inebriety. In general we conclude that the quantity of spirits, wine, etc., imbibed by the patient should be regulated as carefully as that of any other drug, and that they should be used only to the extent in which they aid the digestion and absorption of fats and proteids.

TREATMENT OF PNEUMONIA IN ADULTS.

M. Manges says that the tendency is to forget that this is a general disease in which there may be great disparity between the local signs and the patient's general condition, severe cases sometimes giving evidence of but slight lung involvement and vice versa. So far, the attempts to devise a specific treatment have not been successful, and but little is to be expected in this direction, for the pneumococcus is not always a constant quantity, and various other organisms, including the influenza bacillus, which, of late, has markedly influenced the disease, may be present in mixed infections. The author's detailed discussion of the treatment is subdivided under the following heads: (1) To maintain life. The careful management of the stomach by a suitable diet to prevent distension and the consequent cardiac embarrassment of the highest importance. It is wiser to give too little food than too much and to avoid all carbonated beverages. (2) To support the heart. The best drugs for this purpose are strychnine, caffeine, alcohol, camphor and ergot. If prompt results are not obtained all the drugs should be given hypodermatically and in sufficient amount to exert their physiological action. Views as to the value of large doses of digitalis are still divided. Adrenalin, the precordial ice-bag, cupping and venesection are also useful measures. (3) To control hyperpyrexia. Large, flat ice-bags on the chest will be found useful, but care is necessary to avoid producing intercostal neuritis. Cold sponging and packs are of value, but must be used with caution, and cold baths are contraindicated. The rational use of coal tar antipyretics in small doses may contribute much to the patient's comfort. (4) To relieve suffering. The cough and pain are combated by the use of small doses of morphine hypodermatically, or of heroin hydrochlorate. The Paquelin cautery is of great value for the pleuritic stitches. Oxygen is probably of less value than is generally supposed. Every effort should be made to secure as much sleep for the patient as possible. (5) To control complications. Pleurisy with effusion, empyema, pericarditis, endocarditis, etc., require the treatment ordinarily pursued.—*Medical Record*, December 10, 1904.

EDITORIAL ITEMS.

Inflamed and Prolapsed Hemorrhoids. Ivanoff recommends relieving by painting with tincture of iodine.

Epididymitis. Guaiacol, with twice as much olive oil, is lauded as a local application by the editor of the *Critic and Guide.*

Aortic Aneurysm. Osler relies on rest and restriction of liquids; also ten to twenty grains of potassium iodide t. i. d.

Rupture of Empyema into Bronchus. Eichhorst instructs to use mild narcotics with expectorants if the cough is severe.

For Vomiting of Pregnancy. Peroxide of hydrogen (*Critic and Guide*) a tablespoonful to the quart of water, is good in any quantity.

Mutually Destructive. Says the *Critic and Guide:* Do not prescribe carbolic acid and peroxide of hydrogen in the same mixture.

For Plastic Bronchitis. Eichhorst mentions steam inhalations; expectorants or emetics when casts are loosened; mercurial preparations; and potassium iodide, twelve grains thrice daily in the chronic form.

Gall-Stone Jaundice. Icterus is present in only about half of all cases of gall-stone colic. In chronic impaction the jaundice is of varying degree.

Drug Rashes. Quinine, atropine and turpentine give rise to erythematous rashes (*Medical Record*), the last named being of a blotchy nature.

Physicians in New York City. The 1904 edition of the "Medical Directory of the City of New York" includes the names of 5,909 practitioners in Greater New York.

Hysterical Pneumatosis. Among useful remedies are camphor, valerian, hyoscyamus, musk, iodoform, ether, ammonia, spirits of lavender, lavage, and particularly suggestion.

Pyloric Insufficiency. A diet readily digested by the intestines is commended by Van Valzah and Nisbet; also intragastric faradization; and frequent small meals if diarrhea and intestinal colic.

Acute Esophagitis. Osler directs to use fragments of ice, and demulcent drinks; cold external applications; feeding by rectum only if dysphagia intense.

Paralytic Dysphagia. Pepper advised to nourish the patient, if necessary, through the stomach-tube; also cautios faradization of interior of esophagus, and etiologic remedies.

Dilatation of Esophagus. In this malformation, as in pulsion or traction diverticula, about all that can be done except by operation is to feed by the rectum or through the stomach-tube.

Cancer of Esophagus. Osler recommends milk and liquid diet with supplemental nourishment by rectum or through stomach-tube; esophagotomy or gastrotomy as a last resort.

Feeding in Lost Epiglottis. Wolfenden advises to hang head over side of the bed and suck milk through rubber tubing from a mug on the floor.

Scarlet Fever. Anointing the body of every scarlatinal patient, especially during the peeling period, with olive oil (*Critic and Guide*) should be a routine practice. It limits contagion and prevents colds.

For Alkaline Urine. To neutralize alkalinity the *Critic and Guide* considers benzoic acid, ten to twenty grains three times a day, a pleasant and effective remedy.

Eosinophile Bronchitis. Teichmueller recommends gymnastic exercises, hydrotherapy; potassium iodide in syphilitic cases; cod-liver oil, malt, and iron and manganese peptonate.

Capillary Bronchitis. Shoemaker prescribes: ℞ Ammonii carb. gr. ss.-i; syr. tolu m. xl. liq. ammonii acet. q. s: A teaspoonful every hour or two.

Subacute Bronchitis. Shoemaker prescribes: ℞ Tinct. sanguinariae m. vi; syr. ipecac. m. xxiv; tinct. lobeliae m. vi; glycerini m. xxiv: Take every two or three hours.

Subacute Chronic Bronchitis. Crinon writes for: ℞ Terp. hydrat. gr. lxxx; glycerini, spiritus aa. ℥ iiss.; mellis despumati ℥ ii. tinct. vanillae m. lxxv: Two to four tablespoonfuls a day.

Chronic Bronchitis with Dropsy. Fothergill has employed the following formula: ℞ Syr. scillae ʒi; acidi hydrobrom. dil ℥ss. One dose.

Anal Fissure. Divulse sphincters thoroughly, says Gant, and apply twice a week after cleansing parts, balsam of Peru or silver nitrate, fifteen grains to the ounce. This treatment cures within ten days.

Library Tuberculosis. Mitulescu (*Clinical Review*) has examined for tubercle bacilli a number of books and periodicals from a public library. Those that were worn and dirty showed the presence of virulent bacilli in one-third of the instances.

Thyroid Glands. Stern (*Medical Standard*) fortifies the system against the untoward effects of thyroid administration, by giving at the same time arsenous acid (1–20–1–60 grain) and adonidin (1–11 grain).

For Exophthalmic Goiter. Kirnberger (quoted by Stern in the *Medical Standard*) has obtained good results from ten grams daily of sodium sulphanilate, which he uses on account of its antagonistic effect to iodine. The chief improvement concerned the heart rate, the weight and strength.

To Cleanse Hypodermic Needles. If neglected so that the wire cannot be passed (*Medical Record*), the point may be heated in an alcohol flame to burn out the organic matter. When the wire is rusted in the cannula, the latter should be soaked over night in a neutral oil, and then heated as before.

Ointment for External Piles. Conlson directs to apply twice a day an ointment of one ounce unguntum zinci oxidi with one-half dram each of liquor opii and liquor plumbi subacetatis.

Thrombotic Hemorrhoids. Incise, turn out the clot, apply an escharotic to the inside, and put patient to bed for several hours, keeping the incision open with a small pledget of cotton

Anal Ulcer. Hilton has had good results from the local application of a solution of two grains mercuric chlorid, ten minims of nitric acid and one ounce of water.

Laxative for Hemorrhoids. Roth employs a mixture of equal weights of precipitated sulphur, powdered rhubarb, compound licorice powder and eleosacchar. feniculi: a teaspoonful morning and evening.

Editorial Items continued on Page 394

BOOKS.

PHYSICIAN'S POCKET ACCOUNT BOOK.—By J. J. Taylor, M.D.
Price, $1.00. Published by the Medical Council, 4105
Walnut St., Philadelphia.

From personal use we can commend this handy pocket
account book as meeting every requirement. The readiness with
which accounts are kept and referred to anywhere is almost surprising. Although containing 200 pages, the book is easily
carried in a coat or hip pocket.

LEA BROTHERS & Co., 706–8–10 Sansom St., Philadelphia, and
111 Fifth Ave., New York: It may not be generally known
that there is published, with annual revision, a general catalogue of all medical, surgical, pharmaceutical, dental and
veterinary books in the English language.

This catalogue includes the books of all medical publishers,
and is arranged under subject classification. A more convenient
little book could not well be devised, and a copy should be on the
desk of every physician, surgeon, dentist or druggist. It is furnished gratis, and a postal card request will bring one promptly.

PRACTICAL DIETETICS.—Diet in Health and Disease. By A. L.
Benedict, Buffalo, N. Y., Member of American Gastro-En-
terological Association, Medical Society State of New York,
etc. 12mo, 400 pages. Green Buckram, Gilt Side Title
and Top. $1.50 net. Chicago: G. P. Engelhard & Co.

This little work has been well named, as it is intensely practical and consequently very useful to the clinician. It is philosophic as well as practical, presenting underlying reasons for most
of the methods and dietary applications advocated. The text is
well printed on good paper, and is at ready command through the
medium of a complete index. We recommend the book to our
readers.

SELECTIONS.

UP TO DATE DOCTORS.—A prominent physician in lecturing recently on a case of senile pneumonia at the Philadelphia Hospital, said:

"Hot flaxseed poultices, well made so as to retain their heat for four hours, were kept about the thorax during the day and at night were replaced by a lamb's-wool jacket, for the better part of a week. It is important when poultices are used that they should be well made and should retain their heat for four hours, in order that the patient shall not be continually disturbed to change them. Fever patients need rest, not only sleep at night, but rest during the day. It is rarely wise to wake the patient, either for food, for medicine, for bath, or for any other application. Save in exceptional instances, sleep will do more to favor recovery than the agent for whose sake it is interrupted."

The time was when the above statements would have received the hearty endorsement of all thoughtful medical men. But this is not the ox-cart, candle or horse-car age. We are living in the twentieth century. The old things must be laid aside. They are valuable only as antiques.

We have the cleanly and convenient electric light instead of the greasy candle. Why not antiphlogistine, made of cleanly and aseptic materials and capable of maintaining a uniform degree of temperature for 12 to 24 hours or more, instead of the bacteria-breeding, soggy, clammy linseed and other poultices?

Most up-to-date doctors say: "Yes, we know all about antiphlogistine and use it regularly as routine treatment in all cases where inflammation is present and a local remedial agent is indicated."

Picture an individual with temperature 104° to 105°, pulse 120-140, resp. 40-70. If any one craves and absolutely needs rest and sleep it is such a patient. A linseed poultice affords a very poor means for the continuous application of moist heat, nothing more. It cannot be sufficiently well made to retain a temperature of value for more than a half hour. Antiphlogistine need not be changed oftener than once in 12 to 24 hours during which time a comparatively uniform temperature is maintained. Refreshing sleep is invited, and not hindered.

A New Therapeutic Agent of Value in the Treatment of Epilepsy, with the Report of a Case.—Hugo Erichsen, M.D., L.R.C.P. and S., reports an interesting case in the *Medical Age*, for September 25, 1904. The author says :

"The patient had had nineteen well defined attacks of epilepsy since the summer of 1900. Shortly after the occurrence of the last I took charge of his case. Up to that time he had been taking the bromides at irregular intervals, owing to the fact that his stomach was easily deranged. Eventually they had to be rejected. Even bromide of sodium proved objectionable for this reason.

"About this time my attention was directed to 'brometone.' It proved to be the very thing I was looking for, as the patient had no difficulty in retaining it and it did not give rise to untoward after-effects. After taking what was evidently an over-dose the patient experienced drowsiness during the day, but when the dose was reduced to 5 grains (in capsules) three or four times a day he had no further trouble in this respect.

"Brometone contains about 77 per cent of bromine, and possesses the sedative and other characteristic effects of that agent. It is preferable to the bromides, because it does not excite nausea, vomiting, or alimentary disturbance. Moreover, it does not seem to produce the undesirable systemic depression often resulting from the older bromides. Although my patient has been taking brometone day after day for over a year, he has not been afflicted with skin rashes or any other indications of bromism. Furthermore, he has not had an attack for sixteen months, has gained in weight, improved in appearance, and takes a more cheerful view of the future.

"From my experience with it I am inclined to believe that brometone will prove of service in the treatment of other nervous conditions, particularly insomnia, headache and delirium tremens. It may also prove of benefit in some cases of asthma and may relieve cough of reflex nervous origin."

Sanmetto in Cystitis, Urethritis and in Inflammation of Bladder Neck, Also in Impotency.—By F. M. Abbett, M.D.. Indianapolis, Ind. My experience with sanmetto has been most satisfactory, from the fact that I have been enabled to get favorable results with my patients. I have used it in a variety of cases during the last ten years, as cystitis, urethritis and inflam-

mation of neck of bladder. As a remedy in impotency I know of
nothing of superior efficacy. I do not keep a clinical record of
my cases, so am unable to give reports in full detail. I can, however, heartily recommend sanmetto to the medical profession as a
remedy that has no superior where indicated, if faithfully used
by the afflicted.

AN OLD REMEDY COMBINED WITH A NEWER ONE.—The
Massachusetts Medical Journal recently published the following,
which will no doubt be interesting to our readers:

"We believe that members of the medical profession should
familiarize themselves with the combination tablet of antikamnia
and heroin. The first of these, antikamnia, years ago, established
a prominent place for itself as a most reliable antipyretic, antineuralgic, and general pain reliever, while heroin is, by all odds,
the most efficient of recent additions to our list of remedies. The
advantages of this combination are fully illustrated by a report of
cases submitted to us by Dr. Uriel S. Boone, Professor of Surgery
and Pharmacology, College of Physicians and Surgeons, St. Louis.
We reprint three of said cases, as each has some particular feature
which successfully called into use in a most beneficial manner,
the synergetic action of these two drugs.

"Case 1. J. P., athlete. Suffering from an acute cold. On
examination found temperature 101° with a cough and bronchial
rales. Patient complained of pain induced by constant coughing.
Prescribed antikamnia and heroin tablets, one every four hours.
After taking six tablets, the cough was entirely relieved. Patient
continued taking one tablet three times daily for three days, when
he ceased taking them and there has been no return of the
cough or pain.

"Case 2. Ed. H., aged 30. Family history—hereditary consumption. Hemorrhage from lungs eighteen months ago. His
physician had me examine sputum; found tubercle bacilli. After
prescribing various remedies with very little improvement, I
placed him on antikamnia and heroin tablets, prescribing one
tablet three times a day and one on retiring. He has since
thanked me for saving him many sleepless nights and while I am
aware he never can be cured, relief has been to him a great
pleasure and one which he has not been able to get heretofore.

"Case 3. Wm. S., aged 28. Lost 20 pounds in last 30 days.
Consulted me July 9th. I thought he most certainly would fall

victim to tuberculosis. Evening temperature 101° with night sweats and a very troublesome cough with lancinating pains. Prescribed 1–100 gr. atropine to relieve the excessive night sweats and one antikamnia and heroin tablet every four hours, with the result that he has entirely recovered and is now at work as usual.

"Neither in these, nor in any other of my cases, were any untoward after-effects evidenced, thus showing a new and distinctive synergetic action and one which cannot help being beneficial."

NATURAL SLEEP.—The treatment of sleeplessness in this generation has become somewhat simplified, because it is now recognized as a symptom and not as a distinct disease. It appears in such various phases and is associated with so many disorders that it is conquered with difficulty. But whether the defect is functional or structural it demands correction. It is a mistake to employ sedatives and hypnotics indiscriminately. First of all it must not derange the assimilative system; it must have no depressing effect on the heart and blood-vessels; and must be palatable.

The only preparation which approximates the theoretical hypnotic, because it meets each of these requirements so completely, is Daniel's conct. tinct. passiflora incarnata. Its action is free from the destructive and irritative effects of the gastric mucosa. It is a local anesthetic to the stomach and a sedative to the entire nuclear areas.

COD LIVER OIL.—Various preparations of cod liver oil have appeared in the market during the past ten years, but for palatability and efficiency none of them has surpassed Hagee's Cordial of Cod Liver Oil Compound. This preparation has become a standard with many doctors all over the country, and the results achieved are most satisfactory. The freedom from grease and the fishy odor makes it peculiarly acceptable to patients with weak stomachs.—*Southern Medicine and Surgery.*

CHLOROSIS.—By E. E. Rowell, M.D. Notwithstanding the steady process of hygiene, the number of anaemic women does not seem to decrease perceptibly. The chief cause of this fact is that women either will not or cannot learn how to live rationally. They do not take sufficient or proper exercise, they *will* partake of all kinds of indigestable foods and at all hours, and, last but not least, they *will* follow the most ridiculous dictates of fashion These several causes work them gradually into the first stage of anaemia, which is a mal-nutrition. With the means at our disposal to-day a diagnosis can be readily made when a patient suffering from anaemia applies for treatment, but, unfortunately, the doctor does not as a rule get the case in its incipiency. I will only discuss from a practical view point, a few of the salient features of anaemia and its practical treatment.

The symptoms of anaemia are well known, indeed they are visible to the naked eye in most cases, but there is a peculiar point to which I desire to direct attention. In all cases the condition of the blood is invariably more or less impaired; anyone who will take the trouble to resort to a proper blood examination will readily ascertain the following facts: first, the proportion and condition of the red corpuscles; second, the proportion and condition of the leucocytes and third, the percentage of hemoglobin. This knowledge will be quite sufficient for the busy practitioner. A thorough laboratory examination, however, will invariably denote a diminution of the total quantity of blood in the body with a corresponding diminution of the red corpuscles. The percentage of hemoglobin will be lower, and the red corpuscles will be modified in shape or size; furthermore the albumen may be wanting. As a matter of fact the constituents of the blood play the most important part in the processes of anaemia. It is known that a poverty of iron in the blood constitutes an important feature. It has been proclaimed by many that if the blood was poor in iron it was an easy matter to effect a cure, consequently, various prescriptions have been put before the profession, all of which have more or less virtue, but do not completely cover the field; they all lack what is most desired—a complete and perfect nutrition, as well as tonic and stimulating effects. It is admitted by all authorities that the constituents of the blood cannot be restored to their normal condition in any other way, but through the processes of nutrition, assimilation and elimination. These three processes brought to the normal standard invariably result in a cure. My experience, clinically, shows Bovinine, which is a perfected food tonic and stimulant, to cover the entire field.

HYDROGEN PEROXIDE: HOW BREAKAGE OF BOTTLES CAN BE REDUCED TO A MINIMUM.—The greatest obstacle that lies in the way of producing a sound container for liquids occluding gases under high pressure, as, for instance, solutions of hydrogen peroxide, is the fact that no process for making unbreakable glass has yet been discovered.

Up to the present, the ordinary amber glass bottles have been found totally inadequate and untrustworthy, though a device patented by Mr. Charles Marchand, goes far towards overcoming this delinquency.

This device practically reduces the danger of bursting of the bottles to a minimum. As long as the bottles, having this device, are kept in stock standing up, the pressure resulting from shaking, high temperature in course of transit, etc., will not rise much above four or five pounds to the square inch; and, therefore, though occasionally a bottle may crack or burst, it is not due to pressure, but to the inherent imperfection of the glass, arising either from the lack of homogeneity, or else imperfect annealing, or both, to which we have already referred.

The worst feature of this unreliability in the bottle is, that there is no accurate way of detecting it. A bottle may be submitted to a pressure of a hundred pounds to the square inch, without betraying signs of weakness, yet even with nothing in it, it may burst or crack within an hour.

The only remedy in these conditions as to the bottles, and that is not absolute, is in changing the material from which the containers are made, and substituting, for the unreliable amber glass, a good article of flint glass. While, as we have intimated, this does not absolutely remove the danger of loss by explosion or cracking, it greatly reduces it, and when the flint glass container is closed by Marchand's Safety Valve Stopper, danger is reduced to a minimum, beyond which, in the present condition of the technics of bottle-making, it is impossible to go.

This is exactly what Mr. Charles Marchand, the manufacturer of hydrozone, glycozone, peroxide of hydrogen, etc., intends to do. Just as soon as his present stock of amber glass containers is exhausted, he will use exclusively flint glass, every bottle being corked with an automatic safety valve stopper. By adopting these expedients, Mr. Marchand, having done all in his power to prevent breakage, can go only one step further—to make good any losses from that direction—replace the bottles that get broken from this cause. Beyond this, it would be unreasonable to expect

him to assume further responsibility. The actual danger to life
or limb from the bursting of a bottle of hydrogen peroxide, or
any of Mr. Marchand's preparations, is trivial, as compared with
those arising from the explosion of bottles of beer, ginger ale,
champagnes, and other sparkling wines, or even Apollinaris or
other heavily aerated waters.

When any of these rupture, the fragments are driven, not
only with all the force and energy of the already liberated gases,
but with the augmented energy of the residual gas suddenly set
free, and so may inflict severe, sometimes irrepparable damage.
The safety-valve arrangement in the stopper of bottles of hydrozone, prevents the sudden disengagement of a great volume of gas.

Assuming that through some imperfection of the stopper,
the puncture should close as soon as the pressure from within rose
to a point far within that required for the rupture of the bottle,
the stopper, not being wired, but merely tied down, will be forced
out.

But glass is a proverbially brittle and treacherous substance,
and it is liable to break in the hands of anybody, at any moment,
and without any discoverable or apparent cause, and that whether
filled or not. As a consequence there must always be some risk
·attached to the handling of glass containers. The best that can
be done, as we have suggested elsewhere, is to reduce the risk of
rupture or fracture to a minimum, and this, Mr. Marchand has
done, not only by his safety stopper device, but also by the promised substitution of the stronger flint glass. The retail trade will,
we are sure, welcome this latter change most heartily, since it
completes and supplements the efforts made in the mechanical
direction, and thus removes, as far as lies in human efforts, all
danger arising from handling Marchand's goods.—*Abstract from
the National Druggist of St. Louis. Mo., October, 1904.*

EDITORIAL ITEMS.— Continued.

Spongy Thickening of Nasal Septum at Junction of Cartilaginous Portion with Bones. Coakley instructs to remove with cold snare if projection sufficient. If this is not the case, use linear cauterization with galvanocautery or trichloracetic acid.

Elimination in Chronic Kidney Disease. Moore (*Clinical Review*) claims that he has seen the drowsiness of impending uremic coma overcome time and again by twenty-grain doses of sodium benzoate, best given in tincture of lemon and water.

Thickened, Pendulous Mucous Membrane on Under Surface of Middle Turbinate. This condition shows a movable but very broad attachment running anteroposteriorly. Coakley directs to remove the pendulous portion only with the cold snare.

Early Arteriosclerosis. Stengel calls attention to the symptomatic value of polyuria alternating with ischuria, and of variations in urinary specific gravity without corresponding change in quantity.

Swelling of Posterior Margin of Nasal Septum. As seen posteriorly there is an oval, pale bulging appearance. Coakley recommends the careful application of trichloracetic acid, after measuring exact distance of swelling from anterior nares.

Slight General Thickening of Nasal Mucous Membrane Remaining After Operation. Coakley advises painting the nasal cavity once or twice a week with a solution of five grains of iodine and ten grains of potassium iodide in one ounce of glycerine.

For Caseoue Rhinitis. Kyle advises the removal of septic material by curettement, followed by the use of a solvent (bicarbonate and biborate of sodium), ten or fifteen grains per ounce, and this by irrigation with equal parts of hydrogen peroxide and cinnamon water.

Gastric Atony or Myasthenia. Kuse and Penzoldt employ strychnine, ipecac and sodium bicarbonate; also orexin in doses of two to six grains in wafers or capsules one to three times a day, followed by a drink of beef-tea or cocoa.

The purity of Scott's Emulsion, the excellent quality of its ingredients and their skillful combination, and the excellent work it has done in the thirty years of its existence, make it the standard cod liver oil preparation.

Samples Free.

SCOTT & BOWNE, Chemists, 409-415 Pearl St., New York.

Constipation. W. D. Robinson (*Medical Review of Reviews*) administers ordinary white vaseline with a little water or orange juice, with excellent results. He has had particular success in the severe constipation that often accompanies typhoid fever.

Pericardial Effusion. Osler advises aspiration (fourth interspace at left sternal margin or an inch from left sternal margin) of serofibrinous exudate (common after rheumatism); free incision and drainage if purulent.

Laryngo-Tracheo-Bronchitis of Measles. Ringer employs inhalations of iodine. N. S. Davis prescribed as follows: ℞ Tinct. sanguinariae m. viiss; syr. scillae co. m. xxii; tinct. opii camph. q. s.: A teaspoonful for adults every three or four hours.

Tracheitis. Local soreness and irritation are relieved by the external application of camphorated oil or camphor-menthol, and by the frequent sucking of tablets containing terpene hydrate, codeine and cannabis indica.

Gangrenous Bronchitis. Ferrand directs to inhale powdered iodoform each night and spray bedroom with thymol. Give a quinine wine before each meal, and a tonic diet; also a dessertspoonful t. i. d. of infusion of quinine with syrup of orange and essence of eucalyptus.

For Mucous Patches. Crippe directs to cleanse parts thoroughly and dust with a powder of 20 grains of calomel, 30 grains of iodoform, one dram of zinc oxide, and one-half ounce of starch. Give mercury internally.

Itching Piles. Matthews directs to apply frequently an ointment of one part of ichthyol in eight parts of vaseline. It is also recommenced to apply once daily after defecation, a few drops of colladion on absorbent cotton.

Pile Suppositories. Potter prescribes: ℞ Iodoformi gr. v; magnesial calc. gr. v; oleo theobrom, cerae albae aa. gr. viiss.; balsami Peruv. gr. x: One morning and evening after washing with cold water. Avoid soft seats.

Pile Ointments. The following is a good formula: ℞ Pulv. gallae gr. xxx; pulv opii gr. x; ung. plumbi acet. gr. xl; ung. simp. ʒl: Colson prescribes: ℞ Ung. hydrarg. nif. ʒl; olei amyg. dulc. ʒviii: Use a little several times a day.

Villous Growths of the Rectum. Stretch the sphincters, says Gant, seize tumor with a pair of pile forceps, draw down, transfix base of tumor with a double ligature, cut this and tie both lobes of the pedicle, and cut off tumor when pedicle is long enough.

Treatment of Rectal Ploypi. Gant directs to remove with clamp and cautery, or place a ligature around the pedicle at its attachment and cut off external portion, or twist and snip off with scissors and place some astringent on stump or apply actual cautery.

Iodine as an Antiseptic. In all kinds of contused wounds (*Medical World*), after cleaning as carefully as possible, the introduction of a little tincture of iodine usually suffices to prevent the purulent complications so common in these cases.

Cutaneous Piles (Skin Tags). Says Gant: Seize (after divulsion) with catch-tooth forceps and snip off with curved scissors, taking care not to remove more skin than is absolutely necessary, for fear of contraction. If considerable space is left between the skin and mucous membrane, unite them with catgut sutures.

Anal Papillomata. If large and warty, says Gant, cut off with scissors and cauterize points of attachment. When small apply powdered alum, zinc, tannin and iron. Snip off any cutaneous tags and correct disordered conditions of rectum. Observe strict cleanliness.

Rumination of Mercyism. This curious gastric motor dynamic affection is treated by Van Valzah and Nisbet by moral and suggestive measures; thorough mastication of food; a diet that leaves the stomach rapidly; hydrochloric acid or alkalies in suitable cases; strychnine or quinine to render food bitter.

Spasmodic Dysphagia. Osler advises to pass bougies and pay special attention to the general neurotic condition. In hydrophobia he employs local applications of cocaine. For hysterical form Charles G. Stockton recommends orthoform, one to four of water through an esophageal syringe.

Gastrisoasm. Van Valzah and Nisbet recommend a soothing diet in small quantities, particularly hot milk (gradually increased), and after a week cereals and later meats should be added.

The Family Laxative

The ideal, safe, family laxative, known as "Syrup of Figs," is a product of the California Fig Syrup Co., and derives its laxative principles from senna, made pleasant to the taste and more acceptable to the stomach by being combined with pleasant aromatic syrups and the juice of figs. It is recommended by many of the most eminent physicians, and used by millions of families with entire satisfaction. It has gained its great reputation with the medical profession by reason of the acknowledged skill and care exercised by the California Fig Syrup Co. in securing the laxative principles of the senna by an original method of its own, and presenting them in the best and most convenient form. The California Fig Syrup Co. has special facilities for commanding the choicest qualities of Alexandria senna, and its chemists devote their entire attention to the manufacture of the one product. The name "Syrup of Figs" means to the medical profession "the family laxative, manufactured by the California Fig Syrup Co." and the name of the company is a guarantee of the excellence of its product. Informed of the above facts, the careful physician will know how to prevent the dispensing of worthless imitations when he recommends or prescribes the original and genuine "Syrup of Figs." It is well known to physicians that "Syrup of Figs" is a simple, safe and reliable laxative, which does not irritate or debilitate the organs on which it acts, and, being pleasant to the taste, it is especially adapted to ladies and children, although generally applicable in all cases. Special investigation of the profession invited.

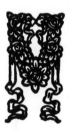

"Syrup of Figs" is never sold in bulk. It retails at fifty cents per bottle, and the name "Syrup of Figs," as well as the name of the California Fig Syrup Co., is printed on the wrappers and labels of every bottle.

California Fig Syrup Company

San Francisco, California.

Louisville, Ky.
New York, N. Y.

Codeine and aconite are of the greatest value. Sedative galvanization and a hot compress may be tied. Vigorous massage is also beneficial.

Gastroplegia. Van Valzah and Nisbet instruct to keep stomach clean and empty by lavage, and nourish body by the rectum. The usual means are indicated to restore the paralyzed muscles or prevent their atrophy. Strychnine hypodermically in large doses is a sovereign remedy for traumatic gastraplegia.

Gastric Hyperperistalsis. Among curative measures mentioned by Van Valzah and Nisbet are rest in bed; indifferent diet; strong intraventricular or epigastric faradization, or preferably anodal sedative galvanization; hudroperapy; good hygiene and reconstituent medication; codeine and electricity for pure neuroses.

Sphincterismus. Kelsey advises attention to the general health allaying nervous excitement; cathartic to empty bowel when spasm is present; anodyne injections, such as twenty drops of laudanum in one ounce of water; introduction and retention of bougie. A cure, he says, is always effected by forcible dilation of the sphincter under ether.

Tubercular Larynigitis. Osler says: Spray ulcers and keep thoroughly clean. Use two or three times a day insufflations of morphine and iodoform, or a four per cent cocaine solution. The distress from these ulcers is quickly relieved, according to Younge, by injecting one minim of pure guaiacol into floor of ulcer by means of a specially curved syringe.

Polyps in the Lower Canliculus. George F. Libby (*Ophthalmic Record*) reports the successful removal of nine polyps the size of grape seeds from this situation, being the fourth recorded case of the kind. There had been localized redness and swelling, a purulent discharge, and pain on reading.

Nitrites in Hemorrhages. The editor of the *Medical Standard* commends amyl nitrite inhalations as an emergency treatment in hempotysis and other hemorrhages. Nitroglycerin prolongs the blood-pressure—reducing action, while atropine may be used to maintain it for a considerable period.

Chronic Furunculosis. Gaucher (*Clinical Review*) recommends an alternating treatment, one week with a tablespoonful of three per cent boric acid solution at meal times, well diluted; the preceding week, tar water, a teaspoonful in half a glass of Vichy water; the following week, a solution of sodium arsenate.

External Piles. A good lotion for frequent application is made with one ounce of fluid extract of hamamelis, four drams of each of fluid extract of hydrastis and compound tincture of oenxoin, one dram of tincture of belladonna, and carbolized (five per cent) olive oil to make three ounces.

Injection Treatment of Piles. Anesthetize, stretches anus, pull down piles and tie with bow-knot (*Journal of American Medical Association*). Then inject about six drops of following mixture: One part of carbolic acid, two parts of eight per cent solution of cocaine and two parts of glycerine. After five or ten minutes untie ligatures and let patient go.

Bronchiectasis. Osler recommends intratracheal injections twice daily of a solution of menthol ten parts, guaiacol two parts, and olive oil 88 parts; also turpentine or terebene and inhalations of corbolic acid or thymol for fetid secretion. Anders prescribes: ℞ Balsami copaibae m. v-x; ammon. chloridi gr. x; ext. glycrrhizae fl. m. ix; mist. ammoniae q. s. A dessertspoonful every four hours.

Organic Stricture of the Esophagus. The syphilitic variety disappears rapidly under iodides. In other forms Tyson advises the careful use of bougies (most useful in children), introducing largest bougies first very gently only as far as obstruction; then try smaller sizes till one is found that will pass, and from this point again larger sizes should be successively employed.

Inflammations and Erosions of Epiglottis. Louis Elsberg directs to anesthetize before meals with a spray of four per cent cocaine solution. Use topical applications of silver nitrate (gr. x.-dr. ii. to ounce); solution of iodine in olive oil (x.-xxv. to ounce, with a few grains of potassium iodide); iodoform in sulphuric ether (dr. i.-ii. ad oz. i); or carbolic acid in glycerine (gr. v. to the ounce).

DENVER MEDICAL TIMES

| Volume XXIV. | FEBRUARY, 1905 | Number 8 |

TUBERCULAR PERITONITIS.*

By C. H. MAYO, A.M., M.D.

Surgeon to St. Mary's Hospital of Rochester, Minnesota.

We may truthfully say that the contagious and infectious diseases have served an important purpose in the development of civilization, by forcing a knowledge of hygienic laws, compelling the world to the isolation of the one and the watchful care of the other, and teaching the lesson that physical and mental development must go hand in hand, would man be near perfection and reproduce a high type of his kind.

History records the terrible ravages of these diseases when transplanted into virgin soil, as shown by the disappearing peoples of the Pacific Islands and the Indians of our own country. We find, also, that the wonderful fecundity of the mixed races, is held in check by their low physical resistance.

Our knowledge of tuberculosis is keeping pace with the general medical and surgical progress of the age. Considering this question we find the surprising reports from those places in which large numbers of necropsies are made, that from sixty-six per cent in the United States, to more than eighty per cent in Germany, of all cases examined, show the presence of active, latent or healed tuberculosis.

These figures are possibly somewhat high for the total population of the countries where taken, as such emaminations would be made most frequently upon those who had seen much hardship and finally terminated life in some charity hospital. The evidence tends to show that while the tubercle bacillus often causes great destruction of tissue, it seldom causes death unless the infection is mixed with other germs, if we leave out of consideration the effect produced in the brain.

*Read before the Rocky Mountain Inter-State Medical Association, Sept., 1904.

Peritoneal tuberculosis was found 184 times in 13,922 necropsies, as collected by Grawitz and Bruin and noted by J. B. Murphy in his recent most thorough monograph upon the subject. Barschke found but two cases which he could consider as primary out of 226 cases, the lungs being involved in 200 of the number. While always due to the tubercle bacillus, it is practically always secondary to tuberculosis in other regions. Although it is possible for infection to be introduced to the peritoneum by the blood stream, the lymphatics or by extension of tissue, we know as a clinical fact that it does reach it most commonly through the tubes, the uterus, appendix or perforating ulcer. In fact it would seem that the peritoneum is more resistant to this than it is in other infections, and when the primary focus, which supplies the local infection, is removed, is capable of wonderful repair. We find about four women afflicted to one man, from the frequency of tubal tuberculosis. The ages most commonly affected are from · 20 to 30 years, although there are some cases in children between the ages of 2 and 5 years.

A tuberculous family history is reported in from thirty per cent to as high as seventy-one per cent, although the highest does not seem excessive when we consider how commonly the disease is found in some form.

From the pathological findings, the peritoneal type is usually classified into miliary with ascites, the adhesive or fibroplastic, the suppurative or mixed infection, and the nodular. Wunderlich analyzed 500 cases which showed sixty-eight per cent exudative, twenty-seven per cent fibro-adhesive and four per cent purulent. Practically the pathological findings vary with the purity of the infection and the resistance of the tissue involved. The great majority of the infections are in the lower half of the abdomen, which is always found most diseased adjacent to the source of infection, the inflammation gradually fading as it gets farther away from the primary focus. This is true of almost all varieties of the disease. Tubal infections usually present the purest type of the miliary variety with ascites, the uterus and appendix next. The mixed infections develop the other forms according to the virulence of the contamination.

Tuberculosis of mucous membranes is a very chronic condition, leading to ulceration and in the appendix to perforation, also occasionally in the bowel. We have seen four cases in the upper abdomen which recovered after laparotomy with removal of the fluid, and in which the source of infection could not be located in the limited examination then made, although many adhesions were found about the region of the gall-bladder, pylorus, and duodenum. The local miliary deposit in the peritoneum and the complete freedom of such condition in the pelvis, would tend to refute the old theory of gravity being a cause of the increased frequency of tuberculosis of the pelvis. One was in a man, the other three were in women. They were all in older individuals, being from 40 to 50 years of age.

Tuberculosis of the peritoneum, as produced by leakage from a local infection of a mucous membrane, is a common cause of ascites. Such cases usually develop exacerbations of temperature from 100 to 103°, with an evening rise, even in the quiescent stage. It is not uncommon to find a history of more or less pain in the lower abdomen, which seem to be increased by peristalsis of the intestine and is relieved when the abdomen increases in size with fluid, just as in the case with tubercular pleurisy. When the infection is in the pelvis the fluid prevents a thorough examination bimanually. There may often be but little pain upon vaginal examination, and a variable amount of movement may be found in the uterus and adnexa. With less fluid there is a more rigid abdomen, which is often board-like in this respect and is, therefore, suggestive of the condition, as it is less painful than the other types of infective peritonitis, and the disease usually has already run a more chronic course.

Many cases of tubal tuberculosis will be found in operating for chronic and subacute appendicitis. It is advisable in women to always gain an idea of the pelvic condition, if possible, when the abdomen is open and the diagnosis questionable; especially is this true if free fluid is found without sufficient active condition of the appendix to account for its production.

In many instances the only diagnosis possible is a tumor or a condition of the abdomen which it will be safer to explore than to leave, without knowledge of the effects of the disease of the peritoneum. However, in most cases, a fairly exact diagnosis is possible and will be made.

Unintentionally, forty-two years ago, Spencer Wells operated upon a case of tubercular peritonitis. The operation was only an incision, diagnosis of the condition and closure of the wound, yet the case went on to recovery. Since then, many hundred similar cases have been subjected to the same treatment with a good percentage of cures. Rouch collected 358 cases with seventy per cent of immediate recoveries and 14.8 per cent of cases lasting more than two years with very many well, although a less period had elapsed. Wunderlich collected 344 cases with 23.6 per cent of deaths and 23.3 per cent of cures over three years. Czerny thinks the cures are between forty and fifty per cent.

The majority of the operations have been by open incision, with a more or less thorough removal of the fluid and closure of the wound without drainage. Occasionally some operators have made a practice of drainage, but with increased risk of mixed infection, intestinal perforations and also ventral hernia. By many, it was considered a good plan to insert a quantity of iodoform emulsion in glycerine at the time of evacuation of the ascitic fluid. Others remove the fluid by trocar, and injected air into the abdomen. The reasons given as to why relief was obtained were various and many. Some said the effect of anesthesia was favorable, others that the operative trauma produced a reparative effect, and that the reduction of nourishment by removal of fluids was influential,—that the removal of fluids and fresh flow of serum was destructive to the tubercle bacillus. Many thought that the air was influential and held the abdomen open for a certain period, while other surgeons allowed the light to enter the incision as freely as possible. However, it was from some or all of these methods that recovery was frequent from one operation, or in many cases, from two or three similar repeated procedures.

It was found by operation, where the condition was general with ascites, that a serious peritonitis was converted into a plastic fibrinous type which walled in the local infection, usually, originally a mucous membrane lesion, and maintained it as a local condition, excluding the general peritoneal cavity from its influence.

In our surgical work upon tubercular peritonitis we have practiced very many of the methods in vogue at the particular time the operations were made; but as some cases required two or three operations and a few relapsed after apparent cure, and others were not cured at all, we were gradually led to search for the original lesion and remove it, leaving the peritoneal condition to cure itself, and closing the abdomen without drainage. We have found the abdominal conditions always to point to the source of disease by the congestion, increased matting of the miliary deposit or increase of general adhesions. There is often a tubercular node of the tube near the horn of the uterus, and the repeated attacks of peritonitis are so many indications of leakage from the tube. A point picked up from a lecture of J. B. Murphy some years ago was that in the tubercular tube the fimbriae are open and turned out while in gonorrhoea or mixed infection they are turned in and closed.

We find that tuberculosis of the vulva, vagina and cervix is not a common disease, and that tuberculosis of the uterus is uncommon during menstrual life, when the mucous lining is naturally thrown off every month; but on the contrary is found before puberty and after the menopause. Tuberculosis of the tube is rather common, and while there is much discussion as to how the infection reaches this location, it nevertheless does and acts upon the mucous membrane as a local lupus. When leakage occurs we have developed an irritative peritonitis, yet not always with peritoneal evidence except the local congestion. The fimbriea being open, the ascites caused by leakage prevents what might become protective adhesions. When the abdomen is open and the ascitic fluid removed by sopping with sponges, the serous peritonitis is converted into a plastic, adhesive variety effectively walling in the tube in the cases benefitted.

It would seem impossible that tubal tuberculosis or lupus would cure itself, except by degeneration of the tubercular deposit and final obliteration. The earlier work done, while favorable as far as it went, did not remove the original focus of leakage, and while primary recoveries occurred in a large proportion of cases many returned for repeated operations and others died within a few months or years of general or local tuberculosis. In fact, Borchgrevink thought the medical treatment as successful as the surgical, reporting twenty-two operative and eighteen medical cases, under the methods at the time in vogue. In our work we have found that the increased percentage of such cases occurring in women is from tubal involvement; we also found occasionally, in tubercular peritonitis, even when the tube appeared in fair condition, that drying the peritoneum and closing the abdomen resulted in a primary cure, yet some later appeared with pelvic masses, and a second laparotomy with the removal of caseating tuberculous tubes resulted in permanent recovery. Such conditions as before stated, led us to attempt the removal of the focus of leakage or infection. In some cases the peritoneum is dried in the usual manner and at a subsequent operation the surgical indications can be accomplished. Of course, cases must be refused operation as their general condition will be such as to render an operation extremely hazardous as well as futile.

In males our incision is over the appendiceal region, while in women it is so arranged as to explore the pelvis. A tubercular appendix in an early stage, before miliary deposits appear, may at times be diagnosticated at operation by the large size of the glands of the mesenteriolum.

The utmost care must be employed not to open the bowel in separating plastic adhesions of the intestine, as they are the most difficult fistulae to close, and usually gradually exhaust the patient. As a rule it is best to keep close to the parietal or pelvic peritoneum, separating as few adhesions as possible, in exposing the region affected. In one case we were only enabled to locate the uterus in the general mass by following the round ligament to its attachment. In some cases the tubal enlargement can be pierced and its entire contents of caseating debris and lupoid material removed, leaving the outer fibrous and peritoneal layers in situ, then applying iodine or iodoform emulsion in glycerine to the diseased area, and closing the abdomen without drainage. We have made this complete operation upon twenty-six (26) cases of tubal origin with only one death.

These conclusions are based upon 144 operations for the relief of tubercular lesions involving the peritoneum at St. Mary's Hospital, where the operative work is. done by W. J. Mayo and myself. There were fifty-nine operations for tubercular peritonitis by the older methods; forty-two were cured, fifteen improved and two died. There were fifty-eight operations for the removal of tubercular tubes with fifty-six recoveries and two deaths, and twenty-seven cases of tubercular appendicitis without a death.

DISCUSSION OF DR. MAYO'S PAPER.

DR. PERKINS. I have nothing to say in discussion, except to compliment the author on his paper. He has reported a very large amount of work; more than all of us here in Denver put together could show in probably one or two lifetimes.

For some time I have thought that the operation for peritoneal tuberculosis should become more common. The cases of tubercular peritonitis on which I have operated have been mostly undertaken without a positive diagnosis of the tubercular condition having been previously made.

In some cases operation has been performed for appendicitis, and some times for tubal or ovarian conditions. But to be able to diagnose the tubercular condition in the early stages, and to operate relieving it is ideal, and it is very much better than to allow patients to go on and suffer for years. I compliment Dr. Mayo very much on his paper.

DR. WETHERILL. In talking with Dr. Mayo about this subject this morning, he made the suggestion that it was an important and interesting one to us, and I replied that peritoneal tuberculosis in Colorado is not as prevalent as the circumstances would lead one to expect. That is, with our relatively large number of tubercular patients we have a relatively small number of cases of peritoneal tuberculosis.

I agree with the statement that Dr. Mayo has reported an experience with tubercular peritonitis such as all of the surgeons of the city of Denver have not had during a similar length of time.

I am very sure that during my experience in an eastern state, I saw two or three cases, perhaps more than that, every year. In looking back over my experience here, I can recall but two cases of turbercular peritonitis in my surgical career of the last ten years in Denver; and in talking with men who have had a larger experience here than mine, I find that these men agree that tubercular peritonitis has been relatively very infrequent. Perhaps the fault has been ours in not recognizing the disease. Dr. Mayo may have acquired some particular skill in the recognition of tubercular peritonitis in the earlier stages that we have not acquired.

If there is any way of recognizing turbercular peritonitis, either of tubal origin or of the region of the appendix, it will be a source of great benefit to the medical profession to know it.

In this connection, I might say, that it is generally conceded in Colorado, that other than pulmonary tuberculosis is not as common here as elsewhere. For instance, Dr. Packard Las told me that bone tuberculosis and other forms of tuberculosis of children are not as common in Colorado, relatively, as he has found them elsewhere; and we all know that Dr. Packard has had considerable experience in the East.   In speaking with our medical men, I find that glandular and other forms of extra-pulmonary tuberculosis are thought not to be so common in Colorado as in sea level places, and this in the face of our having a very large tubercular population.

Dr. HALL.   I have been very much interested in the paper and in the subject in general.   I could claim no such familiarity with the diagnosis of tubercular peritonitis as surgeons with such experience as Dr. Mayo has, and yet I have noticed one point repeatedly in these cases, which I have never mentioned elsewhere, bearing on the matter of diagnosis.   In thin people it is fairly common to find over the abdomen a very slight edema, which leaves a very slight mark as one bears down the stethoscope.

I think a person with a thin abdominal wall and a well developed peritoneal tuberculosis will show its presence by the feeling of the skin.   I have shown it in half a dozen cases at least in the last three or four years to the students at the county hospital. I should be glad to know if, as I suspect, that may be a sign which is recognized by others, and which has escaped me in my reading, and I shall be glad to hear from Dr. Mayo as to that particular point.

I think there is one thing bearing on the general subject of tuberculosis worthy of mention, and it is in accord with what some of the other speakers have mentioned.

I believe from what Dr. Perkins and others have told me, that most forms of extra-pulmonary tuberculosis are less common here than elsewhere.   There is one form here, however, which is wonderfully common, and from what I see of reports from other places, I judge it is more common here than elsewhere.   That is meningeal tuberculosis in the adult.   I have seen six cases recently, all inside of a year, which proved fatal, and it strikes me that is a large number for one to see who is not doing special neurological work.

Dr. D. S. FAIRCHILD.   I think one of the important things in relation to the surgical treatment is to remove the source of the infection itself.   Many operations have been made where the abdomen has been opened and treated by various methods, and the results have not been satisfactory, for the reason that the focus of infection still exists, and the peritoneum is supplied with additional infection which keeps up the continuance of this disease. Now then, if the source of the infection is sought out, and the case is removed, I mean this new infection is removed, then we shall find that the disease does not recur with the same degree of frequency.

Now we know that the peritoneum will take care of a good deal of infection of various kinds if the source of supply is cut off; so it seems to me that one of the most important facts to be taken into consideration is the focus of the infection, which is supplying this infection to the peritoneum, and when this source is cut off, then we may expect very excellent results. That has been my observation and experience covering quite a considerable number of cases.

DR. MAYO. I thank you for the discussion. I had expected upon leaving home that I would find the doctors of this region were having a good deal of experience in the matter of tubercular peritonitis, considering the large number of tuberculous people who come here; and my idea was more in bringing out the point, or at least in dilating upon that point,—that every case of tubercular peritonitis is a secondary process; that it has an original focus, and that this must be searched for, and that, like tuberculosis of the joints and other regions, according to the capacity of the individual that may be taken care of.

In the cases where twenty-two were operated on surgically, and eighteen were treated medically, the results were practically the same. And Fonger, a year before his death, read a paper, which I had the pleasure of hearing, in which he stated he thought that theory was about right; and that we could operate on them and some would live and some would die, and that we could take care of them, and some would live and some would die, and that the result of experience with an even number of cases would be about alike. But in working out the principle that there is a source of infection, and that if we could remove it that the peritoneum part of it would take care of itself, and that tuberculosis is most difficult to cure when we get a mixed infection. The cases that die, are usually of the general miliary type which involves the whole of the body.

The point brought up that we would get a little temporary edema by the use of the stethoscope I have noticed in those cases where there was quite a good deal of pressure from the enlargement and a thin abdominal wall. I have not noticed it so much in the dryer types. Tuberculosis is so varied in its effect upon different individuals, and some persons, apparently, throughout the whole history present the dry type. Some immediately get the ascites, and the only complaint that you have is the ascites, while others will have that period of peritoneal irritation which peristalsis will increase. But if you have that rigid abdomen it is sufficient to operate for, and there is generally something there that wants to be fixed, usually the appendix in men and the tubes in women.

I thank you very much, and I also thank you for the privilege of the floor and the presentation of a paper before this Society. I think this is a Society which is sure to develop. This is the farthest West I have even been and I am sure I have had a very pleasant trip. I thank you.

HYPERCHLORHYDRIA : WITH OBSERVATIONS ON DIET AND GASTRIC ANALYSIS.*

By JAMES RAE ARNEILL, M.D.,

Professor of Medicine in the University of Colorado.

The personal element is an all-important factor in stomach work, both with the physician who diagnoses and prescribes and with the patient who is examined and treated. By this is meant that the physician in his handling of stomach cases, is unwittingly influenced by his own gastric and intestinal idiosyncrasies. Fortunate is the patient whose advice comes from a man with a normal alimentary tract. It is but human nature for the doctor to consider his own stomach and intestines as models of their kind. If they rebel against milk, and are insulted by eggs and are tied up in knots by apple pie, it is only natural to think that if a patient has decent and respectable viscera his ought to do the same thing. We all find ourselves persistently advising against good, sensible, nutritious foods for no other reason than that they disagree with us. As a matter of fact a personal dietetic idiosyncrasy warps one's judgment. I know of many excellent physicians who warn all of their patients against eating eggs, simply because for themselves they are rank poison; others who think that milk is an invention of the devil, simply because their own milk curdling ferment happens to be deficient and they suffer with so-called biliousness if they indulge.

Another doctor raises his voice and hand Munyon like against the time honored luxury of apple pie. He perhaps is an overworked medico with nerves and hyperchlorhydria, in whom the mild acid of the apple, adds fuel to the flame of an acrid juice. This same personal factor exhibits itself in advice given about the number of meals which should be eaten in the course of 24 hours. One physician advises two heavy meals, another five or six light ones, frequently basing judgment on experience with his own peculiar, defective stomach. To illustrate the importance of the personal element in the patient, one has but to call to mind certain cases with supposedly weak or dyspeptic stomachs, who were advised to live on the blandest and most easily digested foods, but who in a rash moment braved the anger of the irate doctor, and satisfied a

---

* Read before the Rocky Mountain Inter-State Medical Association, Sept. 1904.

craving for corn-beef and cabbage—or Welsh rarebit and beer, with the happiest results and a new lease on life. "What is one man's meat is another man's poison." Analysis of the stomach contents with accurate determination of total acidity, combined acid, free HCl, pepsin and lab. ferment, will not decide positively that certain diets will agree with such and such a case. In other words the stomach and intestines are vital tubes not test tubes, and are controlled to a remarkable extent by the personal idiosyncrasies of the patient.

In all stomach work the physician should strive to free himself from his personal prejudices and should never fail to learn the pecularities of the digestive apparatus of his patients; and take advantage of their ripe experience in testing articles of diet. It has been my observation that many patients possess such exquisitely sensitive nervous systems, that their gastric mucosas are irritated by normal stomach juices, with the result that symptomatically and from the standpoint of treatment we are dealing with a case of hyperchlorbydria; while chemically we are dealing with a normal stomach and pathologically with a case of neurasthenia possessing a hyper-sensitive mucous membrane.

Again, in functional stomach diseases, which are by far the most common, conditions change from meal to meal, or day to day. Consequently deductions from *one* analysis may be absolutely wrong. One often has the experience of going over the history of a case very carefully and guessing at the acid contents of the stomach juice and on following this up with an analysis finds much to his surprise (judging from this single analysis), that instead of a hyperchlorhydria he is dealing with a hypochlorhydria. Not satisfied, he tries another different test meal, or perhaps the same kind of meal again, and in the second or third analysis finds his guess of a hyperchlorhydria confirmed. It is because of such experiences that many good men declare that gastric analysis as commonly practiced is uncertain and deceptive; and that they can get better results by taking a good history and guessing at the diagnosis; or by trying the therapeutic tests with acids and alkalis. There is much truth in these contentions, especially where stomach work is not carried out with sufficient detail and accuracy. It is a pleasant mental diversion and one which I always practice, to take a careful history of the patient and then guess on the probability of a hyper- or hypochlorhydria. In the vast majority of cases one can guess correctly. But what of the small percentage in which one is absolutely wrong? On a number of occasions I have secured an excellent history of hyperchlorhydria, but on accurate analysis have found that hydrochloric acid was practically absent, and that the symptoms were caused by a great excess of organic acids.

Notwithstanding the many weak points in modern stomach work, he who argues against gastric analysis, forgets that the chemical question of hyper- or hypochlorhydria may be a very small one, in comparison with the importance of the size of the stomach, its position and its motor power. He also forgets that the chemical and microscopical findings often throw light upon the presence of cancer or ulcer when these cannot be determined by physical diagnostic methods.

An important point recently emphasized by Fischer (*American Journal of the Medical Sciences*, July) and one which I have believed in and followed for a number of years—is that the average gastric analysis may be of rather small value, and may in fact mislead one. This average analysis consists of one test meal of bread and tea, or crackers and water, or a shredded wheat biscuit and water. Such a test meal, though useful as one of a *series* of meals, and excellent for the determination of free HCl, cannot possibly give us the correct idea of the manner in which the stomach would behave when the customary more trying demands of ordinary meals are placed upon it.

We have learned through Pawlow's epoch making investigations upon "The Work of the Digestive Glands," that the secretion of a normal gastric juice is dependent upon a number of factors, outside of the simple presence of food in the stomach. Of these factors an important one not taken into consideration in the commonly used test meal is the effect of appetite, the stimulation of the senses of sight, smell and taste, in producing a so-called psychic gastric juice. To illustrate the importance of the psychic element in the secretion of gastric juice, I will mention one of Pawlow's experiments. By feeding a dog 200 grams of food he secured 135 c.c. of gastric juice. By directly introducing the same quantity of food into the stomach through a fistula, he secured 50 c.c. of gastric juice (sympathetic stimulation). By fictitious feeding of the food he secured 75 c.c. of gastric juice (vagus stimulation).

Troller found that the introduction of food into the stomach through a tube in the human subject produced much less acid secretion than if the same were first masticated. On the other hand the mastication of tasteless substances caused very little acid secretion. The only conclusion to be drawn from these experiments is that the average test meal of bread and water does not furnish a fair test of the stomach's secreting capacity; it *simply* determines the amount of acid which this particular food will stimulate. Inasmuch as the stomach secretion may vary from day to day, one should test several meals; and because each food has its own special acid curve, one should give a variety of meals. A fair series of test meals consists of the following: In the morning give an Ewald-Boas breakfast of bread and water; for the second test allow the patient to eat his average lunch, and for the third meal give him a Riegel test dinner, which consists of a dish of meat broth, a beef steak weighing 5 to 7 ounces, 1½ ounces of mashed potato and a roll. Withdraw in four hours. If the stomach is empty give another Riegel meal next day and withdraw in three fours. With such a series of meals the stomach should be sufficiently taxed to determine the presence or absence of a hyperchlorhydria.

The great influence which the mind wields over the stomach and intestines is a matter of daily observation among physicians. A former student of mine suffered with a very distressing diarrhoea during her senior year, as the result of her dread of the daily quiz. This continued until, at my suggestion, her various instructors assured her that she would not be quizzed, and it immediately ceased. Numerous surgeons have had similar experiences; the worry preceding the operation causing a looseness of the bowels. The analogous effect upon the stomach is to produce in many instances an acute or chronic hyperchlorhydria. Business worry, grief, sorrow, long illness, mental shock of any kind, prolonged physical and mental tax, as in nursing a very sick case, may result in a temporary or persistent hyperchlorhydria. The patient suffering from neurasthenia, hypochondriasis, nervous prostration, and the more profound melancholia is very likely to develop a hyperchlorhydria, which may be a slight or very serious matter. The gastric symptoms may become so pronounced that the patient imagines that all the trouble is located in the stomach, and that the failure of nutrition and the nervous exhaustion are entirely dependent upon the gastric conditions. It is true that a certain percentage of these cases show a hypochlorhydria. It was my experience in a large series of cases of enteroptosis (patients who are notoriously neurasthenic) to find that a majority of them had a diminished acidity. They were drawn largely from hospital practice, however, and from agricultural districts. My belief is that the same number of enteroptotics in private practice would have shown a hyperchlorhydria.

It is difficult to draw accurate conclusions as to the frequency of this condition. To my mind it depends largely upon the class of patients the physician is dealing with. If one's statistics are drawn chiefly from hospitals sought by the poorer laboring classes, he will find among his stomach cases, an excess of hypochlorhydria; if on the other hand they are drawn from literary or social sets, they will almost surely show a great preponderance of hyperchlorhydria. My own records in private practice show a marked preponderance of the latter. I was dealing largely for a period of six years with university students and professors. Riegel, Bouveret, Jaworski, Mathieu, Remond and others hold that hyperchlorhydria is a very frequent functional disturbance. Other authors claim that this symptom is a rare one. Conclusions should be drawn only from cases in which the stomach contents have been analyzed. Symptomatology cannot be depended on for accurate diagnosis. Von Noorden frequently found hyperchlorhydria in cases of melancholia. Some excellent research along this line was done by Dr. Ralston Williams of Rochester N. Y.—working on material furnished by Dr. William M. Edwards, Superintendent of the Kalamazoo (Mich.) Asylum for the Insane. This work was carried out with extreme care and accuracy. Dr. Williams has kindly furnished me with the results of his investigations.

They are as follows: The cases studied were those exhibiting the symptoms of depression or the symptom complex which is commonly designated as melancholia. The patients selected were subjected to a thorough physical and clinical examination and those showing signs or lesions of other disease, which might invalidate the gastric findings were excluded. Special attention was given to the stomach to eliminate, so far as possible, such complications as hypersecretion, gastroptosis, dilatation, carcinoma and ulcer. The stomach in each instance was distended and topographically mapped out by palpation and auscultatory percussion. The Ewald and Riegel test meals and the ordinary hospital dinner were the experimental meals given. The Toepfer method of analysis was employed. In all ten cases were studied.

Summary of Results.

CASE No. 1. Examined nine times. Free HCl values varied from 35 to 70 (Ewald scale) and the total acidity values from 48 to 100. The peptic digestion values by the original Mett method varied from 5 to 16mm (24 hours) and the quantity of the test meal expressed from 25 c.c. to 70 c.c.

CASE No. 2. Nine examinations made. Free HCl values varied from 20 to 77. Total acidity varied from 40 to 102. Peptic values varied from 1 to 11mm. Amount of meal expressed varied from 5 to 180 c.c.

CASE No. 3. Eight examinations made. Free HCl values varied from 8 to 71. Total acidity varied from 25 to 92. Peptic values varied from 0 to 12mm. Amount of meal expressed varied from 5 to 155 c.c.

CASE No. 4. Eight examinations made. Free HCl values varied from 0 to 90. Total acidity varied from 10 to 108. Peptic values varied from 2 to 16mm. Amount of test meal expressed varied from 30 c.c. to 156 c.c.

CASE No. 5. Nine examinations made. Free HCl values varied from 34 to 68. Total acidity varied from 55 to 98. Peptic values varied from 3 to 14mm. Amount of test meal expressed varied from 60 c.c. to 350 c.c.

CASE No. 6. Five examinations made. Free HCl values varied from 0 to 0. Total acidity varied from 2 to 15. Peptic values varied from 0 to 2mm. Amount of meal expressed varied from 10 c.c. to 82 c.c.

CASE No. 7. Five examinations made. Free HCl values varied from 0 to 0. Total acidity varied from 0 to 15. Peptic values varied from 0 to 0. Amount of meal expressed varied from 0 c.c. to 8 c.c.

CASE No. 8. Four examinations made. Free HCl values varied from 36 to 63. Total acidity varied from 50 to 87. Peptic values varied from 9 to 14mm. Amount of meal expressed varied from 24 c.c. to 110 c.c.

CASE No. 9. Free HCl values varied from 30 to 50. Total acidity varied from 67 to 73. Peptic values varied from 7.8 to 15.5mm. Amount of meal expressed varied from 58 c.c. to 170 c.c.

CASE No. 10. Three examinations made. Free HCl values varied from 38 to 48. Total acidity varied from 55 to 68. Peptic values varied from 11 to 12mm. Amount of meal expressed varied from 12 c.c. to 170 c.c.

From the foregoing it will be seen that (1) the range of secretion of free HCl in most of these cases is very great, varying from 10 to 90 degrees, pointing to hyperchlorhydria. (2) The total acidity has likewise a wide range of variation. (3) The peptic values are also extremely variable and in several of the cases are indicative of a marked hyperpepsia. (4) Many of the cases show a disturbance of motor power.

In Case No. 10 this is about all the analysis shows, however, this patient suffered from marked sensory disturbances as did some of the others. In some instances these disturbances were the basis of the delusions experienced.

DIAGNOSIS:—As previously stated these cases can often be diagnosed correctly from a careful consideration of history and symptomatology, especially by those who have frequently followed up the histories of cases with analyses of test meals. The degree of suffering may bear no relation at all to the degree of hyper-acidity, as we find patients with an acidity scarcely above normal complaining most bitterly of the pain, burning and tenderness in the pit of the stomach; also of heartburn and the belching of gas and fluid so acid that it burns the lining of their gullets and sets their teeth on edge. Other patients with most startling degrees of acidity will scarcely complain of a symptom, at most of the merest sensation of uneasiness in the epigastrium. The explanation of these striking inconsistencies lies in the nervous make-up of the patient. The more neurasthenic and hysterical the patient, the more acutely sensitive is the mucous membrane to irritation, and the smaller the power of inhibition and resistance. Cases of hyperchlorhydria usually complain of burning pain or uneasiness in the epigastrium from one-half to several hours after meals. They tell you that they are relieved after eating for perhaps one or two hours or more, depending on the size and kind of meal. Baking

soda or magnesia will also relieve them for a time. It is true
that alkalis may temporarily allay the symptoms of the hyperacidity of organic acids, but to no such extent as in the case of
hyperchlorhydria. On the contrary the symptoms of cases of
organic acid hyperacidity, are more likely to be permanently
relieved by the use of dilute hydrochloric acid.

Food is likely to increase the distress of hyperacidity due to
organic acids. Certain foods like milk, meat and eggs usually
give great temporary relief in hyperchlorhydria, because of their
great hydrochloric acid combining powers.

The relief from symptoms is due to the fact that the food
combines with the free hydrochloric acid, producing a combined
HCl. Consequently there is very little or no distress until all of
the affinities of the food are satisfied and free HCl makes its
appearance in excess.

In certain cases an intense gastralgia may result, associated
with profound nervous symptoms, not relieved by vomiting or
alkalis. Large doses of morphia may be required. Pure cases of
hyperchlorhydria are usually free from symptoms when the
stomach is empty. Physical examination throws very little light
on these cases from the standpoint of differential diagnosis.

The stomach may be normal in size and position and there
may be no points of tenderness. There is usually a diffuse tenderness over the epigastrium. True the stomach may be dilated
and dislocated, but such a condition is very common in hypo- or
anachlorhydria. The crucial diagnostic measure is the analysis
of several varieties of test meals.

DIET:—The diet of hyperchlorhydria has formed the subject
for numerous articles. The diametrically opposite views expressed
by different authorities prove that no arbitrary rules can be laid
down. One authority advises a vegetarian diet, another a meat-
free diet which includes milk and eggs in addition to vegetables;
another advises a proteid diet, and a fourth a mixed diet modified
to suit the individual case.

With all of these excellent results are claimed. The only
method of satisfying one's self of the virtues of these different
diets is to try them on a large number of cases. The writer has
done this and has learned that one can depend upon none of them.
With certain cases the meat-free diet works marvellous results,
but with the very next case one is just as likely to meet with

failure. In many cases the proteid diet gives the most satisfaction and greatest relief from symptoms, while in others it is an absolute failure. Probably the most suitable diet for a majority of cases is a properly modified mixed diet. We learn from experience that there is no specific dietetic treatment for hyperchlorhydria. To obtain success in handling these cases one must treat the patient and his dietetic idiosyncrasies, not the hyperchlorhydria per se. Notwithstanding the great dietetic latitude which these cases demand, certain arbitrary rules must be laid down. We must realize that the patient suffering with this disease has an irritable, morbidly sensitive gastric mucous membrane, which secretes larger or smaller quantities of hydrochloric acid, under comparatively slight provocation.

Consequently the patient must avoid very hot and very cold foods; he must chew his food thoroughly to avoid the mechanical irritation of coarse hard particles. He must avoid those foods which cannot be chewed into small bits, such as gristly fibrous meats and very coarse vegetables and fruits with seeds and stones. The patient must also avoid spices, sauces, salads, acids and sour articles of diet. The supporters of the meat—free and vegetarian diets claim that they stimulate a smaller secretion of HCl than a proteid diet, and that though the symptoms may be temporarily increased because of their smaller acid—combining power, if persisted in will cause a permanent diminution in the secretion of HCl. In opposition to these contentions we have the results of Mayer's experiments. Testing a vegetarian and proteid diet on the same cases of hyperchlorhydria over a long period of time he found that a vegetarian diet finally produced a permanent increase in the secretion of HCl. This was due he thought to the mechanical irritation of the necessarily increased bulk of a vegetable diet. It is a matter of common observation that cases of hyperchlorhydria frequently complain of marked gas formation in the stomach. This is especially severe when the diet contains a large proportion of starchy foods. The reason for this is that in these cases starch digestion is poor. Hydrochloric acid is secreted early and in excessive quantities and quickly stops the action of the diastasic forment of the saliva. Recent experiences convinced me that a vegetarian diet was suitable only in a limited number of cases.

To ILLUSTRATE:—A patient with hyperchlorhydria and gastroptosis did not progress under my care as I wished, so she was placed in the hands of an acknowledged expert in vegetarian diet and physical therapeutics. She grew rapidly worse notwithstanding the additional use of electricity and hydrotherapy. She returned to me and was placed on a modified mixed diet, tonics and alkalis and, with a change of scene in the shape of an eastern trip, improved remarkably. Many cases in which the neurasthenic element is prominent are extremely rebellious to treatment. Diet and medicine may have absolutely no effect and good results are secured only by a complete change of scene and occupation.

As an illustration I will cite the following case:

Patient was a young man of 22, hypochondriacal on the subject of his stomach. He was a confirmed dyspeptic of three years' standing. He thought of nothing but his extreme suffering. His self commiseration was pitiable. He had a fairly marked gastroptosis complicating a high grade hyperchlonhydria.

An Ewald-Boas test breakfast, removed in one hour, showed a total acidity of 80 and free HCl of 50. A Riegel test meal, removed in four hours, showed a total acidity of 130 and free HCl of 50. His Thanksgiving dinner, removed in $4\frac{1}{2}$ hours, showed a total acidity of 90 and free HCl of 30. The motor power was somewhat diminished. He was dieted, given tonics and alkalis, and his stomach was washed with Carlsbad solution. There was no improvement and his mental condition became distressing. I urged a sea voyage. Instead he gave up his position, took a trip to Canada—worked as an ordinary laborer on a ranch and in a short time he was able to eat anything and everything. His stomach regained its motor power, his dyspeptic symptoms disappeared entirely and he quickly decided that life was again worth living. A great many of these cases after apparent recovery still show hyperchlorhydria on analysis. They have regained their nervous force and mental balance for the time being. As a result of any special strain they may again easily develop a pathological increase in HCl. With them a certain amount of hyperchlorhydria is physiological. If this condition is complicated by gastroptosis, dilatation of the stomach, neurasthenia, etc., the treatment naturally differs from that of uncomplicated cases.

Hyperchlorhydria must be differentiated from hyperesthesia, hyperacidity due to organic acids, hypersecretion or Reichman's disease, and from gastric ulcer. The treatment of hyperchlor-hydria may be easy or may tax one's skill to the utmost. The simple—acute—uncomplicated cases are quickly relieved of their symptoms. The chronic cases complicated with neurasthenia—disturbing environments, or with dilatation, etc., may prove one's undoing. Our armamentarium consists of: change of surround-ings—fresh air treatment, massage, electricity, hydrotherapy. Osteopathy and Christian Science may be useful as mental place-bos. Nerve tonics, such as enormous doses of tr. of nux vomica, increasing gradually from 10 drops to 70 drops, t. i. d., after meals. Bismuth and cerium oxalate before meals. Alkalis, such as sodium bicarbonate, calcined magnesia or milk of magnesia at the correct time and in proper dosage after meals. Correction of constipation, with perhaps Carlsbad salts. Lavage is unnecessary in the majority of cases; in a few it is useful. For a diet, one can take his choice of a meat—free—a proteid—or best of all a properly mixed diet, in which proteids predominate, and attention is given to the personal idiosyncrasies of the patient.

At best it will be a matter of experiment. After trial one can eliminate or add certain articles. Coffee, acids, spices, irri-tants both chemical and physical must be eliminated from the start. A large amount of fluid is allowed with the meals, as this will dilute the hyperacid juices. Chemically—hyperchlorhydria is usually limited by certain arbitrary figures. These, however, differ with the variety of the test meal. For instance, in a nor-mal case the total acidity of a Riegel test dinner is always much higher than that of an Ewald Boas' breakfast The acidity also varies with the time of the removal of the meal. For the Riegel test dinner the total acidity varies between 60 and 80 at 4 hours, the free HCl from 10 to 20, the combined HCl from 50 to 60. For the Ewald Boas' test breakfast—the total acidity is about 55 at one hour, the free HCl about 10 and the combined HCl about 45 (Van Valzah-Nisbet). Other authorities allow a little greater latitude for the normal figures. Cases showing an acidity above these figures are called hyperchlorhydria. Therapeutically it is a relative term, as many cases with hyperchlorhydria figures, require no treatment, while other cases with normal juices, but hyper-chlorhydria symptoms, require a well directed therapy.

Cases illustrating comparatively *low* acidity with *severe* symp-toms:

CASE No. 1.   Miss H. A., early twenties, servant girl, Swede, complains of pain in epigastrium, left hypochondrium and bowels, about ½ hour after eating.   At times it lasts all afternoon.   The stomach feels better after eating.   No vomiting, nausea or hematemesis.   Appetite good.   Stomach troubled her as a child and since coming to America it has been worse; not careful of diet, eats great deal of sweets and they disagree more than anything else.   Patient is well nourished.   Chest examination negative— no enteroptosis.   Hyperchlorhydria was suspected in this case. An Ewald-Boas test meal of bread and water was given and removed in one hour.   200 c.c, of bile-stained fluid were obtained— no retention of previous meal.   The analysis showed free HCl of 28 and a total acidity of 44.   The patient was placed on a mixed diet, suitable for a case of hyperchlorhydria, was given increasing doses of nux vomica and milk of magnesia.   Relief from symptoms followed.   I am uncertain whether they continued.

CASE No. 2.   Miss A. C., 24 years of age, servant girl, for the past three years has suffered with a burning sensation at the end of the ensiform. worse from 3 to 5 in the afternoon; also has constantly regurgitated very bitter, sour material.   During the past year has been vomiting two to three times daily, after meals, if not food then a sour liquid.   She gets very hungry, but is afraid to eat as everything hurts her.   She has suffered with sick headaches nearly all her life; these have been extremely severe during the past few years, lasting all day.   Patient is extremely nervous.   Whenever she gets worried she feels it in her stomach. She declares that diet makes no difference in her sensations. Monthly periods very painful.   Has lost in weight from 165 to 140.   Patient is well nourished, of the neurotic type, but no enteroptosis.   I suspected hyperchlorhydria.   A test meal of half a dozen Uneeda biscuits and a glass and a half of water was removed in 55 minutes.   250 c,c. of contents were obtained; this did not smell sour.   The analysis showed a total acidity of 55 and HCl of 14.   A diagnosis of nervous dyspepsia with hyper-esthesia of the gastric mucosa was made and the patient was given bismuth and cerium oxalate before meals and sodium bicarbonate and calcined magnesia after meals.   A mixed diet, suitable for the average case of hyperchlorhydria was ordered.   The patient improved immediately; vomiting, headaches and symptoms generally disappeared.   A series of test meals should have been given, as it is possible that analysis of other meals would have demonstrated a hyperchlorhydria.

ILLUSTRATIVE CASES.

The following histories illustrate cases of extreme hyperchlorhydria, with very slight symptoms:

CASE No. 1. Mr. G. K., age early twenties, tailor. Complains only of a burning sensation in the region of the stomach three to four hours after each meal. This is increased by drinking beer or whisky. Constipation. Patient is slender and wiry, but in good nutrition. Physical examination is negative except that the stomach is somewhat prolapsed. His ordinary dinner was removed in three hours. Total acidity 140, free HCl 50. Four months later his ordinary dinner was removed in $4\frac{1}{2}$ hours. Total acidity 180, free HCl 80.

CASE No. 2. Young man about thirty, senior law student, complained of constipation and indigestion for the past three years. During the last year he suffered with severe headaches at the latter end of the week, sour stomach, belching and occasional vomiting; loss of weight 20 pounds. For one year he washed his stomach with benefit; found food remains 24 hours after eating; ate two meals a day for a while. Distress is more marked when stomach is empty than when full, suggesting hypersecretion. He feels weak in the epigastrium. The greater curvature of the stomach is one inch below the navel. The stomach holds about two quarts. The edge of the liver is felt one inch below the margin of the ribs. The following analyses were made: March 29th, test breakfast of 5 Uneeda biscuits and $\frac{1}{2}$ glass of water; time, 1 hour, amount 250 c.c. Total acidity 72, free HCl 53. March 31st, ordinary dinner; time 4 hours; large quantity. Total acidity 150, free HCl 90. April 27th, 5 Uneeda biscuits, glass of water; time 1 hour; amount 10 c.c. Total acidity 80, free HCl 90. June 1st, test breakfast Uneeda biscuit and water. Total acidity 80, free HCl 60.

Cases illustrating the importance of several test meals of different kinds.

CASE No. 1. Business man, 36 years old, well nourished, but markedly neurasthenic. Has been a dyspeptic for fifteen years; consulted many doctors, among them one of the most eminent stomach specialists in this country. He has tried all kinds

of medicine, has used all sorts of diet and has fasted for many
days at a time. He has never been benefitted and has lost all confidence in physicians. His whole attention is centered on his
stomach. There is belching of much sour gas, beginning one-half
hour after meals and continuing for two hours. He frequently
regurgitates mouthsful of food which tastes sour and fermented.
No pain ordinarily, slight nausea. His chief complaint is that he
feels languid and dopy after meals, cries easily, thinks he has lost
his grip—has felt like committing suicide many times. He broods
over his suffering continually, and magnifies his symptoms many
fold. He is overly sensitive, anticipates trouble, is easily worried
and irritated. He fasts a while and it helps him. He tries it
again and it harms him. Later he will eat everything on the diet
list for periods of two weeks and will feel fine, then he will feel
badly again and diet himself. Melons and berries give him great
distress. Milk acts like a poison with him. Test meal, ordinary
lunch; time $1\frac{3}{4}$ hours. Free HCl 0. Total acidity 30, excess of
lactic acid. Pepsin Mett tube with stomach juice showed no
digestion, tube with juice and two gtts dil. HCl showed 44mm.
Ewald Boas' breakfast of bread and water; time one hour, amount
50 c.c., no retention. Free HCl 30. Total acidity 50. Pepsin
tube with juice 11mm; tube with juice and two gtts dil. HCl
10mm. Microscope showed numerous budding yeast cells.

Riegel test meal; time three hours, 50 cc. Free HCl 20.
Total acidity 80. It will be seen that all three meals showed a
marked variation in free HCl and total acidity and pepsin values.
I have frequently observed in cases of hyperchlorhydria in making
the pepsin test with the Mett tubes that the tubes to which the
dilute HCl is added almost always shows less digestion than the
tube which holds the juice alone.

CASE No. 2. M. J. L., early twenties. Enteroptosis, hypertrophied rectal valves, constipation, nervous dyspepsia, marked
neurasthenic symptoms. Experimental meals. Lunch of lamb
chops and graham wafers; time three hours, amount 250 cc. Free
HCl 44. Total acidity 76. Ewald-Boas breakfast; time one
hour, amount 200 cc. Free HCl 18. Total acidity 38. Microscope shows a few budding yeast cells.

DISCUSSION OF DR. ARNEILL'S PAPER.

DR. MAYO. I have listened with a great deal of interest. I think some of us surgeons, who are devoting our time exclusively to surgery, forget how to use therapeutics. I think that is so with myself; I use less and less medicine every year; so that possibly that point will be carried too far and we will entirely disregard finally the use of remedies. And I have found that these patients do about as well with what they learn concerning their own conditions regarding diet as I could do for them.

I do not find any remedies, which, given for a short period in troubles which are chronic, will do much good except during a temporary period. This class of patients are not content to follow one course of treatment any great length of time. They are the rounders; they make the rounds of all the doctors in the neighborhood, and not continuing any course of treatment long enough, they find they are not being much benefitted and then begin to take care of themselves. They find out from the doctors all about their condition, and find they can do as well with it themselves as any doctor they have tried.

The surgeon's idea, therefore, is that if these patients are suffering with something tangible, in which we can relieve them by an actual surgical operation, why we accept them as patients; but if not, we consider that the time may come in a few years when they will be a proper surgical case, and in the meantime they can take care of themselves pretty near as well as we can take care of them.

DR. ARNEILL. In place of closing the discussion of my paper, I wish to take the time in exhibiting a new apparatus for accurately measuring pepsin digestion in a quantitative way.

This apparatus is a microscope invented by Dr. Cowie, of Ann Arbor, and consists of a stand, millimeter scale, reflector and microscope of small magnifying power. It is used in connection with the Mett tubes.

The following is the method of estimating pepsin digestion by this Mett tube method, which Pawlow, of St. Petersburg popularized. Formerly the pepsin digestion test was made with small discs of egg albumin. By this old method it was absolutely impossible to accurately estimate pepsin digestion. The Mett tube method is a great advance. It is as follows:

"Briefly described, glass tubes filled with coagulated egg albumin are placed in 2–4 cc. of gastric juice and kept in the incubator for ten hours. At the end of this time the tubes are removed and the number of millimeters of albumin digested is estimated. This is ascertained by measuring the portion of the end of the tubes that are clear, including also the clouded or opalescent zone if one be present. For this purpose a scale graduated to .5 mm., a small lens magnifying $\frac{2}{3}$ diameters and a small black glass are employed. With very little practice one can correctly read fifths of a millimeter. The digestion which goes on within the first ten hours, according to Ssamojloff, corresponds to the normal period of stomach digestion. Franz Jung states that from 5.5 to 5.9 mm should be digested in ten hours. However, the results obtained in the laboratory of the University Hospital at Ann Arbor would indicate that these figures are too high and that 3.5 to 4.5 would be more nearly correct.

It has been estimated by Borrissow and Schutz that the amount of pepsin in one juice as compared with another is as the squares of the numbers of millimeters digested are to each other. The foregoing fundamental statements are gathered from Jung's abstracted translation of Pawlow's book, "The Work of the Digestive Glands," (*Jour. A. M. A.*, May 10, 1902) and is the basis of the experiments that follow.

There are several ways of preparing and preserving the Mett tubes. The one employed by the writer is as follows: Thin walled glass tubing, having a calibre of 1.5 mm is cleaned in distilled water and dried. It is then cut into lengths of about 10 cm. convenient for storage for use. These then, are filled by suction with the white of a fresh egg. The egg albumin must be free from air bubbles, one of the chief sources of annoyance and error being the presence of these air bubbles. In filling the tubes, the endeavor is made to secure only the more fluid portion of the egg. This can be done readily by care and manipulation. As each tube is filled its ends are passed slowly through a white gas flame, thus forming small coagulated plugs which serve temporarily to prevent the escape of the albumen. When a sufficient number of these tubes are thus prepared they are placed in a basin of distilled water, supported on glass rods. The water is then heated to a temperature between 90 and 95 degrees C., which is sustained for five minutes. Care is taken to keep an equable temperature throughout the basin. From here the tubes are transferred to a 66 per cent watery solution of glycerin, in which they are preserved.

When it is wished to make a test, a tube is selected, the glycerine washed therefrom and about 10 mm. of one is snipped off, a sharp Stubb's file being employed for this purpose. This piece is thrown away and another about 18 mm. long is taken. In this way a portion is secured free from the action of glycerin, which has an inhibiting effect on the digestion of the egg. This small tube placed in 3 or 4 cc. of gastric juice is put in the incubator and left for either 10 or 24 hours. The digestion in 24 hours is proportionately more. For the reasons before stated, 10 hours is preferred, but usually the 24 hour period is much more convenient, and is therefore used. Frequently in the digested tubes two zones will be seen, one perfectly clear from which the albumin has entirely disappeared, the other hazy and cloudy. In other tubes cone-shaped translucent plugs are formed. The explanation of this is not quite clear, since in the more perfect tubes the digestion is sharply defined, there being only the clear digested and solid or undigested ones. The results may be recorded as the number of millimeters, but for purposes of comparison, these figures should be squared, this being the true index to the amount of pepsin in the sample. (Ralston Williams).

NORMAL OBSTETRICS.

(CHAPTER TEN.)

THE ANTE–PARTUM EXAMINATION — INCLUDING THE DIAGNOSIS OF THE VERTEX PRESEN. TATION AND ITS POSITIONS PER ABDOMEN.

By T. MITCHELL BURNS, M.D.,

Denver, Colorado.

Professor of Obstetrics, The Denver and Gross College of Medicine,

After the study of the maternal changes and the diagnosis of pregnancy should come the ante-partum examination.

Charts.—To facilitate and preserve ante-partum examinations the author has had printed record charts like those at the end of this chapter. These charts show what questions should be asked, what parts should be examined, and for what these parts are to be examined. A physician having a large number of obstetric cases should have charts similar to these printed. If he has only a few cases or does not wish to keep a full record, he can use the outline for questioning and write down only the important deductions in a small book kept for this purpose. If he does not use the charts for writing the answers he should memorize the questions, as otherwise it will appear as if he had to look at the chart to know what to ask. In filling out these charts the writing should be small and abbreviated. It is often convenient to use a check mark "∨" for yes, and a naught "0" for no, and a small straight line "—" for when the question is not asked. After "etc." anything special not covered by the preceding questions is to be written. The outline in reference to the history explains itself, but that in reference to the examination needs explanation, and this will be given under the discussion of the examinations of the first and the second half of pregnancy. The ante-partum examination has been divided into that of the first half and that of the second half of pregnancy, because of the difference in the conditions of early and late pregnancy.

The Examination in the First Half of Pregnancy.—After getting the patient's history as outlined in the printed charts, the examination should be made. It is generally best to make the bimanual examination first, noting the condition of the abdomen, uterus and vagina by touch, and then, as though necessary from the information obtained make an examination of the vulva, abdomen and breasts. All of the symptoms of the first half of pregnancy and abnormal conditions as retroflexion, enlarged tubes or ovaries, should be looked for. The symptoms obtained can be written down on the chart under the following heading: breasts, abdomen, vulva, vagina, cervix, lower segment and pelvic soft parts.

The Bimanual Examination.—Before this examination the bowels and bladder should be emptied. The patient should lie in the dorsal relaxed position, on an examination table or chair or cross-wise of the bed. (The dorsal relaxed position is that position in which the patient lies on her back with her lower limbs flexed and her head and shoulders raised). By the patient being cross-wise of the bed, the abdominal hand can be easily carried from one part of the abdomen to another and per vaginam, first one hand can be used and then the other, if necessary. The patient should be covered with a sheet, and the skirts pushed up above the knees so as not to interfere with the examination. The vulva should have been well washed with soap and water. The doctor's hands should be sterilized, (it may be advisable to see if the cervix is open.) The first two fingers of the examining hand should be anointed with sterilized vaseline. Some only use one finger, but generally a farther reach is obtainable with two. The vulvar opening is found by inspection, or by the hand not used for the examination. The fingers should only be introduced a short distance until the parts relax from the patient getting over the fear of being hurt. To reach as far as possible it is best to press up on the perineum with tLe external fingers well flexed. By this method if necessary the whole hand can be easily carried beyond the plane of the normally situated vulva. It is best to first examine the cervix, next the fundus, upper and lower segment and then the *cul de sac* of Douglas, the broad ligaments, the tubes and ovaries. In England the lateral relaxed position is used. The standing posture is of value in diagnosing prolapsus and it may bring the cervix within easy reach of the finger in some difficult cases. The rectal examination is of considerable value in some abnormal cases. Other points which do not really apply here will be given under the examination for the second half of pregnancy.

The Examination in the Second Half of Pregnancy and the Diagnosis of the Vertex Presentation and Its Positions Per Abdomen.

As has been said, the following charts explain themselves in reference to the history. In regard to the examination the patient's modesty is least offended by examining in the following order: first the pulse, then the heart, next the abdomen and lastly the vagina and breasts if necessary.

The Pulse and Heart.—The pulse may be very fast through the excitement of the ⸱ examination. A pulse of 100 to 120 is not rare. A pulse of a permanent rapidity is due to incomplete hypertrophy of the heart or other disorder. Pregnancy often brings out a slight heart murmur due to previous rheumatism.

The Abdominal Examination.—To the patient should be explained the fact that by the abdominal examination the position and size of the child can be determined, and that for this reason the examination is very important. The patient should loosen all her clothing around the waist so that the abdomen can be freely reached, she should lie in the dorsal relaxed position, lengthwise of the bed, near its edge, or on an examination lounge, chair or table. Her abdomen should be covered with a sheet, or her outer skirt allowed to remain over the abdomen.

Inspection: Under this heading only the size and shape are mentioned, as the presence of striae and pigmentation are only of importance in reference to the diagnosis of pregnancy and can be added under "etc," if desired. (Under the other headings will also be found many omissions, but when of value they can be added at the end, after "etc"). The highest quadrant of the abdomen often contains the back of the fetus.

Palpation: After palpation are written the situation of the different parts of the fetus, the position of the fetus as a whole, the condition of the uterus, the situation of the fundus and of the placenta and cord if felt, the location of tenderness, the presence or absence of cephalic ballottement and anything else that may be noted.

Percussion: If dullness is obtained in any abnormal situation it is mentioned.

Auscultation: Here the situation and character of the fetal heart sounds are given and the presence or absence of the uterine, funic and cardiac bruit, and any other special sounds heard.

Mensuration: It is only used when the abdomen is abnormal in shape or size.

Diagnosis: Here is mentioned the diagnosis deduced from palpation and auscultation of the abdomen.

Summary: Under this heading are outlined the special points of the previous history and examination.

The Special Ante-Partum Record.—This is used when an internal examination is made, when the patient is examined in reference to the condition of the bony pelvis, and when disorders are treated during pregnancy. It seems sufficiently clear to make any explanation superfluous. It is called special ante-partum record because it is not needed in normal cases except for the purpose of study.

THE DIAGNOSIS OF THE VERTEX PRESENTATION AND ITS POSITIONS BY ABDOMINAL PALPATION.

In the diagnosis of all presentations and positions the following method of procedure is the best. The examiner, facing the patient's feet, places his hands beneath the sheet, applies his finger tips to the groins just above the pelvic brim and presses in, i. e., the fingers of the left hand are pressed into the left groin and the fingers of the right hand into the right groin. After careful palpation of the groins the hands are brought upwards and the sides of the uterus palpated and lastly the region of the fundus. (This method of facing the patient's feet, beginning at the brim and working up to the fundus is best, because the situation of the part at the inlet is of most importance and this part cannot be as well examined when the examiner is facing the patient's face, in the method of beginning at the fundus and working down to the brim).

Before taking up the diagnosis of the vertex presentation and its positions, it is best to consider the diagnosis of the different parts of the fetus.

The Diagnosis of the Different Parts of the Fetus by Abdominal Palpation.—The head is diagnosed from the breech by being larger, smoother, rounder and harder, separated from the trunk by a depression, (the region of the neck), and by allowing ballottement. The forehead appears as the largest and smoothest part of the head. The shoulder is round and can be easily grasped by the flexed fingers and lifted up. The back is broad and smooth. The side is not so broad or as smooth as the back, and is contin-uous with the shoulder. The breech is smaller, (unless the lower extremities are included), less smooth and round and softer than the head, is not separated from the trunk by a depression, and does not allow ballottement, i. e., of movement without the whole trunk moving. The extremities are small knob or arm-like ob-jects, which roll or move under the palpating fingers. The body and the smaller parts of the fetus are first gently palpated, then if not recognized they are grasped with some force. Lifting up the fetus sometimes facilitates the diagnosis of its different parts.

The Diagnosis of the Vertex Presentation by Abdominal Palpation.—The flexed head is found in the brim or one of the iliac fossae. The trunk of the fetus is parallel with the long axis of the uterus and the breech is in the fundus.

The Diagnosis of the Positions of the Vertex Presentation, by Abdominal Palpation.—L. O. A., Left Occipito-Anterior Po-sition: The examiner feels in the right groin a prominent, hard object, the side of the forehead, and in the left groin his hand sinks deeply, finally reaching the occiput. The forehead feels larger and more prominent than the occiput, because the head be-ing well flexed causes the occiput to be deeply situated and to project less than the back. The half flexed fingers of the left hand passed upward a little from the occiput and toward the me-dian line, will grasp the anterior shoulder. The right hand may feel the arms to the right and back, nearly opposite the anterior shoulder. The left hand passed up the left side of the uterus will feel the back of the fetus anterior and to the left, while the right fingers by pressing in along the right side will feel the lower ex-tremities in some part of the right half of the uterus projecting to the right and posteriorly. At the fundus the breech will be felt to the left or right side or in the median line, depending upon the amount of flexion of the fetal trunk.

R. O. A., Right Occipito-Anterior Position: This is the same as L. O. A., except that the land-marks are in opposite sides —thus:—the side of the forehead is to the left, the deep depres-sion in the right groin (corresponding to the region of the occi-put), the anterior shoulder to the right near the median line, the back to the right and front, the extremities to the left and back and the breech generally on the right side.

R. O. P., Right Occipito-Posterior Position: A prominent object, the front of the forehead, is the left in groin. The deep depression is in the right groin. The anterior shoulder is opposite the right ilio-pectineal eminence, (i. e., more to the side than in the anterior position). The back is posterior and to the right. The extremities are anterior and to the left.

L. O. P., Left Occipito-Posterior Position: This is the same as the R. O. P., except that the land-marks are in opposite sides, thus:—the front of the forehead is to the right and front, the deep depression is in the left groin, the anterior shoulder is opposite the left ilio-pectineal eminence, the back is posterior and to the left, and the extremities are anterior and to the right.

In posterior positions of the occiput the forehead is more prominent than in the anterior positions, because it is more forward in the former positions. The depression opposite the occiput is deeper because the occiput is more posterior.

THE DIAGNOSIS OF THE VERTEX PRESENTATION AND ITS POSITIONS BY ABDOMINAL AUSCULTATION.

The patient should be length-wise of the bed with the lower limbs extended and the abdomen covered only with a sheet. The ear or stethoscope should be used according to the practice of the examiner or the results obtained. The stethoscope is the more esthetic, but often presses on too small an area to allow close contact with the fetal body without producing too much pain. When the stethoscope is used the sheet is removed from the abdomen. The broad side of the examiner's head can press deeply into the abdomen without causing pain.

The Diagnosis of the Vertex Presentation by Abdominal Auscultation.—In the vertex presentation the fetal heart sounds are heard below the navel and to one side of the median line as a rule, but sometimes when the breech is the part nearest the abdominal wall the fetal heart sounds are heard more distinctly above the navel over the area of the breech.

The Diagnosis of the Positions of the Vertex Presentation by Abdominal Auscultation.—L. O. A., Position: The fetal heart sounds are heard best midway on a line between the navel and the left anterior superior spinous process of the ilium.

R. O. A., Position: The site is the same, but on the right side.

R. O. P., Position: The fetal heart sounds are heard midway on a line between the navel and the right sacro-iliac joint.

L. O. P., Position: The site is the same as in the R. O. P. position, but on the left side.

It must be remembered that sometimes the fetal heart sounds are not heard in these normal positions but may be heard, as mentioned before, over the breech of the fetus, but almost always they are heard on the same side of the abdomen as the back.

The Diagnosis of the Vertex Presentation and Its Position by Vaginal Touch—This will be given under the management of labor as it is often difficult to diagnose the position and sometimes even the presentation before the cervix is dilated and also because as a rule a vaginal examination is not made during pregnancy.

The Diagnosis of the Other Presentations and their Positions.—This will be given under abnormal obstetrics.

ANTE-PARTUM RECORD.

No.. Date..

Name of husband.............................. Maiden name..............................

Occupation of husband.......................... Of self..............................

Address ....

HISTORY

Age..............................

Nationality ....

Married, how long..............................

UTERINE DISEASE

Kind ....

Cause ....

Duration ....

Treatment ....

Result ....

OTHER DISEASES

....

MISCARRIAGES

No. ....

Dates ....

Threatened ....

Incomplete ....

Complete ....

Ectopic ....

How far along..............................

Cause ....

Symptoms..............................

Duration ....

Complications..............................

Treatment..............................

After-effect..............................

Etc. ....

LABORS

No. ....Dr...............................

Dates..............................

Presentations ....

Duration..............................

Weight of Children..............................

Still-births ....

Premature..............................

Forceps ....
Version ....
Retained placenta...........................
Post-partum hemorrhage..........................
Placenta previa............................
Tear..
        repaired...........................
        after effects.........................
Etc. ....

specks ....
blindness..
Sinking of uterus..............................
Bowels..
False Pains..
Diseases during Pregnancy.....................
Prenatal impression.........................
Duration ....
Etc. ....

PUERPERIUM

Up when..............................
Antisepsis...........................
Fever..
Chill ....
Peritonitis..............................
Blood poisoning..............................
FLOW—duration ....
     odor..
     amount ....
BREAST—caked............... lanced...............
Nipples—tender..............................
     treatment..............................
After pains—severity.....................
     duration..............................
Menses while nursing..............................
Backache...............how long...............
Bearing down...........how long ....
When strong......................................
Etc. ....

EXAMINATION

Pulse..
Heart..
Form...................Face..............
BREAST—size...............2nd areola...............
     nipples—size and shape...............
         —tender ....
         —colostrum ....

ABDOMEN

Inspection—shape ....
     size..
     etc...
Palpation—forehead ....
     occiput..............................
     anterior shoulder..............................
     arms ....
     back..
     breech..
     legs ....
     fetus as a whole..............................
     uterus ....
     fundus..
     placenta...............cord...............
     tenderness..............................
     cephalic ballottement...............
     etc...
Percussion..
Auscultation—Fetal heart sounds...............
         situation..............................
         character..............................
         Uterine bruit..............................
         Funic bruit..............................
         cardiac bruit..............................
         etc...
Mensuration ....
Diagnosis ....

PREGNANCIES (present and past)

Last menses..............................
     —character..............................
Fruitful coitus..............................
Menses during pregnancy—No...................
     amount of blood..............................
     duration ....
Quickening—time ....
     site..
Nausea and vomiting—duration...............
         severity..............................
Indigestion ....
Appetite..
Faintness, dizziness and weakness...............
Bladder symptoms..............................
Nervous symptoms..............................
FEET, LEGS AND HIPS—swollen...................
     varicose veins..............................
     numbness ....
     ache..
     tender ....
     pain..
     cramps ....
PAIN—regions..............................
     character..............................
     backache.....................................
     headache ....
Tenderness ....
Bearing-down ....
EYES—weak ....

URINE

Amount in 24 hours..............................
Specific gravity ....
Albumen ....
Sugar..
Casts ....
Urea ....
Etc. ....

SUMMARY

....
....
....

SPECIAL ANTE-PARTUM RECORD.

No................... Date...... ....

EXAMINATION

VULVA

....

VAGINA

Orifice—situation... .
    size ....
    tear . ...
    etc............................. ....
Rectocele...
Cystocele... . ...
Secretion—amount...
    reaction......................................
    consistency .. . .
    color ....
    germs ....
    etc..
Length..
Size ....
Etc. ....

CERVIX

Situation ....
Size ....
Tear...
Consistency.... .. . .
Ext. os—size...
    thickness..
Canal—size..
    shape...
Int. os—size..
Secretion—character...
    germs ....
Presentation and position of fetus.............
....
    felt through os.... ....
    felt through wall of cervix.............

UTERINE BODY

As a whole...
Lower segment...
Upper segment...
Etc. ....

UTERINE APPENDAGES

Cul de sac of Douglas...............................
Tubes...
Ovaries ....
Etc. ....

SOFT PARTS OF BONY PELVIS

Levator ani...
Etc. ....

BONY PELVIS

History—age when first walked.............
    rickets...
    deformity—congenital ....
        acquired ....
    still-births ....
    artificial deliveries...................... ..
    size of children...............................
    etc..................................... ....
Inspection—form......................................
    projecting abdomen.........................
    abnormal spinal curvature.............
    unequal hips.................................
    deformed legs...............................
    ankylosis.................... ....
    increased obliquity.........................
    diminished obliquity.......................
    lumbar triangle ....
    etc...
Palpation—site of vag. orifice.............
    size and shape of pubic arch.........
    size and shape of outlet.............

sacro-coccygeal joint................ .. ..
ischial spines...
sacral curvature....................................
size and shape of cavity.............
promontory...
first transverse line....................
shape and size of inlet....................
other bony prominences...............:.......
tumor ....
etc...
Mensuration (Pelvimetry)... ... .
  External ....
    spines ....
    crests....................................
    conjugate ....
    first oblique...............................
    second oblique................................
    trochanteric ....
    circumference..... R ½ ......L ½ ......
    etc...
  Internal..
    diagonal conjugate.... ....
    Inlet—direct conjugate from
        —diagonal ....
        —extended fingers....................
        —closed fist............................
        transverse........... ....
    Ischial spines................................
    Outlet—transverse........... ....
        antero-posterior ....
    Etc. ....

GENERAL DIAGNOSIS

....

GENERAL PROGNOSIS

....

DIRECTIONS TO PATIENT

Hygiene of pregnancy...............................
Nurse...
Things to have for labor............................
Onset of labor..
Etc. ....

DISORDERS TREATED DURING PREGNANCY

FIRST

Name...
Duration ....
Cause...
Symptoms ....
Diagnosis ....
Prognosis ....
Treatment...
Results ....
Remarks ....

SECOND

Name...
Duration ....
Cause...
Symptoms ....
Diagnosis ....
Prognosis ....
Treatment................................. ....
Results ....
Remarks ....

GENERAL SUMMARY

...................:...
....
....
....

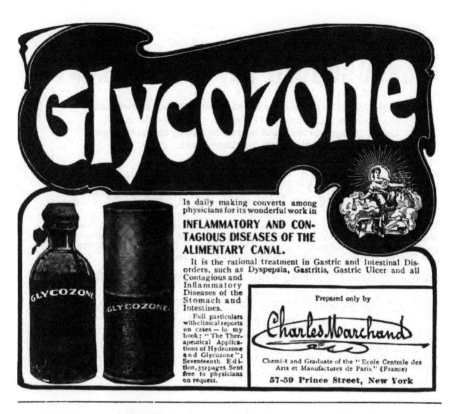

DENVER MEDICAL TIMES

THOMAS H. HAWKINS, A.M., M.D., Editor and Publisher.

COLLABORATORS:

Henry O. Marcy, M.D., Boston.	S. H. Pinkerton, M.D., Salt Lake City
Thaddeus A. Reamy, M.D., Cincinnati.	Flavel B. Tiffany, M.D., Kansas City.
Nicholas Senn, M.D., Chicago.	Erskine M. Bates, M.D;. New York.
Joseph Price, M.D., Philadelphia.	E. C. Gehrung, M.D, St. Louis.
Franklin H. Martin, M.D., Chicago.	Graeme M. Hammond, M.D, New York.
William Oliver Moore, M.D., New York.	James A. Lydston, M.D., Chicago.
L. S. McMurtry, M.D., Louisville.	Leonard Freeman, M.D., Denver.
Thomas B. Eastman, M.D., Indianapolis, Ind.	Carey K. Fleming, M.D., Denver, Colo.
G. Law, M.D., Greeley, Colo.	

Subscriptions, $1.00 per year in advance; Single Copies, 10 cents.

Address all Communications to Denver Medical Times, 1740 Welton Street, Denver, Colo. We will at all times be glad to give space to well written articles or items of interest to the profession.

[Entered at the Postoffice of Denver, Colorado, as mail matter of the Second Class.]

EDITORIAL DEPARTMENT

THE OPERATING ROOM.

When the protective epithelial covering of the body is broken down by accident or surgical intention, the resulting wound is liable to become an infection atrium from which either local or general sepsis may originate. To prevent such septic conditions antiseptic methods must be employed. These measures relate to the patient, the surgeon and assistants, the nurse, the room, clothing, instruments, dressings, and in short, all the environments of the case.

In traumatic emergency cases the wound, if superficial, should be scrubbed out thoroughly with sterilized brush and soap and water, all foreign matter removed and the edges of the wound brought together with sterile sutures, the whole being well covered with a sterile gauze dressing.

All local pus collections should be promptly and freely incised and curetted, then irrigated with alkaline water, hydrogen peroxid and mercuric chlorid, and packed with bichlorid gauze. Deep wounds, as of the chest, abdomen, pelvis or brain, need to be treated on the same general plan as operations for diseased conditions not traumatic in origin.

The operating room should be as nearly sterile as possible,

whether the walls and floor are of wood and plaster, of sheet lead, glass, tiling or some of the patent concretes. In private practice every part of the interior should be scrubbed with 1:2000 bichlorid solution, after removing all unnecessary furniture (pictures, hangings, etc.) from the room. To prevent collapse from cold, the temperature of the room should be kept at 80-85° F. In hospitals glass-topped tables will be used, of course. In dwelling houses an excellent substitute is readily improvised from the ordinary extension table, washed with bichlorid solution and covered with a blanket, rubber sheeting and a sterilized sheet.

An abundance of boiled water, both hot and cold, should be provided in suitable receptacles. The gauze sponges and dressings, towels and gowns, should be sterilized when practicable, by steam heat for 15 minutes at a pressure of at least 40 pounds to the square inch. When steam is not available, the already prepared sponges and dressings should be made into a bundle and baked in the oven for at least a half hour, till the outer part of the package is quite scorched. Instruments are well sterilized by wrapping in a towel and boiling for ten minutes in water containing a dram of powdered sodium carbonate in each pint. The alkali removes grease, dissolves the capsules of germs and keeps the instruments from rusting. All sutures and ligatures, except "catgut," may be sterilized by boiling in plain water. The complete absorbability of catgut renders it an essential in many major operations. This substance can be thoroughly sterilized, after Hofmeister's formula, by first winding on a glass plate and washing in boiling water; second, immersing for 12 to 48 hours in 2 to 4 % aqueous solution of formalin; third, freeing from formalin by immersing in flowing water for at least 12 hours; fourth, boiling in water 10 or 12 minutes; and finally hardening and preserving in a mixture of 95 volumes absolute alcohol and 5 volumes glycerin.

Before any considerable operation the patient should be given a laxative and a general bath. The parts about the incision to be made should be thoroughly soaped and vigorously but carefully scrubbed with a sterilized brush for ten minutes, after which any possibly remaining fat should be removed with pure alcohol or ether. A solution of mermuric chlorid (1:2000) is then to be applied by ablution and as a towel pack covered with dry towels and held in place by a retaining bandage. These preparatory dressings are removed on the operating table and the surface again washed with alcohol and mercuric chlorid solution, the latter being taken up with sterile gauze sponges before using the knife.

The surgeon himself, his assistants and the graduate surgical nurse should all have the instincts of surgical cleanliness well developed and constantly and conscientiously practiced. After sterilizing the exposed surfaces of their own bodies, as far as possible, they should put on sterile uniforms and during the operation, aside from already existing septic conditions in the patient, should handle nothing that is not quite aseptic. The nails should receive particular attention, being cut short and carefully cleaned.

A well-proved method of hand sterilization consists in the following steps: Soaking and scrubbing the hands and forearms for 20 minutes with sterilized soap and a stiff vegetable brush and hot water frequently changed; a second rinsing in running tepid water and scrubbing with a freshly sterilized brush in the direction of the folds of the skin; bathing in ether or pure, fresh alcohol; washing the hands for a few minutes in 1:2000 mercuric chlorid solution.

Since it is impossible to render the hands absolutely sterile, thin, impermeable rubber gloves are coming into vogue with surgeons, being readily sterilized by boiling. In cases in which it has been necessary to immerse the hands in live pus and it is desired to perform another operation at once, Reed states that immediate sterilization can be effected by carefully washing and rinsing the hands, next bathing them in 98% carbolic acid for a few seconds, and then thoroughly neutralizing the acid by washing the hands in pure alcohol. All unnecessary manual contact with the wound should be avoided as much as possible, by the careful use of sterilized instruments.

When there are no contra-indications, well protected surgical wounds are best let alone for about a week—10 to 14 days if buried sutures have been employed. Soiled dressings should be thrown into a paper receptacle and all burned together.

SHOCK.

The neuroparalytic symptoms of operative shock are best prevented by rapid work, warm coverings and hot applications, a warm room, the injection by hypodermocylsis of six or eight ounces of normal salt solution (one dram of sodium chlorid to the pint of boiled water) and the hypodermic injection of strychnine and atropin and perhaps adrenalin chlorid. Very weak patients should

not be further reduced in strength by fasting and by violent catharsis, but should be well nourished on milk and bouillon up to within
a few hours of the operation. It is unwise to administer the anesthetic when shock is beginning. Often too much cleaning is left
until the patient is on the table, and ether and alcohol are sometimes used locally to excess with little effect except chilling.

ANESTHESIA.

The safety or danger of an anesthetic depends much more on
the anesthetizer than on the anesthetic chosen or the condition of
the patient. Chloroform is more pleasant than ether, and less
liable to produce protracted vomiting. The former is contra-indicated in organic heart trouble; the latter in renal and pulmonary
affections. Clover's method of beginning anesthesia with nitrous
oxid and continuing with ether, is perhaps more satisfactory to the
patient. The use of anesthetic mixtures, such as the time-honored
A. C. E., gives additional uncertainty to the procedure.

The preliminary hypodermic injection of a fair dose of atropin and strychnin is a rational measure in preventing the vasomotor
paresis with accumulation of blood in the splanchnic area in chloroform anesthesia. Spraying the nose and throat with liquid vaselin
prior to administering ether, serves somewhat to prevent mucous
irritation. A large cone is best for ether, which should be added
in small quantities very frequently. The conjoint administration
of chloroform vapor and oxygen is much the safest method, in the
writer's opinion. At any rate, plenty of air must be furnished the
chloroformized patient. The anesthetizer must give his undivided
attention to his own duties, watching especially the pulse, the
breathing, the color and the pupils. Shallow or stertorous breathing or irregular pulse, cyanosis and sudden wide dilation of the
pupils are signs of danger. The last mentioned sign, however, may
be due to the patient feeling pain or coming out of anesthesia, in
which event the eyeballs are seen to oscillate. A rather narrow contraction of the pupils, such as is noted in natural sleep, should be
maintained throughout. Holding the lower jaw upward and forward, with the fingers hooked behind its angles, is a very valuable
prophylactic procedure. A tendency to vomit during anesthesia is
sometimes controlled by fresh whiffs of the anesthetic or by fresh
air or oxygen. Post-anesthetic vomiting is best prevented by perfect rest and small sips of very hot water for the thirst; stomach

lavage is having some vogue at present. It is difficult to determine how much objective effect the inhalation of vinegar has in these cases.

PHOSPHO-ALBUMEN.

We beg to call the attention of our readers to announcement of the Phospho-Albumen Company, appearing in this issue, which has the distinction of being the pioneer of all glandular extracts. As a nerve food, tissue builder and blood maker, it stands pre-eminent, and is indicated in all neurasthenias and anemias, as well as in all other morbid and pathologic changes of the nervous and nutritive processes. Liberal samples will be furnished by the company for trial, and we would urge our readers to take advantage of this offer and learn for themselves the merits of Phospho-Albumen.

EDITORIAL ITEMS.

Gastric Sarcinae. For the yeasty vomiting produced by sarcinæ, Butler has found quinine of decided value.

Gastric Indigestion. Potter recommends pepsin, gr. x-xxv before or during meals for vomiting of food after meals.

Indigestion of Infants. Wm. Gay directs to rectify diet, and give bismuth with soda, milk and lime water.

Atony of Stomach. Nux Vomica is useful, particularly when there is constipation.

For Pyloric Stenosis. Hare recommends small doses of opium; pre-digested food; rectal enemata; stimulants; operation.

Ascarides in Stomach. Joseph Leidy says to encourage vomiting until the worm is expelled and give santonin, ⅛ to ¼ grain three or four times a day, followed by castor oil.

Chronic Gastritis. Bartholow utilized the following recipe: ℞ Sodii iodidi, sodii bromidi aa gr. viii; sodii arsenat. gr. 1-30; aquam q. s. A teaspoonful in water t. i. d.

Treatment of Alcoholism. Bechet (*Progressive Medicine*) gradually reduces the alcohol and administers hypodermically 1-30 grain of strychnine and 1-30 grain of apomorphine as frequently as every three hours.

For Tapeworm. Give, says Leger, a dram of spirit of chloroform, diluted with an ounce of syrup and four ounces of water in ounce doses every hour until the whole amount is taken. Before the last dose give a purgative of castor oil or tincture of jalap.

For "Crabs." For the extremely common complaint, pubic pediculi, there is no more efficient and cleanly method, says Landis (*Progressive Medicine*), than the local application of tincture of cocculus indicus.

Rebellious Cystitis. The old method with picric acid instillations, ¼ to 2 per cent. in water, in the treatment of tuberculous and other rebellious cases of cystitis, is recommended by Guillon (*Progressive Medicine.*)

Smallpox in Porto Rico. Smallpox was long prevalent in Spanish-American countries, but since 1900 there has not been a single death from this disease in Porto Rico, says Geo. G. Groff

(*Medico-Chirurgical Journal*). In that year the whole population was vaccinated.

Angina Pectoris Abdominis. Pal (*Progressive Medicine*) states that this condition, as well as tabetic crises and saturnine colic, is probably associated with and caused by spasm of the abdominal arteries, due in the first instance to sclerosis of the vessels.

Prevention of Phosphatic Urinary Lithiasis. Klemperer (*Progressive Medicine*) says that phosphatic deposits are favored by over-excitability of the nervous system, with consequent gastric hyperacidity, and are combated by the ingestion of alkaline waters in large quantities.

Albuminuria of Pleural Effusion. Courmont and Nicola (*Progressive Medicine*) draw attention to the frequency with which slight albuminuria (with excess of chlorides) is seen during the period of absorption of pleural effusions. It may last only a few days, but may persist for many weeks.

Gastric Debility and Depression. For vomiting due to this cause, Hare employs wine of ipecac in drop doses every hour; or tincture of nux vomica, one-half to one drop in cinnamon water every half hour or hour.

Acute Gastritis. Brunton prescribes as follows: ℞ Bismuthi subnit. gr. x; potassii bromidi gr. xv-xx; acidi hydrocyan. dil. m.v; spt. chloroformi m.x; mucil. acaciæ ℥ ii; aquam ad ℥ i; to be taken every three or four hours ten minutes before food.

Gastrectasis. Shoemaker prescribes: Acidi carbol. gr. ½; syr. acaciæ, aquæ cinnam. aa. m.xxx: A teaspoonful before meals. Taylor recommends stomach washing (after emptying) once daily half an hour before the largest meal, with one or two pints of water, pure or containing one or two per cent. of sodium bicarbonate or one per cent of salicylic acid.

Visceral Crises in the Erythema Group. Osler (*Progressive Medicine*) reviews 29 cases of his own characterized by recurring attacks of colic, with vomiting or diarrhea and the occasional passage of blood, in connection only with arthritis, purpura, erythema or angioneurotic edema. The mortality in his series was 24 per cent.

Editorial Items continued on Page 452

BOOKS.

PROGRESSIVE MEDICINE. A quarterly digest of advances, discoveries and improvements in the medical and surgical sciences, edited by Hobart Amory Hare, M.D., assisted by H. R. M. Landis, M.D. Dec. 1, 1904. Lea Brothers & Co., Philadelphia and New York. $6.00 per annum.

The contents of the present volume comprise, "Diseases of the Digestive Tract and Allied Organs," by J. Dutton Steele; "Anesthetics, Fractures, Dislocations, Amputations, Surgery of the Extremities, and Orthopedics," by Joseph C. Bloodgood; "Genito-Urinary Diseases," by Wm. T. Belfield; "Diseases of the Kidneys," by John Rose Bradford; and "Practical Therapeutic Referendum," by H. R. M. Landis. As shown by the numerous extracts we have made for the DENVER MEDICAL TIMES, *Progressive Medicine* is full of practical and helpful memoranda. The surgical section is profusely illustrated.

ANNUAL REPORT OF THE SURGEON GENARAL of the public health and marine hospital service of the United States for the fiscal year 1905.

TEXT-BOOK ON INSANITY BASED ON CLINICAL OBSERVATIONS. For practitioners and students of medicine. By Dr. R. von Krafft-Ebing, late Professor of Psychiatry and Nervous Diseases in the University of Vienna. Authorized translation from the latest German edition, by Charles Gilbert Chaddock, M.D., Professor of Diseases of the Nervous System in the Marion-Sims-Beaumont College of Medicine, Medical Department of St. Louis University, St. Louis, Mo. etc. With an introduction by Frederick Peterson, M.D., president of the New York State Commission in Lunacy. Pages xvi-638, royal octavo. Price, extra cloth, $4.00, net; half-russia, $5.00, net. F. A. Davis Company, publishers, 1914-16 Cherry Street, Philadelphia, Pa.

According to Peterson, there is perhaps no other work on psychiatry which has had the vogue, the wide distribution and the popularity as this of Krafft-Ebing. In the latest edition it is founded on thirty-three years of special study and experience. The text is noteworthy for its clearness and comprehensibility, its particularization and systematic character. Many psychiatric type cases are graphically described, and a special index of them is furnished. An American edition should be appreciated and be quickly taken up.

THE SURGICAL DISEASES OF THE GENITO-URINARY TRACT, VENE-REAL AND SEXUAL DISEASES. A text-book for students and practitioners, by G. Frank Lydston, M.D., Professor of the Genito-Urinary Organs and Syphilology in the Medical Department of the State University of Illinois (the College of Physician and Surgeons); Professor of Criminal Anthropology in the Kent College of Law; Surgeon-in-Chief of the Genito-Urinary Department of the West-side Dispensary. Fellow of the Chicago Academy of Medicine; Fellow of the American Academy of Political and Social Science; Delegate from the United States to the International Congress for the Prevention of Syphilis and the Venereal Diseases, held at Brussels, Belgium, September 5, 1899, etc. Second Revised Edition, illustrated with 233 engravings and 7 colored plates, 6½ x9¾ inches, pages, xv–1008. Extra cloth, $5.00, net; sheep or half-russia, $6.00, net. F. A. Davis Company, publishers, 1914–16 Cherry Street, Philadelphia, Pa.

This work is entertaining as well as instructive; it is indeed good literature. The author has devoted his attention chiefly to these subjects for nearly twenty years, and has consequently many good ideas of his own, which he presents to his readers. His advice on treatment appears to us particularly practical and helpful. The book is complete in itself, and covers a wide field ably and up to date. It contains a fine array of engravings and colored pages, selected for their actual teaching value. Even those who have other good works along the same line, will do well to procure this volume.

GALLSTONES AND THEIR SURGICAL TREATMENT. By B. G. A. Moynihan, M.S. (Lon.), F. R. C. S., Senior Assistant Surgeon to Leeds General Infirmary, England. Octavo volume of 386 pages, illustrated with text-cuts, some in colors, and nine colored insert plates. Philadelphia, New York, London. W. B. Saunders & Company, 1905. Cloth, $4.00, net.

This is a volume that surgeons who operate on the abdomen can hardly do without. The work is founded largely on an extensive personal experience, and is thoroughly trust-worthy and authoritative. The author's account of his operative treatment is complete and accurate. Every phase of cholelithiasis is considered, with abundant illustrative clinical records, and special attention is given to the description of the early symptoms of gallstone disease. The text is copiously and beautifully illustrated.

SAUNDERS' MEDICAL HAND-ATLASES—ATLAS AND EPITOME OF GEN-
ERAL PATHOLOGIC HISTOLOGY. By Dr. H. Durck, of Munich.
Edited, with additions, by Ludvig Hektoen, M.D., Professor
of Pathology, Rush Medical College, in affiliation with the
University of Chicago. With 172 colored figures on 77
lithographic plates, 36 text-cuts, many in colors, and 371
pages of text. Philadelphia, New York, London. W. B.
Saunders & Company, 1904. Cloth, $5.00 net.

This neat atlas is a worthy companion volume to the other
members of the series. The text is concise, yet comprehensive,
and is arranged under circulatory disturbances, atrophy, retrogres-
sive processes, and tumors. The pictorial feature is, of course, the
leading one. It seems to us that the colored plates are as near
nature or perfection as possible. Some of them required as high
as twenty-six lithographic impressions to reproduce the original
painting. We agree with the American editor, Professor Hektoen,
in his opinion that this book will prove even more useful than the
two volumes on special pathologil histology.

DISEASES OF THE LIVER, GALL-BLADDER, AND BILE-DUCTS. By H.
D. Rolleston, A.M., M.D. (Cantab.) F. R. C. P., Physician
to St. George's Hospital, London; formerly Examiner in
Medicine at the University of Durham, England. Octavo
volume of 794 pages, fully illustrated, including seven colored
insert plates. Philadelphia, New York, London. W. B.
Saunders & Company, 1904. Cloth, $6.00 net.

The author has paid special attention to diseases of the liver
for the past twelve years. This product of his literary labors is
the most voluminous treatise on the subject in the English language. He has garnered a wide field of references with great care,
and has shaped up a work which is not only exhaustive, but also
authoritative. He dwells especially upon the underlying morbid
changes, giving thus a sound basis for diagnosis, prognosis and
treatment. Many clinical cases are briefly quoted, serving the
practitioner as a helpful means for comparing notes on his own
patients. The text is handsomely and instructively illustrated.
The subject of liver diseases is of great importance in the practice
of medicine, and the work before us is a noteworthy addition to
our systematic knowledge thereof.

DIET IN HEPLTH AND DISEASE. By Julius Friedenwald, M.D.,
Clinical Professor of Diseases of the Stomach in the College
of Physicians and Surgeons, Baltimore; and John Ruh-
rah, M.D., Clinical Professor of Diseases of Children in the

College of Physicians and Surgeons, Baltimore. Octavo volume of 689 pages. Philadelphia, New York, London. W. B. Saunders & Company, 1904. Cloth, $4.00 net.

This new work has been prepared with special reference to the needs of the general practitioner, the greater part of the text being devoted to the feeding of the sick. Diet for infants and children and diet in relation to surgery are given special attention. The directions for dieting in each disease are explicit and practicable. Many diet lists are interpolated in the section on gastrointestinal diseases. The latter portion of the text comprises much valuable tabular information on hospital dietaries, army and navy rations, the chemical composition of American foods, etc. The introductory sections relate to the chemistry and physiology of digestion, the classes of foods, beverages and stimulants, and various factors in their bearing on diet. The work as a whole may be considered a practical digest of accepted dietary facts and principles of the present day.

A MANUAL OF PERSONAL HYGIENE. Second edition, revised and enlarged. Proper Living upon a Physiologic Basis. By American authors. Edited by Walter L. Pyle, A.M., M.D., Assistant Surgeon to the Wills Eye Hospital, Philadelphia. 12mo volume of 441 pages, fully illustrated. Philadelphia, New York, London. W. B. Saunders & Company, 1904. Bound in silk, $1.50 net.

The present edition has been considerably enlarged by the addition of chapters on physical exercise and home gymnastics, by G. N. Stewart, and on domestic hygiene, by D. H. Bergey; also an appendix, containing methods of hydrotherapy, thermotherapy, mechanotherapy and first aid measures in emergencies. As in the previous edition, Charles G. Stockton contributes the chapter on the hygiene of the digestive apparatus; George H. Fox, the one on hygiene of the skin and its appendages; E. Fletcher Ingals, that on the hygiene of the vocal and respiratory apparatus; B. Alex. Randall, hygiene of the ear; Walter L. Pyle, hygiene of the eye; and J. W. Courtney, hygiene of the brain and nervous system. The articles of these men are marked by the simplicity of authority, and are easily comprehended by any layman of average intelligence. Personal hygiene is applied physiology and a book of this kind will do more to teach people how to live upon a physiologic basis than will all the school text-books on physiology put together.

SELECTIONS.

"GO-SHONO."—In these days of high-class lithography when copies of original paintings are produced so that it requires an expert to detect the difference, we feel at liberty to recommend to our readers the lithograph in eleven colors of "Go-Shono," the Apache Medicine Man, the Tongaline calendar for 1905, which has been issued by the Mellier Drug Company of St. Louis.

This lithograph of "Go-Shono" has been made from an original photograph taken from life and is unquestionably the most wonderful representation of the Apache Indian, the tribe famous for the craft, cunning and brutality of its chiefs.

THE RESPIRATORY LINK.—The truth of the old adage that a "chain is only as strong as its weakest link" is forcibly illustrated in medicine. The constitution of a patient may in most of its relations be normal; yet the chain of health is impaired by one function which is the seat of more or less constantly recurring disturbances.

The most frequent form of this weak physiologic link that confronts the physician is that manifested by the patient who, with the advent of winter, suffers from repeated congestions and inflammations of the respiratory organs. It may be that at all other times of the year the individual is, as far as indications go, in a good state of general health; it is, however, more commonly the case that the skilled diagnostician is able to recognize an impairment of constitutional vigor, which is in reality the cause of the respiratory disturbances. Present-day scientific teaching emphasizes that it is unwise to treat these patients with expectorants, cough syrups and respiratory sedatives; these latter remedies are at the best but palliative and do not reach the cause of the disturbance. It is more rational to endeavor to strengthen this weak respiratory link by restoring its integrity, and the proper way to do this is by treatment directed to the real causative factor, which is an atonic condition of the system.

The experience of many years has taught that these constantly recurring respiratory disturbances may nearly always be prevented or at least reduced in frequency and severity if Gray's Glycerine Tonic Comp. is administered throughout the winter. If, however, this precaution has not been observed and the patient is already suffering from his regular winter cough and bronchial or pulmonary distress, treatment with Gray's Tonic is still the most efficient.

The manner of the action of the remedy in these cases is two-fold: first of all it overcomes malnutrition by stimulating the torpid nutritive functions to assume normal activity; as a consequence the patient's constitutional vigor is strengthened and incidentally the relaxed atonic condition of the respiratory mucous membrane is eradicated.

The second effect of Gray's Tonic in these cases is upon the local disturbances of the respiratory mucous membrane—it has a direct antiphlogistic and tonic influence upon the disordered circulation; it thereby relieves engorgement and restores tone to the relaxed blood vessels.

Gray's Tonic is to be preferred in the management of these acute and chronic respiratory conditions, because it gives the patient *relief* from the very start and if persisted in, overcomes the condition completely. It strengthens not only the weak respiratory link but also the entire claim of constitutional vigor.

LA GRIPPE AND ITS SEQUELAE AGAIN PREVALENT.—The following suggestions for the treatment of La Grippe will not be amiss at this time when there seems to be a prevalence of it and its allied complaints. The patient is usually seen when the fever is present, as the chill, which occasionally ushers in the disease, has generally passed away. First of all, the bowels should be opened freely by some saline draught. For the severe headache, pain and general soreness give an antikamnia tablet, with a little whiskey or wine, or if the pain is very severe, two tablets should be given. Repeat every two or three hours as required. Often a single dose is followed with almost complete relief. If, after the fever has subsided, the pain, muscular soreness and nervousness continue, the most desirable medicine to relieve these and to meet the indication for a tonic, are antikamnia and quinine tablets. One tablet three or four times a day will usually answer every purpose until health is restored. Dr. C. A. Bryce, editor of the *Southern Clinic*, has found much benefit to result from antikamnia and salol tablets in the stages of pyrexia and muscular painfulness, and antikamnia and codeine tablets are suggested for the relief of all neuroses of the larynx, bronchial as well as the deep-seated coughs, which are so often among the most prominent symptoms. In fact, for the troublesome coughs which so frequently follow or hang on after an attack of influenza, and as a winter remedy in the troublesome conditions of the respiratory tract, there is no better relief than one or two antikamnia and codeine tablets slowly dissolved upon the tongue, swallowing the saliva.

A PERFECTED FOOD.—In treating anaemia is it not true that our first thought, and that to which our instinct·should naturally lead us, is a normal blood standard? That there is a deficiency of iron in the blood in most forms of anaemia, is, of course, indisputable; and to endeavor to supply this lack by the administration of iron seems but a common sense procedure. This practice would be sufficient if anaemia were, in reality, nothing more than a condition of iron deficiency; but the profession realize now that the underlying causative factor is a disturbance of the process of nutrition and cell proliferation, and that iron poverty is but one manifestation of this disorder. Ample proof of this fact has been presented to every doctor when he has observed how anaemic conditions persist in spite of the long continued administration of the various preparations of iron. Here, then, iron preparations must be supplemented by such remedies or by such a remedy as had the ability to awaken the depressed nutritive and cell proliferating process. To stimulate, tone up and supply perfect nutrition in all anaemic conditions, I have found Bovinine to meet every indication par excellence.   JOHN GRIGGS, M.D.

TONSILITIS.—Inflammation in any form attacking the tonsilar region gives rise to symptoms of most distressing character and at the same time provides a most favorable soil for the entry into the system of other infections. It is well to remember that at first this disease is only a local disturbance affecting the capillary system and glandular structures and if promptly and efficiently treated will remain local. The constitutional symptoms such as fever, headache, etc., only develop when there is considerable infection taken up.

In treatment the first indication is to increase local capillary circulation. A local remedy must fill two requirements, i. e., a detergent antiseptic and a degree of permanency in effect. Many of the remedies which have been advocated for the varied forms of tonsilitis are antiseptics, but they are not sufficiently exosmotic in their action to increase the circulation or else their effect is too transient. Glyco-Thymoline, frequently applied in a 50 per cent strength with a hand atomizer produces a rapid depletion of the congested area through its well defined exosmotic property, re-establishing normal passage of fluids through the issues, promptly relieving the dry condition of the membrane and giving an immediate and lasting anodyne effect. As a gargle a 25 per cent solution hot may be effectively used providing the process does not cause undue pain. The external application of cloths dipped in hot water and Glyco-Thymoline in a 25 per cent solution greatly increases the venous circulation.

THE DISHONEST DRUGGIST.—Dishonesty of any sort is to be condemned, but there is no language strong enough, no penalty severe enough adequately to denounce and to punish that lowest form of dishonesty by which a man seeks to profit by endangering health and even life itself.

The dishonest maker or retailer of food products may do more or less serious injury to the health of those who buy his impure goods; but the dishonest dispenser of medicine may be directly responsible for the lives of the sick who have depended on him to give them the pure remedies prescribed by their physicians.

There is nothing much lower in the scale of mendacity than the druggist who knowingly sells impure drugs or dispenses inferior substances or substitutes for the ingredients set down in a physician's prescription. In this class also is the druggist who sends to the patient a prescribed remedy deficient in some of its ingredients. Yet what does the record of a recent investigation in this city show?

Prescriptions were sent to 139 druggists, each one calling for pure aristol. Of the dispensed articles twenty-three showed no trace of aristol, sixty-six had 80 per cent of impurity, ten had 20 per cent and nine had 10 per cent. Only thirty-one were found to be pure and as prescribed.

Only two conclusions may be drawn from these tests—out of 139 druggists who daily in dispensing take human life into their hands, 108 are either deliberately dishonest or so careless or incompetent that they are unfit to be intrusted with the dispensing of medicines. Of course, no one will question the unfitness of the dishonest ones.

In this investigation, the results of which have been placed in the hands of the State Board of Pharmacy, it was found that many druggists had bought a "cheap" aristol which chemical tests proved to be an inert substance known as "Fuller's earth." Other brands of the chemical contained a small percentage of aristol and a very large percentage of impurity. It is the business of the druggist to know whether or not he is buying pure drugs. If he does not know how to tell this or does not take pains to find out, then he should not be allowed to dispense.

The dishonest, the careless or the incompetent druggist is a menace to every one. No person can tell when he may be sick, when he may need a physician, when he may have to send a prescription to a druggist. The Board of Pharmacy owes it to the public to prosecute every dishonest druggist, every incompetent or careless dispenser, to let it be known that such men are unsafe, so that persons who have to buy medicines may give them a wide berth.—*Chicago Evening Post.*

Scrofulous Rhinitis.—This form of nasal catarrh is characterized by enlarged glands, anemia, a pinched face; and by excoriation of nasal orifices and crust formation. To effect a cure Kyle recommends outdoor exercise; plenty of fats, beef and other nitrogenous foods; lactate or peptomanganate of iron or the double sulphide of arsenic ($\frac{1}{4}$ to $\frac{1}{8}$ grain); and alkaline cleansing irrigation followed by an oil spray (one grain camphor, three grains menthol, two drops carbolic acid and one ounce of albolene).

Rectal Cancer.—Excision is indicated, says Kelsey, if the growth is in the lower four inches of the rectum—colotomy, when above this point. Keep passages soft but not fluid. Let patient rest in the recumbent posture. Opium or curetting or the cautery or division of the sphincter muscles may be resorted to if needed for pain. Milk is the best diet; cod-liver oil the best medicine. Surgical treatment includes gentle dilation with bougies or removal of part of growth with knife, cautery, finger, curette or electrolysis.

EDITORIAL ITEMS.— Continued.

Diet in Typhoid Fever.—W. Gilman Thompson (*Medical Record*, Dec. 10) is generally favorable to the milk diet, but he says that when tympanites or any other evidence of marked indigestion ensues, milk should be withheld entirely for two or three days, beef juice and egg albumen or broths being substituted. He also uses white of egg, orange juice and light farinaceous gruels. In ordinary cases he commences solid feeding on the day when the body temperature first reaches the normal. About ten per cent of all cases are followed by relapse, no matter what the treatment.

Pyloric Stenosis.—For the benign form Pflaunder advices local anodyne applications, warm compresses. baths and systematic lavage; laparotomy if these measures do not give relief. In malignant stenosis operation is indicated as soon as the condition is recognized. Van Valzah and Nisbet give two meals a day of finely divided, soluble or fluid food.

Prolapsus Ani.—J. C. Da Costa instructs as follows: Avoid straining at stool. Bathe with cold water and replace. Prevent constipation with laxatives or enemata. If prolapse is caught firmly, place patient on knees and chest, wash mass with cold water, grease it with cosmoline, insert finger into rectum and apply taxis around finger, If this fails, cover finger with a handkerchief and try again as before, or invert patient. After reduction apply a compress, to be worn except when at stool. Before each act of defecation give an injection of cold water containing tannin or fluid hydrastis. Excise mucous membrane in bad cases.

Treatment of Rectal Strictures.—Kelsey directs to give a thorough course of mixed treatment for syphilis; also the ointment or oleate of mercury by the rectum. The diet should consist mostly of milk and soups, with toast, crackers and mush. Rochelle or Glauber's salts are useful as laxatives, or one may give enemas of warm water through a long tube reaching above the stricture. Bring about gradual dilation with bougies, leaving in for three or four hours each day or over night. Divulsion may be of service in linear stricture. Other measures are incision with a proctotomy knife (packing rectum tightly with picked lint) or with thermocautery; excision and colotomy.·

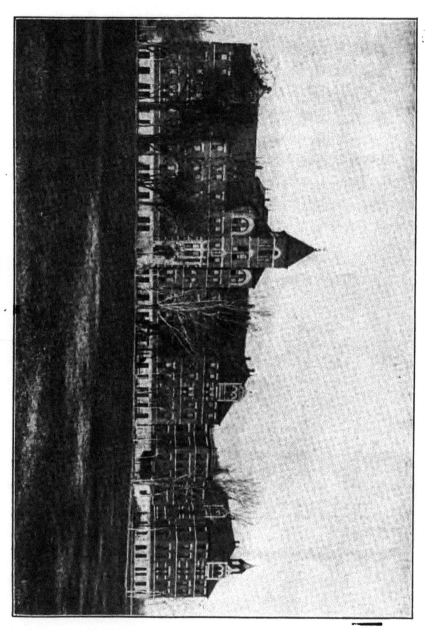

ST. ANTHONY'S HOSPITAL.

Emulsified cod liver oil as contained in Scott's
Emulsion appears in a form so closely resembling
the product of natural digestion—as it occurs
within the body—that it may well be administered as an artificially digested fat food of the
very highest type. In combination with the
other ingredients involved—glycerine being an
emollient of inestimable value—Scott's Emulsion
offers to the physician a valuable, exquisite and
rare accession to his prescription list.

Samples Free.

SCOTT & BOWNE, Chemists, 409-415 Pearl St., New York.

How Much Fluid Should We Allow Patients with General Anasarca?—Thompson thinks (*Medical Record*) the only safe guide is the ratio between the fluid ingested and that which is voided. That is to say, if diminished ingestion of fluid is accompanied by a corresponding decrease in the urinary secretion, more water should be drunk. Upon the whole restriction of drink influences reabsorption of transudates less than does active catharsis.

Edematous Rhinitis.—In this we find serous infiltration of the mucous membrane over the middle or inferior turbinate, unilateral or bilateral and remittent in occurrence, the serum exuding slowly on puncture. J. C. Mulhall states that the best results are obtained by scarification. Nasal deformities, if present, should be removed and attention be paid to the alimentary canal and the general system.

Treatment of Ringworm.—Formalin, a four per cent solution in glycerine (*Clinical Review*), is highly extolled as a remedy in this affection. All grease should be first removed with turpentine, followed by soap and warm water. Then apply the formalin-glycerine, and repeat several times for about an hour. One prolonged treatment of this kind is usually sufficient.

The Chaves Co. Medical Society met at Roswell, N. M., on December 13th, and elected the following officers to serve for the ensuing year: W. E. Parkhurst, President; C. M. Mayes, Vice-President; W. W. Phillips, Secretary, and M. W. Flournoy, Treasurer.

Diet in Arthritis Deformans.—Thompson (*Medical Record*) recommends forced feeding with a full diet of animal food, the fats predominating. The ordinary meals should be supplemented by two or three luncheons during the day. Biliousness can be prevented largely by the use of simple bitters before meals, dilute hydrochloric acid with nux vomica after meals, drinking much water and the occasional use of a cathartic.

Croupous Rhinitis.—This form of inflammation, says Bosworth, often follows operations on the nose. The symptoms include chilly sensations followed by moderate fever with frontal headache, nasal neuralgia, pain in bones, depression and symptoms of acute rhinitis. One can see a pearly white, thin or thick false membrane covering the nasal lining and easily detached without bleeding (diphtheritic membrane leaves a bleeding surface on removal).

Chronic Esophagitis.—Allen A. Jones directs to treat cause; a bland, non-irritating diet; interdict alcohol. Burning after eating is relieved by small doses of bismuth with a drop or two of chloroform suspended in mucilage of tragacanth. Apply silver nitrate (eight grains to ounce of water) with a soft sponge or cotton on an applicator: Pass stomach tube or sound occasionally to prevent stricture.

Paraffin for Fecal Impaction.—Theodore Potter (*Central States Medical Gazette*) lauds the virtues of liquid paraffin, given, by the mouth in the medical treatment of fecal impaction. He reports success in a case where the bowels had not moved for three weeks, giving three ounces of the remedy every three hours. The petroleum hydrocarbons dissolve fecal matter, are neutral, non-irritating and non-absorbable, and cause no griping.

Vesical Ulcers.—Garcean (*Progressive Medicine*) states that the simple ulcer is single, usually circular, often coated with phosphates, and is usually on the posterior vesical wall near the internal border of the ureteral orifice, never encroaching on the trigonum. Tuberculous ulcers are multiple, irregular, seldom encrusted with phosphates, and have a predilection for the trigonum.

Vomiting and Pain of Gastric Cancer.- Ewald relies on lavage an hour before breakfast, followed in a half hour by four drams of infusion of condurango containing 1–32 grain of strychnine sulphate and fifteen minims of dilute hydrochloric acid. He also recommends small pieces of ice with a few drops of chloroform; ice-cold carbonic water in teaspoonful doses; effervescing lemonade or champagne ; morphine, and opium suppositories. Taylor advises the use of ice internally, either alone or with milk; ice applied to epigastrium; effervescing medicines; small quantities of iced champagne; extract of opium 1–6 grain to $\frac{1}{4}$ grain, or morphine $\frac{1}{8}$ to 1–6 grain.

Vomiting and Pain of Gastric Ulcer.—Ewald advises a carefully regulated diet—chiefly milk; drinking large quantities of warm water several times during day; pieces of ice with chloroform. Osler has found lavage most successful. He has also

The Family Laxative

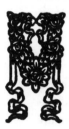

California Fig Syrup Company

San Francisco,
California.

Louisville, Ky.
New York, N. Y.

The ideal, safe, family laxative, known as "Syrup of Figs," is a product of the California Fig Syrup Co., and derives its laxative principles from senna, made pleasant to the taste and more acceptable to the stomach by being combined with pleasant aromatic syrups and the juice of figs. It is recommended by many of the most eminent physicians, and used by millions of families with entire satisfaction. It has gained its great reputation with the medical profession by reason of the acknowledged skill and care exercised by the California Fig Syrup Co. in securing the laxative principles of the senna by an original method of its own, and presenting them in the best and most convenient form. The California Fig Syrup Co. has special facilities for commanding the choicest qualities of Alexandria senna, and its chemists devote their entire attention to the manufacture of the one product. The name "Syrup of Figs" means to the medical profession "the family laxative, manufactured by the California Fig Syrup Co." and the name of the company is a guarantee of the excellence of its product. Informed of the above facts, the careful physician will know how to prevent the dispensing of worthless imitations when he recommends or prescribes the original and genuine "Syrup of Figs." It is well known to physicians that "Syrup of Figs" is a simple, safe and reliable laxative, which does not irritate or debilitate the organs on which it acts, and, being pleasant to the taste, it is especially adapted to ladies and children, although generally applicable in all cases. Special investigation of the profession invited.

"Syrup of Figs" is never sold in bulk. It retails at fifty cents per bottle, and the name "Syrup of Figs," as well as the name of the California Fig Syrup Co., is printed on the wrappers and labels of every bottle.

The advent of the season in which

COUGH,
BRONCHITIS,
WHOOPING COUGH,
ASTHMA, ETC.

Impose a tax upon the resources of every physician renders it opportune to re-invite attention to the fact that the remedy which invariably effects the immediate relief of these disturbances, the remedy which unbiased observers assert affords the most rational means of treatment, the remedy which bears with distinction the most exacting comparisons, the remedy which occupies the most exalted position in the esteem of discriminating therapeutists is

GLYCO-HEROIN (Smith)

GLYCO-HEROIN (Smith) is conspicuously valuable in the treatment of Pneumonia, Phthisis, and Chronic Affections of the Lungs, for the reason that it is more prompt and decided in effect than either codeine or morphine, and its prolonged use neither leaves undesirable after effects nor begets the drug habit. It acts as a reparative in an unsurpassable manner.

DOSE.—The adult dose is one teaspoonful, repeated every two hours, or at longer intervals as the case may require.
To children of ten or more years, give from a quarter to a half teaspoonful.
To children of three or more years, give five to ten drops.

---

employed cracked ice, chloroform, cerium oxalate, bismuth salts, hydrocyanic acid and ingluvin. If the trouble is intractable, the patient must be fed per rectum. Ringer praises dilute hydrobromic acid, m. xxx in water four times a day. Bartholow extolled Fowler's solution in drop cases. Taylor lauds morphine, or bismuth and morphine, effervescing medicines or a few drops of tincture of iodine every hour.

Gastric Hyperacidity.—Bartholow prescribed: ℞ Bismuthi subnit. gr. xx; acidi carbol. gr. ⅓–⅔; mucil. acadiae m. lxxx; aquam menth. pip. q. s.: A tablespoonful for adults three or four times a day. Chambers uses the following formula: ℞ Sodii bicarb. gr. xv; acidi hydrocyan. dil. m. iss; aquae camphorae ℥x: Take t. i. d. after meals. Ringer recommends nux vomica and ipecac simultaneously when there are a creamy-coated tongue and much acidity and heartburn. In the case of infants he adds one-eighth lime water to the milk unless they are constipated, when he employs sodium bicarbonate.

Denver and Gross College of Medicine.—The second regular meeting of the Alumni Association of the Denver and Gross College of Medicine was held at the College Building, 14th and Arapahoe Streets, Saturday evening, December 10th. Dr. Stover read an interesting paper on "Electro-Therapeutics of Acne," and other members reported cases. Thirty members were present. The present officers are: President, Dr. I. B. Perkins; 1st Vice-President, Dr. T. M. Burns; 2d Vice-President, Dr. M. E. Preston; 3d Vice-President, Dr. F. M. McCartney; Secretary, Dr. C. Parsons, and Treasurer, Dr. G. M. Blickensderfer. Regular meetings are held on the first Saturday of each month, except during the summer.

Strychnine as an Evacuant.—In infectious and autotoxemic conditions the sympathetic motor centers are noticeably blunted, with resulting constipation. As a stimulant to these centers Geo. E. Pettey has had excellent results from the use of strychnine. The dose for this purpose varies with age, tonicity of tissues, etc., from ⅛ to 1–30 of a grain, given at intervals of two or three hours until four to six such doses have been given. The drug is satisfactorily combined with salines, mercurials and other purgatives.

Treatment of Capillary Bronchitis.—Dickey advises the use of a cotton batting jacket, three layers over chest, shoulders and back; also sponging with cold or tepid water for hyperpyrexia. He prevents heart failure with one or two drops each of tinct. nux vomica and belladonna every hour or so to a child a year or two old. If pain annoys he uses hot fomentations of capsicum, a half teaspoonful to the quart of water. Ammonium chloride is a reliable expectorant. Turpeth mineral, two or three grains, may be given as an emetic if needed to clear the tubes.

A Series of Foreign Bodies in the Vermiform Appendix Met with in 1,600 Necropsies.—L. J. Mitchell gives a list of true foreign bodies found in the appendix during his service as Coroner's Physician. One or more grape seeds were present in eight cases, one or more shot in three cases, and fragments of bone in two cases. Other objects were a portion of a shingle nail, a globule of solder, a piece of nutshell, a portion of the vertebral column of a small fish, and fragments, apparently, of ash or stone. None of the appendixes containing these bodies showed any signs of inflammation either past or present.—*Medical Record.*

Cardiospasm.—Van Valzah and Nisbet advise etiologic and constitutional measures and cervico-esophageal sedative polar galvanization or intragastric anodal galvanization, or the use of a large flexible esophageal sound as the mainstay—once a day before breakfast instagnation form—before each meal if esophageal retention—smear lower end of tube with cocaine ointment. If there is esophageal dilation, wash out contents at bedtime, or introduce all the food through the stomach-tube. Potassium bromide is often palliative, but is contraindicated in hyperchlorhydria. Extracts of coca and hyoscyamus, washed down with chloroform water, one-half hour before meals, are very beneficial. Control hyperacidity from any cause. Use a non-irritating diet; avoid condiments and acids and half mastication of foods; take no food or water between the regular three meals.

Gastroptosis.—Van Valzah and Nisbet advise to replace and support the stomach with a well-fitted pelvic or hypogastric belt, applied next to skin every morning while in bed and tightened from below upward; also rest, massage, electricity, nutritious diet and gentle laxatives if needed.

DENVER MEDICAL TIMES

Volume XXIV.   MARCH, 1905   Number 9

PREGNANCY COMPLICATED BY TUMORS OF THE UTERUS. *

By D. S. FAIRCHILD, M.D.

Des Moines, Iowa.

The main facts in relation to tumors of the uterus are so well worked out there is little room for profitable discussion, but there is one point in connection with these growths which may be considered worthy of review on account of its great importance, and on account of the great uncertainty which may arise in the mind of the medical attendant as to the wisest course to pursue in an individual case. The low mortality which follows a hysterectomy or a myomectomy leads us to look with favor upon these operations in all cases of growing or mischief-making tumors of the uterus, and while we have no doubt as to the course to be pursued under ordinary circumstances we may not be so clear as to the best course to adopt when pregnancy exists as a complication.

We are familiar with the fact that uncomplicated tumors of the uterus sometimes undergo degenerative changes which makes an operation imperative aside from any mechanical consideration. When complicated with pregnancy nutritive influences may arise from the stimulus of the condition which will hasten such changes, or lead to a rapid growth of the tumor and to dangerous or distressing symptoms or from mechanical influences, as twisting of the pedicle and so impair nutrition as to promote degenerative changes, or even lead to supperation and to acute or chronic peritonitis. Baring these nutritive and degenerative changes which may arise in a uterine fibroid in the pregnant condition, the main questions to be considered are mechanical, and the accidents which may arise should an abortion occur.

It may be assumed that no surgeon will adopt a course of procedure which will interfere with pregnancy unless he is certain that the woman's life is greatly imperiled. It has been repeatedly observed that women suffering from uterine fibroids have safely

---

*Read before Rocky Mountain Inter-State Medical Association, September, 1904.

passed through the various stages of gestation and labor, while on the other hand, others have after great suffering lost their lives.

The factors involved in the complication of pregnancy with uterine tumors will be chiefly mechanical. The tumor may be so located and of such size as to wedge into the pelvis and prevent the escape of the organ into the abdominal cavity as gestation advances, and give rise to serious pressure symptoms which may occur during the first four months of utero-gestation. Large tumors may take on increased rapidity of growth, which together with the enlarging pregnant uterus may cause dangerous abdominal pressure symptoms.

Tumors in the lower segment of the uterus may become impacted in the pelvis and present insuperable difficulties in the passage of the child at the time of labor. All these difficulties may at first be more apparent than real. On first examination when it is discovered that a tumor complicates pregnancy, it may be concluded that only one of two things will save the patient; either the production of an abortion, or a supra-vaginal hysterectomy, but it is finally discovered that gestation passes through its various stages and that delivery is accomplished without serious accident.

Aside from mechanical difficulties which may complicate the first period of pregnancy and the period of delivery, there arise questions in relation to the completion of the normal period of gestation. It may be found in some cases that the uterine wall is so occupied by multiple tumors that there is but a very limited area of normal uterine tissue which is capable of physiologic development. A case of this kind recently came under my care. The woman was said to be three months pregnant. She was suffering from moderate attacks of hemorrhage and some pain. An examination showed that the right side and median portions of the uterus was occupied by a hard resisting body, while on the left side a tumor extended about two inches above the level of the umbilicus which on palpation presented the evidences of a cyst. The symptoms seemed to indicate the approach of an abortion; if, indeed this should not occur the rapid growth would certainly lead to serious abdominal pressure difficulties. The woman was extremely anxious to bear a child. In view of this fact, and with the fear of an abortion and hemorrhage before me, and the danger to the patient if an abortion should not occur, led me to open the abdomen to determine, if possible, what could be done in a surgical way to obviate the danger and to increase the chances of a favorable termination of gestation at full term. It was found that the uterine body was occupied by multiple tumor masses except about the left horn, where normal uterine tissue was advancing in a sac-like form well into the abdominal cavity. It was apparent that full term of gestation was improbable and the greatest safety to the patient depended on a supra-vaginal hysterectomy, which was accordingly done with a satisfactory result. The diagnosis in this case was not complete, in that it was supposed that an ovarian cyst existed in connection with the pregnant fibroid uterus, when in fact the apparent cyst was the thinned out remnant of uterine wall which was capable of physiologic change.

In tumor complications of the extent found in the above reported case, an early spontaneous termination of gestation may be expected. If, however, the tumor has a limited point of attachment to the uterus, it may rise into the abdomen with the enlarging organ and give rise to no serious complication at any stage of gestation, or at the time of delivery, even if of considerable size, unless the circulation becomes disturbed in such a way as to influence nutrition.

The danger from tumors of the uterus complicating pregnancy is not alone during gestation and labor, but may come after delivery. If the tumor is submucous or interstitial, it may interfere with normal contraction of the organ and permit or cause very serious post-partum hemorrhage, which may be difficult or impossible to control.

In view of the fact that any operation on the uterus during pregnancy is almost certainly followed by abortion, the treatment must be either expectant or radical. There may be some exceptions. Mayo Robson removed at the seventh month a fibroma of the cervix of the size of a cocoanut without disturbing pregnancy. He says that when the operation is performed late in pregnancy there may be no interruption in its course. No absolute rule can be adopted and each case must be considered by itself. While this is true, certain principles must govern the surgeon in the management of the individual case. It is desirable that an early diagnosis be made in order to determine the application of the principle involved.

The period of gestation may be divided in two parts, so far as the questions of treatment are concerned. First, the period within the first four months, second, the remaining period of pregnancy. The surgeon will be called upon to consider, first, a conservative course, second, abortion, third, supra-vaginal hysterectomy. The frequent observation that pregnancy passes through its various stages to full term and safe delivery, even when the gravest apprehensions were entertained by the medical attendant as to the results, leads us to look with favor on an expectant course and wait until the later period of gestation has arrived. If, however, it is apparent that the tumor is of such size and so located that an advanced period of gestation cannot be reached, one'of two courses should be adopted, either an abortion or a supra-vaginal hysterectomy. There is much professional opinion to the effect that an abortion should not be performed in this class of cases for the reason that the danger from hemorrhage and infection are greater than the danger from a hysterectomy.

Lefour in 307 cases found 39 abortions ending fatally to the mother 14 times, and in another series of 23 induced abortions observed three deaths. It may, therefore, be properly concluded that if the conditions in the early months of gestation demand any operative treatment, whatever it should be, a supra-vaginal hysterectomy is a safer procedure, so far as the immediate risk to life is concerned. No argument can be offered in favor of preserving an uterus which is so extensively occupied by tumor masses that the condition of pregnancy cannot be allowed to go on undisturbed without great hazard after a most careful consideration of the case.

If it is concluded that gestation can be safely allowed to continue to an advanced stage, the question of treatment will then depend on certain mechanical conditions. If the tumor is so located as to fill the pelvis and offer insuperable difficulties to the passage of the fetus, the medical attendant will be called upon to determine if the pelvis can be sufficiently cleared by an operative procedure, or if the case should go to the time of delivery and be submitted to a Cæsarian section followed by the removal of the uterus. Generally the latter case will be pursued. It may occasionally happen, however, that a tumor will be found attached to the lower segment of the uterus, or to the neck, which may be removed without interrupting pregnancy; as in the case reported by Robson. I am of the opinion that the number of cases in which it may be found advisable to operate before the approach of delivery will be very small. Yet, it may be admitted that if a tumor of moderate size is diagnosed, having a rather limited extent of attachment to the uterus and which is blocking the pelvis, it may be removed at about the seventh month. If at any time it is found that the tumor is undergoing degenerative changes or if tumor masses are suffering from nutritive changes from impaired blood supply from a possible twisting of the pedicle, a hysterectomy should not be delayed. These accidents are not common and may be omitted from the consideration of the case except as a possible contingency, but if it is found that the patient's health is beginning to suffer and no other cause can be discovered, it may be assumed that the condition of the uterus is responsible for it. A careful examination of the woman will, in all probability, reveal evidence to confirm this assumption. Where evidence is presented that degenerative changes are arising in the fibroid uterus, the risk is constantly increasing, for the changes will certainly be progressive and delay in the operation will lessen the chances in recovery.

We may, in conclusion, hold to the view that the discovery of a tumor complicating pregnancy is no certain indication for an an operative procedure of any kind, even when it is at first apparent that mechanical difficulties of very grave nature exist, but a watchful care should be exercised and when it is found in the first four months that the uterus cannot rise into the abdominal cavity or that an abortion is almost certain to occur, the abortion should be left to nature or a supra-vaginal hysterectomy made, but an abortion should not be induced. If the uterus is advancing into the abdominal cavity no interference should be permitted unless grave pressure symptoms should appear as a remote probability amounting to almost a certainty, when a supra-vaginal hysterectomy may be made. If in the latter months of pregnancy a tumor springing from the neck or the lower segment of the uterus threatens to block the pelvis and seriously interfere with delivery, the question of removing it may be considered in anticipation of labor at about the seventh month. In the great majority of cases where the immediate and seeming dangers have passed the case will go on to the period of labor and be treated according to the indications present at the time, either through the spontaneous efforts of nature, or by some operative nature, probably a Cæsarian section and a Porro-Cæsarian.

DISCUSSION OF DR. FAIRCHILD'S PAPER.

DR. OVIATT. I thank you for the courtesy. I am very much interested in Dr. Fairchild's paper, from the fact that only recently I had under my care an almost identical case with the one he described. I have, in fact, had two cases of myofibroma, complicated with pregnancy.

The first woman was brought to the hospital on a stretcher, being between five and six months pregnant and vomiting constantly. We kept her in the hospital a few days trying to get her in better condition before operating. She died three or four days after the operation.

In the last case the pregnancy was only about four months, the tumor filling the basin of the pelvis and there was absolutely no chance for a normal delivery.

I want to endorse every word the doctor has said in relation to this class of cases. He has said all there is to be said, and I believe that many cases of fibroids may be allowed to go on until labor.

Fifteen years ago I attended a woman in confinement with a tumor about the size of a man's fist. I attended her in three or four subsequent pregnancies, each time finding the tumor a little larger, yet causing no bad results as far as labor was concerned. Then a strange thing occurred. After twelve or more years the tumor began suddenly to grow rapidly. This only showed us that we have no reasonable hypothesis to work upon in regard to the growth of fibroid tumors! They may lie dormant for several years, and then suddenly begin to increase in size rapidly. I think Dr. Fairchild has covered the ground thoroughly.

DR. PERKINS. I have been very much interested in that portion of the paper which I heard, coming in, as I did, when Dr. Fairchild had almost finished. I endorse very heartily the ideas expressed in the paper. I think that, in many cases of fibroids of the uterus during pregnancy, the pregnancy would go on to full term and children would be delivered with no trouble. In fact, I know this to be the case.

I call to mind one case where a fibroid larger than my fist was discovered at the time of the birth of the first child. It interfered, somewhat, with the birth of the child, and the child had to be removed with forceps and was still-born. After the patient recovered the first time the tumor shrank very materially, until it was not larger than half a small orange. Two years later she gave birth to another child, and I attended her. This time the tumor was probably a little larger than before, but I had no trouble with it and the result was a living child. I had watched her during the entire term of gestation. Since that time, which was some two or three years ago, she has been delivered of another child by my brother. He spoke of the same tumor, (he was with me in each of the other deliveries), and it seemed a little larger than before. Whether the next time it will give trouble or not remains to be seen.

DR. MAYO. I remember a case which we had a few years ago where a woman, five months pregnant, had symptoms of a cystic tumor; a very large abdomen, as large as she would have been with full term, of an irregular contour, showing the presence of possibly two tumors. She had a temperature which fluctuated from 101° to 103°, during the few days in which we had to examine her before operation. We decided it was a twisted pedicle condition, and could not tell whether it was a fibroid tumor or an ovarian cyst. It was a large fibroid with twisted pedicle which was attached in a great many points in the abdomen, and it was larger than the pregnancy. This was simply excised from the uterus to the opening of the uterine wall, which it nearly went through. In this case it was the patient's first pregnancy. It is a fortunate thing to find this condition in Catholics, as it relieves you of a great deal of responsibility, and in such cases it is best not to interrupt pregnancy unless absolutely pushed to do so by the condition of the patient. She was allowed to go to full term. Another tumor filled the pelvis and lifted itself above the brim of the pelvis, and the patient went to labor without any trouble.

I am often told by medical men of the trouble that they have, being up twenty-four hours with a serious case of fibroid tumor complicating pregnancy; yet how many of these cases are relieved with apparently no more risk, or not so much, as would be involved in presenting to them an abortion. I always fear abortion

complicating such conditions, and unless driven to it by the condition of impending death, I always allow the case to run to full
term, or to natural miscarriage. If driven to it by impending
death the chances are then, possibly, in favor of operating. There
are few cases of these that really run to death, and if we decide
that we must end pregnancy, I believe with the doctor, that it is
safer to go through the abdomen direct than to perform an operation that would leave a condition that is liable to create the same
condition again in the future. Again so many of these patients
have already undergone a few months of suffering and it is their
first pregnancy, and I believe in the cases I have seen, the women
who are thus afflicted are all very desirous of having the child, if
it is possible, and when we let it go on, we generally save both the
child and the woman.

Dr. Niles. I do not feel like letting this subject go by without citing an experience so recent that I cannot help but be deeply
impressed with it.

Less than a month ago I was called, through the courtesy of
Dr. Ewing, to see a case of pregnancy which was complicated by
the presence of a fibroid tumor so as to interfere with the emptying of the bladder, and it became necessary to catheterize the
patient three or four times a day. I do not know whether it was
a coincidence or not, but the nausea during the preceding two
weeks had been very excessive, and it was for that reason she first
consulted a physician, who, not knowing her condition, recommended and carried out a plan of lavage. Later she consulted another physician, who saw fit to give her spirit of nitre without examining the urine or bladder. When Dr. Ewing was called, he
realized the condition, and thinking that surgical measures might
be needed he was kind enough to call me in. At that time she
was further advanced in pregnancy than we thought, being about
three and one-half months, as we discovered afterward. The uterus was not raised from the pelvis, but was jammed down in a
way that it could not be lifted. She had been for three weeks being catheterized.

At this stage, three and one-half months, we did not feel that
these symptoms were likely to be relieved except by operation, as
cystitis was commencing to be developed. She was taken to the
hospital, as we hardly knew what course we might be compelled
to pursue.

I mention this case, as it is possible, or even probable, each member of this Association will meet with some such problem. It so happened that when we opened the abdomen we found a fibroma, perhaps the size of my fist, or a trifle smaller, attached to the anterior wall of the uterus and pressed against the bladder in such a way as to interfere with the emptying of the bladder, and also in such a way as to prevent the likelihood of the uterus being lifted from the pelvis and leave room later for the pregnancy to go on without abortion being produced. This tumor was attached for about two and one-half or three inches, and it was quite easy in removing it to place a pair of long clamps close to the uterus to protect it (since the full strength of the uterine walls was likely to be needed later, and I wanted, if possible, to avoid a miscarriage), and afterwards dissecting for some distance above the tumor on the walls of the peritoneum; doing the stitching with catgut before removing the clamps, and tightening the ligature as the clamps were removed. In that way we scarcely lost a drop of blood. The union was perfect and the pressure symptoms we thought were relieved. On examination we found, however, a number of nodules probably the size of a thumb. As at that moment our only thought was to remove the pressure symptoms, we did nothing with these smaller nodules, knowing that the pregnancy would go on without a complication so far as they were concerned, and that they could be attended to at some future time. She did exceedingly well, and, in fact, wanted to go home on the tenth day, and was certainly quite able so far as the operation was concerned. The operation was completed in perhaps twenty-five minutes; it was very simple, and there were no evidences of an abortion. The urine had been examined quite frequently, not with a view of expecting any kidney trouble, but to notice when the cystitis had subsided. I left the city about that time, and she had, as I say, fully recovered from the operation, and the urine was examined daily from that time on, and no albumen was found, nor were there any indications of kidney trouble. A week, perhaps, afterwards, she had puerpural eclampsia, and in the course of sixteen or eighteen hours died from this cause.

During the attacks the urine had been passed, but the attending physician was very anxious to find out the condition of the kidneys, so he drew some of the urine, and found that there was still no albumen in it. I cannot believe that this unfortunate condition had any connection in any way with the operation, which simply served the purpose of removing the pressure symptoms, and I mention it so that it may be remembered, and possibly there may be a better explanation than I, at this moment, feel prepared to offer.

DR. EWING. As I was interested in this case you speak of, I will say that at the last examination of urine we discovered albumen, and she lay perfectly unconscious all this time, having a spasm about every ten or fifteen minutes. We thought, perhaps, we might relieve the patient by producing abortion, which we did. There was no hemorrhage to amount to anything, and she grew a great deal better. The convulsions ceased and she partially regained consciousness, but never fully, and as the doctor states, she died forty-eight hours later.

DR. FAIRCHILD. I am very much gratified at the discussion which has followed this paper. I was induced to present it on account of the feeling I have that many cases of this kind are not allowed to go along in a physiological way. I have nothing else to offer, as the paper expressed my views on the subject as well as I was able to present them, and therefore, I will not occupy more of your time.

REMARKS ON THE PANCREAS.

By BYRON ROBINSON.
Chicago, Illinois.

Extensive work is being done experimentally, pathologically and chemically in the field of pancreatic diseases. To one familiar with the anatomy of the pancreas, and performing frequently post mortems, many of the current journal articles are superficial and misleading, because the writers are deficient in knowledge. The eyes of the medical world are now directed toward the pancreas. The pancreas began to be of some use to physician and patient when Moritz Hofman, of Altdorf, Germany demonstrated to John George Wirsung, of Padua, Italy, in 1642 that a rooster's pancreas had an exit duct. In 1643 John George Wirsung demonstrated that the pancreas of animals and man possessed an exit duct, and he drew a picture of it, sending it to the Paris Academy through John Riolan, his old anatomic teacher.

For 260 years the pancreas has had a varied history in medicine. Fifty years ago Claude Bernard, of Paris, wrote the most notable monograph on the pancreas. Since that time the notable contributors to the literature of the pancreas have been from Nichalos Senn, Fitz, Balser, Minkowski, von Mehring, Robson, Opie and others. Recently the most significant contributors, to our knowledge of the pancreas, were von Mehring and Minkowski, whose experiments demonstrated that the extirpation of a dog's pancreas was followed by sugar in the urine—diabetes mellitus. Lately many contributions are being made to the literature of the pancreas, notably that of Opie, Lazarus and Kœrter. By inspecting the pancreas in autopsy one is at once convinced of the difficulty, not only of diagnosing any disease which may attack it, but also of the almost insurmountable anatomic factors in surgical intervention. Physiologically its own secretion may induce digestion of its own tissue—fat necrosis. When one considers what are the common diseases of the pancreas it becomes more evident that the diagnosis is frequently impossible medically or surgically.

The pancreas experiences; (a), hæmorrhagic pancreatitis; (b), suppurative pancreatitis: (c), necrotic pancreatitis; (d), pancreolithiasis; (e), pancreatitis cystica. It is difficult in ordinary subjects with pancreatic diseases to make a diagnosis of the exact pathologic condition with the pancreas in the hand and before the eyes. I have inspected in autopsy over 500 pancreases and can say from this experience that gross, palpable pancreatic lesions, with the exception of pancreatitis chronica—a common occurrence in the caput—are, like duodenal ulcers, rare. Half a dozen years ago Kœrter and Olser mentioned the frequent relation of hepatic calculus to pancreatic disease. I present two typical subjects with this article. The diseases of the pancreas met in the intra-abdominal exploration as fat necrosis, hæmorrhagic pancreatitis are difficult of disposition. The surgeon can simply institute drainage. To illustrate the difficulty of diagnosing pancreatic disease within 1904, I listened to four surgeons narrate their experiences. Two cases were diagnosed as disease of the pancreas. On exploratory incision the surgeon could not diagnose the condition with eyes and fingers on the pancreas—he said one case had tubercle in the region of the pancreas, the other case was reported as simply a

dark colored pancreas.   The third case was diagnosed as grave pancreatic disease, an on abdominal incision no disease of any kind
could be observed in the pancreas.   The fourth case was gravely
ill for four to five days and died.   Post mortem showed hæmorrhagic and suppurative pancreatitis, which was not diagnosed by
a surgeon of more than local fame.   Much more study is required

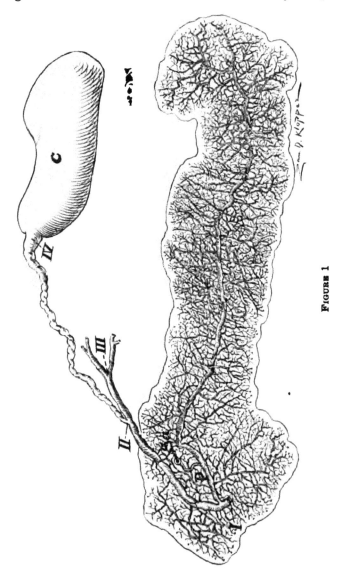

FIGURE 1

to make a diagnosis of pancreatic disease and to make surgery of value in the field of the pancreas. We must be able to recognize some of the diseases of the pancreas after the abdomen is opened.

Figure 1. (Byron Robinson) An X-ray of part of the ductus bilis and ductus pancreaticus of a girl eleven years old. I to II,

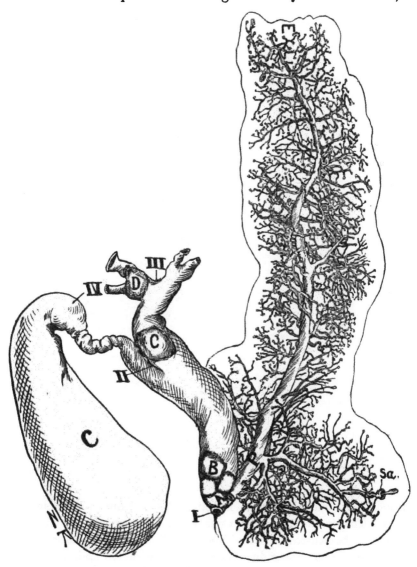

FIGURE 2.

ductus choledochus communis. II to III ductus hepaticus. II, to IV, ductus cysticus. c, cholecyst. It is very easy to observe the segments of the pancreas, viz:—caput, collum, corpus, cauda. In fact, this beautiful accurate illustration establishes the final anatomy. Sa, ductus Santorini functionated as the celloidin projected

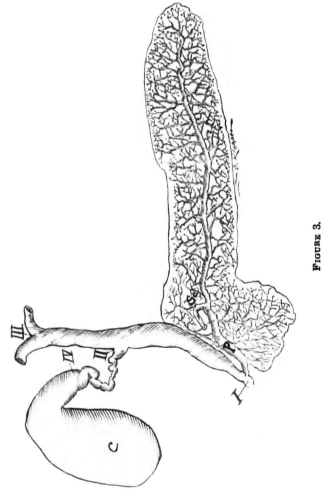

FIGURE 3.

from its exit duct during the injecting of it. Hofman-Wirsung duct. The liver of this patient was advanced in sarcomatous disease, but the pancreas appeared healthy. P, ductus pancreaticus. The liver and pancreatic ducts were injected with red lead, mixed with starch before the X-ray was taken. The intra-pancreatic portion of the choledochus in its natural position.

Figure 2. (Byron Robinson). Roentgen ray of ductus pancreaticus and part of ductus bilis. Contains six hepatic calculi.

From post mortem specimens. I to II ductus choledochus communis, dilated to three-fourths inch in diameter and containng four hepatic calculi (A.B.) in its distal end. II to IV ductus

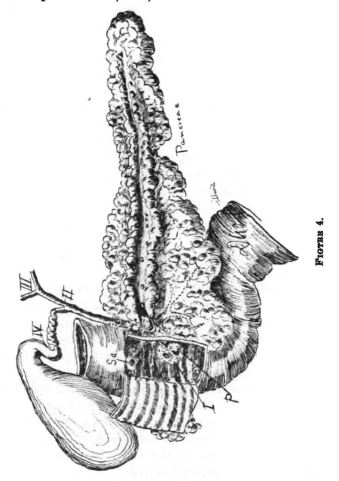

cysticus, dilated to one-third inch in diameter, yet preserving in form six valvulæ Heisterri. II to III ductus hepaticus, dilated to one-half inch and containing a hepatic calculus. (C); cholecyst, normal dimension containing no calculus. P, ductus pancreaticus (ductus Hofmanii-Wirsungii). Sa, ductus pancreaticus accessorius (ductus Santorini). The ductus bilis and ductus pancreaticus are characterized by spirality and irregularity of lumen. The lateral pancreatic ducts end in bulbs or vesicles. This specimen illustrates the facility with which the ebb and flow of infectious waves may travel from the channels of the liver to those of the pancreas and vice versa. For the X-ray the ductus pancreaticus was injected with celloidin and red sulphide of mercury while the ductus bilis was injected with red lead and starch. The presence of calculus had created suppurative chledochitis. The exit of the ductus pancreaticus into the ductus choledochus was widely patulous. I secured the specimen at the autopsy by the courtesy of Dr. W. A. Evans.

Figure 3. X -ray of ductus pancreaticus and part of ductus bilis. The ductus pancreaticus (P) was injected with celloidin and red sulphide of mercury while the ductus bilis was injected with red lead, mixed with starch. The artist, Mr. Zan D. Klopper, reproduced it as a model. The non-uniform caliber of both pancreatic and biliary ducts may be observed. I to II ductus cholodochus communis. II to III, ductus hepaticus. II to IV, ductus cysticus. Sa, ductus pancreaticus accessorius (Santorini). C, cholecyst in living position.

Figure 4. (Byron Robinson). Specimen containing pancreatic calculus.

From a post mortem, man about forty years. I to II ductus choledochus. II to III ductus hepaticus. II to IV, ductus cysticus. Sa, ductus pancreaticus accessorius. P, separate exit of ductus pancreaticus in duodenum. A calculus three-fourths of an inch in length and one-third inch in diameter is incarcerated in the duct of the caput pancreaticum. The calculus of the ductus pancreaticus projects into the lumen of the duodenum. Also six calculi existed in the ductus pancreaticus as noted in sketch. The pancreas was in an advanced stage of suppuration and fatty degeneration. This specimen was kindly presented to me by Dr. A. M. Stober. B. J. Beuker sketched it from the pathologic laboratory of the Cook County Hospital.

NORMAL OBSTETRICS.

CHAPTER ELEVEN

THE HYGIENE OF PREGNANCY AND LABOR DIRECTIONS.

By T. MITCHELL BURNS, M.D.,

Denver, Colorado,

Professor of Obstetrics, The Denver and Gross College of Medicine.

THE HYGIENE OF PREGNANCY.

Examinations.—If any abnormal symptoms, especially those of uterine disease, abortion or kidney disorder, occur, a thorough, gentle examination should be made at once. In all cases the regular obstetric examination of pregnancy should be made at about the end of the eighth month, but it should be made at the end of the seventh month if there is a probability of contracted pelvis.

The Teeth.—The teeth should be kept clean and acidity prevented by the use of a brush and a solution of bicarbonate of sodium. For toughening the gums and preventing toothache, one or two drops of tincture of myrrh on the wet tooth brush, well rubbed into the gums after each meal, is of great value. Toothache is caused by an acid condition of the stomach, malnutrition, and increased irritability of the nervous system, which predisposes to neuralgia. Decayed teeth should be filled, and if the treatment does not stop their aching, they should be extracted under an anæsthetic, preferably chloroform. There is more danger of abortion from severe toothache than from the shock of an extraction under an anæsthetic. (The author has seen premature labor induced by severe toothache, and then stopped by chloroform and extraction).

Food.—The amount of food need not be restricted as long as the general health is good. Often in the first and last months the amount has to be lessened—in the first month from weak digestion and in the last month from lack of room. Any kind of food may be eaten, but preference should be given to easily digested and nutritious foods. Vegetables, fruits and milk are especially indicated. The use of meat should never be excessive, and often nature prevents this by changing the taste so that there is no desire for it. Sugar and starch should be avoided, especially potatoes, as there is a natural tendency to acidity of the stomach, heart-burn, flatulence and colic. A milk diet is of great value in lessening the complications of pregnancy and the duration and severity of labor. "Longings," if within reason, should be satisfied, as the constant refusal is likely to result in more harm than the gratification. Water should be drunk freely, as it aids elimination. Tea, coffee and chocolate may be continued, but they should be taken weak and in small amounts. Alcoholic drinks are not indicated as a beverage, as instead of stimulation, there is generally need of mental and physical rest, and in some there is a tendency to form the habit during pregnancy. In those who have been used to drinking beer or wine it probably would not be best to prohibit these entirely.

A vegetarian diet and the use of distilled water is supposed by some to lessen the amount of bone material, and therefore, to make an easier labor by the bones of the head being softer, but it is more probable that nature will take from the mother all the bone material required, and that the vegetarian diet by causing a more healthy parturient, lessens considerably the severity of labor.

Clothing.—The clothing should not be too light or too warm. In the latter half of pregnancy a little warmer and probably part woolen underwear should be worn, as then the increase in the size of the abdomen removes the skirts from close contact with the lower limbs. Corsets should not be worn unless specially made with elastic sides. The improper use of the corset is said to have stunted and even killed children by interfering with the growth of the uterus.

The Abdominal Bandage.—When the abdominal walls are relaxed, an elastic or other bandage is of great value, if fitted so as to hold up the abdomen without pressing upon the fundus of the uterus.

Bathing.—A general bath should be taken at least once a week during the whole nine months, and during the last month a sitzbath every other night keeps the external genitals clean, and tends to relax the soft parts and the pelvic joints and thereby lessen the duration and suffering of labor. The water should be neither too hot nor too cold, as either extreme tends to excite uterine contractions. (During pregnancy, although hot water may excite or increase pain due to uterine contractions, by increasing the contractions, it generally lessens that due to intestinal colic and may be used for this purpose after other remedies have failed, providing previously a little morphine is given to quiet the uterine irritability).

Innuctions.—Sterilized vaseline, sweet, or olive oil, cocoa butter and other similar preparations ("Mother's Friends"), are of value when applied to the abdomen to relieve tension, and when applied to the external genitals to cause relaxation and relieve itching and other irritation.

The Breasts.—The breasts should not be compressed by corsets, as even in the non-pregnant, one of the frequent causes of deformed nipples is the pressure of the corset. During the last three months of the first pregnancy, and in the subsequent pregnancies if there is any tendency to tenderness, the nipples should be washed with castile soap and then rubbed with witch hazel or alcohol and water. This should be done with some force so as to prepare the nipples for the irritation of nursing.

Air, Exercise and Rest.—The pregnant woman should have an abundance of air and exercise, as she has to furnish them for two. While fresh air and moderate exercise are required to near the point of fatigue, ample rest is also needed and she should lie down at least an hour or two every afternoon and retire early.

Theaters and other crowded places, because of the bad air and excitement, should be avoided, as a rule. Traveling may cause motion sickness and premature pains. Sea voyages are especially dangerous, because of the extreme nausea and vomiting and the long duration of the trip, but much depends upon the patient, as some can do almost anything without harm, while others can hardly move without having a miscarriage. (If a patient has to travel, she may be given codeine or morphine tablets, with directions to use from one-eighth to one-quarter of a grain at a dose for any tendency to pain or sleeplessness and repeat in an hour or so if needed). No pregnant patient should travel on the cars except in a sleeper. A short trip or a street car ride is often of value to those who are inclined to be despondent, but if any pain occurs riding must be stopped.

The Mind.—Because of the unstable condition of the mind, the pregnant woman is easily influenced by her surroundings. Hence there should be no excitement, and all crowds and things that cause worry should be avoided. One of the greatest causes of anxiety is the tales the neighbors tell of difficult and abnormal cases and of instances of maternal marking. The pregnant woman should not listen to any of these remarks of the neighbors and not talk about her condition at all. If she requires any information, she should consult her physician or some reliable book on the hygiene of pregnancy, which her physician recommends.

Under proper care, there is very little danger of maternal death, as not one case in a thousand ought to die in labor or during the puerperal period, and cases of apparent authentic "marking" occur not oftener than once in ten thousand births. (In one thousand cases in which labor directions were given during pregnancy, the labor at term and through the lying-in period were personally attended by the writer, no maternal death occurred).

Sexual Intercourse.—Sexual intercourse should be restricted during pregnancy and should not occur at the time for a menstrual period, or at any time, if there are symptoms of threatening miscarriage or severe nausea and vomiting. In some women the sexual appetite is increased during some pregnancies and diminished during others.

The Bowels.—Constipation should be prevented by the use of fruit, coarse bread and exercise. Prunes stewed with a few senna leaves are of value. A cup of hot water before meals tends to regulate the bowels. If necessary, a cathartic should be used night and morning. Some preparation of cascara is generally to be preferred. Hinkel's cascara cathartic tablets are very good and the following prescription is popular:

R
    Fl. ext. cascaræ sagradæ.
    Fl. ext. cascaræ sagradæ aromaticæ. (P. D. Co.'s.)
    Glycerini.
    Elix. Pepsin. (Fairchild's)   aa ℥ ss.

M. S. ʒi night and morning, if needed for bowels. During the last three weeks it is well to move the bowels thoroughly once a week by giving a teaspoonful of Rochelle salts every two hours until the bowels move twice.

The Kidneys.—The urine of all pregnant women should be examined at the beginning of the ninth month, and sooner if any symptoms of kidney disease. Kidney disease is much more frequent in first pregnancies than subsequently. Frequent symptoms of kidney disease are persistent frontal or occipital headache, epigastric pain, nausea and vomiting, dizziness, spots before the eyes and oedema. The presence of any of these symptoms in the second half of pregnancy calls for repeated careful examinations of the urine. These symptoms in the first half of pregnancy are usually present from the general disturbance caused by the beginning of pregnancy and do not signify kidney disease, which is very rare at this period. Oedema and nausea and vomiting in the second half of pregnancy are frequently due to other conditions than kidney disease, and therefore, should cause no anxiety if the urine is normal. Eclampsia may occur in the last three weeks of pregnancy without any premonitory symptoms, but before this time nearly always the convulsions are preceded by some of the above signs, especially the frontal headache. The examination of the urine is important because if the kidney disorder is not due to chronic Bright's disease, it can almost always be cured and the convulsions prevented.

Measures to Lessen the Severity of Labor.—The severity of labor is more or less diminished by the following measures: (1) Vegetarian diet, especially milk, fruit, lemonade and distilled water, after the sixth or seventh month; (2) warm sitz-baths and inunctions the last month; (3) exercise or work to the point of slight fatigue; rest at the time for menstrual periods; (4) light mental occupation and cheerfulness; (5) bowels regular, especially the last month; (6) strychnine 1-30 gr. t. i. d. if lack of muscle tonus; (7) Lloyd's specific tincture of macrotys, two drops t. i. d. if uterine tension and tendency to pain. These produce a more physiologic pregnancy and labor, and therefore, lessen the pains of labor. By improving the excretions they improve the blood and circulation, and these in turn keep the mind more cheerful and the body stronger, the labor more normal and the getting-up better. The labor after this care may be very painful, but it is quite probable it would have been more so, if these measures had not been employed.

LABOR DIRECTIONS.

Things that the Patient Should Have in Readiness for Labor.—The patient should have in readiness for labor, (1) a fountain syringe, (2) a bed-pan, (3) a piece of rubber or oil-cloth, and *a rubber sheet, (4) three large and *six small hip pads, (5) one dozen sterilized vulvar pads, (6) †six sterilized T-bandages, (7) †three sterilized abdominal bandages, (8) * three breast bandages, (9) * one pair of obstetric or extra long stockings, (10) one pound absorbent cotton, (11) five yards of sterilized gauze or cheese cloth, (12) two cakes of castile soap, (13) a new nail brush, (14) a scrub brush, (15) four ounces of sweet oil or lard, (16) two bottles of vaseline, (17) one box of borated talcum powder, (18) †one or two dozen towels, (19) †one dozen sheets, (20) †six shirts, (21) †six nightgowns, (22) plenty of cloths, (23) one dozen clean newspapers, (24) a diaper and an old piece of flannel or woolen cloth in which to wrap the baby, (25) a piece of rubber or oil cloth, an old piece of carpet or clean gunny sacks to place in front of the bed to protect the carpet, (26) fifty bichloride tablets, (27) two ounces of boric acid, (28) one dozen, 2-grain quinine capsules, (29) a house thermometer, (30) †two dozen large safety pins for abdominal and breast bandages, (31) sterilized pillow slips and a clean box in which to put the above things, (32) the things for the baby, (33) the nurse, (24) the obstetrician, (35) a lady friend or another nurse to assist during the labor, (36) the husband and (37) a good bed-room and bed.

(1) *The Fountain Syringe.*—The best fountain syringes are those made of gray or red rubber. The capacity should be three or four quarts. The combination water bag and syringe is more liable to leak, and the kind having only one opening is an abomination, as the tubing must be detached each time before more water can be added. Before a new syringe is used it should be soaked inside and out in soap suds and then rinsed with plain warm water. Before an old syringe is used for an obstetric case, it should be scrubbed inside and out with plenty of soap and water and a nail brush and boiled ten minutes. Each time after a syringe is used during pregnancy, it should be washed with soap and water and laid away in a clean cloth. At the onset of labor

---

* Can get along without.
† With care may use less—by washing twice a week number used can be lessened one-half.

it should be rewashed and boiled ten minutes. Almost all rubber goods are warranted for one year.

(2) *The Bed-Pan.*—An oblong deep one of granite ware is probably the best, as with it there is little danger of wetting the bed, but the ordinary porcelain bed-pan of large size is very good, if care is used to keep the deep end low. The bed-pan should be washed clean by scrubbing with a brush, soap and water, and if it has been used before, it should be placed in a wash boiler containing hot water and boiled a half hour. After the bed-pan is cleaned, it should be placed in a clean linen bag and put away in a clean box, i. e., the box used to contain all the material for the labor. An ordinary tin wash basin may be used if a regular bed-pan can not be obtained.

(3) *A Piece of Rubber or Oil-Cloth and a Rubber Sheet.*— The whole mattress should be covered with a rubber sheet. The thinner the sheet the better. If it cannot be afforded, it is better to cover the mattress with newspapers. Above this rubber sheet or the newspapers should be placed a linen sheet. To protect the linen sheet, (or the mattress, if the rubber sheet is not used) a piece of rubber sheeting or oil-cloth, a yard and half square, should be used.

(4) *The Hip Pads.*—Three large hip pads a yard square and about one inch thick, or twice as thick as a baby's quilt, should be made of cheese cloth and cotton batting. One of these is to be used during labor, one after labor and the third to replace the second when soiled. If more are needed they may be made when required. The cheese cloth should be boiled before it is used. The pads should be made on a clean sheet and the hands of the maker should be clean. They can be put together with a basting stitch or tacked. They should be baked in an oven until slightly browned or exposed for several hours to strong sunlight. After this they should be put into a sterile pillow slip, that has been baked or boiled and ironed. Good hip-pads can be made of paper, clean cotton batting and cheese cloth. The paper is used as the first or lowest layer so as to prevent the discharge soaking through the pad.

Six small hip-pads should be made about eighteen inches square and half an inch thick. They ought to be made of cheese cloth and absorbent cotton or at least of cotton batting. These are for the purpose of protecting the large hip-pads and while not a necessity, are of value at first, i. e., while the flow is considerable. They should be made thin, as otherwise they would make too much bulk under the patient. In place of them a piece of a linen sheet may be folded and laid on the large pad.

(5) *The Vulvar Pads.*—One to two dozen vulvar pads should be made by passing a piece of sterilized gauze or cheese cloth, about a foot square, round a small roll of absorbent cotton which will easily fit over the vulva and between the limbs. Those for the first day should be made rather thick. The pads should be made with special care to cleanliness, as they are to come in direct contact with the vulva, and after being made should be put in a piece of cheese cloth or a sack and baked. More pads can be made and sterilized during the lying-in as needed. The cotton and gauze pads are probably the best, although many prefer to use sterilized plain or sterilized medicated gauze. Many patients use a folded napkin as when menstruating.

(6) *The T-Bandages.*—Six T-bandages should be made to hold the vulvar pads in place. These are very convenient, as they do away with the necessity of pinning and unpinning the pads in the back, each time they are changed, and the presence of a pin under the patient's hips. The main piece of the bandage should be about three inches wide and forty inches long; the piece to pass between the limbs should be about thirty inches long, at least six inches in width at each end and taper to three inches at the middle, so as to thoroughly cover the vulva and not be too wide between the thighs. The bandages should be sterilized and put away.

(7) *The Abdominal Bandages.*—At least three abdominal bandages are necessary. They should be made of a straight piece of unbleached muslin forty inches long and eighteen inches wide. (A bandage made to fit the shape of the patient is, as a rule, of little value, as the patient's shape changes a little each day, and such a bandage if held down by the vulvar pad may press on the uterus and do harm and if it is not held down it slips up and then is of no value. When the patient gets up from the lying-in period a properly shaped bandage is the best and is often of value.

(8) *The Breast Bandages.*—These should be made of unbleached muslin forty inches long and eight inches wide. The openings for the arms and neck can be easily made by folding the two ends into the middle until they overlap enough for pinning

and then cutting out for the neck and arms through the two thicknesses.

(9) *Obstetric or Extra Long Stockings.*—A pair of sterilized muslin or knit stockings, reaching to the groin are very nice during labor as they keep the limbs clean and warm, and if in the way they can be turned down some. Instead of these long stockings clean ordinary stockings are often used. (Drawers should not be worn as they come too close to the vulva and are in the way).

(10) *The Absorbent Cotton.*—Besides the absorbent cotton used for the pads there should be a pound for use during labor and subsequently for washing and extra pads. The best absorbent cotton is that twice sterilized by the manufacturer and so wrapped in paper that it can be lifted out of the box by an assistant without being touched. The cheaper grades, thirty-five cents a pound, can be used if sterilized by the nurse.

(11) *The Sterilized Gauze or Cheese Cloth.*—The sterilized gauze put up in glass jars or paper packages is easier to keep clean if kept in its container, but if the nurse is careful to sterilize and keep it clean ordinary five cent cheese cloth can be used just as well. Five to ten yards of the gauze or cheese cloth is usually sufficient.

(12) *Castile Soap.*—This soap is for the physician's hands and for washing the mother and baby. Green soap cleanses the hands and vulva better than any other soap, but imported castile soap is less irritating. Ivory soap is clean and about as good as the castile, but a little more irritating. Tar soap is not irritating and is a good cleaner, but it looks dirty. Soap which bites the tongue will irritate the skin or mucous membrane. *Colored castile soaps* are mostly all very poisonous and should never be used. Antiseptic mercurial soaps are antiseptic in name only, as it is impossible to use mercury with soap without producing either an inert or an irritating combination. Lysol soap seems to be all right for the hands and vulva.

(13) *The Nail Brush.*—The nail brush should be new, not have too stiff bristles and should be sterilized at least ten minutes. A colored or varnished brush should not be bought as they are more difficult to sterilize and keep clean.

(14) *The Scrub Brush.*—This should be a small, stiff bris-

tle, cheap (5-cent) nail brush. It is to be used in washing the bowls, pitchers, syringe, bed-pan, etc.

(15–16) *The Sweet Oil, Lard and Vaseline.*—Sterilized sweet oil, lard or vaseline is used as previously mentioned during pregnancy to relieve any tension of the skin of the abdomen and to soften the vulva. During labor sterilized vaseline, and by some sterilized lard, is used to anoint the fingers before an examination, and a few, the author included, use it to lubricate the vagina and vulva to prevent laceration. Vaseline and lard can be easily sterilized by placing the bottle or saucer on the stove, but sweet oil can only be sterilized by a water bath, i. e., by placing the vessel that contains it in another filled with water and boiling the water.

(17) *Borated Talcum Powder.*—Mennen's is mentioned because it is good, and because some of the brands are very poor, almost like sand. Mennen's consists of purified talcum, or silicate of magnesia, boric acid and oil of rose. This powder is used as a general infant powder and may be used for the navel.

(18–22) *The Towels, Sheets, Shirts, Gowns and Cloths.*— Of clean linen there cannot be too much, but with care the amount actually needed can be much less than often mentioned. There should be one dozen towels, one dozen sheets, six shirts and gowns and a dozen large cloths. The mother's shirt should be sufficiently open to allow the baby to nurse. The gowns can be put on more easily if they not only open in the front but also in the back. They should be a little short, so as to avoid getting soiled by an overflow.

(23) *Newspapers.*—These can be used in place of many things which may be absent, viz: rubber sheet, pads, carpet in front of the bed, Kelly pad and the like.

(24) *A Diaper and an Old Piece of Flannel in which to Wrap the Baby.*—The diaper is to keep the flannel clean and the flannel is to keep the baby warm.

(25) *A Piece of Rubber or Oil Cloth an Old Piece of Carpet or Clean Gunny Sacks.*—It is best to have one of these to protect the carpet in front of the bed.

(26) *Bichloride Tablets.*—Tablets of bichloride of mercury with citric acid are to be preferred, as bichloride remains more active in the presence of an acid. Tablets containing chloride of ammonium instead of this acid produce a dirty scum on the water and the bowl, are less soluble and hence, are more liable to be

precipitated and retained in the birth canal and cause poisoning. The prescription for the first tablets is:—

R

       Hydrargyri chloridi corrosivi gr. vii– 3–10
       Acidi citrici   gr. iii. 8–10
       Ft. tabellæ *(P. D. & Co.'s)* No. L.

Sig:—One in a quart of water for the hands *(one to the quart equals 1 to 2000)*, one in two quarts for the vulva and one in three or four quarts for the vagina.

(27) Boric Acid.—This is used in 5 % solution *(half tea-spoonful to half cup of luke-warm water)*, to wash the baby's eyes and the mother's nipples and dry as a powder for the baby's navel.

(28) Quinine Capsules.—One dozen two-grain capsules should be in readiness as they may be needed during the labor or subsequently. During the lying-in they prevent chilling and aid involution of the uterus.

(29) House Thermometer.—Much of the trouble occurring to the mother and the child during the lying-in period comes from the variations in the temperature of the room.

(30) Safety-Pins.—The two dozen safety-pins here mentioned are for the abdominal and breast bandages of the mother. They are often forgotten while those for the baby are remembered.

(31) Sterilized Pillow Slips and a Clean Box in which to Keep all of the Above Things.—This box should be separate from that for the baby's things.

(32) The Things for the Baby.—The clothing for the baby needs slight discussion, as the mother generally knows enough about it. The simpler and looser the better. The belly-band should be about four inches wide and eighteen inches long.

(33) The Nurse.—A trained nurse is very much preferred, but a clean experienced nurse, who is willing to do what the physician desires becomes nearly as good. The obstetrician should always ask the patient if she has obtained a nurse, and if she has not, he should suggest a nurse whom he knows will be congenial and trustworthy and whose charges will be in accordance with the patient's means. Every obstetrician should have several monthly nurse who understand his methods and are willing to follow them. Experienced nurses should be told to wear a dress which can be

easily washed. The eyes of the nurse should be good, for other-wise it is impossible for her to be aseptic, i. e., to see if she gets the patient clean.

(34) The Obstetrician.—The obstetrician should be selected because of his cleanliness, carefulness and skill. The average physician has all the knowledge necessary for 90 per cent of ob-stetric cases. If he is surgically clean he can successfully manage the other ten per cent, provided he is willing to call a consultant when any abnormal condition appears.

(35) A Lady Friend or Another Nurse.—There is always plenty of work for some one besides the obstetrician and the reg-ular nurse.

(36) The Husband.—It is the duty of the husband to help, or at least be present, so that he can appreciate what his wife has to suffer in labor.

(37) The Bed Room.—The bed room should be as nearly aseptic as possible. It should be large, light, warm and well ven-tilated, not connected with the sewer or next to the bath room, and it should not contain heavy curtains and upholstered furni-ture, nor ever have been occupied by a patient with a contagious disease, especially any septic disease. In some houses the bed rooms are quite small, cold, damp, or dark; then it is better to convert the parlor or sitting room into a bed room about one week before the expected time for labor. Though a clean bed room is strongly reccommended it is not absolutely essential to a normal puerpe-rium, for if everything which comes in direct contact with the patient be aseptic, there is little danger of infection. The bed should be strong and clean, especially the mattress, which should at least never have been occupied by a patient with any conta-gious disease, especially puerperal infection, wound infection, ery-sipelas or scarlet fever.

Measures that Should Be Carried Out at the Outset of Labor.—At the onset of labor *(1)* the patient should be pre-pared, *(2)* the bed should be made, *(3)* the pitchers, bowls, etc., that will be needed for labor should be thoroughly cleansed, *(4)* there should be plenty of sterilized hot and cold water, *(5)* all articles that will be needed *(or may be needed)* to put on the bed, the mother or the baby after labor should be placed where they will be warm, clean and easy to find.

(1) The Preparation of the Patient.—A patient ought to be prepared for labor the same as she would be for an abdominal section. Just as soon as the patient realizes that she is in labor, she should have an enema of soap suds; the hands and nails thoroughly cleaned, a general bath and a bath of the external genitals. The enema should be given by putting two quarts of warm soap suds in a clean fountain syringe, hanging the syringe about two feet above the patient, having the patient lie on her left side or back, with the hips higher than the head, allowing the air and cold water to run out of the tubing, putting a little vaseline on the nozzle and inserting it well into the rectum, stopping the flow when any pain and encouraging the patient to use all of the two quarts of soap suds. (It takes from ten to twenty minutes to give an enema.) The finger nails should be cut and cleansed and the hands washed with soap, water and a nail brush. The general bath should be thorough, especially the region of the abdomen and genitals. The external genitals should be shaved or the hair cut short, then the abdomen and genitals washed ten minutes with plenty of soap and water and a piece of sterilized gauze or cheese cloth, and after this bathed with alcohol and water in the proportion of one to four. After bathing the patient should put on a sterilized abdominal bandage, a sterilized vulvar pad, a sterilized T-bandage, a clean shirt and night gown, sterilized leggins or stockings and when up a clean bath robe or a warm wrapper and slippers.

After this preparation the patient should lie down a little while, but after resting she should stay up as much as possible, as staying up and walking about, when the patient is not too weak, facilitates the progress of labor.

The enema should be given even if the bowels have moved several times, as it is very probable that otherwise the bowels will move as the head is being born. Emptying the lower bowel lessens the intra-abdominal pressure, increases the size of the pelvis, and therefore, relieves the "pains" and is a very aseptic procedure. The hands should be thoroughly cleansed so as not to infect, by touching or by thoughtlessly scratching, the external genitals or the nipples. Cleaning of the external genitals is very important, for if the vulva is not rendered surgically clean—a perfect cleansing is difficult—infection may follow. A vaginal douche should not be used, as the vagina in a normal labor is kept aseptic by its own secretions. (In gonorrhea the vaginal secretions are not rendered

aseptic and an eight-quart, one to a thousand bichloride douche-
should be given by the obstetrician after a thorough cleansing of
the vagina with gauze, soap and water.   Vaginal gonorrhea is
diagnosed by finding the secretions alkaline or by the microscope.
In the former method the vestibule is touched with a piece of
cotton and then the cotton is touched with a piece of acid litmus
paper.   If there is much· blood in the flow the vestibule should
be wiped clean with cotton, then touched with a fresh piece of
cotton upon which the litmus paper is to be tried.   The secretions
even when mixed with some blood will generally not be alkaline
if gonorrhea does not exist).

(2) *The Preparation of the Bed.*—The best method of
making the bed is to put on above the mattress first, a large rubber sheet; second, a linen sheet; third, a small rubber sheet;.
fourth, a linen sheet; fifth, a large hip pad; sixth, a small hip
pad; seventh, the upper sheet, and eighth, the blankets.   The
lower sheets should be pinned at each corner to the mattress and
the pads to these sheets to prevent wrinkling.   The large rubber
sheet should cover the upper surface of the mattress completely.
The small rubber sheet should be placed so that it covers the middle of the side of the bed upon which the patient is to lie.   The hip-
pad should be placed on the linen sheet so as to be over the small
rubber sheet.   This method will keep the mattress perfectly clean
and after labor the bed does not have to be changed, i. e., to make
the bed clean, only the pad, one linen and one rubber sheet need to
be removed and a clean hip pad applied.   A simpler method is to
put above the mattress first, newspapers; second, a small rubber or
oil-cloth sheet over the middle of the side of the bed upon which
the patient is to lie; third, a linen sheet, and fourth, a hip pad so
placed on the linen sheet as to be over the rubber one.   In this
method, care should be used to get the rubber or oil-cloth well
over the edge of the near side of the bed so that the edge of the
mattress will not be soiled.   (Most nurses put the oil-cloth about
six inches in from the edge of the bed and as a result the mattress is often soiled.)

The usual hospital method is first, a large rubber sheet; second, an ordinary linen sheet; third, a rubber draw sheet, fourth,
a linen draw sheet; fifth, an ordinary linen sheet; sixth, a rubber
draw sheet; seventh, a linen draw sheet.   The rubber draw sheet
is from a yard to a yard and a half in width, i. e., lengthwise of

the bed and reaches across the middle of the bed. The linen draw sheet is of the same size and situation as the rubber draw sheet, but is made by folding an ordinary linen sheet to one-third of its length. After labor the upper linen and rubber draw sheets and the ordinary linen sheet beneath them are removed. The objections to this method in private practice are the width of the beds and the amount of washing. The draw linen sheets are used in place of the hip pads and have to be frequently changed. If the hip pads were used above the draw sheet, this would be the ideal method.

(3) The Pitchers, Bowls and Other Vessels.—The pitchers, bowls, soap dish, bed-pan, slop jar *(or pail)* and all other vessels that may be needed for the labor should be thoroughly cleansed with scrub brush, soap and water inside and out.

(4) Sterilized Hot and Cold Water.—Plenty of hot, boiled water should be kept in readiness in a teakettle and a pitcher or in some other clean vessels. A pitcher should be filled with boiling water covered with a sterile cloth and placed out of doors to cool so that there will be plenty of sterile cold water.

(5) Articles that will be (or may be) Needed to Put on the Bed, the Mother and the Baby after Labor.—All articles that will be *(or may be)* needed to put on the bed, the mother, or the baby after labor should be placed where they will be warm, clean and easy to find. For the bed, should be placed two linen sheets; for the mother, one large and one small hip pad, several vulvar pads, a T-bandage, an abdominal bandage, a breast bandage, a shirt and a night gown, and for the baby, an old piece of flannel or woolen cloth and a diaper, its clothing and box.

When the Physician Should be Called.—When the "pains" occur every ten minutes and are getting so severe that the patient feels unable to stay up any longer, if the membranes have ruptured, or if there is hemorrhage, the doctor should be called at once. When there is danger of an abnormal condition being present or if the patient has had rapid labors, the physician should be sent for as soon as the onset of labor is determined.

Epithelial Tumors. In a critical study of 468 cases (*Pro-gressive Medicine*) Bloodgood has been struck, first, by the ignorance of patients in delaying to seek advice until a late period after the onset of the tumor; second, the procrastination of the physician in delaying operative intervention. He is also impressed with the frequent applications of various caustics which apparently have aggravated the local condition. Single papillary warts and verruca senilis should be removed whenever they come under the observation of the physician. The multiple papillary warts in the young apparently have no tendency to become malignant, and, as a rule, if left alone disappear. Unusual growth or ulceration is an indication for their removal. Ulceration in multiple areas of keratosis (senile warts) is an indication for their prompt removal.

Occult Blood in the Stools. Hemorrhage too slight to be directly visible (*Progressive Medicine*) is constantly present in cancer of the gastro-intestinal tract; intermittently present in ulcer; occasionally present in organic and spastic pyloric stenosis. To exclude food hematin, keep the patient for several days on a diet free from all sorts of meat and fish, and render the stools soft with some mild laxative, such as Carlsbad salts. Mix two or three gm. of the stools, says Weber, thoroughly with twenty cc. of water, and remove the fats carefully by shaking with twenty cc. of ether. Shake the aqueous residue with one-third its volume of acetic acid, and then with ten cc. of ether—a few drops of absolute alcohol hastens the separation of the ether. To two cc. of this ethereal extract are now added ten drops of freshly made (1:25) tincture of guaaic, with ten to twenty drops of old ozonized oil of turpentine (or hydrogen peroxide) drop by drop. If blood is present, after a few seconds an intense blue (not green or greenish-blue) color will appear in the mixture. Care should be taken that no portion of the ethereal extract touch the skin of the hand, as the fatty acids of sweat give a similar reaction. Boas advises a control test (Klunge's) with the acetic acid and ether extract, the ozonized turpentine and ten to fifteen drops of a solution of aloin in seventy per cent alcohol, getting if positive a bright red color—negative yellow.

DENVER MEDICAL TIMES

THOMAS H. HAWKINS, A.M., M.D., EDITOR AND PUBLISHER.

COLLABORATORS:

Henry O. Marcy, M.D., Boston.
Thaddeus A. Reamy, M.D., Cincinnati.
Nicholas Senn, M.D., Chicago.
Joseph Price, M.D., Philadelphia.
Franklin H. Martin, M.D., Chicago.
William Oliver Moore, M.D., New York.
L. S. McMurtry, M.D., Louisville.
Thomas B. Eastman, M.D., Indianapolis, Ind.
G. Law, M.D., Greeley, Colo.

S. H. Pinkerton, M.D., Salt Lake City
Flavel B. Tiffany, M.D., Kansas City.
Erskine M. Bates, M.D;. New York.
E. C. Gehrung, M.D, St. Louis.
Graeme M. Hammond, M.D, New York.
James A. Lydston, M.D., Chicago.
Leonard Freeman, M.D., Denver.
Carey K. Fleming, M.D., Denver, Colo.

Subscriptions, $1.00 per year in advance; Single Copies, 10 cents.

Address all Communications to Denver Medical Times, 1740 Welton Street, Denver, Colo.
We will at all times be glad to give space to well written articles or items of interest to the profession.
[Entered at the Postoffice of Denver, Colorado, as mail matter of the Second Class.]

EDITORIAL DEPARTMENT

THE CARE OF THE NOSE, THROAT AND EARS.

By far the most prevalent disease in America is naso-pharyngeal catarrh, the causes of which, briefly stated, are a changeful climate, dust and high winds, and the hot-house mode of indoor life of most of the population. Of these three anatomic regions, the nose is nearly always affected first. Nasal inflammation spreads upward to the ears and downward to the pharynx and larynx. Obstructive deformities of the nose lead to mouth breathing, dry throat, the aspiration of air from the naso-pharynx and ear, and eventually more or less deafness. Such anomalies should receive prompt surgical attention.

Adenoids are a common cause of earache and deafness. They obstruct breathing and drainage, lower the physical health, and serve as hotbeds for germs.

In the majority of instances, probably, the nose is the primary portal of infection, and Jacobi's custom of daily cleansing the nasal passage with a simple saline solution of the density of the blood, seems to be an admirable prophylactic measure. In using the nasal douche, the side most obstructed ought to be irrigated first, and care should be exercised not to blow the nose forcibly while holding the nostrils with the fingers, lest mucus be blown into the middle ear and otitis result. The instillation of some bland oil following the douche helps greatly in keeping the air passages open for respiration in the case of acute congestive conditions.

The chief underlying cause of coryza is a depressed state of the nervous system, resulting in sluggishness of the heat-producing centers. In the way of prevention, rational clothing, avoidance of draughts, care of the digestive functions, saline laxatives and the maintenance of nerve tone with strychnin, are recommended. A brisk, dry massage of the limbs morning and evening is an excellent prophylactic measure.

Ear troubles are nearly always due to some dyscrasia or to nasal disorders and neglected colds. The complicating otitis media of scarlatina, influenza and other infections is best prevented by careful antiseptic cleansing of the nose and throat.

Intellectual backwardness in school children is in most instances due to defective hearing. If an infant at the beginning of its second year pays little attention to sounds and shows no evidence of beginning speech, it is pretty surely a deaf-mute and should receive persistent special instruction. The cruel punishment of boxing the ears may cause rupture of the drum membrane and temporary or permanent impairment of hearing. The household usage of pouring sweet oil into the external auditory canal favors the occurrence of myringitis and otitis externa. An eminent aurist once made the sage remark that the layman should never put anything into his ear smaller than his elbow. Inflammation of the middle ear occasionally follows exposure to strong winds or to cold water in bathing. A little plug of cotton in either ear is an effectual preventive, but it should be promptly removed. In case of a perforated ear drum, such a protective barrier might prevent the entrance of water into the middle ear, causing labyrinthine vertigo, or the so-called "swimmer's cramps."

THE PLAGUES.

We of the present civilized places and times can hardly imagine the horrors of those days, some centuries ago, when pestilence stalked unchallenged through the land and counted his victims by the million; when men imprisoned themselves in their own house for fear of contagion; when sons and daughters fled from their own afflicted parents, and in point of fact the dead were left to bury the dead. The cruel quarantine, the starving exiles, the fearful death scenes, and over all the dread of an inscrutable malign divinity, seem now almost like some monstrous nightmare—yet it was all too true. Had not sanitary science discovered in large measure the causes and means of prevention of infectious diseases, the world would be more full of woes than ever before, and dire diseases now almost unknown, would continue to reap their ghastly harvests at more or less regular intervals.

To avert epidemics, says Emmert, the Greeks and Romans erected statues to Apollo and Esculapius. They consulted the Sibylline books, drove nails into the walls of the temple of Jupiter Capitolinus, and performed the Lectisterne ceremonies. Later, in the Christian Era, public seasons of repentance were held and religious structures founded to appease the supposed divine wrath.

Palliative Treatment of External Hemorrhoids. Gant's method is as follows: Avoid stimulants and condiments; keep bowels open with Vichy, Hunyadi, Freidrichshall, etc: calomel parvules, for congested liver; wash parts with castile soap and water. If pile contains a hard clot (thrombotic), apply frequently a lotion (either hot or cold) of three grains of morphine, twelve grains of calomel, one ounce vaseline, four drams liquor plumbi subacetatis, two and one-half drams of laudanum and water to make four ounces. Hot poultices relieve pain and reduce inflammation.

Cough of Beginning Tuberculosis. Ferrand advises the use of repeated sinapisms on sides of chest and back, alternating with revulsive frictions with ammoniacal liniment. Give every hour a mixture of tincture of aconite and syrup of poppy, as needed for cough and insomnia. Apply a blister under the clavicle of the diseased side, and if symptoms are persistent use the actual cautery. Limit diet for a time strictly to soup and milk. Avoid hot, dusty air. Keep the temperature and humidity constant.

EDITORIAL ITEMS.

Mr. E. L. Lomax, General Passenger and Ticket Agent of the U. P. R. R. Co. and his representatives, called on the Editor of the DENVER MEDICAL TIMES and we had a very pleasant visit. We will, through the DENVER MEDICAL TIMES, aid in every way possible, Mr. Lomax and the other officials of the road in bringing a large representation of the Medical Profession to Portland, Oregon to attend the next meeting of the American Medical Association. The surest, safest, most comfortable and elegant way to reach Portland is over the U. P. Road.

For Migraiue. Beale recommends rest, starvation, tea or coffee, acids, warmth and counter-irritation.

Acute Bronchitis. Tyson finds Dover's powder a useful remedy in the dose of $2\frac{1}{2}$ grains every two hours.

First Week of Whooping Cough. Thornton prescriber one-eighth grain of thymol in a dram of aromatic elixir in water three times a day.

Pressure Cough. Gelsemium is said to be beneficial in reflex coughs from irritation of the laryngeal nerves.

For Quinsy. Easby prescribes sodium salicylate, gr. viiss.-x in syrup of acacia and cinnamon water every three hours.

For Uterine Cough. Shoemaker prescribes potassium bromide gr. v-x in two drams of wild cherry syrup every four to six hours.

Coughs Due to Pregnancy. Jewett gives sedatives, such as a pill of valerianate of iron, quinine and zinc after meals; or cannabis indica or bromides.

Rheumatic Cardiac Hypertrophy. Thomson reccommends tincture of chloride of iron with strychnine, or potassium iodide and arsenic.

Vomiting in Measles. Louis Starr advises the drinking of tepid water until the stomach is cleaned out, then apply a weak mustard plaster to the epigastrium. The diet often needs to be carefully restricted.

Vesicular Emphysema. Ringer recommends tincture of cubebs, one-half to one dram in a half tumbler of linseed tea thrice daily.

Chronic Catarrhal Pneumonia. Butler lauds the use of apomorphine, 1–40 to 1–20 grain every three or four hours, for the dry, hacking cough.

Nicotine Poisoning. When alarming symptoms of depression occur in those learning to use the "weed," Tyson advises the recumbent posture and the use of strychnine, heat and stimulants.

Meningitis. Thos. S. Latimer recommends a dark room and perfect quiet; morphine hypodermically; bromides; light food; stimulants per rectum.

Shock and Collapse. Warren uses opium hypodermically or by the rectum; nitroglycerine in doses of 1–200 grain; strychnine; aromatic spirit of ammonia.

Stomach Symptoms of Cerebrospinal Meningitis. Delafield gives dilute hydrocyanic acid m. ii-v and sodium bicarbonate gr. v every three or four hours.

Uvulitis. Levy prescribes a teaspoonful every two hours of a solution of one dram of tincture of iron to the ounce of glycerin. Scarification may be needed for edema.

Coryza. Potter states that a spray of five per cent carbolic acid solution in a steam atomizer often prevents as well as cures a cough due to a common cold.

Relaxed Palate and Uvula. Sajous orders a lozenge every three hours, composed of two grains of alum, one grain of borax, two grains of rose leaves and sufficient sugar, acacia and black currant paste.

Subacute Laryngitis. Sajous gives every three hours a lozenge containing one-half grain of cubebs, two grains of Dover's powder and sufficient licorice, sugar and acacia.

For Beginning Pneumonia. Shoemaker prescribes: ℞ Vini antimon. m. iv; vini ipecac. m. viii; syrupi tolu m. xxvi; aquae laurocerasi m. xvi; aquam chloroformi q. s.: A dessertspoonful every four hours.

Mediastinal Tumors. In addition to the symptomatic use of anodynes, arsenic, says Anders, may influence sarcomatous and ymphadenomatous growths favorably though temporarily.

Hepatic Colic. Tyson mentions with approval the administration of succinate of sodium, five grains t. i. d. between attacks of hepatic colic.

Exophthalmic Goiter. Tyson advises rest and protection from excitement; bromides and digitalis (or aconite if no cardiac lesion and pulse is good and strong); ergot—a rational remedy; iron, if anemia.

Neurasthenic Nausea and Vomiting. Ewald recommends small pieces of ice with two or three drops of tincture of nux vomica; potassium bromide and iron; Neptune's girdle; galvanization of sympathetic.

Vomiting from Cardiac Weakness. A. V. Meigs recommends morphine sulphate, 1–16 grain with two minims of chloroform in a dram of compound tincture of cardamom every two hours. If the vomiting is persistent, Osler says stop the solid food and give small bits of ice.

Pertussis. In severe whooping cough, to prevent vomiting Kilmer advises the use of an abdominal belt. Ringer gives two to six grains of alum every three hours. Hare recommends a teaspoonful or so of milk after each paroxysm of coughing.

Dietl's Crises. For acute attacks of pain and vomiting from twisting of ureter in floating kidney (*Gould and Pyle's Cyclopedia*), place the patient in bed, use hot applications over the abdomen, order opiates, and try to replace the affected organ.

Cyclical Vomiting of Children. For this toxic neurosis, Pepper employed calomel and bismuth, or potassium bromide or chloral, or small doses of laudanum by the rectum; hot brandy for collapse; weak mustard or spice plaster for pain.

Cerebral Tumor. Thornton recommends the saturated solution of potassium iodide, ten drops in water after meals, rapidly increasing to full physiologic effects. In syphilitic cases he employs the oil of mercury (gray solution), five minims hypodermically every second day.

Acute Dilatation of Stomach. Bruce advises supportive measures; the use of the stomach-tube one or more times as early in the case as possible; rectal feeding—nothing by the mouth till the vomiting is nearly or quite controlled.

Gastric Crises of Tabes Dorsalis. Tyson mentions phena-cetin, acetanilid, exalgin, antipyrin; cocaine (1-6 to ¼ grain) or extract of cannabis indica (¼ to ½ grain) hypodermically; morphine as a last resort.

Vomiting in Fevers. This symptom, says Waring, is often effectually relieved by small blisters over the epigastric region. Weak solutions of hydrochloric acid or effervescing soda powders are sometimes quite effective.

Hysterical Vomiting. Weir Mitchell emphasizes firmness and suggestion and he orders enemata to move the bowels if needed. Bartholow employed the following recipe: ℞ Ext. belladonnæ, ext. physostigmatis, ext. nucis vomicæ, aloini aa. gr. ¼; ferri sulphat. exsic. gr. i: One pill at bed time.

Opium Sickness. According to Garrod, this annoying drug-effect is best relieved by tea, coffee, caffeine and effervescing salines. Passiflora is said to be useful alike for this condition and after excesses in liquors.

Early Acute Bronchitis. Hare favors the use of mucilage of acacia with flaxseed infusion, licorice and lemon juice for hacking cough in children or adults. In more chronic cases he has the supraclacicular spaces painted with tincture of iodine.

Hacking Cough of Incipient Pulmonary Tuberculosis. Knopf directs to suppress this dry, tickling cough by discipline or by sips of cold water, orange juice, or milk, small pieces of ice or tablets of Iceland moss, or by holding the breath. Apomorphine in small doses is also effective.

Laryngeal Tuberculosis. A favorite method with Levy has been to spray with two per cent cocaine or eucaine; insufflations of orthoform and of ten grains morphine sulphate with one dram each of iodoform and powdered acacia; lactic acid frictions for ulcerations.

Chronic Laryngitis. Levy directs to remove any nasal cause, and improve local and daily hygiene. Locally cleanse with spray of alkaline solution, followed by swabbing with a solution of silver nitrate, gr. x-xl. ad. ʒi. solution.

Nasal Irritation. This is the most common cause of night coughs in children. Cleanse the nose with alkaline wash or with milk containing a little salt, then instil a dropperful of some bland oil into each nostril.

"Stomach Cough" of Pharyngeal Catarrh. This is manifested by frequent hacking and expectoration of tenacious mucus containing dark particles. It usually occurs in alcoholic subjects. Ewald advises to neutralize or lessen the acidity of the stomach contents.

Acute Pharyngitis. Biddle swabs the throat with alum solution fifteen to twenty grains to the ounce of water. Sajous has used lozenges of sodium borate and potassium chlorate, two grains each with sufficient acacia and black currant paste: One every two hours when throat is dry.

Edema Glottidis. Eichhorst advises the sucking of ice, and ice compresses to the throat; vigorous catharsis in hydremic edema; scarification with a curved bistoury covered with adhesive plaster as far as tip, or tearing of mucous membrane of epiglottis with sharp finger nail; tracheotomy and artificial respiration if need be.

Spasmodic Croup. J. Lewis Smith has recommended demulcent drinks; warm mustard foot baths for restlessness; syrup of ipecac (ten drops) and paregoric (two drops) every half hour for three or four doses for cough; inhalations of a spray of glycerine and water; camphorated oil rubbed over the neck.

Alimentation in Scarlet Fever. Milk is the best food (*Gould and Pyle's Cyclopedia*) three to four ounces every three hours—diminish the quantity and dilute with barley water or Vichy if tympanites and undigested casein in the stools. If there is distaste for milk, substitute koumiss, matzoon or farinaceous gruels.

Varices of Lingual Tonsil. Kyle describes these as bluish, tortuous cords, most frequent in alcoholics and with menstrual disturbances or in pregnancy or at menopause. The patient complains of a peculiar sensation like a moving body in the throat. He directs to relieve underlying causes of venous stagnation, and puncture dilated vessels here and there with the galvanocautery.

Laryngismus Stridulus. Bartholow claimed to abort or prevent attacks by a full dose (five to fifteen grains) of chloral. Hosmer A. Johnson recommends hot wet cloths applied to neck and chest or a hot bath with cold wet cloths on the head; non-depressant emetics; sodium bromide, three to five grains every three to six hours to prevent recurrence.

Hydronephrosis with Acute Symptoms. *Gould and Pyle's Cyclopedia* directs to aspirate—on left side, just below last inter-costal space—on right side, midway between last rib and crest of ilium. When repeated aspirations fail, nephrotomy is indicated —stitch edges of kidney to surface—and nephrectomy if the one kidney is extensively damaged and the other is in fair condition, or if a permanent suppurating fistula is present.

For Neurotic Vomiting. Meisl employs 1–10 grain of menthol and ten grains of sodium bicarbonate in capsules t. i. d. Quinine hydrobromate (Dad's pills), two to eight grains per dose, is sometimes useful. Wm. Gay commends the shower bath and valerian and other anti-spasmodics. Beard and Rockwell utilizes galvanization of the sympathetic or the pneumogastric (cathode over stomach, anode on last cervical vertebra) or strong faradiza-tion through the stomach.

Chronic Granular Pharyngitis. The glycerite of tannin locally applied at short intervals for a considerable period often gives relief. Causal conditions should be corrected. Brunton recommends the occasional use of blue pill. As an alterative treatment, Thorowgood prescribes liquor sodii arseniatis in two minim doses in plain or Vichy water; it may be combined with two or three grains of sodium iodide.

Persistent Vomiting from Any Cause. Hare recommends a mustard plaster over the stomach or an ice-bag to the nape of neck, lumbar spine or epigastrium; peptonized milk or milk and lime-water freely, or koumiss in teaspoonful or dessertspoonful feedings every fifteen minutes to an hour; iced champagne; nutri-ent enemas when vomiting is absolutely persistent.

Dry Pleurisy. To abort an incipient attack Bartholow relied on a dose of $\frac{1}{4}$ grain of morphine and fifteen or twenty grains of quinine. When established he gave every hour or two in water two drops of tincture of aconite root and six drops of deodorated tincture of opium. Butler lauds coniine in the dose of 1–10 to one minim. Hartshorne prescribes: ℞ Hydrarg. chlor. mitis gr. ss.; pulv. opii. gr. $\frac{1}{4}$–$\frac{1}{2}$; antimon. et potass. tart. gr. $\frac{1}{8}$: A pow-der every three to five hours.

Reflex Coughs. Bruce recommends ammonia and squill for cardiac valvular disease. Bartholow has found potassium bromide serviceable in renal coughs. Brunton employs dilute hydrocyanic acid for reflex cough arising from gastric irritation. Bartholow uses cerium oxalate (dose two to five grains in pill or suspended in mucilage) for cough associated with vomiting. In mitral regurgitation with cough, said Loomis, one-half ounce of infusion of digitalis every two hours for twenty-four to forty-eight hours, is often required.

Pleurisy with Effusion. Generally speaking, paracentesis is required in from ten days to three weeks. A favorite remedy is sodium salicylate, sixty to ninety grains daily, adding caffeine in case of weak heart. Ringer recommends cantharidal collodion, applied over a small area and repeated after healing. Shoemaker gives ten grains of potassium iodide in thirty minims each of glycerine and syrup of iodide of iron four times a day. In chronic cases Bartholow employs potasssium iodide, five grains in milk every four hours, and painting one-third of the affected side each day with tincture of iodine.

Acute Laryngitis. Bartholow employed a trituration of equal parts of chloral hydrate and camphor, painted over the larynx to allay spasmodic cough. Hare prescribes: ℞ Acidi hydrocyan. dil. m. iis; morph. sulph. gr. 1–12; syr. pruni. virg. q. s.: Levy recommends heroin, 1–12 grain every four hours; a spray of Dobell's solution, followed by a one per cent. spray of suprarenal extract, or insufflations of equal parts of powdered suprarenal extract and powdered acacia. He has the patient use inhalations of three grains each of powdered camphor and menthol to the cup of steaming water, and later gives an expectorant mixture of five grains ammonium chloride, twenty m. paregoric, and syrup of licorice to make a dram—to be taken every three hours.

Uremic Vomiting. Huchard advises lavage, saline purgatives and hot baths. Taylor recommends effervescing mixtures and dilute hydrocyanic acid or tincture of iodine, m. iii-v every hour. Bruce directs to withhold food entirely for a time and give only water (sometimes in effervescing form with a little spirit when pulse is very low, or as iced water taken through a glass tube); thereafter koumiss or peptonized milk by the teaspoonful or tablespoonful, or enemas of peptonized milk and weak milky tea. As stomach sedatives he employs dilute prussic acid, creosote, tincture of iodine in water, or nitro-glycerine; also two grains each of calomel and sugar of milk under the tongue, and epigastric applications.

Chronic Vomiting of Infants. Goodhart and Starr advise careful restriction of diet (artificial human milk, digested milk, milk and lime water, milk and barley water, whey and cream or cream alone, veal broth, etc.—everything cold); patient, persistent trial of each kind of food; spoon feeding of very little food in worst cases; calomel, 1–16 grain on tongue every three or four hours; Fowler's solution ½ drop in a dram of water t. i. d.; five drops of brandy every hour in bad cases.

Peritoneal Bands and Adhesions. Lejars calls renewed attention to those not infrequent cases where gastrointestinal symptoms followed some time after an apparently slight injury to the abdomen. These symptoms include rebellious colics, vomiting, constipation or diarrhea, without other evidences of organic disease. When the presence of adhesions simulates ulcer, gall-stones, etc., operation with loosening of the adhesions is indicated.

Hyperexcitability of Gastric Mucous Nembrane. Hare recommends cocaine, two or three drops of a four per cent, aqueous solution every fifteen minutes until ten drops are taken, or tincture of aconite, two to five drops in a little water every thirty minutes until pulse shows weakness—patient should lie down; or a powder every half hour of eighteen grains of bismuth subnitrate and two or three drops of tincture of aconite.

Primary Tuberculosis of the Hypertrophical Pharyngeal Tonsil. Donald M. Barstow (*Medical Record*, Oct. 7), reports a case probably of this nature. The patient had a throaty cough of two years standing with chest pains, sweating, and a large number of tubercli bacilli in the sputum. After removal of the tuberculous adenoid, there was immediate improvement of the symptoms and disappearance of the bacilli.

A Coated Tongue. A practical and important point, says J. Dutton Steele (*Progressive Medicine*) is that the lingual dermatitis giving rise to a coated tongue may persist for some time after the original disturbance has subsided; hence we need not always wait for the tongue to clear before commencing a more liberal diet.

Gastrutus if Chronic Alcoholism. Ringer recommends drop doses of wine of ipecac every hour or thrice daily. Shoemaker prescribes: ℞ Tinct. belladonnæ m. i; tinct. nucis vomicæ m. iiss; tinct. dioscoreae villosæ m. x; syr. zingiberis q. s.: A teaspoonful in water every four hours. After an alcoholic debauch, Thornton employs ten to sixty drops of dilute hydrochloric acid in water every two hours.

Chronic Gastric Catarrh of Infants. A. D. Blackader instructs to give no food by the mouth; remove all extraneous sources of irritation; sedative enemas containing small doses of opium or bromide with chloral hydrate twice daily for nervous erethism; lavage of stomach, or a combination of Rochelle salts with a small amount of sodium bicarbonate in hot water early every morning, or equal parts of Vichy and hot water once or twice daily.

Morphine in Chronic Renal Disease. In the discussion of the treatment of chronic renal disease at the last meeting of the British Medical Association *(Progressive Medicine)* most speakers alluded to the dangers which might follow the use of morphine, but at the same time pointed out that it was of great service in the treatment of some forms of uremia, especially uremic convulsions.

Overloaded Stomach in Infants. Goodhart and Starr advise to empty stomach, if not already so, by emetic of ipecac (one dram of wine or five grains of powder), followed by a dose of castor oil or one-half grain of calomel and one grain of rhubarb. Give also equal parts of cinnamon water and lime water, a dram at a dose. Restrict diet for several days, giving a little sodium bicarbonate and potassium citrate three or four times a day.

Irritable Stomach. Bartholow used the following formula: ℞ Acidi carbol. gr. ss.; bismuth subnit. gr. xv; mucil. acaciae ʒi; aquam menth pip. q.s.: A tablespoonful every two to four hours. When due to improper feeding in children, Shoemaker employed: ℞ Bismuth subnit. gr. iii; sodii bicarb., pulv. rhei aa. gr. i.: A powder every four hours.

Editorial Items continued on Page 508

BOOKS.

PRACTICAL PEDIATRICS.. A Manual of the Medical and Surgical Diseases of Infancy and Childhood. By Dr. E. Graetzer, Editor of the "Centralblatt Fur Kinderheilkunde" and the "Excerpta Medica." Authorized translation, with numerous Additions and Notes, by Herman B. Sheffield. M.D., Instructor in Diseases of Children, and Attending Pediatrist (O.P.-D.) New York Post-Graduate Medical School and Hospital; Visiting Pediatrist in the Metropolitan Hospital and Dispensary, etc. Pages XII.-544. Crown Octavo. Flexible cloth, Round Corners. Price, $3.00 net. F. A. Davis Company, Publishers, 1914-16 Cherry Street, Philadelphia.

This compact volume comprises a vast amount of useful instruction on the diseases of infants and children, arranged systematically, and clearly presented by the American translator, who has made many interpolations of his own. The text is noteworthy for attention given to deviations from type. Also deserving of special mention is the extensive second part of the book, which deals with the materia medica and therapeutics of infancy and childhood. To the younger practitioners this work should prove particularly helpful.

A PRACTICAL TREATISE ON NERVOUS EXHAUSTION (NEURASTHENIA), Its SYMPTOMS, NATURE, SEQUENCES, TREATMENT. By George M. Beard, M.D., A.M. Edited, with notes and additions, by A. D. Rockwell, A M., M.D., Professor of Electrotherapeutics in the New York Post-Graduate Medical School and Hospital. Fifth Edition. Enlarged. Price, $2.00. New York. E. B. Treat & Co., 241-243 West 23rd street. 1905.

This standard monograph of the late Dr. Beard on the "American Disease" has been revised and enlarged by Dr. Rockwell, who, *inter alia*, adds a chapter on the neuron theory in relation to neuroses. He makes more clear the distinctions between lithemia and neurasthenia. He is a strong advocate of electrical treatment, both for its psychic effect and because of "its ability to restore the conductibility of the neuron that has become resistant to the nerve current."

BACTERIOLOGY AND SURGICAL TECHNIC FOR NURSES. By Emily M. A. Stoney, Superintendent of the Training School for Nurses, St. Anthony's Hospital, Rock Island, Ill. Second Edition. Thoroughly Revised and Enlarged by Frederic Richardson Griffith, M.D., of New York. Illustrated. Price, $1.25. Philadelphia, New York, London. W. B. Saunders & Co. 1905.

The reviser found little to alter in this excellent *vade mecum* for nurses. Among the additions are numerous illustrations; a chapter upon certain minor procedures, one dealing with obstetrical nursing, another upon bandaging and dressings, and a final chapter concerning the nurse herself. A glossary of the technical terms and phrases used throughout the text has been added also.

A TEXT-BOOK OF LEGAL MEDICINE. By Frank Winthrop Draper, A.M., M.D., Professor of Legal Medicine in Harvard University; Medical Examiner for the County of Suffolk, Massachusetts. Octavo volume of 573 pages, fully illustrated. Philadelphia, New York, London. W. B. Saunders & Co., 1905. Cloth, $4.00 net.

This is one of the best books on the subject of legal medicine for the use of general practioners. The author has had an exceptionally large experience in medical matters, in his service as Medical Examiner for the City of Boston for the past twenty-six years, his investigations during this period having covered nearly eight thousand deaths under suspicion of violence. His long teaching career, moreover, has enabled him to present facts and procedures clearly and concisely. The interest and value of general statements are much enhanced by frequent details of illustrative cases. The work is quite up to date, as shown by the attention given to special tests for human blood. Many of the illustrations have been prepared expressly for this volume.

A COMPEND OF THE PRACTICE OF MEDICINE. By Daniel E. Hughes, M.D., Late Chief Resident Physician, Philadelphia Hospital. Seventh revised edition, edited, revised and in parts rewritten. By Samuel Horton Brown, M.D., Assistant Dermatologist, Philadelphia Hospital. Illustrated, 12mo. 779 pages. Price, $2.50 net. Philadelphia. P. Blakiston's Son & Co., 1012 Walnut Street, 1904.

The seventh edition of this deservedly popular work has been completely revised, rewritten and reset, with considerable enlargement. Introductory notes have been placed at the beginning of each section, and several specialties on clinical and physical diagnosis have been added. The contents are fully indexed. The book as it now stands is very comprehensive, including a section on mental diseases and another, quite complete under the circumstances, on skin diseases.

A COMPEND OF THE DISEASES OF THE EYE AND REFRACTION, INCLUDING TREATMENT AND SURGERY. By George M. Gould, A.M., M.D., Editor of *American Medicine;* and Walter L. Pyle, A.M., M.D., Assistant Surgeon to Wills Eye Hospital, Philadelphia. Third edition, revised and corrected, 109 illustrations, several of which are in colors. Price, $1.00 net. Philadelphia. P. Blakiston's Son & Co., 1012 Walnut Street. 1904.

This is one of the best of Blakiston's quiz compends. Facts are carefully stated, and the book contains a great deal of useful matter, and is handsomely illustrated, considering its low price.

PNEUMONIA AND PNEUMOCOCCUS INFECTIONS. By Robert B. Preble, A.B., M.D., Professor of Medicine, Northwestern University. Illustrated. Price, $1.00. Chicago. Floyd J. Head & Co., 40 Dearborn Street, 1905.

This brochure deals with an extremely important subject, and is well worth a careful perusal by every general practitioner. The author is wisely conservative, and has no specific treatment for disease, yet he reminds us of many valuable points, diagnostic, therapeutic, etc. The text is illustrated with a number of instructive clinical charts.

A BOOK ABOUT DOCTORS. By John Cordy Jefferson, Author of "The Real Lord Byron," "The Real Shelley," "A Book About Lawyers," etc., 1904. The Saalfield Publishing Co., New York, Akron, Ohio, and Chicago.

The writer of this volume of the already celebrated "Doctor's Recreation Series" has collected and here presented in a highly attractive and readable form a great mass of quaint and curious medical ana. The following titles of a few of the twentyseven chapters that make up the contents of the book will suffice in a measure to show the general nature of the text: Something about Sticks and rather less about Wigs; Quacks; Fees; Bleeding; Imagination as a Remedial Power; The Quarrels of Physicians;

The Loves of Physicians; The Country Medical Man. On the whole the work may be ranked with the elder Disraeli's "Curiosities of Literature."

ANNALS OF SURGERY. The December, 1904 number of this standard publication completes the twentieth year of its existence, always under the editorial management of Dr. Lewis Stephen Pilcher. This memorial number contains nearly 300 pages of valuable original matter, many of the articles being accompanied by colored plates and other drawings. The *Annals* has ever been a mirror and exemplar of modern scientific surgery.

Hepatic Insufficiency. Abbott (*Alkaloidal Clinic*) says that cases of hepatic insufficiency should receive a mixed diet consisting largely of vegetables, bread stuffs and cereals, with well-cooked meat, not more than once a day, plenty of eggs and milk, as little fat as possible, and no spices, condiments or alcoholic beverages.

Absorption from the Stomach. K. H. Baas (quoted in *Medical News*) seems to prove that the old salivary test for absorption from the stomach with a capsule of potassium iodide, is of no value. Morphine causes a spasm of the pylorus, and on giving a moderate dose of this drug before administering the iodide, the iodine reaction is greatly delayed, showing that the potassium salt is absorbed from the duodenum, and not from the stomach.

Vomiting of Cardiac Origin. Bruce says: Stop usual drugs for several hours or a whole day, trusting entirely to a teaspoonful of brandy and water at intervals, or feed by the bowel and give digitalin and strychnine tentatively under the skin. Allow small sips of very hot water or champagne, and the cautious administration of dilute prussic acid, bismuth subnitrate, cerium oxalate or calomel. In less urgent cases use strong meat essences, peptonized milk or koumiss in small quantities frequently repeated, stimulants in sparkling forms, effervescing potassium bromide and small doses of calomel. Do not give up digitalis lightly, but change form of preparation or substitute strophanthus or caffeine.

SELECTIONS.

NUTRIENTS.—Nutrition spelt with a big N should be one of the largest words in the vocabulary of the physician. The weak, the delicate, and those who are below par from overwork or imperfect development should be nourished oftentimes to the point, almost we were disposed to say of "stuffing." Of course the proper nourishment of our patient at all stages of disease is important, and in the acute period for a time the proper nutrition really means judicious starvation or the withholding of food until the digestive tract can be placed in a condition to do its work. Beef tea, time out of mind, has been one of the chief stand-bys of the sick room, but as a matter of fact, we know now that which we should have known long ago, that the average beef tea is a fraud, and that it is no more nutritious than a weak toddy would be; that it is practically nothing but water with a few soluble salts of the beef contained therein.

The only way that we can hope to give the elements of nourishment in a concentrated form, represented by beef fibre, is to order a commercial extract of beef, and in doing so we should be sure that the product which we order is made by a skillful pharmacist. The Charles N. Crittenden Company has for years been furnishing to the profession a most efficient product of beef under the name of Colden's Liquid Beef Tonic, which is most valuable in all forms of wasting diseases and in some cases of convalescence from severe illness. It is indeed a food medicine, which is promptly assimilated, and which interrupts and prevents the breaking down of vital tissues; and one great advantage to the patient is that it is agreeable to the taste and acceptable to the most delicate stomach.

Dr. Geo. E. Pettey, who had a retreat in Denver for the treatment of alcoholic and drug addicted cases, has opened a similar institution in Oakland, Cal., with Dr. C. L. Case as Medical Instructor. Dr. Pettey is conducting his business along strictly ethical lines and is entitled to the respect and support of the medical fraternity.

Hagee's Cordial Cod Liver Oil Compound is very highly recommended for all cases of lung trouble, as a restorative in children, as well as adults, after pneumonia and la grippe. In bronchitis in old people it is excellent. It is palatable, easily assimilated, and is a good tissue builder. Often where other preparations of cod liver oil have been taken without the least benefit, Hagee's will be found to do the work.

THE CARABANA PRIZE CONTEST.—*To the Editor:* Believing that many of your readers are keen critics of the advertising columns of your valued journal, it has occurred to us that they might be willing to enter into a little contest which we are organizing and for which we shall award $50 in cash prizes, as follows:

A committee of three physicians will award, not later than July 1st, a first prize of $25, a second prize of $15, and a third prize of $10, to the doctor sending in, prior to June 1st, the best five reasons why physicians should and do daily prescribe our Carabana aperient water. The five reasons should be stated as concisely as possible, not exceeding twenty-five words each. All that is necessary for your readers to qualify will be that they are personally familar with the various uses in which Carabana water is put, and that they write from personal experience.

In order to ensure fairness, physicians competing must sign their reasons with a "nom de plume," and in a separate envelope enclose their professional card, on which the "nom de plume" should also appear. Address: Carabana Contest, 2 and 4 Stone Street, New York.   Yours very truly,

GEO. S. WALLAU.

ACUTE CATARRHAL RHINITIS.—Inhaling alcohol, ammonia or menthol crystals will frequently aid in reducing the nasal swelling. A spray composed of menthol and cocaine ten grs. each, to albolene one oz., applied to the nasal cavities three or four times at intervals of one or two hours will usually cut short, or materially modify the attack if used during the period of watery discharge. On the other hand, if used when the discharge is thick, I believe it serves to prolong the attack. When the cocaine is used it is unwise to inform the patient of the fact.

G. H. QUAY, M.D., Cleveland, Ohio.

AMERICAN ANTI-TUBERCULOSIS LEAGUE.—The next meeting of this society will be held at Atlanta, Ga., on April 17, 1905.

Dr. Geo.'Brown, president of the association, together with the other officers, extend a hearty invitation to the Colorado physicians to be present. An unusually good time is promised, together with "A hot time in the old town."

A CASE OF PNEUMONIA FOLLOWING SEVERE TYPHOID:—RE-COVERY.—From a correspondent in Florida. J. B. W., white, male, age 30 years, was recovering from a severe case of typhoid. On the thirty-sixth day his temperature was normal. On the thirty-ninth day it again began to rise and in a few days had reached 104.5, the pulse 140. A severe cough and consolidation of the right lung told the story of a complicating pneumonia. After the long and severe drain upon his resources incident to the typhoid his condition presented a very alarming, not to say, desperate situation.

Counsel was called and it was decided that his only hope lay in the generous use of Antiphlogistine. A "Large" package was secured and heated by placing the sealed can in hot water. The temperature of the room was brought up to about 80°. A cotton lined cheese-cloth jacket, open upon the shoulders and in front, was prepared and warmed. Uncovering the patient's thorax, Antiphlogistine as hot as could be borne was spread upon the skin about one-eighth inch thick over as much of the thoracic walls as could be reached (back, front, side and over the shoulder). This was covered with the jacket. Turning the patient over, the other side was dressed in the same way. The jacket was then drawn together over the shoulders and down the front with stout thread. It is proper to say the entire contents of the 34½ ounce package (large) was used for the one dressing.

The effect was surprisingly prompt. In a few hours, the temperature had declined to a point of safety and the pulse to 120. A similar dressing was applied fresh every twenty-four hours. The improvement was steady and marked and in six days the patient was again convalescent, thanks to Antiphlogistine.

The brilliant outcome in this case taught me the importance of careful attention to detail in the use of Antiphlogistine. Like every thing else worth while, it must be properly used if the best results are to be obtained.

EDITORIAL ITEMS.— Continued.

Bronchial Ast ma. Phillips praises aconite in the short, dry cough of asthmatics with a full strong pulse. Shoemaker uses the following formula in the latter part of the attack: ℞ Tinct. sanguinariæ m. vi; ammonii brom. gr. ix; spt. etheris nitrosi m. xxiv; syr. pruni virg. q.s.: A dessertspoonful in water every two or three hours.   In the intervals he prescribes; ℞ Potassii iodidi gr. xii; liq. potass. arsenitis m. iii; ext. grindeliæ m. xxx; tinct. euphorbiæ fl. m. x; ext. yerbæ santae fl. q.s.: A teaspoonful three times a day.

Penile Pain.   Bennett (*Medical Record*) says that pain in the glans penis may be due to any of the following conditions: Stone impacted low down in the ureter; phimosis with a single small adhesion; anal fissure; rectal polypus; sarcoma of the inguinal region; tuberculous testis.

Gastrosuccorrhea.   For the acid form Benedict directs to give the stomach rest, feeding by the rectum; interdict salt; use only distilled water as a drink; hot air baths to remove salines through sweat ducts; tonics and hygienic measures for an overwrought nervous system. Milk and lime water are of some service.

Chronic Catarrhal Pharyngitis.   It is a matter of every day experience, says Levy (*New York Medical Journal*, Dec. 17, 1904) that patients in whom no nasal cause can be found for this affection, present sufficient evidence of gastric catarrh to warrant treatment of the latter affection, and to base the prognosis of the pharyngeal affection upon that of the gastric.

Nervous Coughs.   Ringer states that gelsemium is of value when there is excessive excitability of the respiratory center. Hare asserts that belladonna is our best remedy in these cases. Phillips gives chamomile oil gtt. ii-viii in coughs due to heightened reflex irritability, especially in hysterical women.   Macfarlan orders tincture of nux vomica in drop doses every five minutes for laryngeal couch of neurotic origin.   Potter affirms that the frequency and violence of nervous coughs can be controlled by a determined effort of the patient's will.   Shoemaker prescribes fifteen minims of tincture of hyoscyamus in syrup of wild cherry every third or fourth hour.   Strychnine, particularly the valerianate, is recommended for neurotic periodic night coughs.   In neurotic children near puberty correction of habits and hygiene,

plenty of outdoor exercise, cold shower baths, and a short course
of bromides are indicated.

To Make Sweat. The best method of inducing diaphoresis,
says Stern (*Medical Standard*) is by the application of uniform
heat, whether steam or dry heat or the hot wet pack, for from
fifteen minutes to one hour. Before the heat is applied take
a large draught of a freshly made, hot but weak infusion of lin-
derae cortex (spice-bush bark), or of hot lemonade. Dangerous
diaphoretics, like pilocarpine, should only be resorted to when
other means have failed.

The Pains of Flat-Foot. Often the greater part of the pain,
says S. C. Baldwin (*Medical Sentinel*), is felt in the calf of the
leg or under the knee, and sometimes even in the hip or back.
Sometimes the severest pain is felt over the peroneus longus and
brevis. Tenderness on pressure may be elicited under the anterior end of the os calcis, or less often under the schaphoid or at
the base of the metatarsals between the third and fourth; also
with swelling under the malleoli, more frequently the external.

"Knock-out Drops." These means for criminal ends have
generally been stated to consist of chloral hydrate. Carel (*Clinical Review*) calls attention to the use of cococlus indicus in this
connection, looking in whiskey like the extract of hazelnut kernel
sometimes employed by barkeepers to improve the flavor of the
liquor. The symptoms of the active principle, picrotoxin, are dizziness, deep sleep, epileptiform convulsions, tonic or clonic spasm,
dilated pupils, delirium, coma, paralysis, and finally death.

Acute Inflammatory Bronchitis in Adults. Ferrand gives
his patients an abundance of hot emollient drinks and a diet of
milk and soups. He applies fifteen to twenty dry cups to the
thorax, and four wet cups to its base. He paints with iodine between the shoulders, or applies a large blister for six hours, then
poultices. He administers a purgative of one ounce of sodium
sulphate in an infusion of 150 grs. of senna, keeping the bowels
open thereafter with pills of rhubarb and aloes each $\frac{3}{4}$ grain and
1.6 grain of extract of belladonna.

Pylorospasm.—Van Valzah and Nisbet counsel to improve
tone and strength and allay irritability of the nervous system.
Use a soothing, easily evacuated, non-ferme ntable diet; cervico

Carabana the Ideal Aperient Water.—In a very interesting brochure Dr. E. Monin, secretary-general of the French Society of Hygiene, gives a detailed description of the valuable properties of the Spanish mineral water, carabana, known as La Salud (Health.) Carabana water is derived from the province of Madrid. This water is highly esteemed by Spanish physicians and has received the endorsement of the French Academy of Medicine. The composition of carabana renders it of peculiar efficacy. It contains the sulphate and the sulphite of sodium, the sulphate of magnesium; the chlorides of sodium, magnesium, and calcium; the phosphate of sodium, and a trace of alum. It is remarkably constant in composition; is a clear, transparent, and limpid fluid of an alkaline reaction, entirely free from organisms. Carabana is a cathartic, sanguifacient, antiseptic and antipyretic. It likewise promotes the nutritive processes. The comparatively small proportion in which magnesia is present permits the use of carabana by those predisposed to the formation of ammonio-magnesian calculi. In patients suffering from disease of the bladder and urinary passages carabana is a preferred laxative. Carabana water is markedly beneficial in visceral congestions, secretory disorders in general; moist skin diseases, as eczema and herpes; and in lymphatic and herpetic diathesis. Carabana is of no value in the management of rheumatic and syphilitic patients. more particularly when these have abused the salicylates, arsenic, iodides and mercury. Carabana leaves no disagreeable bitter taste, dryness in the mouth or thirst, and does not produce lassitude. Its laxative action is rapid but gentle. It does not give rise to sickness of the stomach or griping pain. In small doses it has a sedative and antiphlogistic effect. In fractional doses it is serviceable in those of languid circulation and depressed nutrition as well as in convalescence attended by gastro-intestinal failure. Carabana is an admirable remedy in many forms of dyspepsia, whether of gastric or intestinal origin. It produces regular evacuations, while at the same time it gives tonicity to the muscular coat of the alimentary tract. It acts likewise as a reliable intestinal antiseptic. It is of particular advantage in atony of the stomach, relieves gastralgia, and arrests the gastrorrhea of drunkards. The special utility of carabana is in constipation; but when we reflect upon the diverse and numerous morbid conditions engendered by habitual constipation we readily recognize the wide range of the usefulness of this natural water. Constipation is the fruitful source of auto-intoxication and of different forms of depravity of the blood. In diseases of the bowels carabana is no less valuable than in those of the stomach. In affections of the liver carabana has been found of signal efficacy. Its influence is exerted both upon the biliary and the sanguifacient functions of that organ. It allays catarrh of the biliary passages. It relieves engorgement of the liver and jaundice. In the more remote troubles which depend upon disturbances of the functions of the liver carabana may be used with excellent effect. It is directly beneficial in anemia, affections of the heart and lungs, in neuralgia due to retentions of excrementitious material, in nephritis, dropsy of various forms and in obesity. In short, carabana may be advantageously employed in those multitudinous pathological conditions which are dependent upon or associated with inactivity of the gastro-intestinal apparatus. Analysis of the water showing its superiority over other aperient waters. Official analysis:

(In grains per U. S. gallon, 231 cubic inches at deg. Beaume.)

Sulphate of Sodium	5,831,800
Sulphide of Sodium	2,910
Sulphate of Magnesium	179,101
Chloride of Sodium	93,309
Chloride of Magnesium	27,841

The tonic and nutritive properties of Scott's Emulsion are strikingly proven in the case of rickety children and pale, delicate girls. The ease with which it is assimilated makes Scott's Emulsion especially valuable in the treatment of malnutrition.

SCOTT & BOWNE, Chemists, 409 Pearl St., New York.

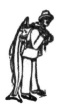

gastric galvanization; Winternitz or hot compress during digestion. Silver nitrate is valuable, if the stomach is morbidly sensitive or secretes excessively. Extracts of coca and belladonna may
be given before each meal; and codeine phosphate hypodermically
or chloral hydrate per rectum, if much pain.

Eructatio Nervosa. Change of scene, rest, hydrotherapy,
electricity and strong moral control and suggestion are advised by
Van Valzah and Nisbet. Bromides sometimes do good in non-
neurasthenic cases. The intragastric spray is the most valuable
single remedy, using warm water alone, or warm water followed
immediately after its removal by cold water, or a solution of silver
nitrate five grains to the pint of distilled water. Prolonged paroxysms may be cut short by twenty grains of chloral hydrate per
rectum.

American Electro-Therapeutic Association. At the Four-
teenth Annual Meeting of this Association, held at St. Louis, Mo.,
September 13, 14, 15 and 16, 1904, the following were elected,
viz.: Emil Heuel, M.D., President, 1 West 94th St., New York,
N. Y. Charles Hamilton Hughes, M.D., First Vice-President,
3857 Olive St., St. Louis, Mo. Morris Weil Brinkmann, A.B.,
M.D., Second Vive-President, 54 W. 90th St., New York, N. Y.
Richard Joseph Nunn, M.D., Treasurer, 5 York St., Savannah, Ga.
Clarence Edward Skinner, M.D., LL.D., Secretary, 67 Grove St.,
New Haven, Conn.

*Marked Mental Improvement Following Operation for De-
pressed Fracture of the Skull.* B. Van D. Hedges describes the
case of a boy of eight years who, four years proviously, had been
struck on the head by a brick, which had caused a marked depression in the bone at the seat of the injury. From time to time
there was evidence of a change in his mental and moral make-up.
Intellectually he was at a standstill, and all moral· sense appeared
to be lost. Over a year ago the author removed the area of depressed bone, and since that time the boy's mental and moral
condition has become normal. The depression was about one inch
in diameter, one-quarter inch in depth, and situated in the median
line along the course of the sagittal suture, the center of the depression being one inch and a half anterior to the vertical point
and four and one-half inches to the glabellar point.—*Medical Record,* January 28, 1905.

Stenosis of Main Bronchus. This anomaly, usually due to syphilis, is characterized at times by laryngeal cough and stridor, and by thick, viscid sputum. Powell states that small, regulated doses of chloroform for inhalation relieve the spasmodic cough and aid expectoration. For bronchial and tracheal stricture Taylor advises active antisyphilitic treatment by means of mercury and potassium iodide.

Infectious Bronchitis. Ferrand prescribes a pill t. i. d. of pulv. scillæ gr. ⅓, ammoniæ gr. ¾; ess. eucalypti gtt. If these fails he orders: ℞ Creasoti m. 1–13: ess. citroni m. 1–20; syr· aurantii flor. m· xii; aquam q. s.: A teaspoonful every two or three hours. He also utilizes sulphurous inhalations, a glass of quinine wine (glycerine may be added) before each meal—alcohol at end, and tonic diet.

Internal Piles. The palliative treatment (Gant) includes the following measures: Reduce protruded tumors; correct errors in diet and living; recumbent position if inflamed, applying constantly astringent ointments or lotions or poultices; if not large or strangulated, apply pure nitric acid to bases; wear a pile supporter; correct constipation. In operative treatment thorough divulsion, followed by the use of the clamp and cautery, is probably the best procedure.

The Bacteria of the Stomach. E. Palier (*Medical Record,* Nov. 19) finds that carcinoma ventriculi is characterized by the vibrio geniculatus ventriculi, many staphylococci and no fungi (mycelia) In euchlorhydria or hyperchlorhydria there are present yeast and mycelia and a small, Gram-negative, ammonia-producing bacillus. In subnormal acidity with stasis, he usually found yeast, mycelia and the vibrio geniculatus. For clinical purposes he employs sugared agar.

The Limitations of the Office Treatment of Rectal Diseases. C. B. Kelsey discusses the rectal operations which it is feasible to perform in the office under local anesthesia. The author states that a very large proportion of all cases of piles, fissures, superficial ulcers, and pruritus, and a certain proportion of abscesses and fistula, may be radically cured in one's office without resorting to ether or confinement to bed, but much judgment is necessary in selecting the proper cases. In general it may be said that it is often simpler in the end, and safer and more comfortable for the

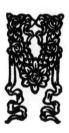

patient. to do at home or in the hospital an operation which might have been performed in the office.—*Medical Record*, Jan. 28, 1905.

Geheimrath Dr. Dettweiler.—Eulogy pronounced on the occasion of the first anniversary of his death.—S. A. Knopf, who was for a time assistant to Dr. Dettweiler, points out the great part played by this physician in developing the modern sanatorium treatment of pulmonary tuberculosis. In the performance of his duties as military surgeon he contracted tuberculosis and was compelled to resign from the army. Regaining his health, he made the treatment of this disease his lifework, and the sanatorium he founded at Falkenstein is still the Mecca for students of phthisiotherapy from all over the world.—*Medical Record*, January 28, 1905.

Gluttony as a Cause of Symptomatic Epileptic Convulsions. W. P. Spratling describes a type of epilepsy due to errors of diet which is fairly common and is generally amenable to treatment. The patients are usually middle-aged men of plethoric physique, leading inactive lives, and eating and drinking to excess. The primary cause of the convulsive attacks in these cases seems to lie, first in the weak stomach, and second in some obscure disorder of metabolism, The type of convulsion induced is usually of the *grand mal* variety, though *petit mal* seizures are also observed. The treatment is that of the toxic state induced by the metabolism and is mainly dietetic and hygienic.—*Medical Record*, January 28, 1905.

Treatment of Croupous Rhinitis. Kyle advises to use a warm alkaline solution douche of eight grains each of borax and sodium bicarbonate to the ounce of water, followed by hydrogen peroxide diluted with an equal amount of cinnamon water. Repeat the alkaline solution and remove carefully with cotton on probe any particles of caseous material still adherent. Then dry surface carefully and apply to site of membrane, by means of cotton carrier, not more than three times daily, Loeffler's solution (36 parts tolluo, 60 absolute alcohol, 4 parts liquor ferri sesqui-chloridi). Give calomel (1-10 grain with one grain of sodium bicarbonate) every hour for ten doses, followed in three hours by citrate of magnesia; repeat this course on second day. Tinct. chloride of iron in ten to twenty drop doses. Bromide of quinine (two to five grains) and extract of nux vomica

($\frac{1}{8}$ grain) may be given every four hours in pill or capsule. In the fibrinoplastic variety detach membrane forceps and touch bleeding areas with fifteen per cent chromic acid solution after cleansing with hydrogen peroxide and a simple alkaline wash.

Fatty Stools. Mayo Robson (*Practical Medicine Series*) has the following to say of fatty stools: Fat occurs in the stools in three forms:—as fat driblets; as fatty acid crystals; as soap crystals. The capacity for digestion and absorption of fats is limited; if therefore, fat be taken in large quantities it is found in the stools. Steatorrhea occurs in some cases of jaundice, in some cases of interitis, and in some affections of the pancreas, but in none of these constantly. When jaundice and interstitial pan-creatitis coexist, there is a great excess of fat in the stools. The presence of and excess of fat in the motions, in the absences of jaundice and diseases of the intestine, is suggestive of pancreatic disease. If the cammidge pancreatic reaction be found in the urine along with steatorrhea, some affection of the pancreas is almost certain. If azotorrhea be found along with steatorrhea, it is almost certain that the pancreas is diseased; and if the pancre-atic reaction in the urine, diabetes, and an epigastric tumor be present the diagnosis is certain.

WHERE TRUE QUALITY IS SHOWN.—The excellence of Scott's Emulsion is recognized by the highest authority. The *London Lancet* said of it: "The value of the hypophosphites combined with cod liver oil, especially in wasting disease and debilitating conditions, is well known. In addition to these constituents, Scott's Emulsion also contains glycerine, which is well recognized as assisting very materially in the absorption of oils and fats. We have examined the preparation with care, and find that it fulfills all the requirements and presents all the conditions of a very sat-isfactory emulsion. In appearance and consistence it is not unlike cream, and under the microscope the fat globules are seen to be of perfectly regular size and uniformly distributed. In fact, the preparation, microscopically examined, presents the appearance of cream. So well has the oil been emulsified that even when shaken with water the fat is slow to separate, the liquid then looking like milk. The taste is decidedly unobjectionable and is pleasantly aromatic and saline. We had no difficulty in recognizing the presence of the hypophosphites in an unimpaired state. The Emulsion keeps well even when exposed to wide changes of tem-perature. Under the circumstances just described the Emulsion should prove an excellent food as well as a tonic."

DENVER MEDICAL TIMES

| Volume XXIV. | APRIL, 1905 | Number 10 |

NEURASTHENIA IN PULMONARY TUBERCULOSIS.*

By J. E. COURTNEY, M.D.

Denver, Colo.

The condition of morbid hopefulness; the spes phthisica of the old authors certainly does not pertain today to the same extent as they describe, or as popular belief in the unfailing cheerfulness of the tubercular might lead one to suppose. This must be due to the much more widely diffused popular information regarding pulmonary tuberculosis, its often progressive tendency, even without pain, in fact with a comparative sense of well being, and the greater candor of physicians to friends and patients on the subject of the disease.

In any event the condition of nerve exhaustion and depression and the accompanying train of subjective and objective symptoms known as "neurasthenia" pertains quite frequently as a result or leading complication in pulmonary tuberculosis. While neurasthenia in this condition might be regarded as only an accompaniment, yet the prominence of the symptoms even when the pulmonary condition is so ameliorated as to be no longer the imperative trouble; and as the train of symptoms come at the time of life and in the individuals constitutionally liable, it seems fair in such cases to regard the neurasthenia as the disease requiring attention and treatment, tuberculosis being regarded as the aetiological factor. It is surprising that the nervous system is not oftener and more seriously affected by the slow and prolonged absorption of toxine generated in the tubercular process. This might well be expected to produce neurasthenia; let alone the excessive expenditure of energy in the impaired functions of respiration and digestion. It would seem that tubercular toxins have not a predilection for nervous tissue compared to toxins generated in other processes; in diphtheria, for example. On the other hand they do manifest

*Read before the Rocky Mountain Inter-State Medical Association, Sept. 1904.

a predilection for nephritic tissue—witness the great frequency of Bright's and the numerous forms of tubercular kidney. I will give a brief history of a few cases of neurasthenia in pulmonary tuberculosis who presented themselves at the clinic for "nervous diseases," Denver and Gross College of Medicine.

CASE 1. Samuel S., age 24, tailor, came to Colorado from New York City for the climate two months ago, nothing notable in family nor his own early history. For the last six years says he has had stomach trouble; sometimes dysenteric symptoms. Three or four months ago had pneumonia or bronchitis or·grippe, not certain which. At present has sick stomach once in a while; complains that he is irritable, slight noises annoy him excessively, has singing and whistling sounds in the ears, worse if speaking; pains and "pricking and sticking feelings" in the legs, worse if he walks much, has a sensation in the knees as if something wet was about them; sleeps poorly; no deafness; complexion very white; lips excessively red, very little cough or expectoration; no bacilli.

CASE 2. H. E. W., insurance solicitor, age 36, native of Massachusetts; last 12 years in Chicago, 9 months in Colorado for the climate; father and mother living and well, four sisters living, one brother died of consumption at 17½ years; maternal grandmother died at 22 of consumption. Diagnosis of tuberculosis made one year ago and bacilli found. At present coughs and expectorates a little mornings; no bacilli. Color and weight good; is very nervous, cannot sleep well, easily confused, forgets very familiar things, almost loses himself at times; quite depressed, tires out easily, head feels too muddled to do insurance soliciting, appetite fair; bowels regular and often contain gas. After nearly two years and great improvement in general condition and in material prospects, the neurasthenic symptoms are still present more or less.

CASE 3. William Z., 23 years old, coachman, German parentage, born in U. S. A.; in Colorado for the climate 18 months; father living and well, mother died of cancer at 36 years; two sisters, one brother well. Pulmonary tuberculosis two years, neurasthenia for a year; says he has palpitation of the heart, sudden smothered feelings, dizzy sensations, specks floating before the eyes, hot flashes, cannot remember as well as he used to, has had some nocturnal emissions which worry him greatly, numb feelings in left arm and leg; dermographia forearms, does not sleep well, dejected in pose and expression, constipated.

CASE 4. Nathan L., 25 years old, tailor, Hebrew German; 4 years in U. S. A., 4 months in Colorado for the climate; came from Boston; family history incomplete. He dates his pulmonary tuberculosis from 2 years back; very nervous; face, hands, lips and tongue tremulous, various fleeting disturbances of sensation; felt happier East; evidently a large element of nostalgia in the case; some insomnia; blepharitis, gums spongy, patella reflexes are active; a little cough and scant expectoration mornings.

CASE 5. Alfred J., tailor 26 years; from Chicago, 3 weeks in Colorado for the climate. Mother died at 50 of consumption, father at 57; three brothers, two well; one thought to be consumptive; three sisters, all died of diseases of childhood. Pulmonary tuberculosis of 6 months duration, present symptoms insomnia, pains in the head, bad dreams, pains in the legs and hips, legs and hands "get numb." Troubled with night emissions; palpitation of the heart, gets dizzy; very much alarmed for fear he will "go out of his head." Cannot keep his mind off his sickness, some photophobia; tongue coated, patella reflexes dull.

CASE 6. A. Q., 35 years old, Russian Hebrew, tailor; in U. S. A. 18 years; here from Boston for the climate 6 weeks. Eleven months ago had grippe; was in Boston City Hospital, tubercular bacilli found; in Hebrew National Home, Denver, for a short time. For last six months very nervous, aching in top of head and also the body, weak feelings and is much discouraged about himself has prickling and tingling sensations all over like electric wires, shakings and tremors at times, no bacilli in sputum; patella reflexes very active.

CASE 7.—Cassell G., age 33, tailor, German Hebrew, here from New York City 7 months for the climate; family and early personal history negative; sick 3½ years; nervous symptoms demanded attention for the last two months, frontal headache, burning and weakness in right forearm, fingers feel as if asleep at times; again like pins and needles pricking; depressed; tired and "don't care" feelings; often weak and feels like falling; some of the symptoms in this case were those of an occupation neurosis.

I have selected these from the card index of the clinic as illustrating these cases. A summary of the symptoms, head pains, paresthesia, insomnia, fear, anxiety, vaso-motor disturbances and psychical depression generally, constitute the accepted syndrome of neurasthenia; one will note the striking uniformity of the subjective and physical symptoms. I am not able to fix upon any definite percentage of persons suffering from pulmonary tuberculosis, who present this group of symptoms to a degree classing them as neurasthenics. The chronic, or at least quiescent and non progressive stage of pulmonary tuberculosis rather than the initial acute or the late terminal stage is the period at which I have seen the cases cited. I cannot but think that those are cases of neurasthenia directly caused by pulmonary tuberculosis. I do not think the frequency of the cases here is a matter of altitude or other climatic conditions nor that the percentage of cases is larger here than may be explained by the fact that many who come to Colorado have often made great social and financial sacrifices. These factors might naturally be operative in causing a lowering of tone in addition to that induced by the pulmonary condition. The treatment and prognosis of this type of neurasthenia, while in the main the same as in the ordinary cases must be modified by the pulmonary condition and improvement or retrogression therein. The very serious question sometimes arising is whether the neurasthenia be but a stage in the development of some of the psychoses, enough cases of insanity in tubercular subjects having appeared to create a large literature and even give a name to one subdivision in some classifications of insanity. Neurasthenics like these should be treated for this trouble and the symptoms not passed by as inevitable accompaniments of pulmonary tuberculosis.

GENERAL SEPTIC PERITONITIS—REPORT OF A CASE.*

By I. B. PERKINS, M.D.

Denver, Colo.

In the short time allotted me for the presentation of this paper, I shall not attempt to do more than to speak of a few of the more important points connected with the subject, and these will principally be on diagnosis and treatment.

An early diagnosis is of the greatest importance; for if we fail in this particular, we miss practically, our only opportunity of applying remedies at a time when we may reasonably expect favorable results.

The cause of the trouble is usually the sudden entering of bacteria into the free abdominal cavity. This may occur in the form of leakage from a fallopian tube or the rupture of a tubal or appendix abscess or the sloughing of an appendix where an abscess has not been formed. Rupture of the gall bladder, or perforation of a gastric or intestinal ulcer, frequently gives rise to the disease. It is very common in the gangrenous type of appendicitis for two reasons; first, because the advance of the disease is so rapid that sloughing takes place before the appendix is surrounded by adhesions, and second, because no adhesions will be formed at a gangrenous point. A general septic peritonitis may also occur in inflammatory conditions of the abdominal viscera, by the pathogenic organisms penetrating the tissues and thus reaching the free peritoneal cavity without there being a perforation present.

Some investigators claim that in 10 per cent. of the cases there are no germs present. If this be true it may account for some recoveries which we have heretofore credited to different medicines or modes of treatment. There appears to be a great difference in the virulence of different kinds of bacteria as well as a great difference in the resisting power of different portions of the peritoneum. The pelvic peritoneum appears to be more tolerant than any other portion, while that portion in the upper part of the abdominal cavity and especially that covering the diaphram appears to possess

*Read before the Rocky Mountain Inter-State Medical Association, Sept., 1904.

the least resisting power. This is probably largely due to the fact that the absorbing power of this part of the peritoneum is very much greater than that of other portions. That of the small intestine probably is second in power of absorption. The glandular openings are larger in that portion which covers the diaphragm and through them, not only more rapid absorption takes place, but absorption of larger particles occurs and these are carried direct to the glands of the anterior mediastinum. The entire peritoneum presents a surface for absorption which is almost if not quite equal to that of the entire integument of the body, and from this vast surface is said to be capable of absorbing in one hour, from three to five per cent. of the entire weight of the body.

The bacillus coli communis is probably the most virulent of the types usually seen, while the gonicoccus and the tubercle bacillus are not nearly so active or destructive. Immediately following the absorption of bacteria from the peritoneal cavity the system begins to show symptoms of toxemia, the extent of which depends upon the virulence of the poison and the rapidity with which it is absorbed. This makes it necessary for us to make the earliest possible diagnosis in a case of septic peritonitis. If the cause in a given case is from sudden perforation of some organ, sharp pain in the region of the perforation is apt to be the first symptom noticed, and symptoms of shock are present. The temperature will be below normal and the pulse will be slow and depressed. Soon following this the pain becomes general, tympanites is present and the temperature begins to rise. In a short time, however, there is little or no pain, due perhaps to the poison having reached the nerve centers, producing toxic paralysis.

If the disease is slower in its onset, the symptoms will be less severe in character and may even be so mild as to entirely mislead the attendant as to the conditions present.

I have seen general peritonitis with a temperature almost if not quite normal and yet operation would show large quantities of pus in the free abdominal cavity. Rigidity, however, is almost invariably present, especially after the first few hours of the onset of the disease. Every surgeon can call to mind cases of peritonitis where the diagnosis was not made until after the abdomen had been opened, showing the subtleness with which the disease sometimes advances.

The prevention of peritonitis is one which should elicit our most careful attention. We are powerless in most cases, it is true, to foresee this possibility, but in conditions where it is possible to do so, it is the point of wisdom to try to prevent peritonitis by removing the cause before the disease has reached so advanced a stage. This can often be done in pelvic abscesses, gall stones, gastric ulcers, as well as appendicitis in the early stages. These should all be operated early when the possibility of effecting a cure of this much dreaded disease would be greatest.

When from any cause a case has reached this deplorable condition our remedy must be promptly applied if favorable results are expected.

The abdomen should be immediately opened and the cause quickly removed if possible, and the cavity as thoroughly cleansed as it is possible to do without injury to the peritoneum. When flushing is used the temperature of the water should be from 110 to 115 degrees F. It is well in the course of the flushing to introduce into different parts of the abdomen three or four ounces at a time of hydrogenperoxide and follow in a few moments with salt solution. Large drainage tubes should be placed in different parts of the cavity and especially down into the pelvis. These tubes should be placed in pairs, and one should not be perforated so that water can be carried to the bottom of the cavity it is intended to drain. If the patient is a female, it is well to incise the vault of the vagina and introduce a double drainage tube into the pelvis. The patient is then placed in bed with the head of the bed elevated to an angle of from 30 to 45 degrees, for the purpose of allowing the remaining infection to drain to that portion of the cavity that has the greatest resistance and away from the diaphragm which would drink up the fluids fastest. Having removed what poison it is in our power to remove, and having prepared for subsequent removal of myriads of new colonies of germs, which we will yet have to encounter, our attention must now be turned to ridding the system of the poison already absorbed, and this is considered by most clinicians the most difficult part of the work.

The treatment which appears to the writer to promise the greatest results in these cases can best be described by reporting the following case:

Mr. C. S., aged 20 years, blacksmith, was taken ill the afternoon of November 10, 1903, while working in his shop. He first complained of pain which was not very severe and was distributed over the entire abdomen. He went home, but did not go to bed nor did he call a physician until about 11 o'clock the next day. On arriving at the bedside of the patient the physician at once diagnosed acute appendicitis of the severest type and removed him to the hospital. Temperature was a little under 100° and pulse 120, weak and thready. Rigidity was marked all over the abdomen, a little more on the right side. Abdomen was scarcely distended at all. Operation was decided upon and was performed at once. Incision was made on the right side a little inward from Mc-Burney's point. On cutting through the peritoneum quantities of pus poured out at the wound. The appendix was gangrenous and had sloughed along one side, emptying fecal secretions into the free cavity. Appendix was removed. The peritoneum had lost its lustre and lymph had begun to form on the intestines. Large quantities of pus and sero-purulent fluid were washed from the pelvis, from the left side of the abdomen, and from the right side high up above the incision. The abdomen was freely washed with salt solution and peroxide of hydrogen, a pound of the latter being used in the washing. Care was taken not to remove the intestines from the abdominal cavity, thereby lessening the shock. Infusion of salt solution was given during the operation. Eight drainage tubes were used, some of them a half inch in diameter, and were placed in different parts of the abdomen, one pair going deep into the pelvis. Of each pair the larger tube was freely perforated to admit of free drainage, and the smaller one was not perforated in order that water might subsequently be carried to the bottom of the cavity. Loose packing was put about the tubes and in the open wound and no attempt was made to close any part of the incision. Patient was then placed in bed with the head of the bed elevated to an angle of about 40 degrees and was given strychnine hypoderatically one-thirtieth grain every two hours, and every two hours an enema composed of 1 ounce of whiskey, 3 ounces of coffee and 4 ounces of salt solution was given. Every four hours a pint of salt solution was given sub-cutaneously. As soon as the patient could swallow, he was given two cathartic capsules every hour until he had taken ten. The capsules each contained Ext. Colocynth Comp. gr. 2, Ext. Hyoscyamus gr. ½, Ext. Jalapæ gr. 1, Ext. Leptandra gr. 1/5, Res. Podoplyllin gr. 1/10.

The following day the patient began to vomit in the characteristic manner common in these cases. He received frequent high enemata, some of salts and some of soap suds, but with no results. He was taken to the dressing room and on removing the loose packing from the wound and examining with the finger, it was found that few if any adhesions had yet taken place. The abdomen was again flushed through the tubes, several gallons of water being used. The stomach was washed with several gallons of hot water, each quart of which contained one ounce of sulphate of magnesia. After washing for a considerable time the water ran clear, but a few moments later a portion came that was very much colored, showing that the water was pentrating deeper into the intestines. The temperature of the water was about 110 degrees F. at first and was gradually increased to about 112 degrees. On finishing the stomach lavage, and before the tube was removed, a pint of water was introduced into the stomach containing an ounce of magnesia sulphate.

The stomach washing was grateful to the patient and the stomach had become tolerant of the salts used and readily retained the ounce left in the stomach when the tube was removed. There was considerable more that had been left in the intestines by the washing, besides the amount that had been absorbed during the treatment, which required half an hour.

Before leaving the dressing room the bowels began to show signs of life and within an hour after being placed in bed a copious stool was the result. At this time the patient began to take broth and convalesced rapidly.

At the end of about four weeks the discharge from the abdomen had ceased and an anaesthetic was given, the wound scarified and closed with interrupted sutures of silk-worm gut placed close together. Recovery was without incident and there has been no hernia or trouble of any kind.

From observation of this and other cases the following conclusions have been reached:

First.—That the earliest possible diagnosis should be made in these cases and operation should usually be performed at once.

Second.—That free flushing of the abdominal cavity with removal of all poison possible is of the greatest importance when the infection is general.

Third.—That an elevated position, draining the contents of the abdomen into the pelvis, the point of greatest resistance is of great benefit.

Fourth.—That in these profoundly septic cases where general infection is present adhesions form slowly, allowing frequent subsequent flushings of the abdominal cavity with hot salt solution, which can do no harm and will aid materially by removing large quantities of toxic material from the 'abdomen.

Fifth—That the subcutaneous or intravenous use of salt solution is valuable in that it dilutes the poison and lessens the toxemia and stimulates the kidneys to free action.

Sixth.—That free catharsis should be obtained at the earliest possible moment and should be kept up during the entire convalescent period, thereby aiding in the elimination of much septic material which has been cast into the bowel and which would be reabsorbed if left alone. Also troublesome adhesions are less liable to form if the bowel is kept active.

Seventh.—That the use of some cathartic salt in the water when the stomach is washed aids materially in establishing peristalsis.

DISCUSSION OF DR. PERKINS' PAPER.

DR. COFFEY. I am glad to hear Dr. Perkins speak of peritonitis in the way he does, namely, in giving a cause. In so doing we practically eliminate the words "primary general peritonitis." In considering this subject the question is: Do we always have a general peritonitis when we have symptoms that lead us to believe that we have? For instance when there is a case of acute appendicitis, or rupture of the appendix. There we have the symptoms of general peritonitis, yet by close investigation we will find that only a small section of the abdomen is involved. It is upon this fact that the so-called Ochsner treatment has probably been based. By limiting the field the abscess becomes circumscribed.

I believe that the doctor's principal point, however, is in the main correct; that we do not have general peritonitis *per se;* at least, we say, in very rare instances. The two principal points in the treatment of this condition are brought out by the doctor; washing and draining. These are questions in which I believe I would, to a certain extent, differ from the Doctor in reference to some points. First, as to washing. If we know that we have a general peritonitic condition throughout the abdomen, which I consider is in but a very small per cent. of cases, then the washing is all right; but in the great majority of cases, as in the rupture, we do not have a general peritonitis. In a rupture of the appendix, unless there is a large abscess already in existence, we do not have a general peritonitis; it is a local condition. The same may be said also of certain perforations of the gall bladder. Then another thing I believe we should consider in the matter especially of drainage that there are certain cavities with the patient lying on his back; there are at least three points in which fluid will accumulate. Put the cadaver at a level and you will find that there are certain cavities in addition to the pelvic cavity which will hold quite a considerable quantity of fluid. I refer to the flanks just below the kidney regions. It is these things we sometims forget. Therefore the position would have a great deal to do with it.

As to the drainage, this is a subject upon which I have done a great deal of experimenting, and am still going a great deal. I disagree with the doctor in the use of a drainage tube. If you will take any kind of a vessel, or put the tube inside of cotton or gauze that is thoroughly wet with solutions, you will find that tubal drainage is of absolutely no avail; while you may take capillary drainage and, if properly placed, almost a quart of fluid will easily be raised from the pelvis without any effort whatever in a few minutes, and the pelvis will be found to be perfectly dry, as shown by experiments on the cadaver. It is surprising what an amount of fluid will be lifted in this way.

If we take a roll of gauze the size of your little fingers, and put it into a cavity containing fluid we will find that fluid will be emptied, we will say, in one hour. If we put thirty of those drains into the same cavity, we will find that that fluid will be emptied drain, and use a small drainage; the body has absorbed enough to thirty times as rapidly. So that if you drain with a capillary practically produce death.

I differ from the doctor relative to washing in all cases, but would limit washing to cases where we have positive evidence that the condition is a general peritonitis. But where we have this condition due to the rupture of a large abscess, we find in such cases that we have the entire peritoneal cavity infected. Therefore in that case wash very thoroughly.

I believe the differentiation between the use of the drainage tube and drainage gauze is in this fact; the drainage tube will drain provided you have a circumscribed cavity in which there is a constant upward pressure, but will not drain in an open peritoneal cavity to any great extent. Capillary drainage will drain as well if not better, up than down, and will drain any kind of a cavity.

If we have a general peritonitis, I will say drain at the point of infection as near as possible.

Now as to the matter of drainage, I believe that we can use not only one but fifty or sixty drains the size of the finger. This is not simply done by pressing the drainage down among the intestines, but first hold the intestines away and begin at a point and gradually circle around them, and then when through give your patient a position in accordance. For instance in appendicitis I believe drainage is very much helped by giving the patient the elevated head position, and turning the patient to the right side. Do not remove capillary drainage short of five days. A small amount of gauze drainage will obstruct; a large amount will not.

DR. FAIRCHILD. I have had a good many misfortunes arising from this class of cases. As long as 35 years ago I saw a child who undoubtedly had an attack of appendicitis. I opened the abdomen and drained it and let the pus run out. Twenty-five years ago I saw another case of a similar character. I did not treat it in the beginning but saw it three or four weeks afterwards, and found the abdomen was full of pus. This was opened and the pus was allowed to run out. Both these cases got well. Since then I have opened the abdomen with the diagnosis of acute general peritonitis and washed out the abdomen very carefully. I have opened the abdomen in a number of cases where there was pus present, and have drained it, and some of the patients have gotten well.

Now then, my conclusion is that it is not so much the question of the treatment of the case as it is the kind of infection you have that produces death in this class of cases. A certain kind of infection will kill whether you flush the abdomen or not, whether you put in sixty or seventy drains.

If I had treated today the two cases I mention as having been treated so long ago, I would have flushed out the abdomen very carefully, and I would have ascribed the patients' recovery to the fact that I had been diligent in the washing out of the abdominal cavity; yet those cases both got well, and I did nothing but let the pus run out. So I think when we come to canvass the whole situation, consider the whole case, those that we have washed out and the cases that we have drained, that we will come to the conclusion it is not so much what we do for them as it is the kind of infection that produces death. In those cases where the abdomen is opened, the patient should be elevated high enough so that the pus will run out through the wound that is low down. It is not the flushing that counts so much as letting the pus drain out.

DR. MAYO. I am always glad to hear any method discussed by the result of which the patient is saved. A man who is doing surgical work can tell more from his own statistics than the rest of us can, because we cannot always see things from his point of view, and he cannot always describe things actually as he does them, so that we will understand.

The point that comes up is this: Dr. Fairchild states that there are different varieties of infection, and we know very well that there are different stages of the same infection. We know that very often the nature of an infection changes very materially even in twenty-four hours. We know that very often if serious cases run along from seven to ten days without death that the pus gets thick and it has then lost its virulent character. Therefore the particular stage in which an operation is made makes a great deal of difference.

If we "butt" in when nature is trying to do something with this infection, and allow to escape by drainage the very cells that nature can control itself, if we operate at the wrong time, we may only do harm.

The question comes up about flushing and draining. There

are various solutions used for washing that will prevent absorption; others favor it. If we flush them and do not drain them out absorption will take place; therefore if we are going to shut up the cavity we should leave in it a saline solution.

With reference to the capillary drains; if there is much pus —much fibrin, according to the stage of the peritonitis, they will block in a short period of time.

I think this term "general peritonitis" is a poor one. We should say diffuse peritonitis. If the patients die, call it general peritonitis, if it is such, afterwards. I think I have operated on cases, which, to use the old term, they were called general peritonitis, yet they were not.

Now after draining that, if we operate twenty-four or thirty-six hours after the primary onset, in most cases the chances are that recovery will take place. If we do the same thing on the third, fourth or fifth day it may possibly be followed by death in the severe cases.

Glass being smooth, and the bowels still having a little lustre, is good material for a drain, as it is not blocked by fibrin.

Now comes Fowler with his position: That is all right, but when we lift the head of the bed two feet and a six-foot person lies on it, the sixteen inches of the abdomen is only lifted one and one-half inches, which is not enough to drain the abdomen. Do this much and more by sitting them upright, with a rack behind for support.

Dr. Perkins. In closing the discussion, I will say that the first speaker misinterpreted me altogether if he thinks that I would flush the abdominal cavity in all cases.

In the case I described there was a large amount of pus in the pelvis; also there were large amounts in all parts of the cavity. There was probably as much as a quart of pus altogether.

Where the infection is known to be general, I think the best results are to be gotten by free flushing; at least my best results have been gotten by this method. Where infection is local I would not flush.

As regards drainage tubes, a drainage tube of gauze will drain serum, but it will not drain pus or blood, and if I were to use a gauze drain I would use a tube as well.

One object in using drainage tubes is to have a means for after-flushing.

The absorption that takes place while flushing is not so great, I think, as we formerly believed. And by flushing the abdomen you remove much of the poison, thereby preventing it from being absorbed. I think flushing removes little or none of the lymph. I would not wipe the lymph off, for by so doing you nearly always open up fresh surfaces for infection.

I think it quite true that, as Dr. Fairchild remarked, our cases of recovery may often be due to nature and not to our methods. The mortality is so great in this class of cases, that we should try every possible means to get some method by which we can get better results.

It is probably true that pus becomes less virulent if let alone. However, I would feel very nervous, to say the least, if I knew that there was a quart of pus in an abdomen, and I did not make the best effort I could to get it out.

DR. MOLEEN. The matter of neurasthenia is one in which the profession has been subjected to a good deal of criticism in the use of that term, and only recently I saw quite a caustic article in relation to the use of the term "neurasthenia," in which the stand was taken that the use of such a term was merely an evasion of a deeper and more thorough examination and diagnosis. While that may be true, I think in the absence of any more thorough data we must accept the symptomatic term for the naming of such a symptom so complex as we find it in the cases we have seen fit to term "neurasthenics."

The cause of neurasthenia is undoubtedly widespread. I think that the later work of Van Noorden on the metabolic disorders gives a great many cases of neurasthenia.

I take it that the application of neurasthenia to tubercular patients, as has been cited, may be somewhat dependent upon its condition. We well know how hard it is to get a tubercular case to eat fats. The nitrogenous foods we can scarcely get them to take, and, as has been well shown by Van Noorden and his classes, with the carbo-hydrates, including starch and sugar, we have the urid acid intoxication, the oxybutyric and the acetic, and it is to them and their irritant effects that a good many of the irritant neuroses have been attributed. I simply mention this in connection with the excellent paper of Dr. Courtney on neurasthenia occurring in tuberculosis.

NORMAL OBSTETRICS.

(CHAPTER TWELVE.)

THE PHYSIOLOGY OF LABOR.

By T. MITCHELL BURNS, M.D.,

Denver, Colorado.

Professor of Obstetrics, The Denver and Gross College of Medicine,

The Synonyms for Labor.—The synonyms for labor are childbirth, confinement, parturition and travail.

The Definition of Labor.—Labor is the process by which the ovum or the fetus and after-birth are expelled from the uterus.

The Frequency of Labor.—Of married women about 85 per cent have children. The average number of children to each mother is four.

The Classification of Labor.—Labor is divided into normal or natural—eutocia (u to' ke ah), abnormal or difficult labor—dystocia (dys to' ke ah) and artificial. Abortion is labor before the formation of the placenta or before the end of the fourth lunar month. Miscarriage or immature labor (partis immaturus), is labor after the formation of the placenta, but before viability of the fetus, i. e., from the end of the fourth to the end of the seventh lunar month. Premature labor (partis prematurus), is labor after the fetus is viable, but before the end of the natural duration of pregnancy, i. e., before the end of the tenth lunar month. Labor at term (partis maturus), is labor at the end of the tenth lunar month. Postponed labor is labor at the end of the tenth lunar month. Missed labor is postponed labor with the fetus dead at the onset of the labor.

The Time of Labor.—A frequent time for "labor pains" to begin is between 10 and 12 P. M., and twice as many cases end at night, i. e., between 9 P. M. and 9 A. M., as in the day.

The Stages of Labor.—Besides the premonitory stage, labor has three definite stages, namely:—The first stage or the stage of dilation of the cervix, the second stage or the stage of expulsion of the fetus, and the third stage or the stage of the expulsion of the after-birth and the retraction of the uterus.

The Duration of Labor.—The exact duration of labor is not really known, for in some dilation of the cervix begins long before any "pains" are present, while in others "pains" begin before there is any apparent dilation. The extremes in the duration of labor are from a few minutes of bearing down sensations or slight "pains" to three or four days of severe "pains." In the latter case the duration is sometimes ended by the mother dying from exhaustion. The average duration of labor in the primipara is about eighteen hours and in the multipara about nine hours. Hence, the average duration of labor in multips is about half that of primips. The duration of labor is shorter in multiparæ because of the previous stretching of the birth canal. The longer the interval between the labors, the longer the labor as a rule, for the relaxation produced by the previous labor has been obliterated. Labor is said, by the majority, to be longer in very young and elderly primiparæ, but the practice of some men (Dr. Davis of Philadelphia and myself) does not confirm this in reference to the very young. Elderly primips do have a harder time than the average primip, because of the rigidity of the birth canal, lack of strength or nervous irritability. The duration is often relatively longer in stout women, muscular women, frail nervous women and in society women. Abnormal presentations, large and sometimes small fetuses prolong labor by interfering with the engagement of the presenting part. The duration of the different stages of labor is as follows: In primiparæ the first stage averages sixteen hours, the second stage one and one half hours, and the third stage one half hour. In multiparæ the first stage averages seven and one half hours, the second stage one hour and the third stage one half hour. It is very difficult to estimate the duration of a given case of labor, as often very good "pains" die away or an apparently rigid cervix suddenly dilates.

The Conditions Usually Necessary for Normal Labor.—The conditions usually necessary for normal labor are 1st, a normal relation between the fetus and the mother, i. e., as to the size, shape, presentation, position and attitude of the fetus and the condition of the birth canal; 2nd, normal, acting urine and abdominal forces; and 3d, a normal mother and fetus. As an exception easy labors occur without all of the preceding conditions being present. A rare example of this is the case, mentioned by Lusk, of the woman who, while suffering from paraplegia, had an easy labor.

The Causes of Labor.—These are divided into predisposing and exciting. The Predisposing (or Determining) Causes: They are those conditions which prepare the way for labor, viz., (1) increasing uterine irritability or contractions especially marked at cause the onset of labor. What this exciting cause is has not been that which produces the increased uterine contractions, which the time for each menstrual period; (2) increasing tension of the fully developed uterine walls—effects easily noted in cases of excessive distention of the uterus, as in twins; (3) changes in the placental decidua—thinning and loosening from fatty degeneration, obliteration of sinuses from thrombi and formation of young connective tissue; (4) changes in the placental blood—increase of carbon dioxide and other waste products and diminishment of oxygen—resulting from changes in the placenta, certain changes in the fetal circulation and accumulation of some non-used substance from the fetus when it is fully developed; (5) changes in the placental and uterine circulation from the above changes in the decidua and from the beginning closure of the ductus arteriosus and venosus and foramen ovale, and (6) the gradual relaxation of the cervix. In brief, we may say changes in the uterine irritability, contractions and tension, the placental decidua and blood, the placental and uterine circulation and the cervix.

The Exciting (or Efficient) Cause: The exciting cause is determined. The author believes that labor and menstruation are rhythmic processes like the action of the heart and bowels, and that labor is excited by the irritation produced at that time for a menstrual period, generally the tenth, which corresponds most closely with the complete ovular development, that when the ovum is ripe it acts as a foreign body as do the contents of the distended rectum, and that the irritation which converts the ovum into a foreign body is the waste material from the ripe placenta, and possibly from the fetus, and that the irritation acts on the sympathetic ganglia of the uterus. (Waste products from the placenta because when certain premature changes occur in the placenta before the tenth lunar mouth, the ovum is expelled and when these changes do not occur the placenta continues to be retained in the uterus, even though the fetus is dead.) All believe that in some cases any extra exertion, strain or emotion may act as the exciting cause. Whether the normal exciting cause acts through the sympathetic, the cerebro-spinal or both systems is not known, but it has been determined that from certain centres in the sympathetic and cerebro-spinal systems, uterine contractions, powerful enough to cause labor, can be artificially produced. In the sympathetic system irritation of the cervical ganglia by the finger, pressure of contractions in the pregnant and non-pregnant, and after the uterus the presenting part or electricity increases or produces uterine has been removed from the body irritation of the ganglia in the cornua may cause uterine contractions. In the rabbit, if the pregnant uterus, adnexa and pieces of the aorta and vena cava are removed together, the blood vessels cleaned of blood with Locke's saline solution and these organs kept in a properly prepared moist container, labor will take place apparently as it does when the uterus is connected with the cerebro-spinal system. In the cerebrospinal system there is a center in the medulla and a center in the lumbar region of the cord. The center in the medulla acts reflexly and directly. It acts reflexly from the irritation of the spinal nerves, e. g., from rubbing the breasts. It acts directly from change in the circulation in the medulla. Impure or anemic blood produce, contractions, while strong emotions produce or stop them. The center in the lumbar region of the cord acts reflexly, only.

The Characteristics of the Uterine Contractions ("Labor Pains").—1. Involuntary, but affected by mental impressions. The coming of an unknown physician may stop "labor pains," while the confidence felt by the presence of the family physician may increase them.

2. Intermittent but increasing in frequency from every thirty to every five minutes. The duration of a contraction is about one minute. Each contraction increases up to a maximum and then

declines. This intermittency prevents the parturient becoming
exhausted and the fetus asphyxiated. Constant contraction of the
uterus would stop the placental circulation by compressing the
uterine blood vessels. It is only during a contraction that any
labor is done, but the interval of rest prepares for the effort of
the next pain.

3. Peristaltic. The contraction begins at the fundus and
passes so rapidly to the cervix that it seems as if the whole uterus
contracted at once, but a hand in the uterus can feel the contraction start at the fundus. (Playfair).

4. Painful. The amount of pain varies greatly with the
individual, the conditions present and the stage of labor. The pain
begins after the contraction commences and ends normally before
it is finished. At the beginning of the first stage of labor the
pains are dull and colicky with a pressing down sensation, and
near the end of this stage cutting or tearing. These pains are felt
in the lumbo-sacral region and radiate around into the groins and
at times down the front of the thighs. In some cases they are felt
first in the lower abdomen and then in the back. (In such cases the
labor is generally easier). In the second stage bearing down pains
occur which culminate in a terrible tearing sensation, as the head
passes the vulvar orifice. In this stage the pain is situated in the
lumbo-sacral region, pelvic joints and the parturient canal, (i. e.,
the lower uterine segment, the cervix, vagina and vulva). The
pain is due to the pressure on, the stretching and tearing of the
nerves of the lower segment, the cervix, vagina, vulva and neighboring structures.

5 and 6. Change the form and position of the uterus. Between contractions the uterus is relaxed and flattened antero-posteriorly. When the patient is standing, if the abdominal wall is
relaxed, the uterus is ante-flexed ,but if the abdominal wall is
firm it is flexed backwards and rests upon the spinal column, as it
does when the patient is in the dorsal position. During a contraction the uterus becomes more cylindrical, i. e., the axis of the
fundus, body, cervix and the pelvic inlet correspond, and the fundus so markedly bulges the abdominal wall that it can be easily
seen.

7. Powerful. The power depends upon the resistance, the

frequency of the uterine contractions and the presentation and position of the fetus. It is most powerful in the L. O. A. position. This power is independent of the general strength of the parturient. The independency of this power is shown by the great force exerted by the uterus in some weak women.

8. Cause, aided by uterine retraction, expulsion of the uterine contents. Mechanism in brief: When the uterus contracts its whole area squeezes on its fluid contents, but because the lower uterine segment is thinner and, therefore, less contractile and retractile and because there is an opening in the cervix, the contractions and retractions of the upper segment gradually dilate the lower segment and the cervix from above downwards, and then pushes the uterine contents into and through the lower segment and the cervix.

9. Form the "forewaters." 10. Rupture the membranes and 11. Detach the placenta and membranes. The formation of the forewaters, rupture of the membranes and detachment of the placenta are aided by uterine retraction. Their mechanism will be given in the physiology of the different stages of labor.

THE PHYSIOLOGY OF THE PREMONITORY STAGE OF LABOR.

Time.—This stage begins from one day to three weeks before the real onset of labor.

Cause.—It is due to the sinking of the uterus. (See "Sinking of the Uterus" under chapter eight, "Maternal Changes").

Symptoms.—Its symptoms (precursory symptoms of labor) are sinking of the fetus and uterus and their concomitants, frequent micturition, leucorrhoea, swelling of lower limbs, vulva and their veins, difficult locomotion, constipation, freer respiration and less gastric distrurbance. The last two constitute what is called "lightening" (to cheer up, i. e., to feel better).

The Size of the Cervical Canal and Its Ora.—In the premonitory stage and in the last month of pregnancy, in primigravidæ, the finger can generally be introduced into but not through the internal os, and in the multigravidæ one or two fingers may be introduced into the external os and often one into the interior os, and sometimes even two. This is not due to any expulsive effort caused by the uterine contractions. It is due to the relaxed condition of the cervix from local congestion and lacerations, and to the distention of the uterus. It does not indicate that the external os begins to dilate before the internal, but it does show that the internal os is a much more powerful sphincture.

The Condition of the Anterior Lip of the Cervix.—The anterior lip of the cervix in the premonitory stage is usually stretched much more than the posterior. This is due to the presenting part pressing more upon the anterior lip, the cervical canal being posterior to the centre of the pelvic cavity. This difference in the lips occurs more often in the primigravidæ because of the early descent of the presenting part. If the presenting part is pushed up the stretching of the anterior lip will disappear, showing that it is not due to a permanent retraction of the cervix.

THE PHYSIOLOGY OF THE FIRST STAGE OF LABOR.

The physiologic phenomena which occur in this stage are the formation of the "bag of waters," the dilation of the cervix and the rupture of the membranes.

The Forewaters—Synonym, "Bag of Waters."—Definition: That portion of the liquor amnii in the membranes below the presenting part is called the forewaters. Cause: The forewaters are due to each uterine contraction pushing the liquor amnii and fetus towards the cervix but not perfectly corking the lower segment with the presenting part. Some say it is formed by the ball-valve action of the presenting part. Size and Form: The size and form of the bag of waters depends upon the amount of the liquor amnii, the presentation, position and engagement of the presenting part. presenting part, it is large and wide, except in some cases where (In abnormal presentations, from imperfect engagement of the it projects through a partially dilated cervix, then it is long and narrow.)

The Dilation of the Cervix.—Cause: The cervix dilates from above downward by the contractions and retractions of the upper segment being greater than those of the lower segment and the cervix, as previously mentioned, but there are other conditions which assist dilation of the cervix, viz:—The presence of a large bag of waters and softening of the cervix. A large bag of waters dilates the cervix by its hydrostatic action, which is more perfect than the pressure of the presenting part, and by its softening effect, due to its pressure checking the venous return in the cervix and causing an exudate of serum. Softening of the cervix is due to the intra-abdominal pressure acting on the blood vessels of the abdomen and not upon those of the pelvic cavity, to sinking of the uterus and fetus, and to the presence of a large bag of waters. Abdominal contractions may assist dilation of the cervix but they are not normal until near the end of the first stage, as they tend to cause exhaustion of the patient if long continued. Time: Nearly all now believe that the cervical canal does not really begin to dilate until term. (See "The Maternal Changes." The author believes that the lower segment does dilate during pregnancy. See "Changes in the lower segment" under "The Maternal Changes.")

The Condition of the Edge of the External Os: During the first half of the dilation of the cervix the external os becomes thin, and often in primiparæ feels like a thread or the edge of a sheet of paper, later it becomes thick, especially in multiparæ, in whom it sometimes becomes thicker than the little finger.

The Changes in the Thickness of the Wall of the Cervix: At the beginning of dilation the wall thins, like the edge of the external os, but later, as the cervical canal dilates, the wall thickens from retraction, and may become as thick as it was at the beginning of labor. This retraction is what causes the external os to thicken.

The "Show."—This is the term applied to the blood-streaked leucorrhoea which is present in the first stage of labor. This blood is due to slight lacerations of the cervix, the result of rather rapid dilation (and possibly at times to slight separation of the placenta).

The Rupture of the Membranes.—The increasing tension of the expanding membranes opposite the cervix causes them to rupture. The tear generally begins opposite the opening of the cervix, as here there is the least resistance to the expansion or stretching of the membranes. Normally only the liquor amnii in front of the presenting part escapes. As the tension in the "bag of waters" becomes sufficiently strong the membranes rupture. This is normal at the time of complete dilation of the cervix. Premature rupture,

i. e., rupture before the cervix is dilated is not rare. It is due to the contraction being abnormally powerful or to the membranes lacking the normal resistance. *"Dry Labor,"* i. e., a dry birth canal, results when the membranes rupture at the beginning of dilation and most of the liquor amnii escapes. The liquor amnii escapes because of the imperfect engagement of the presenting part. Dry labor causes prolonged labor from lack of fluid for the uterus to contract upon, and lack of fluid for dilation and lubrication. *Late rupture* occurs when the membranes do not rupture until they begin to pass through the vagina or vulva. This is not rare and is normal if it does not delay labor. Very rarely the membranes do not rupture, the ovum being born with the sac entire. As a rule the presenting part follows the "bag of waters" in its passage through the vagina, but when the presenting part does not engage, as frequently is the case in abnormal presentation, and there is considerable liquor amnii, the "bag of waters" may descend to the vulva and the presenting part still remain within the cervix.

The "Caul."—This is the term used to express the fact that the child is "born with a vail," i. e., with a piece of the membranes over its face. (In these cases a circular rent occurs in the membranes, probably by the opening in the membranes opposite the occiput being small, while the nose or chin makes a rent posteriorly as the head is expelled from the vulva, and then the two openings uniting laterally, leave a piece of the membranes over the face.) Many laymen believe that the "caul" signifies that the baby will be a clairvoyant or a seer, but obstetricians cannot see any connection between the two.

Nausea, Vomiting and Shivering.—Nausea, vomiting and shivering frequently occur together or separately, in the first stage of labor. The nausea and vomiting are reflex from pressure. The shivering is generally reflex, i. e., nervous, but it is often due to sweating and subsequent chilling between "pains."

The Physiology of the Second Stage of Labor.

The physiologic phenomenon of this stage is the expulsion of the fetus, i. e., its passage through the birth canal. When the cervix is completely dilated the presenting part begins to pass into the vagina. In the expulsion of the uterine contents the uterine contractions and retractions, previously mentioned, are greatly aided by the contractions of the abdominal muscles.

The Action of the Abdominal Muscles.—The abdominal muscles are under the control of the will until near the end of the second stage, when the head begins to press upon the rectum and stretch it. The mechanism of the action of the abdominal muscles is as follows: The parturient takes the bearing-down attitude and holds her breath, i. e., she presses her feet firmly against some object, brings her shoulders forward, flexes her legs, grasps something with her hands, holds her breath and contracts the abdominal muscles. After the contraction she relaxes her muscles, straightens out and breathes rapidly for a while. The action of the abdominal muscles tends to push the whole of the abdominal contents into and out of the pelvis, but the pelvic floor and uterine ligaments hold the uterus and other organs back so that, as a result, only the uterus is pushed more or less into the pelvis and through the opening in the pelvic floor. At times, especially in primiparæ, when the contractions of the abdominal muscles are very strong, the uterus is pushed more or less into the pelvis. The action of the abdominal muscles in labor is the same as in defecation. (Prolapsus of the uterus and hernia may result from contraction of the abdominal muscles in lifting.)

The Action of the Uterine Ligaments.—The uterine ligaments contract with the uterus, hold the uterus forward and against the pelvic brim and, as stated above, prevent the descent of the uterus.

The Action of the Vgaina and Pelvis.—As the fetus passes through the cervix it meets the resistance of the vaginæ and pelvic walls, the former is quickly overcome by stretching, but as the latter is solid, the fetus has to mould itself to correspond in shape with the shape of the pelvic canal, and, as a result, goes through a wonderful mechanism before the uterine contractions expel it through the pelvis. This mechanism will be studied at the end of this chapter.

Recession of the Fetus.—With each utero-abdominal contraction the fetus advances a little. After the contraction it recedes some from the relaxation which follows a contraction. This relaxation prevents the child being asphyxiated by constant compression.

The Mechanism of Dilation of the Perineum and Vulva.—
This is similar to the dilation of the lower uterine segment and
the cervix, first stretching then retracting. When the presenting
part begins to press upon the pelvic floor the vulva begins to dilate.
As the force is mostly directed against the lower part of the posterior vaginal wall, it stretches the perineum to a length of four
or five inches, between the anus and the vaginal orifice. Then the
presenting part is thrown fully forward into the vulvar opening
by the posterior resistance of the pelvic floor and the perineum
itself. As the presenting part enters the vulvar orifice it pushes
the whole orifice forward and stretches it, and when the orifice
is dilated nearly to the size of the presenting part, the whole vulva,
but especially the perineum, retracts and passes over the presenting
part. As the tension in the perineum often becomes very great,
from expansion, it frequently tears, especially in primiparæ, when
the head is large and is expelled rapidly or the posterior shoulder
is delivered last.

*The Expulsion of the Fetus from the Vagina and Vulva
After It Leaves the Uterus.*—This is mainly due to the contractions of the abdominal muscles, as the uterus has nothing on which
to contract. The contraction of the vaginal muscles may produce
some effect.

Lacerations of the Perineum and Vulva.—Frequency: According to the author's experience in every case of labor carefully
examined, abrasions of the perineum or vulva may be found. Of
all primiparae 90 per cent. are torn sufficiently, either externally
or internally, to warrant repair (Auvard, out of one hundred primiparæ, found the vulva intact only in five). At least 20 per cent.
of all multiparæ are torn sufficiently to warrant repair. (Older
writers give the frequency as 30 per cent. in primiparae and 10
per cent. in multiparae).

Effect: Tears within the vaginal orifice, in the region of the
vestibule and labia minora generally heal kindly without repair if
not extensive, as their walls are generally in apposition. Tears
of the perineum tend to gap and offer a good field for infection
and predispose to prolapsus of the uterus by breaking the pelvic
floor. (Prolonged excessive stretching of the perineum without
tearing is according to the author's experience more liable to cause

prolapsus of the uterus than is a good-sized tear repaired, i. e., the latter leave the vagina smaller).

Situations and Varieties: The tear generally occurs in the perineum and a little to the right or left of the median line and extends more or less externally towards the anus and internally up the posterior wall of the vagina. At times it extends laterally from the fourchette to the labia minora. It may form a transverse slit. Rarely the tear extends into the rectum. Small tears in or near the vestibule are very frequent.

Causes: They are in order of importance, thin and tense perineum, rapid exit of the head, delivery of posterior shoulder last, incomplete flexion, small pubic arch, small vulvar orifice, large head, wide shoulders, improper pressure of the hand or the dorsal decubitus of parturient. Pushing the head toward the pubes tends to slightly increase tearing of the vestibule but it greatly diminishes tearing of the perineum.

THE PHYSIOLOGY OF THE THIRD STAGE OF LABOR.

This stage is characterized by the detachment and expulsion of the placenta and the complete retraction of the uterus.

The Detachment and Expulsion of the Placenta.—Mechanism: As the fetus is expelled the uterus retracts upon the placenta. In from 5 to 30 minutes the uterine contractions fully return and, as before, acting more strongly on the upper uterine segment, detach and finally expel the placenta into the vagina, and then the abdominal and vaginal contractions expel it out of the vulva. Separation occurs in the meshy degenerated portion of the maternal part of the placenta, leaving a varying portion still adhering to the endometrium which is finally absorbed or passed off in the lochia. The placenta folded once upon itself, generally makes its exit from the cervix edgewise, but if for any reason the card has been pulled upon, it comes centre first and, being less compact, more than fills the cervix and often delays delivery and by allowing blood to accumulate between it and the uterine walls favors post-partum hemorrhage.

The Amount of Placental Tissue Remaining Adherent to the Uterus After Delivery of the Placenta.—In apparently normal cases, the maternal surface of the placenta, looking unbroken, varies from practically none—the placental site being as smooth as the rest of the endometrium, or slightly honeycombed—to a definite amount, causing a raised well honeycombed area marking the site of placental attachment. (Deduction by the author from Caesarian sections, post-mortem examinations and explorations of the uterine cavity immediately after labor).

The Retraction of the Uterus.—As soon as the placenta is expelled the upper segment retracts, followed by the lower segment and the cervix, and all the torn blood vessels caused by the separation of the placenta are closed by this retraction and by the formation of thrombi in the ends of the sinuses. After the fundus is properly retracted it is generally just below the navel and firm.

The Amount of Blood Lost.—Normally the amount of blood lost does not exceed in amount one-half the size of the placenta, or about two pounds and is mostly venous. After the placenta is expelled there is normally very slight, if any continuous flow of blood from the vagina. Any amount which affects the parturient is abnormal.

Nausea, Vomiting and Shivering.—The shivering is much more frequent than the nausea and vomiting. The shivering is partially due to exposure, loss of blood and the cessation of muscular exertion.

THE EFFECTS OF LABOR UPON THE MATERNAL ORGANISM.

The temperature is increased from one to two degrees by the uterine contractions, i. e., the muscular exertion. The respirations are slowed or stopped during contractions, but between the contractions are increased in frequency. The pulse increases with the contractiones until the acme is reached, then the pulse may stop from the general muscular tension. Just after the acme, the pulse is rapid, but subsequently to this it gradually resumes the normal. The author has seen a pulse which was only 60 between contractions rise to 120 just before the acme. (These changes in the pulse were given under "The Maternal Changes"). The arterial tension is increased and as a consequence urination is frequent and profuse and the perspiration free. Congestion of the head and extremities occurs during contractions in the second stage from the increase of intra-abdominal pressure forcing the blood out of the abdomen into the extremities. A loss of weight occurs, independent of the loss of the fetus and its appendages, from the increase of waste due to muscular exertion, loss of blood, perspiration and urination.

THE SYMPTOMS OF LABOR.

These will be given under the management of labor.

THE PLASTIC PHENOMENA OF LABOR.

The Caput Succedaneum.—This is a serous swelling, which often forms upon the centre of the presenting part during the second stage of labor and sometimes during the first, from the pressure upon the rest of the head causing an exudate of serum into the non-pressed area.

The Moulding of the Presenting Part.—As the fetus is pushed by the force from behind through the pelvic canal, the resistance offered by the latter causes the head or other presenting part to mould itself to correspond with the shape of the canal. The moulding differs in the different presentations and causes considerable change in the diameters of the head. These changes will be studied under the different presentations. In the vertex presentation the O. F., S. O. F. and S. O. B. diameters are diminished while the O. M. diamater is increased. These changes in the shape of the head in the vertex presentation will be understood by imagining the changes produced by pushing the head into a cylinder, which is a little smaller than the head.

THE MECHANISM OF LABOR.

Definition.—The manner in which the fetus passes through the pelvic canal.

Similarity.—It is similar in all presentations, but most perfect in the vertex.

Review.—It would be better if at this time the anatomy of the bony pelvis, the pelvic soft parts, the attitude, form, lie, presentations and positions of the fetus and the diameters of the fetal head and trunk are reviewed.

The Mechanism of the Vertex Presentation.

The Six Stages.—The six stages are flexion, descent, rotation, extension, external rotation and expulsion, or to be more explicit, (1) flexion of the head, (2) descent of the head and trunk, (3) internal anterior rotation of the occiput, (4) extension of the head, (5) external rotation of the head and internal rotation of the shoulders and (6) expulsion of the trunk.

Descent and the Other Stages.—Descent accompanies all other stages, but especially flexion and expulsion of the trunk.

Accommodation.—All these stages are movements of accommodation, i. e., changes to facilitate the expulsion of the fetus. In other words motion in the direction of the least resistance.

The First Stage—The Stage of Flexion of the Head.— (Flexion and Descent: Many authors give descent as the first stage but as flexion is present to a considerable extent before labor begins, i. e., is a part of the attitude of the fetus, we believe that flexion should be given as the first stage in the mechanism of labor.)

Cause: (1) The normal *attitude* of the fetus causing partial flexion of the head. (2) The lever action of the head—the forehead, being the long end of the lever, the occiput being the short end and the atlas being the fulcrum; equal forces, or resistances, e. g., the lower segment of the uterus or the pelvic brim,—acting on the ends of the lever from below would cause bending of the forehead toward the trunk, i. e., flexion. (Here the head is "a lever of the first kind." (3) The *moulding* of the head—(Pajot's law—when a solid body is contained within another, the sides of which are slippery and a little angular, the inner body under motion tends to conform to the shape of the container).

Site: In the lower uterine segment, (especially in primiparae), the inlet, the pelvic cavity, or on the perineum or not at all, depending upon the situation and amount of resistance.

Value: (1) It substitutes a lesser for a greater diameter, i. e., it causes the head to enter the pelvis with the S. O. B. diameter parallel with the plane of the inlet, instead of the S. O. F. or O. F. diameter. (2) It converts the fetus into an immobile rod, i. e., it places the chin firmly against the chest so that the head cannot move. Continuance: Flexion continues until the head reaches the perineum.

The Second Stage—The Stage of Descent of the Head and Trunk.—Cause: (1) The normal attitude of the fetus, i. e., flexion of the head, (2) anterior rotation of the occiput, (3) anterior position of the occiput, (4) moulding of the head and trunk, (5) The *visa tergo,* the uterine contractions and retractions and the abdominal contractions. The entrance of the head into the inlet: In the vertex presentation the long diameter of the head, the antero-posterior, the S. O. B. diameter, enters one of the oblique diameters parallel with the plane of the inlet, while the B. P. diameter enters the opposite oblique diameter parallel with the plane of the inlet. (The rule in all presentations is that the long diameter of the presenting part always enters the pelvis in the long diameter of the inlet.) Continuance of the head in the axis of the inlet: The head follows the axis of the superior strait until the pelvic floor is reached.

The Third Stage—The Stage of the Anterior Rotation of the Occiput.—Cause: (1) The complete flexion of the head or the occiput being the dependent part. (Flexion assists because, as will be seen the more dependent the presenting part—the lower end of the lever, the occiput, and the higher the other end of the lever, the forehead—the easier the rotation), (2) the resistance of the perineum and probably the sacrum, posteriorly and below near the outlet, and to a much less extent the resistance of the pelvic side wall anteriorly and above near the inlet. The resistance of the perineum causes that which descends first, i. e., the most dependent part, in the vertex presentation, the occiput, to be pushed, i. e., rotated, anteriorly while the part remaining high up, the forehead, is pushed backwards. (That the perineum is the main cause has been proven by pushing a fetus through the female cadaver. As long as the perineum remained firm the occiput rotated anteriorly even in the posterior positions.) (3) Anterior position of the occiput: This assists because it makes the mechanism shorter, instead of the occiput having to travel three-eighths of a circle it has only to travel one-eighth of a circle and because the occiput is where the force is more directly forward, and the forehead, where the force is more directly backward. Continuance: Anterior rotation continues until the A. P. of the head diameter is into, or nearly into the A. P. diameter of the outlet.

The Fourth Stage—Extension of the Head.—Cause: (1) The attitude, for extension to occur there must be some flexion; (2) the resistance posteriorly of the pelvic soft and hard parts, especially the perineum; (3) the lack of resistance anteriorly at the vulvar orifice; and, (4) the impingement of the back of the neck against the subpubic ligament. Time: Extension of the head begins when the occiput gets below the subpubic ligament.

Description: After the occiput rotates anteriorly, the resistance of the perineum, still acting, throws the occiput forward beneath the pelvic arch until finally the back of the neck rests against the subpubic ligament. Then as the back of the neck cannot advance any more the forces from above and the resistance of the perineum posteriorly causes the forehead to be pushed forward—i. e., the head to extend—the back of the neck pivoting on the subpubic ligament, while the forehead describes the arc of a circle, whose radius extends from the back of the neck to the forehead; thus, the bregma, then the forehead, the face and the chin pass over the perineum and are delivered. Briefly, the occiput enters the vulvar orifice, the back of the neck pivots on the subpubic ligament and the head is born by extension, the forehead appearing over the perineum, then the nose and lastly the chin. (It is very probable that the chin does not begin to leave the chest until the neck rests against the subpubic ligament.)

The Fifth Stage—The External Rotation of the Head.— Rule: The occiput turns toward the side it occupied at the inlet. (In all presentations the short end of the lever turns toward the side it occupied at the inlet.) Cause: (1) Internal rotation of the shoulders, one shoulder, (generally the anterior) being lower than the other. (2) Restitution. Description: When the occiput rotates anteriorly the shoulders rotate nearly into the transverse diameter. As the head is born the shoulders reach the pelvic floor and the anterior shoulder rotates anteriorly as a rule, because it is the lower. This brings the shoulders into the antero-posterior diameter of the pelvis and by necessity rotates the head externally from the antero-posterior diameter to the transverse. Restitution: If the shoulders do not rotate into the transverse diameter, when the occiput rotates anteriorly, the neck is twisted and when the head is born, being free, the neck untwists and the occiput turns toward the side it occupied at the inlet. This is called restitution. An exception to the rule: Sometimes the posterior shoulder is the lower, then it rotates anteriorly and as a result the occiput, instead of turning toward the side it occupied at the inlet, turns toward the opposite side.

The Sixth Stage.—The Expulsion of the Trunk.— Cause: (1) Uterine contractions and retractions. (2) Abdominal contractions. (3) The normal relation between the size and shape of the trunk and pelvis. Description: The anterior shoulder passes under the subpubic ligament upon which it pivots, while the posterior shoulder is passing over the perineum. This mechanism is often imperfect, both shoulders being born together, or the anterior before the posterior. The trunk undergoes lateral flexion and is rapidly delivered in a spiral direction. The breech is delivered the same as the shoulders.

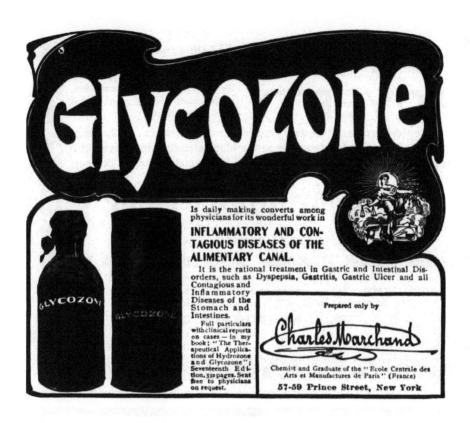

DENVER MEDICAL TIMES

THOMAS H. HAWKINS, A.M., M.D., EDITOR AND PUBLISHER.

COLLABORATORS:

Henry O. Marcy, M.D., Boston.
Thaddeus A. Reamy, M.D., Cincinnati.
Nicholas Senn, M.D., Chicago.
Joseph Price, M.D., Philadelphia.
Franklin H. Martin, M.D., Chicago.
William Oliver Moore, M.D., New York.
L. S. McMurtry, M.D., Louisville.
Thomas B. Eastman, M.D., Indianapolis, Ind.
G. Law, M.D., Greeley, Colo.

S. H. Pinkerton, M.D., Salt Lake City.
Flavel B. Tiffany, M.D., Kansas City.
Erskine M. Bates, M.D:, New York.
E. C. Gehrung, M.D, St. Louis.
Graeme M. Hammond, M.D, New York.
James A. Lydston, M.D., Chicago.
Leonard Freeman, M.D., Denver.
Carey K. Fleming, M.D., Denver, Colo.

Subscriptions, $1.00 per year in advance; Single Copies, 10 cents.

Address all Communications to Denver Medical Times, 1740 Welton Street, Denver, Colo.
We will at all times be glad to give space to well written articles or items of interest to the
profession.
[Entered at the Postoffice of Denver, Colorado, as mail matter of the Second Class.]

EDITORIAL DEPARTMENT

THE AMERICAN MEDICAL ASSOCIATION.

The greatest gathering of medical practitioners ever held west of the Rocky Mountains will be the meeting of the American Medical Association at Portland, Oregon, on July 11-14 of the present year. Oregon has an ideal summer climate, and the grand scenery of the Columbia river will be a leading attraction to intending visitors. To appreciate nature's charms at her best, it has been arranged to hold one day's session of the delegates on barges.

The Portland physicians propose to entertain socially visiting members of the Association on a large and elaborate scale. The general sessions will be held in Festival Hall, a building erected especially for such purposes. This building is within the grounds of the Lewis and Clark Exposition, which will be under way at the time the medical convention meets. A hotel within the same grounds will accommodate 600 people. On account of the exposition the railway companies are offering special rates to Portland— much better rates from distant points than ever before for a similar event. The tickets will be good for 90 days and will provide almost unlimited stopover privileges. Yellowstone Park may be visited en route and it is expected that arrangements will be perfected whereby a person may go one way by a northern route and the other through California. It is thought that at least 2,500 members of the Association, with their families and guests, will take advantage of this unequaled opportunity for combining science and pleasure.

VALEDICTORY ADDRESS AT JOHNS HOPKINS UNIVERSITY.

The Journal prints in full, March 4, the valedictory address of Dr. Osler of Johns Hopkins University, which has been quoted and misquoted in the daily press. He deals with some of the problems of university life and states that at times the loss of a professor may be of benefit to a university. He stated that to a man of active mind too long attachment to one college is apt to breed self-satisfaction, to foster a local spirit, and to promote senility. He said that much of the phenomenal success of the Johns Hopkins University has been due to the concentration of a group of intellectual men, without local ties, whose operations were not restricted and who were willing to serve faithfully in whatever field of action they were placed. Dr. Osler advised the interchange of teachers, both national and international, and even advised the changing of college presidents now and then "for the good of the exchequer." He said that intellectual infantilism and progeria were two appalling maladies due to careless habits "of intellectual feeding." As a prophylactic measure he advises visiting other universities and colleges, both at home and abroad. He said that it is a very serious matter to have all the professors in a university growing old at the same time, and said that there should be a fixed period for the teacher, either of time of service or of age. He spoke of the comparative uselessness of men above 40 years of age, and said that to modify an old saying, "A man is sane morally at thirty, rich mentally at forty, wise spiritually at fifty—or never." He said that the young man should be encouraged and afforded every possible chance to show what is in him, and that the chief value of the teacher, who is no longer a productive factor, is to determine whether the thoughts which the young men are bringing to the light are false idols or true and noble ideas. He said that it would be of incalculable benefit, in commercial, political and professional life if men would retire from work at the age of 60. He said that the teacher's life should have three periods, study until 25, investigation until 40, profession until 60, at which age he would have him retired on a double allowance. He went at some length into the history of the Johns Hopkins Medical School, mentioning the strict entrance requirements and the scientific training in laboratory work especially. He dwelt on the necessity for practical training in the hospital wards as well as in the laboratories and class rooms. He said that the faculty of Johns Hopkins University has been blessed with two remarkable presidents, who had been a stimulus in every department, and that the good fellowship and harmony among the faculty has been delightful.

THE COUNCIL ON PHARMACY AND CHEMISTRY OF THE AMERICAN MEDICAL ASSOCIATION.

The board of trustees of the American Medical Association have created an advisory board to be known as the Council on Pharmacy and Chemistry and consisting, in addition to Dr Simmons, of fourteen of the leading American professors of pharmacy and chemistry. The purpose of the Council is to supply to physicians, through the medium of the Journal of the American Medical Association and by means of a book to be published, necessary and desirable information concerning those new and now unofficial proprietary remedies which it considers unobjectionable. This information will comprise composition, indications and uses, dosage, etc., much along the lines of the U. S. Pharmacopeia. The idea seems to us rational, and, if impartially executed, should prove an onward movement both in medicine and in pharmacy.

KIDNEY FAILURE FOLLOWING SURGICAL OPERATIONS.

At a recent meeting of the Clinical and Pathological Society Wetherill broached this important subject. His experience had shown him that while subjects of renal diseases sometimes bear operations and chloroform anesthesia well, cases in whom previous urinary examinations revealed no lesions of the kidneys would not infrequently develop post-operative albuminuria and suppression of urine, occasionally fatal. As to the causes of these serious complications a number of suggestions were made, including impure anesthetics, prolonged anesthesia, toxins from inflammatory foci, vasomotor paralysis, etc. After consideration, it seems to the writer that the principal cause of albuminuria with casts and later suppression in these surgical states, excluding pressure on or direct trauma to the urinary organs, is in lowered general blood pressure from shock and deficiency of fluids. The urinary condition would therefore be comparable to that observed in the renal ischemia of cholera and severe diarrheas, albumin escaping through the cells impaired by relative dehydration, and also being formed from these injured cells by maceration, as in the urine of chronic cystitis and in that retained within the bladder of dead persons. If these views are correct, albuminuria and urinary suppression after operative procedures are an accompaniment rather than a cause of failing vital forces, the phenomena being of the same nature as those noted toward the fatal end of non-surgical cases. Rational deductions for practice are to have plenty of fluid in the body and to prevent undue lowering of blood pressure, by short operations and by the free use of strophanthus, strychnine, digitalis, apocynum cannabinum, and particularly by the systematic injection of physiologic salt solution. Here as elsewhere and now as ever the heart is the mainspring of life, and its action must be considered first of all and in due season.

CHRONIC NASOPHARYNGEAL CATARRH.

This condition may depend on atrophic rhinitis, enlarged pharyngeal tonsils, the exanthemata, alcoholism or chronic Bright's disease. The patient complains of "dropping in the throat, hawking, hemming," swallowing and nasal secreatus, sometimes with nausea and vomiting in the morning after breakfast, and frequent headache. The symptoms are much worse in cold, damp weather. Inspection shows a constant, more or less profuse, thick, yellow, mucopurulent discharge from the vault of the pharynx. Posterior rhinoscopy reveals a large amount of thick, inspissated mucus in the vault and behind the palate; also a projecting gland-mass back of the vault. The mucous membrane is thickened and dull red in the simple relaxed form; dry and glazed in dry catarrh (hearing improved during running stage of a cold); with scattered millet-seed-like elevationns and injected vessels in granular catarrh.

For the simple form of the disease Kyle advises local applications of a solution of one drop of carbolic acid, five grains of borax and twelve drops of glycerine in one ounce of water; or of 1/2000 trichloracetic acid, or two to five per cent. zinc chloride solution or zinc sulphocarbolate solution (eight grains to the ounce), or a one to three per cent. formalin solution. In making these applications the probe should be curved so as to mop the back part of the soft palate. In the atrophic form the author directs to use freely a tepid alkaline antiseptic solution with the post-nasal syringe, followed by hydrogen peroxide and, if need be, the curved applicator with cotton to remove crusts. For excessive dryness he sprays every two or four hours with six drops each of oil of cassia and of sandalwood to the ounce of liquid albolene or benzoinol. The compound tincture of iodine is recommended for internal use. In the case of children Jacobi injects carefully into the pharynx twice a week a solution of one-half or one grain of silver nitrate in one ounce of water, using a dram of sodium chloride to the pint of water several times a day by insufflation.

BATHING.

Man should be a clean animal, both within and without. The external use of water is often or more benefit by way of its neurotonic effects than for mere cleanliness. For most adults a daily morning cold shower bath is a most excellent preparation for the day's work. Children, invalids and the aged may be given tepid baths, making better the night's rest. The cool tub bath is an important prophylactic against infantile summer complaint. Russian and Turkish baths are luxuries rather than necessities. Surf bathing is an invigorating pleasure. Strongly alkaline soap should not be used on the body. Infants and little children should be well massaged while in the bath. The duration of a bath ought seldom to exceed ten minutes, lest reaction be slow and difficult. When the full bath is impracticable at the time, it is well at least to bathe the feet and other parts most used or exposed to dust and friction. A cold bath morning and evening is of service as a prophylactic against heat prostration.

CLOTHING.

Two important sanitary factors are equal pressure and equal warmth. The extremities should be especially protected. Infan-

tile colic is frequently due to refrigeration, from allowing the
child to walk or sit on a wet floor, or lie in a wet diaper or with
the abdomen exposed to a draught of cold air.

On account of its being relatively a non-conductor and a good
absorber of moisture, wool is generally the best cloth for clothing
at all seasons. Of secondary value are silk and linen-mesh goods.
into extra-sensitiveness by wearing mufflers and "chest protectors."
Rubber articles hinder natural evaporation, and should be used
only in hot weather. The chest and neck should not be coddled
Much of the baldness of men is doubtless due to their tight un-
ventilated hats. Leather footwear should be comfortably loose,
with broad toes, low heels and soles of fair thickness. Even China
is awakening to the calls of hygiene, and the Dowager Empress
has issued an edict prohibiting foot-binding in the kingdom.
White clothing is much worn in tropical countries, to reflect the
sunlight and so reduce the effects of the great heat.
duce displacements of the womb and paresis of the diaphragm.

Corsets and other waist-constricting devices are a predisposing
cause of gall-stones and enteroptosis. The follies of fashion pro-
It should be added, however, that the corset is passing, for the time
at least, and the "Greek girdle" now largely worn is so narrow
that it cannot be injuriously tightened without making the parts
above and below bulge so much as to render the wearer ridiculous.
Indiscretions at the menstrual period are a prolific source of future
suffering from endometritis and sterility.

EXERCISE.

Parts and organs that are not used must atrophy. Daily systematic exercise, preferably in the open air, is conducive to health
and longevity. Walking is perhaps the best exercise for most
people, and a total of ten miles per day is a proper average. The
use of the bicycle has done much good and a little harm. Hamilton said, "The best thing for the inside of a man is the outside
of a horse." Athletic sports are frequently overdone, and the
victors become eventually physical wrecks. The rational object of
exercise is not to develop muscular lumps and humps, but to keep
the human organism at its highest working efficiency. Girls
should be encouraged to exercise as fully and freely as boys.

EDITORIAL ITEMS.

Pulmonary Gangrene. Sajous uses inhalations of carbolic acid, m. iii-vi to a half pint of boiling water.

Fibroid Phthisis. Hare recommends the continuous employment of arsenic.

For Pneumonic Cough. Preble employs carbonate of guaiacol in 5- grain doses, either with or without apomorphine, 1/20 grain.

Constipation of Infants. Ringer recommends sodium bicarbonate, one-half to one drachm to the pint of milk.

Gall-Stone Vomiting. Bartholow used to give a few drops frequently of ether or chloroform.

Acute Perihepatitis. Tyson recommends cuppings, sinapisms, fomentations; surgical intervention if suppuration.

Volvulus. Anders advises gastric lavage every four hours; no food for some hours; hydrostatic or pneumatic pressure or celiotomy.

Pulmonary Apoplexy. Tyson advises absolute rest, counter-irritation over the area involved, and anodynes to relieve pain.

Anemia. Brunton praises the ammoniocitrate of iron (dose 2 to 5 grains) as a medicine for young women.

Rectal Polpi and Large Hemorrhoids. Sulphur as a remedy is particularly valuable. It may be given as the compound licorice powder.

Senile Bronchorrhea. According to Hare, strychnine is the best remedy. Opiates and other sedatives are contra-indicated.

Bronchial Asthma of Children. Garrod employs chloral hydrate, 2 to 5 grains each hour during the asthmatic fit.

American Medical Association. Physicians going to Portland in July to attend the A. M. A will have to go by way of the Union Pacific Railway if they want solid comfort.

For Habitual Constipation. Roth prescribes: R Ext. cascarae fl., syrupi zingiberis, aq. dest. aa. partes equales; one to two teaspoonfuls at night as required.

Acute Constipation With Autointoxication. Thornton advises to take six ounces of liquor magnesii citratis and repeat in six hours if necessary.

For Passive Pulmonary Congestion. Shoemaker prescribes: R Ergotinae gr. 1/3; ext. digitalis gr. 1/4; pulv. ipecac co. gr. ii; one pill every three or four hours.

Vomiting of Appendicitis. John Ashhurst, Jr., employs calomel (1/20 to 1/12 grain) with bicarbonate of sodium (1 or 2 grains) in repeated doses.

Vomiting of Typhoid Fever. Charles W. Earle furnishes the following: R. Bismuthi subnit. gr. iv; acidi carbol. m. ⅛; glycerini m. viii; aquam q.s. A teaspoonful every two to four hours.

Pneumokonioses. Anders advises change of occupation or several hours' exercise daily in the open air. Treat supervening chronic bronchitis and emphysema or tuberculosis.

Neurotic Cough in Children Near Puberty. Correct habits (masturbation, etc.) and hygiene. Take regular outdoor exercise and cold shower baths, and bromides for short periods.

Hope's Dysentery Mixture. R Acidi nitrosi ℨi; mist. camphorae ℨvii; tinct. opii gtt. xl. A fourth part to be taken every three or four hours.

For Lead Colic. Morphine should be administered hypodermically; magnesium sulphate and dilute sulphuric acid may be given by the mouth.

Vomiting of Acute Pancreatitis. Louis Starr has the patient swallow lumps of ice; also iced carbolic acid water and effervescing draughts.

Sick Stomach Due to Constipation. Hare employs a pair of seidlitz powders, one-fourth of each paper in half a wineglassful of water every fifteen minutes till all is taken.

For Chronic Constipation. Da Costa prescribed: R Aloini gr. 1/12; strych. sulph. gr. 1/60; ext. colocynth. comp. gr. 1/12; hyoscyami gr. i. One pill after each meal.

Gastric Disturbances of Nephritis. Osler says: Restrict amount of food; suck ice; take drop doses of creosote, also iodine and carbolic acid, dilute hydrocyanic acid with bismuth.

Great Fecal Accumulations. Bartholow recommended three parts of tinct. aloes et myrrhæ and one part of tinct. nucis vomicæ. Fifteen to twenty drops two or three times a day.

Pleuritic Adhesions. Pain and dyspnea due to these adhesions are best overcome by lung gymnastics, climatotherapy, tonics and nutritious diet.

Stricture of Trachea. Elsberg advises the use of soothing inhalations and dilation through the natural passages or tracheotomy. For syphilitic stenosis potassium iodide and mercuric chloride are specific curatives.

Fibrinous Bronchitis. E. Clifford Beale recommends inhalations of a spray of lime water. Emetics and mercury and potassium iodide are useful in some cases.

Typhlitis Stercoralis. Hughes prescribes: R. Magnesii sulph. dil. m.v.; tinct. opii deod. m.x.; spt. chloroformi m.v.; aquam menthæ pip. q.s.: A teaspoonful, diluted, every hour.

Acute Bronchitis. To establish secretion in the early stage Thornton prescribes: R Syrupi ipecac. m.x.; potasii citrat. gr. v.; syrupi limonis m.x.; aquam q.s.: A teaspoonful every four hours.

To Prevent Chill. The administration of ten grains of quinine after urethral instrumentation *(International Journal of Surgery)* often prevents a severe chill.

Chronic Intestinal Obstruction. Osler directs to wash out the stomach three or four times a day, and get thorough irrigation of the large bowel with injections.

Constipation with Dilated Colon. In this condition there may be enormous distension and marked tympany of the abdomen. For relief of symptoms Tyson advises a high enema along with calomel, one-fourth grain or more hourly.

Recurrent Vomiting in Children. Rachford *(Archives of Pediatrics)* recommends careful restriction of diet, relief of constipation and the continued use of wintergreen, sodium salicylate or sodium benzoate with essence of pepsin and peppermint water.

Esophageal Cancer or Stricture. The American Text-Book of Surgery directs to pass a small rubber catheter once or twice a week. Give liquid and finely minced solid food, or feed by rectum. Gastrostomy or esophagotomy may be required.

Infantile Constipation. The most common cause is relatively great length of the large intestines with flexures. By way of treatment Jacobi advises washing out bowel with warm water daily, and waiting for time to remedy the anatomic defect.

Chronic Interstitial Pneumonia. To promote resolution Thornton prescribes as follows: R. Potassii iodidi gr. iv.; hydrarg. chlor. corros. gr. 1-32; tinct. ipecac et opii m. ii.; syr. sarsaparillæ comp. m. xv.; aquam. q.s.: A teaspoonful in water after meals.

Umbilical Protusion. This defect may give rise to neurotic cough and other symptoms, which are readily remedied by replacement and compression with adhesive plaster over a large button in a pad.

Acute Attacks of Intense Dyspnea in Phthisis. Knopf advises the use of a hypodermic of morphine and the inhalation of oxygen or Walton's compound oxygen (two parts of oxygen, one part nitrous oxide, and one per cent. ozone).

Pneumonic Dyspnea. Turpentine stupes or hot poultices usually give much relief. Butler lauds aspidosperma, five to thirty drops of the fluid extract. Roth recommends the inhalation of chloroform for several minutes—about thirty drops every half hour or hour.

For Shortness of Breath in Pulmonary Tuberculosis. Thornton prescribes: R. Strychninæ sulph. gr. 1-20; quininæ hydrochlor. gr. i; sodii arsenat. gr. 1-20; ext. gentianæ gr. i: One pill t.i.d. after meals.

Bronchopneumonia. J. A. Coutts has had excellent results from the administration of extract of belladonna, one-fourth grain every three or four hours at any age. Flushing of the skin or a scarlet rash usually accompanies this medication.

Editorial Items continued on Page 565

BOOKS.

Eye, Ear, Nose and Throat Nursing. By A. Edward Davis, A.M., M.D., Professor of Diseases of the Eye in New York Post-Graduate Medical School and Hospital, and Beaman Douglass, M.D., Professor of Diseases of the Nose and Throat in the New York Post-Graduate Medical School and Hospital. With 32 illustrations. Pages XVI-318. Size, 5½x7⅞ inches. Extra cloth. Price, $1.25, net. F. A. Davis Company, publishers, 1914-16 Cherry Street, Philadelphia.

So far as we can recollect, this is the first book in the English language devoted exclusively to eye, ear, nose and throat nursing. The importance of skillful nursing in these conditions is at least as great as in any other. In this volume special attention is given to asepsis and antisepsis, and explicit directions are furnished for the preparation of sterile solutions and dressings and the application of remedies. Postures, devices and protective dressings are amply illustrated with figures in the text. The book should prove of service to students and practitioners as well as to nurses, for whom it is primarily intended.

First Annual Report of the Henry Phipps Institute. For the study, treatment and prevention of tuberculosis.

Practical Manual of Diseases of Women and Uterine Therapeutics. For students and practitioners. By H. Macnaughton-Jones, M.D., M.Ch., Master of Obstetrics, Royal University of Ireland; formerly University Professor of Midwifery and Diseases of Women and Children in the Queen's University; Ex-President of the British Gynecological Society. Ninth edition. New York. Wm. Wood & Co., 1905.

The first edition of this work was published in 1884. The present edition has been practically rewritten to conform with recent advances. The author's aim to furnish a reliable digest of gynecologic practice has been attained in the most satisfactory manner. His personal contributions are of considerable importance, and the style in which the various subjects are presented favors their easy comprehension. The 1044 octavo pages of the book comprise a vast amount of valuable matter, clinical reports and quotations being printed in small type. The text is handsomely illustrated with 63 drawings and over one hundred plates. Students and practitioners who anticipate doing gynecologic work will do well to have this volume close at hand.

THE INFLUENCE OF GROWTH ON CONGENITAL AND ACQUIRED DE-
FORMITIES. By Adoniram Brown Judson, A.M., M.D., Or-
thopedic Surgeon to the Out-Patient Department, New York
Hospital, 1878-1903; formerly President of the American
Orthopedic Association. Twelve mo.; 276 pages. Profusely
illustrated. New York. Wm. Wood & Co. 1905.

The author has had an unusually extensive personal experi-
ence as an orthopedic surgeon, and the views which he promulgates concerning the relation of growth to deformities are worthy of careful consideration. Among the subjects presented in a new light are the application of the weight of the body for the reduc-tion of club-foot, the use of the equine position of the foot to in-crease the length of a shortened limb, the adoption of symmetrical movements and correct rhythm for removing deformities and ex-cluding lameness, and the manner in which misleading tumors are produced by the rotation of lateral curvature. The text is always lucid and readable without effort and the details of mechanical treatment in particular are made plain by the numerous illustra-tive figures.

THE DISEASES OF SOCIETY. (The Vice and Crime Problem.)
By G. Frank Lydston, M.D., Professor of Genito-Urinary
Surgery, State University of Illinois; Professor of Criminal
Anthropology Chicago-Kent College of Law; Surgeon to St.
Mary's Samaritan Hospital. Philadelphia and London.
J. B. Lippincott Company. 1904.

In this, his latest literary effort, Dr. Lydston goes deep down into the underlying factors of vice and crime, and the methods for their cure and prevention. In his usual racy style he flays with cold facts, the hypocrisy and stupidity of society and the law. He advocates the spaying of criminals to prevent their reproduction, condemns capital punishment and believes in the treatment of the criminal by confinement and moral and industrial measures rather than revengeful punishment of crime. He would make no dis-tinction between the tramp and the dude, and holds that true nobility abides with the workers. The text is profusely illustrated with typical skulls and photographs of criminals.

THE LAW AND THE DOCTOR. VOL. 2, THE PHYSICIAN AS WITNESS. Arlington Chemical Company, Yonkers, N. Y.

This brochure, prepared expressly for gratuitous distribution to physicians by the enterprising company above mentioned, is a brief but comprehensive guide to the physician unskilled in court procedures, whenever he may be called as witness in court of justice.

In its new series the ECLECTIC MEDICAL GLEANER makes quite an imposing appearance. It is issued bi-monthly from the Lloyd Library, Cincinnati. The editor is Harvey Wickes Felter, M.D.

INTERNATIONAL CLINICS. A quarterly of illustrated clinical lectures and especially prepared original articles on Treatment, Medicine, Surgery, Neurology, Pediatrics, Obstetrics, Gynecology, Orthopedics, Pathology, Dermatology, Rhinology, Laryngology, Hygiene and other topics of interest to students and practitioners. By leading members of the medical profession throughout the world. Edited by A. O. J. Kelly, A. M., M.D., Philadelphia. Volume IV. Fourteen series. 1905. Philadelphia and London. J. B. Lippincott Company. 1905.

The twenty-one articles of the latest volume of this standard quarterly are all deserving of a careful perusal. Among the more noteworthy contributions, from the viewpoint of the reviewer, are: "The excessive use of drugs in the treatment of chronic diseases, with reference to medicinal intoxication", by George Hayem; "Indications for dechloridation treatment", by Adolphe Javal; "The treatment of patients who seem desperately ill in consequence of accident, hemorrhage or infection", by F. Lejars; "The clinical significance of albumosuria", by H. Senator; and "Recent investigations concerning the pathology of the infectious diseases", by Aldred Scott Warthin. The article on radium and the section on surgery are copiously illustrated.

ONE HUNDRED YEARS OF PUBLISHING—A BRIEF HISTORICAL ACCOUNT OF THE HOUSE OF WILLIAM WOOD & Co. Illustrated. New York. William Wood & Co. 1904.

This tasteful brochure gives a modest account of the progress from 1804 to 1904 of the firm of Wood, which with the exception of the Methodist Book Concern, is the oldest publishing house in New York. The founder of the house was Samuel Wood. Since about 1817 particular attention has been given to medical publications, and this firm has published the most extensive medical works in America.

ATLAS AND EPITOME OF OPERATIVE OPHTHALMOLOGY. By Dr. O. Haab, of Zürich. Edited, with additions, by George E. de Schweinitz, M.D., Professor of Ophthalmology in the University of Pennsylvania. With 30 colored lithographic plates, 154 text-cuts, and 377 pages of text. Philadelphia, New York, London. W. B. Saunders & Co. 1905. Cloth, $3.50, net.

This new volume concludes the excellent series of atlases on the eye prepared by Professor Haab. The colored illustrations are unsurpassable and the directions for the preparation and the use of instruments in ophthalmic operations are as clear and accurate as thirty years of practice as an oculist can make them. The editor, Dr. de Schweinitz, has enriched the text with valuable additions. This book, it seems to us, is almost indispensable to men and women who do or expect to do operations on the eye.

GYNECOLOGY—MEDICAL AND SURGICAL OUTLINES FOR STUDENTS AND PRACTITIONERS. By Henry J. Garrigues, A.M., M.D., formerly Professor of Gynecology and Obstetrics in the School for Clinical Medicine and Professor of Obstetrics in the Post-Graduate School and Hospital. 461 pages, with 343 illustrations. Price, $3.00. Philadelphia and London. J. B. Lippincott Company. 1905.

This handsome volume is designed by the author for the use of medical students and as a guide to general practitioners. It is essentially medical in scope, and has all the valuable features which a lifetime of special practice and teaching can impart. Minor operations are described in detail. The text is copiously and instructively illustrated. The book is well worth the price asked for it.

. THE MEDICAL EXAMINATION FOR LIFE INSURANCE AND ITS ASSOCIATED CLINICAL METHODS—With chapters on the Insurance of Substandard Lives and Accident Insurance. By Charles Lyman Greene, M.D., St. Paul, Professor of the Theory and Practice of Medicine in the University of Minnesota. Second edition. Revised and enlarged. With 99 illustrations. Price, $4.00. Philadelphia. P. Blakiston's Son & Co., 1012 Walnut Street. 1905.

This book has been out of print for two years, and has been thoroughly revised and considerably enlarged for the present edition. The author, who was formerly medical director of the Minnesota Mutual Life Insurance Company, is a master of the subject of this treatise. He presents diagnostic and prognostic considerations with clearness and accuracy. The side-notes on each page and the general arrangement of the text conduce to prompt and satisfactory reference. The numerous diagrams are very helpful. The work should prove invaluable to those for whom it is intended.

List of Fellows, Members, Extra-Licentiates and Licentiates of the Royal College of Physicians, London.

Active Congestion of the Lungs. W. S. Christopher recommends poultices, cotton and oil-silk jacket; fraction with camphor or an ointment of turpentine and lard; sweet spirit of nitre by the mouth. Venesection is indicated, says Bruce, when cyanosis obtains.

Acute Miliary Tuberculosis. Tyson uses moderate doses of antipyretics, three to five grains of phenacetin being probably the best. He employs also anodynes to quiet cough and secure comfort, and supporting food and stimulants.

For Pneumonic Dyspnea. When seen during the first 48 hours, before hepatization is complete, nothing, says Preble, is so efficient as a free blood-letting (18 to 20 ounces), provided the patient is robust and full-blooded.

Fecal Impaction. Anders uses high rectal injections, preferably with warm saline solutions or olive oil, with patient in inverted position and methodical kneading of the abdomen. No cathartics should be given until the main mass is moved.

Vomiting of Dyspeptic Diarrhea. For that of infantile indigestion A. A. Smith gives wine of ipecac, one minim every ten or fifteen minutes. In simple infantile diarrhea he gives gray powder 1-24 grain every fifteen or twenty minutes.

SELECTIONS.

Every physician requires almost daily a reliable calmative to replace the many injurious narcotics and anti-spasmodics now in general use—something that possesses a pronounced specific action as a nerve sedative and hypnotic and that will induce tranquility and equilibrium of the nervous system. They have found in Daniel's Conct. Tinct. Passiflora Incarnata the properties that contribute to this result and remove conditions resulting from impaired nerve function. And while Passiflora's action is potent and invariable, its superiority lies in the delightful after effect produced. The opiates, bromides and several so-called calmatives, insure sleep, but leave the patient with nerves strained and exhausted, while Passiflora gives rest without reaction and the patient feels the refreshing exhilaration of a night's sound slumber.

Passiflora is unequaled for Insomnia, Hysteria, Convulsions and kindred diseases.

LISTERINE DERMATIC SOAP.—The Lambert Pharmacal Company has lately inaugurated a new venture in the way of an antiseptic soap which possesses the virtues of Listerine in so far as a soap may. It is only a matter of recent years that especial attention has been given to producing soaps which shall possess a degree of curative power in diseases of the skin and in the care of surgical conditions. A considerable variety of such soaps is now on the market and the mission of the lot is wide; it is safe to say that Listerine Dermatic Soap will prove one of the most serviceable, and will soon make itself a popularity with the profession in keeping with that which has been established by Listerine.— *Medical Fortnightly, Jan. 25, 1905.*

CLINICAL TRIALS OF THE ACTION OF DIURETIN.—By Professor Gram, Copenhagen.—From very numerous trials the author concludes that Diuretin possesses a very powerful diuretic action, and that this is due to a direct influence on the kidneys. Diuretin is readily absorbed into the system and is wholly non-toxic, as only in one case was slight vertigo experienced. The ordinary daily dose is about 90 grains, which is given in single doses of 15 grains

each. The quantity of urine is frequently increased by administration of Diuretin more than five fold.—*Therapeutische Monat-
shefte.*

"LIQUOZONE".—To the Secretary Douglas County Medical
Society, Lawrence, Kan.: Dear Sir—At the request of your society I have made an examination of a sample of Liquozone,
brought to me by your representative, Dr. E. Smith. The bottle
when opened smelled strongly of sulfur dioxid. The solution contained:

	Per cent. by weight.
Sulfur dioxid	0.24
Sulfuric acid, free and combined	0.76
Total solids (mineral matter)	0.034

Yours truly,   E. H. S. BAILEY,

Journal of the Kansas Medical Society, Oct. 12, 1904.
—Extract from *The Medical World, Jan. 1905.*

THE THERAPEUTIC VALUE OF PEPTO-MANGAN (GUDE)—By
Dr. Vehmeyer, Haren, Germany.—1. Pepto-Mangan (Gude) is
incontestably a blood-forming preparation, and in this respect is
fully equal to every other preparation.

2. Its use is therefore recommended in all those diseases in
which, through an increase of blood and improvement of its quality, a cure or a beneficial influence upon the organism is to be expected; as for instance, in chlorosis, anæmia, leukæmia, in chronic
diseases of the respiratory organs, in many digestive disorders,
especially after diarrhœas, and in convalescence from various
diseases, especially in weak and anæmic women after childbirth.

3. Owing to its great palatability and tolerance this preparation does not require any correctives, and is adapted especially in
obstinate and protracted disease, in nervous, neurathenic, and all
other persons who are unable to take other iron preparations even
for a short time. In people who require iron and are afflicted
with nervous dyspepsia Pepto-Mangan (Gude) is not only by far
the best ferruginous preparation, but at the same time a stomachic
which has a most favorable influence upon the secretory functions
of the stomach.

4. Its blood-forming and in general curative properties depend both upon the direct introduction of iron and upon its power

of stimulating the appetite and digestion. Owing to its fortunate
composition this preparation deserves a general symptomatic employment.

5. Unpleasant by-effects are excluded.

Pepto-Mangan (Gude) therefore constitutes a valuable addition to our list of remedies. I prefer this preparation, which has
never left me in the lurch, to all similar products, and am persuaded that within its field of indications it will prove of equal
service to others. As regards the dose, it is advisable in general
to follow the printed directions, although in individual cases it
may be exceeded without the least untoward effects; for it is one
of the prominent advantages of the preparation, that while exhibiting in full its curative effect, it never satiates or becomes
repugnant, but permits of administration according to requirements, for a short period as well as many months, and that it is
equally well tolerated by children and adults of both sexes without
exciting the least aversion.

No More Poulticing in the U. S. Army.—In a recent
notification by the Surgeon General of the U. S. army, it is as-
serted that all the good results from poultices can be obtained in
a more cleanly way by the use of wet hot compresses. Hence the
order of the army surgeon to drop linseed and linseed meal from
army medical requisitions—*Virginia Medical Semi-Monthly.*

We supposed that every one in this enlightened age was using
Antiphlogistine in all such cases because of its advantages over
everything else in permanency, efficiency and cleanliness.

A Spring Medicine.—In the spring the organs of elimination do not possess their usual activity on account of having become
clogged by the accumulation of poisonous and perverted secretions
during the winter months when the skin neglects its duties and
the kidneys are overworked.

Where there are indications of any excess of uric acid, Tongaline and Lithia Tablets (tongaline 5 grs., lithium salicylate 1
gr.) will be found much more effective and satisfactory that lithia
alone or lithia waters.

In Tongaline all the salicylic acid is made from the purest
natural oil of wintergreen, the only kind that should be adminis-

tered internally, as the synthetic weakens the heart and depresses the entire system.

THE TREATMENT OF EXOPHTHALMIC GOITRE WITH THE BLOOD OF THYREOIDECTOMIZED GOATS.—In 1894, Lantz treated two exopthalmic-goitre patients with milk from thyreoidectomized goats. The results were so favorable that the treatment was applied to four other patients, all of whom as a consequence showed marked improvement and gain in weight.

In 1894 Drs. Ballet and Enriquez took the blood of thyreoidectomized dogs that had lived long enough to experience the blood changes which loss of thyreoid function is sure to entail,—and injected that blood into patients suffering from exophthalmic goitre. The results were so encouraging that other practitioners soon adopted the method, or a modification of it. The *Deutsche Medicinische Wochenschrift*, No. 38, 1899, contained a report of three cases of exophthalmic goitre, in the practice of Dr. Burghart, that improved under the treatment, two of them decidedly. Dr. Burghart did not confine himself to the use of injections, but administered a dried alcoholic extract of the blood.

Later, a Darmstadt chemical house prepared a serum from the blood of thyreoidectomized sheep, which, administred to patients who had exophthalmic goitre, produced a good effect; it was given both per os and subcutaneously.

A patient of Schultes (*Munch. Med. Woch.*, No. 20, 1902) in whom the symptoms of exophthalmic goitre had been in evidence for four years, with pronounced psychic disturbance at times, is said to have been completely cured in two months by the use of gradually increasing doses of the serum (from the blood of thyreoidectomized sheep.)

In 1901 Mobius (*Munch. Med. Woch.*, Jan. 27, 1903), proposed the preparation of a serum from the blood of sheep, from which the thyreoid gland had been removed, to be used in the treatment of exophthalmic goitre. He first injected 1 gramme of serum subcutaneously, but subsequently found that better results could be obtained by giving it internally. In his patients, all of whom had been treated for years with various remedies, the circumference of the neck was reduced, the goitre became smaller, and the patients slept better and were less agitated. It is not presumed that a cure can be established by this mode of treatment, but there seems to be sufficient ground to hope for beneficial results.

Messrs. Parke, Davis & Co. have perpared a dried product of the blood of thyreoidectomized animals, called "Thyreoidectin," which appears to produce the effects observed by Lantz, Möbius et al., much relief from reslessness, tremor, insomnia, and the usual train of nervous symptoms so generally observed. A gradual reduction of the pulse-rate and in the size of the gland was also noted.

THE USE OF GLYCOZONE IN A FEW GYNECOLOGICAL CASES— By C. H. Powell, A.M., M. D., St. Louis, Mo.—It is surprising how physicians fall into habits regarding the use of certain agents in their practice, and how loth they are to resort to something new. No doubt this fact exemplifies the maxim: "Be not the first by whom the new is tried nor yet the last to lay the old aside." This saying, were it put into active practice, would interdict the use of any new drug or remedy, as from the very nature of things a leader must be acknowledged, and the leader would himself violate the above maxim. In the treatment of uterine and ovarian diseases the well-known glycerole of tannin tampon, or the use of glycerine and Goulard's solution, or glycerine with other astringents, has been for years recognized and appreciated by gynecologists over the entire world. In the clinics solutions of these agents are ever at hand, and habitually are ensconsed into the vaginal canal with very little regard as to the scientific results that will accrue. It has often occurred to the writer that many of the solutions used by gynecologists favored the development of bacilli, and no doubt contributed in no small degree to the lighting up of attacks of pelvic peritonitis so frequently encountered by gynecologists. Glycerine no doubt is without peer in successfully treating a long range of diseases that afflict women, as the well-known hygroscopic qualities of the remedy bring about a local blood-letting from the hyperæmic structures which, when followed by hot douching, is usually relied upon to reduce many inflammatory complications of the uterus and its adnexa. Not being satisfied, for the reasons above given, with the usual formulæ of glycerine in gynecology, a sample bottle of glycozone which came to my desk several months ago, although not referred to in the treatment of diseases of women, appealed to me. Accordingly, in view of the highly oxygenated properties of the remedy, which I believed would necessarily possess bactericidal properties, I was induced to try glycozone in my gynecological practice; the results were so pronounced, and the beneficial influence of the remedy so decided and permanent, that I have for several months past persistently resorted to glycozone in preference to anything else in my local work. I will outline the following clinical cases as indicating its usefulness in the conditions stated:

Chronic Endometritis with Profuse Leucorrhoea.—This case was one of long standing; the lady had been treated by several physicians not only in connection with a hospital but on the outside, and curettage had been twice performed, the old trouble invariably recurring. I concluded it would be a good case to test the instillation treatment of glycozone upon, and accordingly used this remedy alone in that manner, together with its local application upon the tampon to the cervix uteri. This lady improved at once, and after the very first application. I had her under my care, and reapplied the remedy for about two weeks all told; she not only recovered absolutely during the time stated, but over three months have now elapsed without the slightest evidence of any recurrence of her former difficulty. I could report many other cases of the utility of glycozone in diseases of women, and I use the remedy to the exclusion of others where particularly glycerine is indicated. It surely will bring about results that cannot be obtained by the use of anything else, and I feel certain that a trial will satisfy the most skeptical of its merits.—Abstract from *New England Medical Monthly*.

EDITORIAL ITEMS.— Continued.

Vomiting of Enterocolitis. The main indications are for lavage of stomach and bowels, and abstinence from food for 12 to 24 hours. Hughes recommended calomel 1-8 grain, sodium bicarbonate 2 grains, and saccharum lactis 2 grains, every hour or two dry on the tongue.

Management of Intestinal Carcinoma. W. W. Johnston prescribes a diet chiefly of milk, eggs, soups, broths and readily absorbed animal substances. He gives gentle laxatives and procures frequent flushings of the bowels with copious clysters of warm salt water, a dram to the pint.

Floating Liver. Einhorn advises the use of a well fitted abdominal bandage to support the lower half of the abdomen in an upward direction; general massage, hydrotherapy, and gymnastic exercises in the open air; more food for weakly individuals— less for large eaters.

Cause of Appendicitis. Freeman thinks that the principal cause is kinking of the appendix, leading to defective drainage and favoring the growth of concretions. He estimates that eighty per cent. of his cases have shown this kinked condition.

Dietetic Regimen in Asthma. Thorowgood advises judicious depletion of the abdominal viscera by a course of mineral waters in gouty bronchitis and asthma. Reduce the allowance of meat and withhold stimulants.

Electricity for Constipation. Bartholow relied on faradization of the intestines, with an insulated electrode in rectum, and large sponge-covered rheophore well moistened and passed over abdomen along course of intestines.

Tracheal Dilation. Louis Elsberg recommends methodical and continuous compression by applications of astringent collodion or by mechanical means. Tracheotomy should be resorted to if indicated by suffocating attacks.

Bronchitis Depending on Cardiac Lesions. Mays prescribes: R. Strych. sulph. gr. 1-32; quininæ sulph., acetanilidi, caffeinæ citrat. aa. gr. 1 1-4; ferri sulph. gr. ss.; pulv. digitalis gr. 1-3; acidi arseniosi gr. 1-128: One capsule four times a day.

Isn't It True

that fats are spontaneously emulsified in the body by the chemical action of the intestinal secretions?

Is it probable that emulsions prepared by purely mechanical methods are as fit for absorption as those produced by the chemical or physiological process?

Hydroleine presents a fat—the purest Lofoten Cod-Liver Oil—which has been subjected to an exact laboratory duplication of Nature's method of fat emulsification. That's only one of the many reasons why Hydroleine produces immediate and positive results when the ordinary emulsions are ineffective. Write for literature.

Sold by all druggists.

THE CHARLES N. CRITTENTON CO.
SOLE AGENTS,
115-117 FULTON STREET, NEW YORK

PASSIFLORA

In Nerve-Starvation Daniel's Conct. Tinct. Passiflora Incarnata acts as a stimulating and invigorating food, as well as a sedative and hypnotic. Nerves are quieted and restored by nourishing and strengthening the depressed vital organs. In the hysteria of nervous women it regulates the heart action, urges composure and gives natural rest. Passiflora is unequaled in its power to control the nervous system.

Write for Literature.
Samples Supplied,
Physicians Paying Express Charges.

LABORATORY OF
JNO. B. DANIEL,
ATLANTA, GA.

Enlarged Bronchial Nodes. Syrup of iodide of iron, cod-liver oil, guaiacol and hypophosphites are serviceable remedies. The patient should be given a liberally large nitrogenous diet and should be plentifully supplied with fresh air and sunshine.

Retroflexion with Incarceration of Impregnated Uterus. Lusk has directed to catheterize the bladder and replace the uterus by pressure with two to four fingers in the vagina, the patient being in the knee-elbow posture.

Sleeplessness in Pneumonia. Preble says that sleeplessness can generally be combated by securing quiet for the patient, but if it persists it may seriously injure the patient and should be controlled, preferably by a small dose of morphine.

Typical Bronchial Asthma. For such cases Von Noorden recommends atropine, 1-130 grain daily, increased by same amount to 1-16 grain each day. Gradually diminish the dose after some time, continuing medication four to six weeks.

Alkaloidal Treatment of Lobar Pneumonia. According to Waugh, it consists in one mgm. amorphous aconitine, one-half mgm. veratrine and one mgm. digitaline given together every one-fourth to two hours for sthenic symptoms, substituting one-half mgm. strychnine arsenate for veratrine when asthenic conditions begin.

Vomiting of Peritonitis. J. Henry Fruitnight directs to stop all food and drink by the mouth, using nutrient enemata instead—later, predigested food by the mouth; give ice pills and iced champagne in small doses frequently repeated; use soft flannel cloths saturated in solution of tincture of iodine in castor oil and applied over belly.

Persistent Vomiting of Cholera Morbus. W. W. Johnston mentions carbolic acid, hydrocyanic acid, bismuth, sodium bromide, and small doses of calomel. Withhold food, he says, as long as possible; then give iced barley water, followed by milk and lime water in very small quantities at short intervals.

Intestinal Indigestion of Infants. Louis Starr directs to withhold milk for a time and give instead equal parts of veal broth (one-half pound of meat to the pint) and barley water; or equal parts of whey and barley water, sweetened with milk sugar; or a teaspoonful of raw beef juice every two hours.

Scott's Emulsion is a scientific pharmaceutical preparation, the medicinal ingredients of which are pure cod liver oil, with hypophosphites of lime and soda and glycerine. In this preparation the oil has been artificially digested by mechanical processes, thus preparing it for immediate absorption into the circulating fluid and supplying what deficient digestive ferments fail to supply. The utility of this expedient in the dietetic management of many morbid states has received the approval of high authority.

Samples free.

SCOTT & BOWNE, Chemists, 409-415 Pearl St., New York.

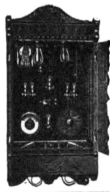
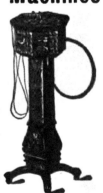

Vomiting of Cholera Infantum. J. Lewis Smith had good results from carbolic acid, 1/8 drop in a teaspoonful each of lime water and milk p.r.n. Also from the following recipe: R. Bismuthi subnit. gr. iiss; spt. ammonii arom. m.ii-iv; syrupum et aquam q.s.: A teaspoonful every half hour or hour.

Torpid Liver. Small doses of podophyllin are recommended by Hare. After excesses in eating or drinking, Hughes gave a good dose of calomel, ipecac and soda, followed by a saline or sodium phosphate till free catharsis. To children with clayey stools, Ringer gives gray powder, one-third grain with sugar of milk dry on the tongue every two hours.

For Gastralgia. Tyson recommends equal parts of spirit of chloroform, compound tincture of cardamom, aromatic spirit of ammonia and brandy: A teaspoonful every fifteen or thirty minutes till relief occurs. A few drops of deodorized tincture of opium may be added to each dose for its anodyne effect.

Bronchial Asthma. Chloroform inhalations, says William Ewart, gave immediate relief. Stramonium fumes are usually specific for the attack. Potassium iodide is of use in loosening the tenacious secretions of bronchiolitis exudativa. Systematic purgation should be employed if it does not dangerously lower the strength of the patient.

Foreign Body in the Larynx or Trachea. This is characterized by marked dyspnea and a whistling or wheezing sound that stops at the obstruction. The body moves on violent coughing and there is a small area of dullness. Irrigation of the nasopharynx may cause expulsion by reflex action. If not, one should use the laryngeal forceps or perform tracheotomy and remove the intruding object.

Deficient Intestinal Peristalsis. Napheys states that podophyllin is useful when there is torpor of the upper portion of the bowel and may be continued indefinitely in small doses. Meigs prescribes: R Ext. belladonnæ gr. 1-12; ext. nucis vonicæ gr. 1/4; ext. colocynth. gr. ii: One pill three times a day.

Inhalations for Bronchitis. Four to six drops of creosote are recommended by Sajous when there is profuse discharge. The same author employs inhalations of five minims of oil of pine for the torpid chronic bronchitis of phthisis. In bronchiectasis he advises inhalations of one minim of oil of thyme and three minims of oil of anise.

Mechanical Treatment of Constipation. An old and tried method consists in massage of the abdomen with a cannon ball of three to five pounds weight, covered smoothly with flannel or chamois skin, to be rolled over the course of the colon for ten minutes by the patient with knees drawn up, in the early morning while in bed and after evacuating the bladder. The Scotch douche (alternate hot and cold water) directed against the abdomen is a good tonic measure for daily use.

Impacted Feces. Taylor uses large and frequently repeated enemas, followed by careful diet, exercise and electric treatment or massage. J. Henry Fruitnight recommends irrigation of the bowel through a rectal tube, with four drams of ox-gall to the quart of water—also one dram of turpentine and four drams each of tincture of asafetida and castor oil. For fecal accumulations in children I. N. Love gave a dram of castor oil, with lemon juice or in hot milk flavored with nutmeg.

Gastrointestinal Catarrh with Constipation. A. D. Blackader gives some preparation of cascara regularly at bedtime in doses sufficient to secure a daily movement of fair consistence, also daily massage of large bowel and regulated habits. Hughes prescribed: R Magnesii sulph. ℨi-ii; sod. et potass. tart. ℨss.-i; acidi tart. gr. xx: Dissolve in a glass of water and drink effervescing an hour before breakfast.

Pulmonary Collapse. Treat the primary disease (capillary bronchitis usually), says Anders, and try to prevent this complication by full inspirations at regular intervals and by frequent change of position. Other means of relief are cold water poured over the neck; compressed air inhalations; tonics, stimulants, nourishing diet; tepid baths in kyphoscoliosis, and cardiac stimulants if required.

Gastrointestinal Disturbances Accompanying Endometritis. Audhorii prescribes: R Ext. nucis vomicae gr. ¼, ext. belladonnae, ext. opii aa. gr. 3/20: One pill at night. Tyler uses this formula: R Liq. bismuthi et ammon. cit. ℨ ss.; acidi hydrocy.

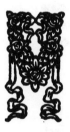

dil. m. iii; sodii bicarb. gr. viiss.; tinct. lavand. comp. m. xx; aquam q.s.: An ounce twice daily.

Dr. E. S. McKee, 19 W. Seventh, Cnicinnati, has been asked to recommend "a young, unmarried, competent Christian doctor" to go to Egypt to act as assistant to an American medical missionary for two years. A small salary and traveling expenses will be paid. The doctor says all the men he knows who would fill the bill are married.

Intestinal Ulceration. Aside from etiologic remedies, Anders advises to keep stools soft and bowels flushed out from below and with salines. He also employs antiseptic astringents, such as thirty grains of bismuth and five grains of salol every four hours; also enemata of silver nitrate (gr. 1/4 ad ℥ i) or creolin (two per cent.) The same treatment is indicated for duodenal as for gastric ulcer.

Volvulus of Bowel. After median incision, Greig Smith instructs to follow the most dilated and congested portion in direction of increasing distension and congestion, to find obstruction. Unravel the twist if possible; if not reducible, pull out distended intestine and open part of curve, empty of contents and try again to reduce, suturing bowel afterwards if successful. This second attempt failing, make an artificial anus in the first convenient piece of gut above the volvulus.

Intestinal Stricture. To produce mushy stools Thornton directs to give twenty grains of washed sulphur and ten grains cream of tartar in a cachet night and morning. The American Text-Book of Surgery advises enteroplasty for narrow circular strictures; intestinal anastomosis if stricture is wide or there are several near together; enterectomy only if necessitated by pathologic state of bowel at seat of obstruction.

Incarcerated Hernia. Roberts directs to reduce at once by gentle taxis (lift tumor and press slightly, then push back first the part which escaped last, raising pelvis at same time), continued only for a few minutes. Rectal enemas, ice or ether locally and morphine internally, and a hot bath, may make the rupture reducible after a few hours. Immediate herniotomy should be performed if taxis fails. If the intestine is gangrenous, notch the constricting band and incise gut, establishing an artificial anus or fecal fistula.

Intussusception. The American Text-Book of Surgery directs to withhold food by the stomach and give opiates. Distend bowel (under anesthesia) below obstruction with hydrogen or filtered air, after washing colon with two to four quarts of warm water. This failing, resort at once to laparotomy and reduction, or if patient is too weak, enterostomy or colostomy. If irreducible after abdominal section, employ anastomosis or resection of invaginated portion, and circular enterorrhaphy or formation of an artificial anus.

Cough of Habit or Sympathy. Bartholomew prescribed: ℞ Ammon. muriat. gr. viiss; mist. asafetidæ ℥iv. One dose as necessary for after-cough from habit. For the night cough of habit Boyland gives two grains of terpene hydrate at bedtime and in the early morning. For the nervous cough of mothers during whooping cough in the household, Bartholow prescribed: ℞ Acidi hydrocyan. dil. m. ii-iv; syr. tolu m. xxx-lx; aq. laurocerasi q.s.: A teaspoonful or two every three or four hours.

Dyspnea of Phthisis. Napheys advises the use of dry cups or a croton oil liniment to the surface of the chest. When the dyspnea is greatly aggravated by coughing spells, inhalations of chloroform will sometimes check these. Inhalations of hyoscyamus vapor (five grains of extract to pint of boiling water) are also recommended. The compound spirit of ether, in the dose of one-half to one dram, is serviceable in all forms of dyspnea.

Edema of the Lungs. Calomel, says Thomson, is of great use in cardiac dilation—one-half to two-thirds of a grain three times daily for several days—stop at the first indication of mercurialization. Wet cupping sometimes gives great relief, according to Bruce. For chronic affections with excess of secretion, Sajous recommends inhalations of ten minims each of oil of tar and oil of cubebs, ten grains light carbonate of magnesium and one-half ounce of water: A teaspoonful in a half pint of boiling water.

DENVER MEDICAL TIMES

| Volume XXIV. | MAY, 1905 | Number 11 |

INTRACEREBRAL INJECTIONS OF ANTITETANIC SERUM IN TRAUMATIC TETANUS.*

By S. D. HOPKINS, M.D.

Denver, Colo.

Neurologist to the Denver City and County Hospital, St. Anthony's Hospital and Mercy Sanitarium.

Tetanus is strictly a localized infection. In the wound only a small number of the bacilli are found, and they rarely reach the blood or any of the distant organs.

The toxin has been proven to have a particular affinity for the central nervous system, especially the ganglion cells of the anterior horns of the spinal cord and medulla, with which it unites with such firmness that it is difficult to separate it. Its presence has been demonstrated in the cerebro-spinal fluid. Roux and Borrel conclude that antitoxin injected subcutaneously remains in the blood, and is therefore unable to reach the toxin which is fixed in the nervous system.

Experiments by Meyer and Ransome also support this conclusion, explaining as they do the variation in time (from four to fourteen days) elapsing between inoculation with the toxin and the appearance of symptoms.

It would seem that tetanus toxin does not reach the spinal cord through the blood stream, but by slowly passing along the axis cylinders of motor cells from their terminations. Apparently the myelin sheath acts as a quite impervious membrane, and the toxin enters at the end of the neuron where it is not provided with this sheath. Sensory nerves do not transport the toxin to the cord. The toxin enters the nerve-endings from two sources; the first is at the site of the infection, where the toxin is most concentrated, and this probably explains why tetanic spasms frequently begin in the vicinity of the infected part, or are most marked at this point. The rest of the toxin is taken up by the blood and lympth

*Read before the Rocky Mountain Inter-State Medical Association, Sept., 1904.

and distributed, to enter the motor nerve-endings in small quantitise all over the body, and by passing along the motor fibers to enter the cord diffusely, leading to the generalized spasms. The latent period that elapses after injection of the toxin before symptoms appear is occupied by the passage of the toxin along the motor fibers to the spinal cord; if the toxin is injected directly into the spinal cord symptoms appear at once.

From the pathology it is therefore seen that the intracerebral injection of the antitetanic serum is the correct method of treatment for this disease. The following cases tend to confirm this conclusion:

Case 1. F. M., age twenty-one years, occupation shoemaker. Family and previous history negative.

Present Illness. On May 8, 1903, while working in a livery stable, he stepped on a rusty iron nail, which entered the left great toe. The following two days no symptoms were noticed, except that the wound was tender to the touch. During the fourth day the patient complained of severe headache, associated with stiffness of the posterior neck muscles, which gradually increased in intensity. About 11 a. m. the next day trismus developed and at the same time he complained of pain in the masseter muscles and cramps in the legs.

In this condition he presented himself at police headquarters, and while there he had his first tonic spasm. At first the spasms came on about every fifteen minutes, but became more frequent, and at the time of admittance to the County Hospital they occurred every two or three minutes. The convulsions were so severe that the patient's body was in complete opisthotonos, although during these attacks consciousness was unaffected. At the time the operation was performed the temperature was 99° F., pulse 115, respiration 24. Had difficulty in swallowing and was unable to talk on account of the jaw being locked.

Examination. May 12, 1903. Patient was conscious of his surroundings and his condition. All deep and superficial reflexes were increased. There was marked spasm of the masseter muscles causing lockjaw, the teeth being separated about one-half inch and the lower jaw immovable even with the greatest pressure.

During the examination he had a convulsion in which all the

muscles of the body were affected, including those of respiration. All special senses normal. The pupils equal and responding to light and accommodation. Fundi normal.

On May 12 at 6 p. m. Dr. C. B. Lyman and Dr. J. K. Swindt made a small trephine opening in the right frontal bone and injected 20 c.c. of antitetanic serum into the right frontal lobe of the cerebrum. At 6:30 p. m., while under chloroform, he had a convulsion. At 1 a. m. May 13, he had a slight convulsion, with marked trismus. Chloral hydrate grs. xxx was ordered at this time on account of the severe twitching. At 7 a. m. May 14 slight twitching, rigidity of masseter muscles very much less than in previous attacks. After this convulsion chloral hydrate grs. xxx, sodium bromide grs. xl were given every six hours.

The trismus, which was constant before the antitetanic serum was injected into the cerebral tissue, continued after the operation for seventy-two hours, when it ceased, as did the spasms. He remained in the hospital until May 26, 1903, when he was discharged after making a complete recovery.

CASE 2. E. F., a boy, ten years of age, while playing with a toy pistol on July 4 last, exploded a blank cartridge, the wad of which took effect in the palm of the left hand, inflicting a somewhat lacerated wound and burying itself deeply in the tissues. He was taken to the police station, where the wound was dressed and subsequently cared for until it had entirely healed.

On July 23, nineteen days after the injury, Dr. I. B. Perkins saw the patient in consultation with Dr. A. A. Clough, who had just been called into the case. Marked trismus was present. During the tonic spasms, which came at short intervals, the jaws set tightly together. The posterior muscles of the neck, as well as the muscles of the back, became rigid, and the boy appeared to experience great pain. In the interval between the spasmodic attacks, the muscles of the jaws were not so rigid, but they did not relax sufficiently to allow the jaws to be separated. The muscles of the neck and back relaxed slightly in the interval, but contracted instantly on the approach of the spasms, drawing the head firmly backward.

Tetanus was diagnosed and immediate operation decided upon. While on the way to the hospital slight jars of the vehicle caused severe spasmodic attacks. While being anesthetized, and after he was unconscious of his surroundings the rigidity of the muscles remained and the jaws could not be separated until he was completely anesthetized. When coming out of the anesthesia the trismus returned and was quite marked before the return of consciousness. Roux's point was selected for injecting the serum into the brain-substance. The patient being right-handed, a flap one inch in diameter was made over the right frontal bone, with the open portion of the shoe directed toward the temple. The periosteum was lifted with the flap, and a trephine button one-fourth inch in diameter was removed. The needle of the syringe was introduced into the brain-substance to a depth of two inches, with the point directed downward and toward the median line, and 10 c.c. of antitetanic serum was slowly injected in the same manner with the point of the needle directed forward and downward, and not toward the median line. The tissue flap was then sutured in position. The button of the bone was not replaced.

An incision was made in the hand at the point of injury and several small pieces of the wadding were removed.

Reaction following the operation was prompt, and although the trismus returned on the return of consciousness the spasms were not nearly so severe and subsided altogether after forty-eight hours.

Immediately following operation, sodium bromide grs. x and chloral hydrate grs. v were given by enema. This was repeated at varying intervals for several days, and then small doses of the bromide and chloral were given by mouth, sufficient being used to keep the patient sleeping most of the time. The temperature was 99° F. at the time of the operation, and did not go above 99° F. at any time. The highest rate of pulse was 108.

There was some stiffness of the limbs on first attempting to walk, which was two weeks after operation. This was not more marked on one side than on the other, and disappeared in a few days. At this time the patient appeared to be in perfectly normal condition, having made a complete recovery.

CASE 3. A. C., aged twelve years, schoolboy. Always en_ joyed good health. On July 4, 1903, while playing with a revolver, it exploded, the contents of the blank cartridge entering the right knee. He was cared for by his mother for fourteen days after the accident, but the symptoms became so alarming that Dr. J. M. Perkins was called to see him.

On examination it was found that he had had headache, cramps and stiffness of the muscles for the past two days. During the examination the patient had a general convulsion on an average of every fifteen minutes. While transporting him from his residence to the hospital the spasms occurred so frequently that it became necessary to use chloroform. On arriving at the hospital the pulse was 150, temperature 101° F., respiration 50. Twenty cubic centimeters of antitetanic serum were injected into the right frontal convolution.

Patient died two hours after operation.

In the three cases reported a trephine opening was made in the right frontal bone half way between the outer angle of the orbit and a point on the vertex, at the juncture of the line crossing over between the two auditory canals. The trephine opening should be small; a small slit made in the membranes and the needle introduced two inches into the cerebral substance of the frontal lobe of the brain. In these cases the right frontal lobe was selected for the injection because the patients were right-handed, for if any paralysis followed the injection of the serum the center of speech would not be involved. The needle is directed forward and slightly downward.

The mortality of cases of traumatic tetanus treated by the ordinary medical means is very high, averaging about 9 per cent. In 147 cases treated by the intracerebral injection of antitetanic serum the mortality is 61 per cent.

The total quantity of antitoxin injected into the brain varies from 5 to 70 c.c. at any one time. In the three cases reported 20 c.c. were injected into the cerebral substance at once, and it is the belief of the writer that the success of this method of treatment depends upon the use of large quantities of the serum.

The danger in using serum intracerebrally is due to the fact that it acts as an irritant, and may cause a meningitis, cerebritis or a cerebral abscess. In a number of cases hemorrhages have occurred.

DISCUSSION OF DR. HOPKINS' PAPER.

DR. MOLEEN. I was astounded with the rapidity with which the symptoms developed. There was no question that it was a case of tetanus. It is gratifying to know in this connection that the warning which was published a year ago in the Journal of the American Medical Association has been effective in reducing the number of cases to a great extent. Some four hundred and fifty cases were reported in the United States one year ago, and since the publication of this article warning different municipalities regarding the use of the firecracker and the cap-pistol it is interesting to know that only 105 fatalities were reported this year.

A RECURRENT PERINEPHRITIC ABSCESS, OF 26 YEARS STANDING, AND PRESENTING A CLINICAL PICTURE OF ADDISON'S DISEASE.*

By GEO. A. MOLEEN, Ph.G., M.D.

Denver, Colo.

Last year I presented before this association a case by which I aimed to show the importance of a complete examination and detail record in the study of cases, and I take pleasure in citing to you at this time one more forcibly emphasizing these points.

It is not often our good fortune to take a history of a malady extending over a quarter of a century, interposed with numerous diagnoses and prognoses and by the "lancing of a boil" veritably annihilate the seemingly fatal symptom complex; yet such in brief is the case about to be presented.

It is not the purpose at this time to discuss the various theories regarding the pathology of Addison's disease any more than to call to mind the summary of the recorded morbid anatomical lesions of the adrenals and adjacent sympathetic structures of Rollison, as follows:

1. Fibro-caseous due to tuberculosis.
2. Simple atrophy.

*Read before Rocky Mountain Inter-State Medical Association, September, 1904.

3. Chronic interstitial inflammation, leading to atrophy.

4. Malignant disease invading the capsule, including Addison's case of malignant nodule compressing the suprarenal vein.

5. Blood extravasated into the suprarenal bodies.

6. No lesion of the bodies themselves, but pressure or inflammation involving the semilunar ganglia.

Nor does it seem wise to dilate upon the possibility of unilateral pressure as a cause of this remarkable symptom complex, since three out of Addison's original eleven cases were apparently due to lesions of the gland on one side. It does, however, seem important at this time to emphasize the fact that in this case the mischief was apparently due to pressure and probably without interstitial or parenchymatous change in the gland itself as indicated by the rapid dissipation of the characteristic symptoms and also by the remissions, to which reference will be made later.

When first seen this case was suffering from dysentery and this fact, taken with the asthenia, emaciation, small rapid pulse and apparent anemia pointed to a "snap" diagnosis of tuberculosis dysentery.

Subsequent inquiry revealed the fact that he had been told that he had an incurable "muscular wasting." The peculiar bronzing of the face and hands was however something more than a cachexia. The following record was then taken:

Mr. J. A. M., aged 45, born in Ohio; been in Colorado a little over one month; came on account of his health though not lung trouble.

Family History.—His mother and father were born in Ohio; both are dead, the former as a result of rheumatism and the latter from apoplexy, at 72. He has two sisters and three brothers living in good health. One brother dead (cause unknown); one sister died of "croup." Negative as to tuberculosis, tumor or cancer and other chronic diseases, including nervous and mental disease.

Previous History.—He enjoyed good health as a child outside of the usual diseases of childhood, of which he remembers especially whooping cough. He did not have scarlet fever or diphtheria. He states that his growth and development was that of the average child of his age, and he is quite certain that he was not noticeably fat. In 1876-'77 he had an attack of "fever and ague" and in '78 he had a congestive chill (?). About eighteen years ago he passed some gravel.

Present Condition.—About twenty-six years ago he noticed that his left eye-lid began to droop and later the right, and that at the same time his arms and hands were becoming weak; he first noticed that he "had no grip in his hands." This weakness increased gradually, progressed very slowly, finally involving his legs, which like the arms became very weak though they did not diminish in size to any great extent.

In May, 1893, while eating he suddenly became unable to swallow, which difficulty persisted until about November of the same year, when with the slow return of this faculty he became stronger. Previous to this attack, however, though weak, he worked though he would frequently drop things, e. g., he could not milk, or when ploughing he would have to use both hands at the corners.

After the onset of these attacks he would become weaker and weaker for two or three months, then to gradually improve, very slowly, reaching his climax in about two years. He has had three attacks (previous to the present one) about four years apart and in the interval he would become quite strong, though his hands would never regain their proportionate strength and he states that in the present attack his hands are stronger than in the beginning.

He became exceedingly well two years ago, and believing himself to have recovered, he was married.

The present attack began February, 1903, as before by a drooping of the left eye-lid, followed by the right, and at the same time noticed a "drawing sensation" in the calves of both legs; from this time he grew gradually weaker until June, 1903, when he suffered a chill resembling a malarial attack, i. e., chill, sweat, vomiting, followed by sleep. He was in bed about twelve days, then up and around until the last of September, when while in the yard he fell as though struck on the head and in falling did strike the back of his head; he was unconscious for about five minutes. He recalls having fallen once before. He knew he was falling each time but could not avoid it, and he thinks the unconsciousness was due to the fall. While considerably weaker after this he was in the main the same as before, and in October and November he seemed stronger. In November he contracted a "grippy" cold which he states responded unusually well to treatment. ·

In January, 1904, he began to complain of pain in the right side, especially in the lumbar region, accompanied by a chill and a difficulty in speech; he could but mumble on attempt to speak. He had also during this time some difficulty in swallowing. Some time later he indicated a desire for a drink which when brought he found he could swallow and later to speak clearly and has done so ever since.

Until a dysentery began, about May 30, he was gradually improving. He has had several similar attacks of dysentery.

Examination. June 15, 1904. He is a man about six feet tall, well built and shows no marked atrophies in any muscle or group of same, though they are not as firm as usual and could be readily acocunted for by disuse. There is a seeming wasting of the thenar eminenes, though the adductors of the thumbs show as much strength as the rest of the hand muscles. He shows a slight bronze tint especially on the face and dorsal surface of the hands, and very slight of the entire body. He is anemic in appearance and the sclerotics are bluish white in color.

There are no evidences of disease in either lung.

The heart is normal in size and position, the action is regular, though markedly weak and rapid and without murmur. Pulse is small, running in character and very weak. Rate of pulse, 102. Temperature, 100.5.

The liver dullness in the mammillary line begins at the right nipple and extends two inches below the rib. There is considerable tenderness in the right hypochondrium though not as great as in the right lumbar region.

He responds to all inquiries promptly and with clear enunciation.

In walking he moves slowly on account of weakness and the pain from which he is suffering in his right side, though there is no ataxia to be seen in his gait. He stands without swaying with his eyes open or closed. Dynamometer: R. 49; L. 20. He is right-handed. Reflexes: Knee joints, R. present and also on reinforcement; L. same. Ankle clonus, absent. Tendo achilles, R. present; L. same, not as great as right. Deep reflexes of the forearm; R.

present; L. same, and about normal, as are also the biceps, triceps and deltoid. Masseter, absent. Tongue is protruded in the median line. Mouth is retracted equally and he is able to whistle, though at times, he states, he has been unable to do so.

Special senses: Eyes—All external ocular motion is normal and equal; pupils are equal and respond equally to light and accommodation. Fields are apparently normal. Discs are clear in outline and normal in color; the veins are slightly larger than the arteries. Hearing—(Watch) R. 12-24, L. 1-24. Tuning fork is heard best in the left ear. Aerial conduction is almost equal to that of bone in the left ear. R. normal (i. e. Rinne positive). Speech is at present unaffected. Taste is present and equal, and there is apparently no disturbance in smell.

Sensory Phenomena—All forms of sensation, including tactile, pain, pressure, postural, joint and thermic are present and equal. Urine—Very turbid and yellow in color when filtered. Odor foul and pungent. Acid in reaction. Sp. Grav. 1028; No albumen, sugar or bile. Microscopically—Almost entirely pus with very few blood corpuscles. Cover slips stained with carbol fuchsin and methylene blue revealed no tubercle bacilli, but there were staphylococci and a few chains of streptococci. The quantity excreted in twenty-four hours was 48 ounces. Urea (in 24 hours) 28.8 Gms. (644.3 Grains). A blood count was not made and record of blood pressure was likewise omitted.

A diagnosis of perinephritic abscess was made and he was referred to Dr. Sherman T. Brown for operation, whom I have asked to state to you his findings.

Considering the myasthenia, tachycardia, pigmentation, especially of the hands and face, and its absence in the mucous membranes and sclerotics, the gastro-intestinal symptoms, and in the absence of persistent bulbar disturbance one must admit the resemblance to a case of Addison's disease. The transient attacks of ptosis and aphasia, while not usually a part of such a clinical history, do occur as shown in the case cited by Philips (of simple atrophy of the adrenals verified by autopsy).

The remissions, to which reference has been made, were accounted for by the recurrence of the abscess, which at the height of each attack, in all probability, ruptured into the pelvis of the kidney and consequently drained through the bladder and which was in progress when examined, though the urine at the previous examinations, I am informed through the kindness of his former physician, Dr. Pickard, contained no pus when examined by himself and Dr. Church, of Chicago.

The chills mentioned as malarial in character, and the congestive chills spoken of as supposedly pleuritic were, one or other, noted some time in each attack. These with the increased liver dullness, pyuria, and the finding, by cystoscopic examination that this pus was coming from the right kidney only, were reasons for the diagnosis of perinephritic abscess.

At the operation, the numerous old adhesions and the extent and course of the burrowing bore testimony to its having existed a great length of time.

Since operation the improvement has been rapid, steady and continuous, the pigmentation, however, remains; his rapid increase in strength is remarkable, he having walked 26 squares in a forenoon two months after. He has been taking ferruginous tonics with strychnia to which it was deemed advisable to add two-grain doses of desiccated suprarenal substance.

In the study of this case it was observed that the same general symptoms are present in nearly all conditions involving the ductless glands or their sympathetic ganglia. Most noteworthy, in the present case, is its similarity to a case of asthenic bulbar paralysis or myasthenia gravis, in which, however, there is seldom if ever, pigmentation. Hun states the important positive symptoms in establishing a diagnosis to be (1) a chronic paresis affecting muscles supplied by many motor nerves, both spinal and cranial (ocular and bulbar); (2) rapid tiring; (3) variation in the intensity of the symptoms; and (4) the electrical myasthenic reaction. Of almost equal importance are the negative symptoms: The absence (1) of fibrillation; (2) of muscular atrophy; (3) of the electrical reaction of degeneration, and (4) of sensory symptoms.

The pathological findings in this interesting symptom complex seem to have excluded the central nervous system, though changes in and about the thymus gland are becoming more constant as is shown in Hun's case as well as in that of Weigert. A case of Oppenheim's, a sarcoma of the anterior mediastinum and that of

Golfram's, in which a lympho-sarcoma of the upper lobe of the lung was found, are interesting, and since Weigert's work a considerable proportion of autopsies have shown conditions similar or analogous to the conditions described by him.

Anther condition apparently closely related is that of exophthalmic goitre or Basedow's disease. Nine cases of myasthenia reported by Kalischer, Goldfram, Karplus, Charcot and Marinesco, Murri, Hey, and Finzio presented symptoms of Basedow's disease more or less pronounced (exophthalmia or goitre or both).

On the relation between Addison's disease and Basedow's disease Gowers states that an affection of the abdominal sympathetic, similar to the constant affection of the cervical sympathetic, would explain the pigmentation, and the occasional watery diarrhea seems also to show that the abdominal nerves are sometimes involved.

The heart action in all conditions is seemingly increased in rate and in exopthalmic goitre the volume is increased; in myasthenia little afiected, sometimes increased, while in Addison's it is almost constantly lowered.

The foremost symptom, myasthenia, which in itself would presuppose an electrical myasthenic reaction as described by Jolly, may under the light of future investigation prove to be an expression of disease of the ductless glands, or their sympathetic communications, and with the association of the ocular, or more particularly the palpebral symptoms, the character of circulatory disturbance, the presence or degree of pigmentation, with the gastro-intestinal symptoms, we may definitely localize the seat of such disturbance.

In closing there may be added to these observations two queries: Has the languor or fatigue so frequently observed in chronic Bright's disease an explanation in the sympathetic communication of the renal plexus? and, may not the asphyxia which so often closes the scene in these cases as in the diseases under discussion be as likely due to this association as to uremia.

REFERENCES

1. Philips, Journ. Experimental Medicine, Vol. iv., p. 581.
2. Hun, Albany Medical Annals, 1904, Jan., p. 51.
3. Oppenheim, Die Myesthenische Paralyse, Berlin, S. Karger, p. 114.
4. Kalischer, Zeitschrift fur Klinische Med., 1896, Bd. xxxi., p. 93.
5. Goldfrom, Deutsche Zeitschr. f. Nervenheilkunde, 1893, Bd. iv., p. 332.
6. Neurologisches Centralblatt, 1902, Bd. xxi., p. 97.
7. Karplus, Jahrbuch fur Psychiatrie u. Neurologie, 1897, Bd. xv., p. 330.
8. Charcot and Marinesco, Comptes Rondes Hebdomaire, 1895, p. 131.
9. Murri, Il Policlinico, 1895, Vol. ii., pp. 441, 458.
10. Hey, Muenchener Med. Wochenschr., 1903, Bd. i, p. 1867.
11. Finizio, La Riforma Medica, 1898, No. 1, xiv., 589.
12. Gowers, Diseases of the Nervous System, 2nd Ed., Vol. ii., p. 890.

A SUPPLEMENTARY REPORT.

By R. C. COFFEY, M.D.

Portland, Oregon

In the January number of THE DENVER MEDICAL TIMES an article of mine was published under the title, "Surgical Treatment of Displacements of the Uterus," in which was described an operation which I have been using for nearly three years. I have had an opportunity to see its results in a case which is reported below.

On Aug. 9th, 1904, I operated upon Mrs. X. for extreme retroflexion and partial prolapse of the uterus. A certain amount of salpingitis and oophoritis existed, accompanied by some adhesions. The round ligaments were completely stretched, much attenuated, and temporarily paralyzed as far as action was concerned, the broad ligament also relaxed. Condition had existed seven years. Operation: Removed cystic portion of left ovary and enucleated a cyst from the right; tubes while inflamed were not disturbed; the operation here described for shortening the round and broad ligaments was performed, also amputation of cervix and perineorrahaphy. Patient went home, but soon began to notice pain in her left side, and considerable soreness was experienced in the pelvis. March 31st, 1905, nearly seven months after the first operation, she returned. Examination showed tumor on right side in ovarian region. On opening the abdomen, a cyst was found in the right ovary the size of an orange. The left tube was markedly inflamed, and was covered in by omentum and intestines which had formed a wall around the inflamed tube back of the uterus. The folds of the broad ligament which had been plicated had blended absolutely, making a broad ligament as smooth as a normal broad ligament, and had blended with the uterine peritoneum exactly as sutured at the time of the operation. There were no inflammatory adhesions at the site of suturing of the broad ligaments. The uterus was held in place more firmly than by a normal broad ligament, but was freely movable. The round ligament had apparently straightened itself out as soon as the catgut had absorbed, had assumed its normal position and had regained its normal size. The result in this case as far as the support was concerned was better than my most sanguine anticipations,—in fact, was perfect. The case proved to my mind more thoroughly than I have ever been able to prove in any other way the propositions which I have been trying to demonstrate:

First—*"The peritoneum is the universal suspensory support of the abdominal and pelvic organs."*

Second—*"Two peritoneal surfaces brought together firmly and held together in an aseptic state will blend and become as one."*

Third—*"The connective tissue or outer side of the peritoneum cannot by any known means be made to permanently adhere to a muscle, connective tissue redeveloping and loosening it from its moorings as soon as the agent holding it is removed."*

Fourth—*"The muscular ligaments of the uterus act exactly as muscles in other parts of the anatomy, namely,—to contract and produce motion, and will under no circumstances bear any considerable weight constantly."*

According to my friend, Dr. S. C. Baldwin, the well-known orthopedist of Salt Lake City, a muscle which has been overstretched for a long time becomes temporarily paralyzed and useless. If the tension is removed, it shortens to its normal length and regains its normal power. In discussing this paper, Dr. Baldwin believed this to be the case with this operation. I scarcely thought it possible until I saw that it did actually occur in this case. Apparently as soon as the catgut holding it was absorbed, the weight of the uterus being held by the folded and blended peritoneum, the round ligament began its contraction and soon straightened itself out in the connective tissue under the peritoneum, and at the same time regained its normal size and appearance.

THE TREATMENT OF GASTRO-INTESTINAL DISEASES IN CHILDREN.

By D. T. QUIGLEY, M.D.

North Platte, Neb.

The gastro-intestinal diseases of children under six months of age are almost invariably associated with the presence of pathogenic bacteria, and the disease process usually depends on the production of toxins due to putrefactive and fermentative changes in the contents of the canal; toxins are absorbed and cause the fever, depression, etc. There is another condition which is always present in greater or less degree, and may be overlooked; that is an inflammation existing in the mucous lining of the stomach and bowels, as a result of direct contact with the acrid products of decomposition. These conditions are more frequent in the child under six months, because the stomach of the baby of that age secretes very little hydrochloric acid, which in an older child protects the organ to a certain degree on account of its antiseptic action.

The necessary steps in treatment are, therefore, (1) speedy evacuation of the bowels; (2) the use of antiseptics; (3) something to counteract the acidity of the bowel-contents and have a soothing effect on the inflamed mucous membrane. The first indication I meet by the injection into the rectum of a solution of bicarbonate of soda, followed by a 1:1000 solution of Acetozone. The second is met by giving the solution of Acetozone (1:1000) in teaspoonful doses every half hour, if the stomach will tolerate it that often. Given this way it not only kills bacteria but destroys the toxins by oxidation. The third indication will require, in many cases small doses of bismuth subnitrate, which may or may not be combined with calomel (gr. 1/20). In many cases the bismuth will not be needed on account of the healing effect of the Acetozone.

NORMAL OBSTETRICS.
(CHAPTER THIRTEEN.)

THE DIAGNOSIS AND MANAGEMENT OF LABOR.

By T. MITCHELL BURNS, M.D.

Denver, Colo.

Professor of Obstetrics, the Denver and Gross College of Medicine.

The Obstetrician's Clothing and Person.—The obstetrician's clothing and person should be clean and neat. His hands and gloves should be kept especially clean. While an obstetrician should not attend an infectious case, especially scarlet fever, diphtheria, infected wounds or puerperal infection, he may do so by using due precaution in the matter of disinfecting when called to an obstetric case. After attending a septic case, he should render his hands aseptic by the permanganate method, take a general bath, shampoo his head, change all his clothing, and have those worn at the septic case disinfected by sunlight or formaldehyd.

Calls.—All calls to confinement cases should be answered immediately. Before going, the physician should write and leave the address or telephone number of the patient, so that if another important call comes in while he is gone, a message may reach him. He should also carefully examine his obstetric satchel to see that it contains everything he may need. The things which are liable to be missing, through their being all used or left at a previous case, are bichlorid tablets, chloroform and inhaler, ergot, vaseline, boric acid, nail brush, manicuring scissors, sutures, umbilical cord ligatures and the uterine irrigator.

The Obstetric Satchel.—The best obstetric satchel is the cabin style. It is the best because it holds the most for its size, and because the contents may be easily seen. It is a little too large to carry on a wheel. The lining of the satchel should be made of tanned leather, so that it may be disinfected easily with formaldehyd or turpentine or cleaned with gasoline. Some use a detachable linen lining which can be boiled, but probably the tanned leather lining is just as good. (The author has used both.) The interior of the satchel should be touched as little as possible when the hands are not clean. To keep the exterior of the satchel clean and attractive, it should be blackened once a month with shoe polish.

The Contents of the Satchel.—A perfectly equipped obstetric satchel should contain all articles herein enumerated, but many of these (see asterisks) are not necesary in ordinary practice. Instead of carrying all in one large satchel, it is better to place the aprons, Kelly pad and fountain syringe in the sterilizer or in pans for sterilizing, or in wrapping paper. Antiseptics: Tr. green soap, 1 oz., or castile soap 1 cake; bichlorid of mercury tablets, 50 (bichlorid 7.3 gr., citric acid 3.8 gr., P. D. & Co.'s); *permanganate of potash ½ oz.; *oxalic acid 2 oz.; alcohol 2 oz.; protargol, 2% solution, ½ oz. Lubricant: Sterilized vaseline. Anesthetics: Chloroform, Squibbs, 4 oz.; chloral 2 dr.; morphine and atropin and morphine tablets. Oxytocics and stimulants: Ergot, Squibb's fl. ext., 2 oz.; quinin capsules, 5 gr., 1 doz.; strychnin tablets, hypodermic, gr., 1/30; ammonia, aromatic spirit, 1 oz. Cathartics: Croton oil, ½ dr. Dressings: Absorbent cotton ½ lb.; gauze, plain, one yd., iodoform, 1 yd.; sterilized towels (Seabury & Johnson's.) Instruments: For anesthesia—inhaler Schimmelbusch's folding mask; drop bottle, ordinary 1 oz. corked vial. For sterilizing—sterilizer or two pans, 15x8x3. For physician's hands and clothing—rubber gloves, sterilized in a rubber pouch; manicuring scissors; nail file; unvarnished brush; *rubber apron; linen or cambric apron. For irrigation—fountain syringe, 3 qt., gray rubber; Kelly pad, uterine irrigator, Glasgow's inner tube or Burns' postpartum irrigator. For catheterization—catheters, soft rubber, 2 No. 10 A. For curettement—above instruments for irrigation; tenaculum forceps, Schroeder's (with an assistant Skene's is better); vaginal depressor, Porter's (may use bivalve speculum); uterine sound, Simpson's; uterine dilator, Goodell's latest aseptic; curettes, one or more sharp, with flat handle, Sims or Thomas'; uterine dressing forceps, Bozeman's. For tears—needle holder, Richter's; 6 needles, full curve No. 7 and 8, or Emmet's taper point full curve No. 1; silk-worm gut sutures, medium size, one skein; scissors. For umbilical cord—hemostatic forceps, 2 pairs Pean's long jawed 5-inch; surgeon's twisted silk No. 12, one reel, or ordinary grocery twine; umbilical scissors, plain blunt pointed, or American pattern with serrated edges. For artificial delivery—

Simpson's forceps; *Smellie's scissors; *combined hook and crochet, Budd's. (*Collyer's pelvimeter should be kept in the office. *Instruments for the Caesarian section and Porro's operation—scalpel, 6 hemostatic forceps, 2 tissue forceps, 2 retractors, hysterectomy clamps, ligature carrier, sponge holder, large and small size chromicized catgut sutures, sterilized gauze sponges, dressings, gowns and towels—should be in another satchel at home, where they may be easily found.) For hypodermic injection—hypodermic syringe and needles. For subcutaneous injection of normal salt solution—2 aspirating needles. To hold small instruments—pocket case. To hold large instruments—pieces of gauze.

The contents of the satchel in the main, need little description, as they will be described under other headings. Antiseptics: Some good soap should be carried in the satchel, as it is not to be found in every house. The permanganate of potash and oxalic acid are of special value only when the hands have been contaminated by a septic case or are stained. Anesthetics: Squibb's chloroform is known to be absolutely reliable, as are all of his goods, hence it should be used. At least 4 ounces should be carried and, if in the country, 8 ounces, as cases of eclampsia and some of difficult labor require much chloroform. Hypodermic tablets of morphine are needed for eclampsia, of morphine and atropine for false pains. Oxytocics and stimulants: Quinin, strychnin and ammonia are used to increase the patient's strength and to increase uterine contractions during any stage of labor. Ergot is used to aid retraction of the uterus after delivery of the placenta. Cathartics: The croton oil is for eclampsia. Dressings: The dressings are to be used only when the patient has none. Iodoform gauze is often needed in placenta previa and post partum hemorrhage. Instruments: Schimmelbusch's folding mask is the best, because it gives plenty of air and so fits the face that it does not have to be held in place. The two tin pans are nearly as good as a sterilizer and will heat very quickly. The rubber gloves should be sterilized in a rubber tobacco pouch so that they may be used at once in an emergency. The small manicuring scissors used by ladies are the best, as they are very strong and will cut the nails short. A cheap brush for the hands is just as good as a costly one. An unvarnished brush may be sterilized with other instruments without soiling them. The rubber apron should be as light as possible and cover only the front of the body, as otherwise it is very warm. The linen or Lonsdale cambric apron should cover all the clothing and have short sleeves which tie above the elbow. (Duck aprons are too heavy and are bulky to carry.) A Kelly pad may be made out of newspapers and be covered with a sterilized cloth. (See The Management of First Stage.) The inner tube of a Glasgow uterine irrigator makes an excellent catheter when a rubber one can not be secured and may be better than the rubber when the head is offering considerable resistance against the urethra. Porter's depressor is preferred, as the groove in its handle prevents the hot water used in uterine irrigation from touching the external parts. A sharp curette is all that is necessary, as by using it gently it will do no more harm or denuding than a dull one. Richter's needle holder holds the needle firmly, but if the needle is grasped near the eye it will be broken. A little smaller needle is needed for vaginal and rectal work than for the external perineum, hence two sizes are given. Emmet's taper point needles do not wound the tissues as much as other needles. Ordinary blunt pointed scissors are as good as cord scissors. Dull scissors tend to prevent secondary hemorrhage from the cord. The probabilities are that secondary hemorrhage follows much less frequently when the cord is tied with real heavy silk or ordinary grocery twine than with tape. Simpson's forceps are preferred because, while not being as powerful as the Elliot, they are strong enough for general use and do not tend to mar the head nor lacerate the maternal parts as does the Elliot instrument, but in some difficult cases the author has found the Elliot necessary. A pair of large household scissors can be used in place of Smellie's scissors, and the forceps may be used instead of the cranioclast and basiotribe. It is best to have two hypodermic syringes, as one may not work.

The instruments for curettage, except the fountain syringe and Kelly pad, should be in one piece of gauze, those for the cord and tears may be wrapped together or separately. (In primips both sets are always to be boiled and in multips both may be needed.) The obstetric forceps should form one package and the other instruments for artificial delivery, another. Several drugs and instruments necessary in post-partum work have not been mentioned here, as it is much easier to carry them in a small post-partum satchel. (See chapter fifteen, "The Post-Partum Satchel.")

THE MANAGEMENT OF THE FIRST STAGE OF LABOR.

Preparation and Antisepsis.—The following method is that used by the author and may be used under any conditions with slight modifications. Upon arriving at the house, the obstetrician should inquire about the condition of the patient and if all the measures to be carried out at the onset of labor have been performed as directed in chapter XI under "Labor Directions." If they have not been performed, the obstetrician should direct the nurse in reference to them. He should be particularly careful about his directions in regard to the preparation of the patient and bed. If the bowls, pitchers, soap dish, fountain syringe, etc., are not washed clean by the nurse, the obstetrician should order them rewashed or rewash them himself.

As soon as the water and bowls are ready, the obstetrican should remove his coat, vest, necktie and collar, roll his shirt sleeves well up above his elbows, put on a clean house apron, wash his hands with soap and water—to remove the superficial dirt and soften his nails—then wipe his hands and cut and clean his nails.

The satchel is opened. A bottle of vaseline is put on the stove. A nail brush is put in a little pan of water to boil ten minutes. A teaspoonful of ergot is poured into about two tablespoonfuls of water in a cup. The chloroform inhaler is unfolded and a clean cloth placed in it. A common, one or two ounce vial is converted into a drop bottle by cutting a groove in the cork, inserting a tooth pick or the point of a safety pin between the cork and the bottle. The ergot, chloroform and inhaler are carried to a convenient place in the bedroom.

The bedroom and bed are examined to see that they are properly arranged. If the room is very small and there is time, it is better to remove the bed to a larger room. If the obstetrician has not brought a Kelly pad he should make a drain pad out of newspapers. Six sheets of newspaper, unfolded, are placed one upon the other, the two corners of one end brought together and overlapped to form the spout and the other end and its sides folded in to form a ridge like that of the Kelly pad to prevent any overflow into the bed. The end corners, where the sides overlap, should be pinned to keep the folds in place.

The instruments for the cord (2 pieces of silk or twine 6 inches long, 2 hem. forceps and scissors), the uterine irrigator (used for vagina and uterus), the instruments for tears (needle holder, 2 needles, 10 silk-worm gut sutures and scissors), a nail brush and if no gauze or cotton, a dozen cloths, 6x6 inches, are placed in a clean pan. At once or near the end of the first stage enough hot water is poured into the pan to cover the instruments and cloths, a tablesponful of baking soda added, and the pan covered with a tin, cloth or paper lid, is placed on the stove and allowed to boil five minutes. The fountain syringe is thrown in and the water boiled five minutes more. (Boiling a rubber syringe more than five minutes may injure it, if it is made of poor material). A nail is ordered driven into the wall so that the syringe may be hung near the bed. A clean cloth or newspaper is hung about the nail so that the syringe will not touch the wall. (A piece of heavy cord is often fastened to the syringe before the latter is boiled so that the syringe can be hung on a post of the head of the bed).

The obstetrician, having prepared everything, leaves on the house apron or puts on a rubber apron or a clean surgeon's linen or cambric apron, and renders his hands and forearms aseptic as for a surgical operation by washing with soap, water and nail brush five minutes, rinsing with plain water followed by alcohol and then soaking in bichlorid solution (1 to 2,000) for five minutes. If the hands have been in contact with anything septic the permanganate method should be used. It is the same as the preceding, except that in place of the alcohol the hands are first soaked in a saturated solution of permanganate of potash and then in a saturated solution of oxalic acid. If the obstetrician has a sterile apron, it is now put on over the rubber or house apron. If it is necessary to move chairs or open doors, the obstetrician may do so by the use of elbows or feet and if anything else has to be touched, which is not aseptic, it is best to use the palm of the hand or the little finger, i. e., the parts which are farthest from the examining fingers.

The nurse is directed to dissolve a bichlorid tablet in a cup of boiling water. The obstetrician lifts the fountain syringe out of the pan and holds it, while the nurse fills it with hot water and throws in the bichlorid solution. He attaches the uterine irrigator and drops it into the bag and hangs the syringe on the wall. Care is used that neither the nurse nor anything else touches the syringe.

If the obstetrician believes that the patient's lower abdomen and external genitals have been thoroughly cleansed as directed, the vulvar pad is removed and the parts bathed with bichlorid (1 to 2,000), but if there is any doubt, the obstetrician cleanses these parts. The patient is brought into the obstetric position—i.e., crosswise of the bed, hips well over the edge on the Kelly pad, feet on chairs which face each other and are separated enough to allow room for the slop jar or pail, with knees sufficiently apart to permit the obstetrician, who sits upon a chair, to easily reach the vulva. The lower abdomen and vulva are left bare, but the legs are covered with obstetric stockings or sheet. (The author has the nurse so draw the sheet that is over the patient, that it drops below the knees and is taut from the knees to the upper abdomen). The wash bowl of water, the sterilized gauze, cotton or cloths, soap and scissors should be conveniently at hand. The vulvar hair is cut short, the lower abdomen and genitals washed ten minutes with plenty of soap and water, using sterilized gauze or cheese cloth, and then a solution of bichlorid let run over the parts from the fountain syringe or from a small pitcher, or by applying a pad saturated in the solution. In the obstetric position the crevices of the labia, vestibule and vaginal orifice are more thoroughly cleansed, than if the patient is lengthwise of the bed upon the bed pan. A vaginal douche should not be used, as the vagina in normal labor is kept aseptic by its own secretions, but in cases of gonorrhea the vaginal secretions are not aseptic and an eight-quart, one to two thousand bichlorid solution should be given by the obstetrician after a thorough cleansing of the vulva as above described. (Because of the possibility of gonorrheal or other infection being present, the author believes that if a strictly vaginal douche could be given at the onset of labor it would always be preferable).

Care is used to prevent the irrigator or the tubing next to the irrigator touching anything but the hands of the obstetrician, the interior of the vagina and the syringe. During the irrigation, the perineum is pressed backwards a little so as to favor the return flow of water and to dilate the vaginal folds. In operative cases nearly all authorities cleanse and douche the vagina.

The Vaginal Examination.—The vaginal examination should be made as soon as the cleansing is completed and if the patient is in the obstetric position, the examination is very much more satisfactory. Before each examination the hands should be rewashed and soaked in bichlorid solution. The number of examinations should be as few as possible, not to exceed three, and as a rule not more frequent than once an hour. (It is well not to make a vaginal examination, if the abdominal examination indicates that everything is natural and the pains continue normal. Where there is delay, it is not considered a wise procedure, for it is impossible to determine the cause by abdominal examination and the patient will not think the accoucheur is döing his duty. Some German obstetricians and a few others, deliver the great majority of their patients without any internal examination, using abdominal palpation, assisted in the second stage by the fingers pressed upwards against the perineum to note the descent of the head). The method of introducing the fingers, reaching the cervix and examining the pelvic landmarks, described in chapter ten, under The Examination of the First Half of Pregnancy, should be adopted.

By vaginal examination the presence or absence of the onset of labor, cervical dilation and the rupture of the membranes should be determined; then the presentation and the position of the fetus should be diagnosed and, if a vertex presentation, the presence or absence of the caput succedaneum, engagement, complete flexion, descent and rotation of the head determined. If necessary the membranes should be ruptured and the duration of labor estimated. In the first stage of labor the presentation and position of the fetus can not always be determined, the caput succedaneum is rare, engagement, complete flexion and descent may not be present and rotation is infrequent, but as they may be present it is best to consider their diagnosis here.

The Diagnosis of the Onset of Labor.—This is made by finding increasing painful uterine contractions, increasing dilation of the cervix or escape of the liquor amnii. A discharge of bloody mucus, i. e., the "show," generally indicates a rapid onset. The patient's word must not be taken as evidence that the liquor amnii has escaped. A positive diagnosis of the presence of labor should often not be made until at least an hour ofter the first examination. (See False Labor Pains, under Abnormal Pregnancy.)

The Diagnosis of the Amount of Dilation of the Cervix.— The exact amount of dilation of the cervix should be determined by considering how many finger-breadths its diameter equals. The capability of introducing three fingers if the opening is circular, or four if it is only a transverse opening, indicates that the cervix is half dilated. The width of three fingers is furnished by separating the first two fingers enough to allow one finger between them—the latter equals about half the width the fingers will separate. Complete dilation is present when the cervix and vagina form one continuous canal, i. e., when the cervix is as large as the pelvic cavity. At times when the cervix is very thin, as in primiparae, feeling the edge of the external os is difficult, but by remembering that the border may feel like a thread (or the edge produced by the overlapping of a sheet of paper) its situation ought to be always readily determined and the error of mistaking the thinned cervix for the membranes prevented.

The Diagnosis of the Presence or Absence of the Bag of Waters.—If the bag of waters is present, the examining finger will feel during a uterine contraction a smooth, tense membrane; between the contractions a wrinkled one and often, some forewaters. If the membranes have been ruptured, the conditions present will be just the opposite, viz., during a contraction there will be felt the wrinkled scalp; between the contractions, the smooth scalp, and if the hand is passed up between the head and the cervix, as a rule the liquor amnii will escape. Very rarely a speculum may have to be introduced to determine the presence or absence of the membranes. Frequently, when the bladder empties involuntarily, the patient thinks that the bag of waters has ruptured. The escape of "external or false waters," i. e., fluid from between the amnion and chorion or the chorion and endometrium sometimes makes a like error. After the bag of waters has been found to be present, its size, shape, and tenseness during and between pains, should be determined.

The Diagnosis of the Caput Succedaneum.—The caput succedaneum may be mistaken for the bag of waters. It pits on pressure, .does not fluctuate and remains the same during and between pains, except growing a little larger during pains, and the examining finger can be passed beyond it on the non-edematous portion of the presenting part.

The Diagnosis of the Presentation and Position.—In making an examination it is important to keep the first two fingers, the hand and forearm parallel, as otherwise, the fingers may unconsciously extend into another quadrant of the pelvic cavity.

Often, when a position is diagnosed with one hand and then an examination made with the other, the second diagnosis will not agree with the first. This is due to the difference in the flexion of the fingers and hands and to the fact that the sense of location is better developed in one hand than the other, usually the less used hand.

The Diagnosis of the Vertex Presentation.—This is made by feeling a hard, round, smooth body which nearly fills the inlet and presents sutures and fontanelles. The vertex can generally be easily diagnosed through the membranes, and sometimes through the cervix, but in the latter case, the sutures and fontanelles can very rarely be felt.

The Diagnosis of the Position of the Vertex Presentation.— This is not made, as a rule, until after rupture of the membranes.

L. O. A., Left Occipito-Anterior Position: The posterior fontanelle is to the left and front, opposite the left ilio-pectineal eminence, i. e., in the left anterior quadrant of the pelvic inlet; the anterior fontanelle is high up to the right and back, opposite the right sacro-iliac joint, i. e., in the right posterior quadrant of the pelvic inlet; and the sagittal suture is in the first oblique diameter.

R. O. P., Right Occipito-Posterior Position: The posterior fontanelle is to the right and back, opposite the right sacro-iliac joint, i. e., in the right posterior quadrant of the pelvic inlet; the anterior fontanelle is high up to the left and front, opposite the left ilio-pectineal eminence, i. e., in the left anterior quadrant; and the sagittal suture is in the first oblique.

R. O. A., Right Occipito-Anterior Position: The posterior fontanelle is to the right and front, opposite the right ilio-pectineal eminence, i. e., in the right anterior quadrant of the pelvic

inlet; the anterior fontanelle is high up to the left and back, opposite the left sacro-iliac joint, i. e., in the left posterior quadrant;
and the sagittal suture is in the second oblique.

L. O. P., Left Occipito-Posterior Position: The posterior
fontanelle is to the left and back, opposite the left sacro-iliac joint,
i. e., in the left posterior quadrant of the pelvic inlet; the anterior
fontanelle is high up to the right and front, opposite the right ilio-
pectineal eminence, i. e., in the right anterior quadrant; and the
sagittal suture is in the second oblique.

Diagnosis of the Engagement of the Head.—This is done by
finding the head fitting the inlet and passing into the pelvic cavity.
(Davis says the head is engaged when the most dependent part is
on a level with the subpubic ligament.) The head is not normally
engaged in the vertex presentation, unless the head is well flexed.

Diagnosis of Complete Flexion.—When the posterior fontanelle is consideably lower than the anterior, near the centre of the
pelvic cavity, and the anterior fontanelle is hard to reach, there
is complete flexion of the head. When the anterior fontanelle is in
front, it seems lower than when it is back as it is nearer the vulva.

Diagnosis of Descent.—Descent of the head is estimated by
noting at intervals the distance of the head from the subpubic
ligament. This is determined by marking with the unemployed
finger, on the vaginal index finger where the latter touches the subpubic ligament. The obstetrician may be in error as to the progress of the birth, from the descent of the head still enclosed in
the cervix, (the cervix being so thin as to resemble the membranes)
from the descent of the bag of waters without the head, or from the
descent of the caput succedaneum.

Diagnosis of Rotation.—This is made by feeling the rotation
at the time it occurs, or noting the new position of the posterior
fontanelle after it has taken place.

The Abdominal Examination.—If there is time, an abdominal examination may be made to confirm the one made during
pregnancy and the vaginal examination. Because of the severity
of the uterine contractions during labor, it is generally more difficult and annoying to the patient, but at times, the uterus relaxes
more between labor contractions than between those of pregnancy.

The Patient's Clothing.—As is is not known when the membranes will rupture it is best to have the patient's clothes so arranged that neither her gown nor her shirt will subsequently be soiled. Her gown and shirt are therefore, to be carefully rolled up to the axillary region, and if she is to be up, a sheet should be so folded that it will reach from the arm-pits to below the knees, be pinned to the rolled-up gown, and ave its opening in front, or to the right side, if the patient is to lie on her left side.

The Patient's Position.—As sitting up, walking and change of posture increase the force of the uterine contractions and favors the engagement of the presenting part, they should be encouraged. If the patient is not able to sit up, she should change her position in bed often, and keep her limbs extended as much as possible.

Bearing Down.—Bearing down should not be 'allowed, because it not only weakens the patient but does little good. This is not the stage of expulsion and the effort is liable to cause laceration of the cervix by stretching it too rapidly.

Food and Drink.—Light food, water, tea or coffee may be given, if desired, as they keep up the patient's strength and courage.

Estimations on the Duration of Labor.—Care should be used not to make a definite answer as to the duration of labor, especially not to state that labor will not occur before a definite time; for frequently labor will end before the time stated. If one says it will occur in a couple of hours and it takes longer, this error is not so objectionable, for the patient will think it is said to ease her mind. It is best to say that all depends upon the pains, or that if the pains continue as they are, the labor will probably be over in so many¯hours, estimated by the conditions present.

Simple Measures to Lessen the Duration and Suffering of the First Stage of Labor.—While the first stage of labor should be left as much as possible to nature, there are certain things which may be used to advantage. Keeping the patient up, letting her eat a little, having her change her position frequently, quiet, but cheerful attendance, talking about little things to keep her mind from her pain, moral suasion, ten grains of quinin, a little brandy or whiskey, aromatic spirit of ammonia and one-thirtieth grain of strychnin, are of value. While chloroform diminishes the suffering, it frequently lessens the force of the uterine contractions, hence, its use should be restricted as much as possible. Two to five drops may be given at the very beginning of a pain, but no more until the next pain begins. (It is sometimes necessary to aid dilation of the cervix by very gentle manual assistance, but this is not considered a part of the management of normal labor, hence, it will be discussed elsewhere.)

The Care of the Fetus.—In this and the next stage, the fetal heart sound should be noted, especially if the labor is long; as they indicate the conditions of the fetus, and "to be forewarned is to be forearmed."

The Presence of the Obstetrician.—The less the accoucheur is present during the first stage of labor, the better. When the obstetrician is present the patient is apt to think labor will soon end. She naturally worries and asks, "How long will it be?" When the pains are not less than ten minutes apart and the cervix is not dilated more than three fingers, the obstetrician may be away, but he should be near and be called when the water breaks, blood appears or the pains occur every ten minutes and are more severe. Much depends upon distance and the patient.

Treatment of Delayed Rupture of the Membranes.—Always, before rupturing the membranes, a careful diagnosis of the presentation and engagement should be made and abnormal conditions corrected. (Malpresentations are more easily changed before rupture than after, because of the presence of the liquor amnii. Imperfect engagement of the presenting part in the vertex and other presentations, should be corrected before rupture of the membranes, as otherwise, prolapsus of the cord or of an arm, may follow.)

If there is no advancement half an hour after the cervix is completely dilated, the membranes should be ruptured. A sterilized hairpin or one of the hemostatic forceps used for the cord, is introduced between two fingers, and at the height of a contraction is pushed by the fingers of the other hand into the most dependent part of the bag of waters. Then one or two fingers are introduced into the opening to enlarge it to the size of the cervix. The membranes are rarely so tense that a scalpel is required, while in other cases, the finger is sufficient.

Treatment of Delayed Engagement, Incomplete Flexion. Abnormal Presentations and Other Causes of Delayed Labor.—(See Abnormal Labor.)

(To be concluded next month.)

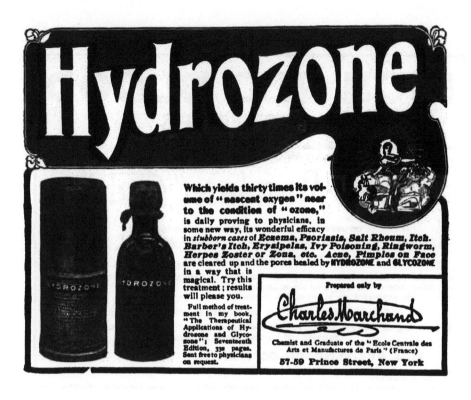

DENVER MEDICAL TIMES

THOMAS H. HAWKINS, A.M., M.D., EDITOR AND PUBLISHER.

COLLABORATORS:

Henry O. Marcy, M.D., Boston.
Thaddeus A. Reamy, M.D., Cincinnati.
Nicholas Senn, M.D., Chicago.
Joseph Price, M.D., Philadelphia.
Franklin H. Martin, M.D., Chicago.
William Oliver Moore, M.D., New York.
L. S. McMurtry, M.D., Louisville.
Thomas B. Eastman, M.D., Indianapolis, Ind.
G. Law, M.D., Greeley, Colo.

S. H. Pinkerton, M.D., Salt Lake City.
Flavel B. Tiffany, M.D., Kansas City.
Erskine M. Bates, M.D;. New York.
E. C. Gehrung, M.D, St. Louis.
Graeme M. Hammond, M.D, New York.
James A. Lydston, M.D., Chicago.
Leonard Freeman, M.D., Denver.
Carey K. Fleming, M.D., Denver, Colo.

Subscriptions, $1.00 per year in advance; Single Copies, 10 cents.

Address all Communications to Denver Medical Times, 1740 Welton Street, Denver, Colo.
We will at all times be glad to give space to well written articles or items of interest to the profession.
[Entered at the Postoffice of Denver, Colorado, as mail matter of the Second Class.]

EDITORIAL DEPARTMENT

PROGRESS IN SURGERY.

The frightful mortality from "blood poisoning" was up to about 25 years ago the terror of surgeons, who feared especially to do operations on the viscera, and who expected "laudable pus" in all successful operative cases. In the charnel houses known as military hospitals many more died of infection than directly from battle wounds. Frequently and over wide areas of territory, as Park remarks, epidemics and endemics of puerperal fever would result in the death of almost every lying-in woman. It was the American author-physician, Oliver Wendell Holmes, who first called attention to the contagiousness of puerperal fever.

The "germ theory" is by no means new as a theory, but is rather recent, in fact. Addison, in the *Spectator,* affirmed that everywhere in the body and without, there abounded innumerable minute organisms. Leuwenhoek in 1675 discovered living rod-like bodies with the microscope. In 1849 Pollender and Davaine discovered anthrax bacilli. Pasteur, about 1865, taught that fermentation is always due to microscopic plants or animals, and assumed there was a special germ for every disease. Pasteur, Tyndall, Voit, Pettenkofer, Cohn, Klebs and Koch, elaborating the researches of Appert, Schwann, Schroeder and Dusch, proved the nature of infectious material in air, water and dust, and overthrew the ancient myth of spontaneous generation. They also showed that heat and filtration rendered innocuous the minute impurities or germs in air and liquids. Bacteriology was first made an exact science by Koch's discovery of differential culture methods. Protective inoculation with bacteria whose virulence had been lessened by cultural methods, was first practiced by Pasteur, and applied successfully in chicken cholera and the charbon of sheep and cattle.

Concerning antiseptics, it should be added that Jules Lemaire led the way in 1863 by a comprehensive work on the use and action of an emulsion of coal-tar, first prepared by Le Boeuf in 1850. But the new epoch really began four years later with Lister's first article upon this subject.

Lister and his coadjutors erroneously considered the air the chief medium of infection, and in addition to scrupulous care in cleansing hands, instruments and the site of operation, and treating dressings and ligatures with strong germicidal solutions, they used a cumbersome and somewhat dangerous spray of carbolic acid during the course of the operation.

The original method of Lister has been greatly simplified and largely replaced by aseptics, that is by cleanliness so nearly absolute as practically to exclude germs. Lawson Tait was the chief exponent of aseptic surgery. The irritating and even necrotic effects of strong antiseptic solutions have led to greater care in their employment and a widening of the scope of the dry method of treating surgical and accidental wounds. The occlusive first-aid dressings used on and by wounded soldiers on the battle-field mark a distinct advance in prophylactic surgery.

The solidarity of scientific interests is nowhere more strikingly exemplified than in the seemingly irrelevant relations of the little yeast cells that Pasteur studied and the wonderful life-saving results accomplished daily by the surgeons of the present.

Before the eighteenth century surgery was in low repute, and was entrusted to barbers, cobblers, tinkers, farriers and swinespayers. The striped barber pole thus represents both blood and lather. According to Wilder, even Ambroise Pare, the inventor of sutures and ligatures, was a barber, and in the old Prussian army it was the duty of the regimental surgeon to shave the officers. In

1745 the two callings of barber (blood-letter and dentist) and surgeon were definitely separated by an act of the English parliament.

ANESTHESIA.

The first clinical use of ether as an anesthetic was by a Georgia country doctor, Crawford W. Long, who on March 30, 1842, removed a small cystic tumor from the jaw of a young man named Venables, under anesthesia, without causing the slightest pain.

The man who deserves the credit of demonstrating publicly the use of ether as an anesthetic was the Boston dentist, William T. G. Morton, who on October 16, 1846, administered ether for a surgical operation by Dr. J. C. Warren at the Massachusetts General Hospital. A patent was issued to Morton on Nov. 12, 1846, but these rights were later nullified by the government itself, and Morton died in 1868, a poor and bitterly disappointed man. Of his three chief rivals for reward, Jackson, Wells and Marcy, the first went insane, and the second took his own life. Dr. Horace Wells, a Hartford dentist, was the first (1844) to use nitrous oxid (on his own person) to prevent the pain of tooth-pulling.

Chloroform was introduced as an anesthetic by James Y. Simpson in Scotland in 1847. The terms anesthesia and anesthetic were suggested to Morton by Oliver W. Holmes. The impetus which anesthesia gave to surgery was exceeded only by antisepsis.

Compare the painless amputations of the present day with those of a few centuries ago when a limb was cut off with a sickleshaped knife and a saw, and the bleeding stump dipped in boiling pitch or oil or seared with a red-hot iron—and all without anesthesia.

MODERN MIRACLES.

At a recent meeting of the Denver Clinical and Pathological Society, Levy presented a woman 75 years of age who, two years before, had been examined by himself and Freeman. One nostril was then filled with a large mass, which, on histological examination by Mitchell, of Denver, and Welch, of Baltimore, proved to be a round-celled sarcoma. Prolonged use of the X-Rays, by

Stover, had no appreciable effect. Levy removed the tumor from
the nostril, but after a few months it recurred on the other side of
the nose and was so bad that further operation was deemed inad-
visable.

The patient concluded to try what "Christian Science" could
do for her. After some time the mass in the nose disappeared,
along with four out of six tumors on the lower limb—the other two
are increasing in size, and new ones are developing. Now it is
such rare and anomalous cases as this which provide an apparent
basis for the various moonshine cults of healing. To give the
credit of this partial cure to Eddyism, would be to depose our
common sense. Even the well-known effect of the mind on the
body could hardly come into play here since, owing to her age, the
patient's mentality is enfeebled considerably. Simply stated, the
unexpected phenomenon was a spontaneous trophic change, the
exact nature of which is thus far beyond the horizon of our knowledge.

Whether, as is not improbable, this lady again grows worse
and dies from multiple metastases, or whether her departure is due
to old age, the Eddyites are certain to herald the case as a complete and remarkable cure "after she was given up by all the doctors." Which reminds me that a neighbor of mine who had been
"cured" of consumption by "Christian Science" died in the Christian Science Temple from a pulmonary hemorrhage.

WHOOPING COUGH.

This disease now ranks ahead of diphtheria and scarlet fever
in its mortality, largely by reason of complicating bronchopneumonia. It is thought to be due to the presence of the bacillus tussis
convulviivae, which can be readily discerned in the mucous sputum, after staining with eosin. It is about one-third the length
of the tubercle bacillus and is apparently sporeless.

On its first appearance pertussis closely resembles a common
cold. In a week or so when the paroxysmal stage begins, and
before the pathognomonic whoop is heard, one must distinguish
this disease from bronchitis, which can generally be done by the
absence of fever and rales in the former. Vomiting and epistaxis

after coughing are characteristic of whooping cough. In young children convulsions may accompany the paroxysms or even replace them, as in a case of Kilmer. Among the dangers to be dreaded, aside from bronchopneumonia, are wasting, anemia, enlarged bronchial glands, emphysema, atelectasis, pleurisy, pneumothorax, phthisis, pericarditis, paralysis, acute nephritis and hernia.

The duration of typical cases is from six to twelve weeks, and in severe epidemics treatment does not seem to shorten this period to any appreciable degree. The great number of remedies recommended for pertussis shows how little each of them is worth. The chief therapeutic considerations seem to be fresh air, light nourishing food and avoidance of chill to the body surface. The benefit derived from the vaporization of formaldehyde or carbolic acid is somewhat problematic. Severe paroxysms may be limited by the use of antipyrin during the day and chloral at night. The nose should be douched and oiled one or twice daily. A firm belly band aids in preventing vomiting and hernia. When the weather is dry and windless, the child should be warmly clad and kept out of doors most of the day.

Venereal Diseases. Geo. M. Kober, Washington, D. C. (*Journal A. M. A.,* March 11), points out the terrible prevalence of venereal diseases among the general population. He quotes statistics showing that in large cities from 12 to 15 per cent. of the population are afflicted with syphilis and a still larger proportion with gonorrhea. While he does not think that public regulation of the evil is advisable in this country, he maintains that the state should enforce laws against solicitation and seduction, and that health boards should recommend the enactment of sanitary regulation of all occupations by which extragenital syphilis may be conveyed, and special examinations should be made of wet nurses, etc. He believes that these measures would be of great educational value and suggests that a general educational campaign be instituted against these disorders.

EDITORIAL ITEMS.

Gouty Constipation. W. W. Johnston gives the wine of colchicum, five drops or more three times a day.

Membranous Enteritis. W. W. Johnston advises the persistent use of an exclusive milk diet.

Constipation Following Diarrhea. J. Henry Fruitnight recommends strychnine, alone or in combination with iron and quinine.

Stomach Trouble With Sore Mouth. Dessar prescribes: ℞ Pulv. rhei gr. iiss; sodii bicarb. gr. iv; tinct. gent. co., aq., menth. pip. aa. m. xxx: A teaspoonful three times a day after meals.

Lavatives in Puerperium. Castor oil is the best laxative in the puerperal period, aided if need be by enemas. Salines are indicated for fever or congested breasts.

Venous Pelvic Congestion. Bruce recommends a saline draught mornings with a hematinic or other tonic during the day; or an aloes and iron pill at bedtime.

Constipation in Typhoid Fever. A. B. Palmer prescribes: ℞ Olei ricini, mucil. acaciae, aq. camphorae aa. ℥ i; sacchari albi ℨ ii: Three to six teaspoonfuls at a dose.

Constipation in Measles. Louis Starr uses enemata or glycerine suppositories and calomel in broken doses or milk of magnesia with aromatic syrup or rhubarb.

Simple Peritonitis. Perhaps the best medical treatment consists in the administration of full doses of salines along with the judicious use of opiates.

Colonic Dyspepsia. The compound rhubarb pill, alternated in special cases with extract of nux vomica or belladonna, is recommended by S. G. Armor.

Unpleasant Effects of Digitalis. Hecht states that the unpleasant effects of digitalis on the stomach *(Clinical Review)* may be avoided by combining it with strychnine and quinine.

Yeast in Vaginal and Uterine Catarrh. Caronbach (quoted in *Chicago Clinic*) states that in vaginal and uterine catarrh, especially in gonorrhea in pregnant women, yeast is of great value.

Constipation with Uterine Disorders. Goodell has prescribed: ℞ Ext. colocynth. comp. gr. ii; ext. belladonnae gr. ss.; ext. gentianae gr. i; oler carui gtt. ss.: One pill at bedtime.

Atony of Abdominal Muscles. This condition may depend on ascites, obesity, senility or repeated pregnancies. Osler writes favorably of the use of an abdominal bandage to support the muscles of stout persons or women with pendulous abdomen.

Acute Appendicitis. The most important point, says Ochsner, is to avoid peristalsis by exclusive rectal feeding with any concentrated food dissolved in three or four ounces of normal salt solution, and given through the rectal tube every three to six hours.

Fissure of Rectum in Infants. This causes much pain, manifested by crying on bowel movement, and predisposes to constipation. A good method of cure is to stretch the sphincter gradually with the fingers and massage the abdomen.

Constipation of Sedentary Persons. Osler recommends moderate exercise; friction or regularly applied massage in more chronic cases; enemata of tepid water (with or without soap), olive oil or glycerine; and the use of a metal ball weighing four to six pounds, rolled over the abdomen every morning for five or ten minutes.

Constipation of Senility. W. W. Johnston combines strychnine, iron, quinine or gentian with aloes, colocynth, rhubarb or podophyllin. When flatulence accompanies the costive state, Thornton prescribes one or two pills at bedtime of one-half grain aloin and two grains of asafetida. For great torpor of the intestines Ringer recommends a grain of ipecac every morning.

Oral Treatment of Hemorrhoids. Shoemaker prescribes: ℞ Massae hydrarg. gr. ii; ext. rhei gr. i; ext. colocynth. co. gr. ii; saponis gr. 1/6: A pill to be taken at bed hour, followed in the morning by a teaspoonful of Rochelle salt in water before breakfast. A teaspoonful of compound licorice powder at bedtime renders the stools soft and is particularly useful in the hemorrhoids of pregnant women.

Treatment of Sciatica. Lange (quoted in *J. A. M. A.*) has used, with surprisingly good results an injection of a solution of from 70 to 100 cc of beta encaine in 8-1000 salt solution. The injection is made through the muscle down to the sciatic nerve at its point of emergence from the sacro-sciatic foramen.

Local use of Alcohol for Superficial Pain. When the skin is intact the *Clinical Review* recommends to sprinkle four or five layers of cheesecloth well with alcohol and spread the cloth upon the painful area. Where the skin is comparatively thick and insensitive, the cheesecloth may be well covered over with some close material.

Poultices Out of Date. By order of the Surgeon-General of the U. S. Army, Medical Dept *(Clinical Review)* linseed and linseed meal have been dropped from army medicines. It is held that any good effects that might accrue from poulticing, can be just as well secured by simple hot wet compresses.

The Life of Vaccine. The *Clinical Review* says: As a result of experiments carefully carried out it has been found that average commercial vaccine can be depended upon for not more than three months from time of manufacture, in winter, while in midsummer it holds its activity scarcely beyond one month.

Cold Feet and Colic. Louis Fischer *(Dietetic and Hygienic Gazette)* calls attention to the relations of these conditions. He frequently insists on the use of cocoa-butter rubbed into the soles and feet of children suffering with cold extremities and has seen good results therefrom.

Chronic Enterocolitis. Four to eight ounces of sweet oil may be injected through a colon tube (inserted full length) every second or third night. Small enemata (one-half pint) of cool water or a pint of warm water containing four grains of alum or zinc sulphate thrown high up once daily, are likewise useful. W. W. Johnston recommends the use of mineral waters, alternated with aloin, strychnine and belladonna.

Dyspepsia With Costipation. In gastric hyperacidity alkalies and a non-stimulating diet are indicated. For children with constipation and indigestion Earle directs to correct diet and give pepsin and hydrochloric acid and cascara or compound syrup of taraxacum. Following an alcoholic debauch Thornton corrects the prima via with five grains of calomel and twenty grains of powdered jalap, in one dose taken dry on the tongue. For severe constipation Einhorn prescribes: ℞ Podophyllin. gr. 1/6; ext. nucis vom.; ext. physostig. aa. gr. ¼; ext. gentianae, pulv. glycyrrhizae aa. q.s.: One pill t. i. d.

Plumbic Obstipation. This form of constipation, being caused by spasm of the intestinal musculature, presents the paradox of being in some cases relieved by opium or tobacco. The following measures are advised by W. R. Hobbs: An enema of soap-suds thrice daily; calomel and soda or epsom salts; if these fail, give a capsule (up to five) every two hours containing one minim of croton oil, two minims of fluid extract of belladonna and sufficient sodium bicarbonate at same time with enema of salts or of olive oil containing five minims of croton oil; also strychnine, gr. 1/30 hypodermically twice a day; and potassium iodide after bowels move, 15 to 30 grains in a bitter tonic t. i. d. after meals. Beef tea and chicken soup form the best diet during the acute symptoms.

Laryngismus Stridulus. Osler directs to dash cold water into the face if attack is severe and lividity great—or thrust the finger far back into the throat. In a severe case place the child in a warm bath two or three times a day and sponge back and chest thoroughly for a minute or two with cold water. If the gums are hot and swollen, lance freely. Regulate bowels carefully and give a nourishing diet and cod-liver oil.

Chronic Bronchitis. For paroxysmal attacks of cough and dyspnea Bruce prescribes: ℞ Spt. etheris m. xxx; spt. ammon. arom. m. xxx; tinct. aurantii amari m. xx; aquae camphorae ℥ iv; aquam dest. ad ℥ i: Take when required. He also recommends counter-irritation to the chest with four drachms of chloroform liniment, eleven ounces of turpentine, two drachms of glacial acetic acid and eleven drachms of camphor liniment.

Chronic Bone Sinuses. The method of Von Mosetig *(International Journal of Surgery)* is to apply a constrictor, remove the sinus and all diseased bone, then chisel out more bone with fresh instruments until an entirely healthy surface is exposed. Cleanse cavity and wash thoroughly with one'per cent. formalin solution, dry with swabs and hot air and fill with sterilized melted mixture of sixty parts each of spermaceti and oil of sesame.

The Personal Influence of the Physician in Venereal Diseases.—H. D. Holton, Brattleboro, Vt., *(Journal A. M. A.,* March 11), calls attention to the great good that might be accomplished by physicians giving personal instructions to patients concerning the prevention of venereal diseases. He quotes circulars discussed at the 1903 meeting of the State and Provincial Boards of Health of North America, which are issued by the various boards to physicians in their jurisdiction.

Intussusception. John Ashhurst, Jr., recommends extracts of opium and belladonna (1/12 grain of former and 1/24 of latter for child of two years) by suppository every hour or two to put bowel at rest. He uses large injections (one to six quarts) of warm water or warm olive oil with a long rectal tube and a fountain syringe (eight feet above patient if an infant), keeping patient etherized and semi-inverted, and preventing escape of fluid with an india rubber collar and cotton or lint. Other methods of treatment are inflation with air, hydrogen or carbonic acid gas; abdominal taxis; enterotomy or laparotomy.

Non-Medical Treatment of Constipation. Gant directs to divulse sphincter (Wales bougies for gradual dilation—numbers 6 to 12); frequent abdominal massage, ten to twelve minutes every other day—metal ball of three to five pounds covered with cloth; copious high warm water injections, a half gallon or more in beginning of treatment; a regular hour of evacuation; simple diet, much fruit; abundance of water—a glass of cold or hot water before breakfast; out-door exercise; daily cold bath before breakfast; warm dress in winter, cool in summer; temperance; change of occupation.

Patriotic Polyuria. Dr. E. S. McKee, of Cincinnati, in his duties as physician to the Society Francaise de Secours Mutueles de Cincinnati reports that there came under his care a battle-scarred veteran of the '70's who showed symptoms of diabetes. He asked him before his return to the office to measure the amount of urine passed in 24 hours in some convenient vehicle. He returned hte following Sunday and said: "I passed four of Frenches quart milk bottles full." The French are as patriotic as polite.

Cardiac Failure of Pneumonia. For this chief danger Preble advises, when symptoms arise, an ice-bag constantly over the precordium, or the use of digitalis or digitoxin (1/500 grain) Strychnine, caffeine, camphorated oil, ammonia, and alcoholics carefully regulated are likewise of service. Cases with vulvular lesions should receive digitalis from the onset, and those present-ing evidence of chronic myocarditis, or arteriosclerosis should be kept under the influence of nitro-glycerin. As a last resort, parti-cularly when signs of pulmonary edema supervene, venesection is ad·isable, and in a certain low percentage of cases will be a life-saving procedure.

Locomotor Ataxia and Paretic Dementia. While speaking before the City and County Medical Society on these diseases Dr. H. T. Pershing called attention to their close relationships. Both are practically always post-syphilitic in origin, and locomotor ataxia not infrequently passes over into general paresis. In this event the "lightning" pains and crises of tabes are apt to amelior-ate somewhat, perhaps because the toxic element is not abundant enough to "go around" the whole nervous system.

Gonorrhea as a Cause of Death. Joseph Taber Johnson, Washington, D. C. (*Journal A. M. A.,* March 11), reviews the opinions of authorities as to the effects of gonorrhea in producing female sterility and disease, and states his belief that if the mor-tality from this cause could be ascertained it would be found to equal that from either typhoid fever, pneumonia or tuberculosis, and that possibly it might be found to exceed the mortality from all three diseases. He thinks that gonorrhea is the cause of at least 30 per cent. of the deaths among prostitutes, and that through its later effects on the generative organs it may be the cause of death in a very large number of virtuous married women.

Acute Intussusception in an Infant; Resection of Gangrenous Intussusceptum; Murphy Button Anastomosis; Recovery. E. W. Peterson reports what he believes to be the first successful operation on an infant, for the relief of intussusception in which resection of the gut was performed. The patient was an infant of four months and twenty days, with typical symptoms pointing to an intussusception of about thirty hours' duration. Four inches of the ileum, the cecum, and an inch of the ascending colon were resected and an end-to-end anastomosis made by means of the Murphy button. Convalescence was stormy, but the patient was discharged on the fifteenth day. The button was expelled on the fourth day. The author considers that it is of importance to avoid the systematic use of opium in the postoperative treatment of these cases, owing to the risk of the drug's aggravating the enteritis and toxemia usually present.—*Medical Record,* March 4, 1905.

Senile Constipation. Charcot and Loomis mention as important daily punctuality at water closet; abdominal friction or galvanic current; a diet largely vegetable, prunes, figs, oatmeal with molasses; a goblet of fresh, cold water just before retiring or on rising; laxatives (always combined with tonics)—colocynthin, gentian and quinine, or aloes, rhubarb and strychnine or iron, or podophyllin. In very obstinate cases begin with compound extract of colocynth, scammony and one-sixth drop of croton oil, one or two pills before dinner or at bedtime. Purgative enemata are useful as adjuvants to all forms of treatment.

Intestinal Obstruction by Cicatricial Contraction of Bands. Greig Smith directed to tie peritoneal adhesions of omental cords close to points of attachment and cut off short between. An adherent Fallopian tube may be divided as a simple band. If the appendix is the cause, liberate the bowel by dividing adhesions, or if this is impossible, cut through appendix, double inward and close by suturing peritoneal surfaces. If the gut is much distended, incise and empty at some distance from point of constriction; if gangrenous or about to perforate, excise this part.

Editorial Items continued on Page 628

BOOKS.

THE INTERNATIONAL MEDICAL ANNUAL. A Year Book of Treatment and Practitioner's Index. 1905. Twenty-third year. Price, $3.00. New York. E. B. Treat & Co., 241-243 West Twenty-third street.

Within the limits of 644 pages one finds a vast amount of useful and timely information, collected, condensed and presented by thirty-five leading American and British practitioners. The book is in fact a library in itself. Full references are given at the end of each subject discussed. A novel feature consists in sixteen stereograms representing diseases of the eye. Piroplasma hominis, the hematozoon of Rocky Mountain spotted fever, is shown pictorially in colors, as is likewise the Gambian trypanosome.

THOUGHTS FOR THE OCCASION: FRATERNAL AND BENEVOLENT. Reference Manual of Historical Data and Facts; helpful in suggesting themes, and in outlining addresses for observance of timely or special occasions of the various orders, compiled by Franklin Noble, D.D., editor of the *Treasury Magazine*. Price, $2.00. New York. E. B. Treat & Co., 241-243 West Twenty-third street. 1905.

American fraternal organizations are said to enroll six million persons among their members, fully half of whom are included in the insurance fraternities, which have sprung up mostly within the past quarter of a century. In the present volume the author furnishes a brief outline of the history of each of the principal of these social and benevolent brotherhoods, beneficiary and fraternal orders, reformatory and religious fraternities, and various other orders and societies. The greater portion of the text consists in celebrated addresses, sermons and excerpts from literature bearing on the subject of the different fraternities. The book will prove helpful to anyone preparing an address along these special lines.

STUDIES IN THE PSYCHOLOGY OF SEX—SEXUAL SELECTION IN MAN. I, Touch; II, Smell; III, Hearing; IV, Vision. By Havelock Ellis. 6⅜x8⅞ inches. Pages XII-270. Extra cloth, $2.00, net. Sold only by subscription to physicians, lawyers and scientists. F. A. Davis Company, publishers, 1914-16 Cherry street, Philadelphia.

The problem of sexual selection as conditioned by sensory stimuli is worked out by the author of the forelying volume in his usual thorough and painstaking way. He has drawn his data from a great number of sources, both ancient and modern, and his personal observations make up an important portion of the text. In the appendix are considered the origins of the kiss tactile and olfactory, and some autobiographic histories of sexual development.

DISEASES OF THE HEART. A Clinical Text-Book for the Use of Students and Practitioners of Medicine. By Edmund Henry Colbeck, B.A., M.D., B.C., F.R.C.P., D.P.H., Physician to Out-Patients at the City of London Hospital for Diseases of the Chest; Physician to the Metropolitan Dispensary. With forty-three illustrations. Second edition, revised and enlarged. Price, $2.00. W. T. Keener & Co., 90 Wabash avenue, Chicago. 1905.

This book is an admirable one for practical clinicians. The author knows his subject at first hand, and presents it with logical clearness from etiology to prognosis. He distinguishes with precision the various factors that enter into the symptomology of cardiac diseases, both organic and functional. His advice as to the treatment of each affection is rational, and is evidently based on a large personal experience.

CONSERVATIVE GYNECOLOGY AND ELECTRO-THERAPEUTICS.—A Practical Treatise on the Diseases of Women and Their Treatment by Electricity. By G. Betton Massey, M. D., Attending Surgeon on the American Oncologic Hospital, Philadelphia; Fellow and Ex-President of the American Electro-Therapeutic Association; Member of the Societe Francaise d'Electro-Therapie, American Medical Association, etc. Fourth edition, revised, rewritten and greatly enlarged. Illustrated with twelve (12) original, full-page chromo-lithographic plates; twelve (12) full page half-tone plates of photographs taken from nature, and 157 half tone and photo-engravings in the text. Pages XVI-468. Royal octavo. Extra cloth, beveled edges. Price, $4.00, net. F. A. Davis

Company, publishers, 1914-16 Cherry street, Philadelphia.

This valuable volume gives the other side of the question as contrasted with the exclusively surgical view of diseases of women. The author is master of his subject, and the successive editions have permitted him to improve the work in many ways and bring it quite up to date. Four new chapters on the treatment of cancer by electrolysis and sterilization have been added to the present edition. While the use and application of electric modalities in the treatment of the pelvic diseases of women form the main portion of the text, several lucid chapters are devoted to the rudiments of medical electricity. The appendix comprises a table of one hundred and ten consecutive cases of fibromata, with details of treatment and ultimate results. The colored plates and other illustrations add much to the value of the book.

PROGRESSIVE MEDICINE, VOL. I, MARCH 1905. A Quarterly Digest of Advances, Discoveries and Improvements in the Medical and Surgical Sciences. Edited by Hobart Amory Hare, M. D., Professor of Therapeutics and Materia Medica in the Jefferson Medical College of Philadelphia. Octavo, 298 pages, 10 engravings and full-page plate. Per annum, in four cloth-bound volumes, $9.00; in paper binding, $6.00; carriage paid to any address. Lea Brothers & Co., publishers, Philadelphia and New York.

The first volume of the present year comprises a resume of the past year's literature on the surgery of the head, neck and thorax; infectious diseases (including acute rheumatism, croupous pneumonia and influenza); diseases of children; larnology and rhinology; and otology. The compilers in order are Charles H. Frazier, Robt. B. Preble, Floyd M. Crandall, Charles P. Grayson and Hobert L. Randolph. The present volume is as valuable as its predecessors to the progressive practitioner of medicine or surgery.

A TEXT-BOOK OF MEDICAL CHEMISTRY AND TOXICOLOGY. By James W. Holland, M.D., Professor of Medical Chemistry and Toxicology, and Dean, Jefferson Medical College, Philadelphia. Octavo volume of 600 pages, fully illustrated, including 8 plates in colors. Philadelphia and London. W. B. Saunders & Co. 1905. Cloth, $3.00, net.

Professor Holland has had thirty-five years of experience as a teacher of chemistry and medicine, so is amply qualified to know what and how to write on the subject of this volume.

The work is quite comprehensive, embracing the newer facts of physiologic chemistry, and is particularly strong on toxicology, water supply and the clinical chemistry of milk, urine and gastric contents. The colored plates of color reactions are among the best we have seen, and certainly the author has spared no pains and the publishers no expense to make the book take place in the front rank of its kind.

AMERICAN EDITION OF NOTHNAGEL'S PRACTICE, DISEASES OF THE BLOOD. Diseases of the Blood (Anemia, Chlorosis, Leukemia, Pseudoleukemia). By Dr. P. Ehrlich, of Frankfort-on-the-Main; Dr. A. Lazarus, of Charlottenburg; Dr. K. von Noorden, of Frankfort-on-the-Main; and Dr. Felix Pinkus, of Berlin. Entire volume edited, with additions, by Alfred Stengel, M. D., Professor of Clinical Medicine, University of Pennsylvania. Octavo volume of 714 pages, fully illustrated. Philadelphia and London: W. B. Saunders & Co. 1905. Cloth, $5.00, net; half morocco, $6.00 net.

This volume on diseases of the blood is the ninth of Nothnagels Practice to be published in English. The subjects considered include anemia, chlorosis, leukemia, chloroma and myeloid leukemia, and each condition is treated with characteristic German fullness and thoroughness. Dr. Alfred Stengel, the editor of the series, is the individual editor of this volume, and he has contributed many valuable additions, particularly to the histology of anemia. The work is handsomely illustrated and a very copious bibliography is appended to each chapter. The publishers anticipate issuing the three remaining volumes of this great enterprise within a short period.

THE EYE, MIND, ENERGY AND MATTER. By Chalmers Prentice, M.D., Chicago. Published by the Author. 1905.

As near as we can gauge Dr. Prentice's literary production, it is a brief for the conjoint use of physical culture, mental dedicine and conservation of energy in the cure even of incurable diseases. He has considerable to say about eye-strain, which he treats largely by the use of prisms, base in for esophoria. Altogether the author emits a number of striking thoughts which are quite at variance with the accepted theories of modern science.

THE OPEN-AIR TREATMENT OF PULMONARY TUBERCULOSIS. By F. W. Burton-Fanning, M.D., Physician to the Norfolk and Norwich Hospital. Price, $1.50. Chicago. W. T. Keener & Co. 1905.

This little volume embodies the personal conclusions derived as to the treatment of pulmonary tuberculosis in the author's experience with the Kelling Sanatorium and the Mundesley Sanatorium, and in private and hospital practice. The author favors simple methods of housing and regime, and emphasizes the fact that the majority of the inmates of a sanatarium require life-long care and assistance if their recoveries are to be maintained. He therefore advocates and explains methods for helping the consumptive working man after leaving the sanatorium. The book has been carefully thought out and clearly written, and should prove of service to all general practitioners.

MALFORMATIONS OF THE GENITAL ORGANS OF WOMAN. By Ch. Debierre, Professor of Anatomy in the Medical Faculty at Lille. With eighty-five illustrations. Translated by J. Henry C. Simes, M.D., Emeritus Professor of Genito-Urinary and Venereal Diseases in the Philadelphia Polyclinic. Price, $1.50. Philadelphia. P. Blakiston's Son & Co., 1012 Walunt street. 1905.

This monograph fills a void in English medical literature. It is both interesting and instructive, as are all well-written accounts of teratologic phenomena. The philosophy of these anatomic perversions is being opened forth as never before.

A HAND-BOOK OF NURSING. Revised Edition for Hospital and General Use. Published under the direction of the Connecticut Training School for Nurses, connected with the General Hospital Society, New Haven, Conn. Philadelphia and London. J. B. Lippincott Company. 1905.

This hand-book has the unique distinction of having been commended in writing by two presidents of Yale College, Porter in 1878 and Woolsey in 1898. It is well arranged, simply set forth and full of the best advice and directions. Family hygiene and the management of emergencies until the doctor comes, are considered at some length. The present revision has been carefully accomplished by the attending staff of the hospital and of the medical college, besides others.

SAUNDERS' QUESTION COMPENDS: ESSENTIALS OF THE PRACTICE OF MEDICINE. Prepared especially for students of medicine. By William R. Williams, M.D., formerly Instructor in Medicine and Lecturer in Hygiene, Cornell University; Tutor in Therapeutics, Columbia University (College of Physicians and Surgeons), New York. 12mo. of 461 pages. Philadelphia and London. W. B. Saunders & Co. 1905. Double number. Cloth, $1.75, net.

In this new volume of the S. Q. C. S. the student is furnished with a book of great practical value. Special stress is laid on characteristic symptoms and differential diagnosis, and the remarks on treatment are worthy of careful study. For the convenience of students, a short list of questions is appended to the discussion of each particular subject.

SAUNDERS' AMERICAN YEAR-BOOK FOR 1905. The American Year-Book of Medicine and Surgery for 1905. A Yearly Digest of Scientific Progress and Authoritative Opinion in all branches of Medicine and Surgery drawn from journals, monographs, and text-books of the leading American and foreign authors and investigators. Arranged, with critical editorial comments, by eminent American specialists, under the editorial charge of George M. Gould, A.M., M.D. In two volumes. Volume I, including Genral Medicine; Volume II, General Surgery. Two octavos of about 700 pages each, fully illustrated. Philadelphia and London. W. B. Saunders & Co. 1905. Per volume: Cloth, $3.00, net; half morocco, $3.75, net.

The 1905 issue of Saunders' American Year Book of Medicine and Surgery fully maintains the high standard of accuracy and utility set by its predecessors. The eminent editor and his large staff of able collaborators have executed their individual labors with the most conscientious thoroughness. They have skimmed the cream of medical and surgical literature for the past year and present it all ready for the doctor's mental digestion. The work is invaluable to every progressive practitioner, who can imagine, though he can hardly appreciate, the great saving of mental effort and tedious research which its possession implies.

LEA'S SERIES OF MEDICAL EPITOMES. Edited by Victor C. Pedersen, M.D.

HOLLIS' EPITOME OF MEDICAL DIAGNOSIS. A Manual for Students and Physicians. By Austin W. Hollis, M.D., Attending Physician to St. Luke's Hospital; to the New York Dispensary, etc. In one 12mo. volume of 319 pages, with 13 illustrations. Cloth, $1.00, net. Lea Brothers & Co., publishers, Philadelphia and New York. 1905.

Accurate diagnosis is the key to genuine success in the practice of internal medicine. This compact little volume has been prepared in accord with the best and latest methods of diagnosis, and should prove of special service to medical students and young practitioners.

THE PRACTICAL MEDICINE SERIES OF YEAR-BOOKS. VOL. 1, GENERAL MEDICINE. Edited by Frank Billings, M.S., M.D. and H. H. Salisbury, M.D. Series of 1905. Price of this volume, $1.00; of series of ten volumes, $5.50. Chicago. The Year-Book Publishers, 40 Dearborn street.

The editorial staff remains the same for the present series as for the one just completed. This review of medicine comprises 374 pages of condensed information on practical subjects with valuable editorial interpolations.

THE PRACTICAL MEDICINE SERIES OF YEAR-BOOKS. VOL 2, GENERAL SURGERY. Edited by John B. Murphy, M.D., Professor of Surgery, Northwestern University Medical School. Series 1905. Price of this volume, $1.50; of series of ten volumes, $5.50. Chicago. The Year-Book Publishers, 40 Dearborn street.

In his resume of progress in surgery, Dr. Murphy goes more extensively into details than most compilers. He quotes fewer authors, but at greater length. The greatest surgical advances during the past year have been related to the stomach, duodenum, pancreas and gall-bladder. These and other noteworthy matters are considered authoritatively in the forelying volume, which is illustrated with 76 drawings.

THE DOCTOR'S WINDOW. Poems by the Doctor, for the Doctor and about the Doctor. Edited by Ina Russelle Warren. With an introduction by Wm. Pepper, M.D., L.L.D. 1904. The Saalfield Publishing Co., Chicago, Akron, O., New York.

This anthology of medical verse was first published in 1897, and is now republished in a more attractive form. About all the striking lubrications of the medical muse, whether humorous or pathetic or quaint and curious, are here set forth. Like the other members of the Doctor's Recreation Series, this one will please and hold the patient in the waiting room.

THE VERMIFORM APPENDIX AND ITS DISEASES. By Howard A. Kelly, A.B., M.D., Professor of Gynecology in the Johns Hopkins University, Baltimore. With 399 original illustrations, some in colors, and three lithographic plates. Price, in cloth, $10.00; sheep or half morocco, $11.00. Philadelphia and London. W. B. Saunders & Co. 1905.

This splendid octavo volume of 827 pages contains the latest and fullest word on the subject of greatest interest to most surgeons —for as Richardson says, appendicitis is the cause of more deaths than any other acute abdominal lesion—and all the diseases of the appendix are considered here. With great care and thoroughness the authors have gleaned through the immense literature of this organ, and so present composite conclusions, exemplified by clinical reports. Kelly's masterly mind has also been reinforced by the direct aid of many of his surgical friends. The work is probably the most sumptuously illustrated medical volume ever published, the drawings having been done by the artists Horn, Becker, Brödel and Mrs. Brödel. The book is one that every surgeon at least should possess.

Report of Three Cases of Intestinal Anastomosis by the Connell Suture. H. H. Sinclair describes three cases in which he performed intestinal anastomosis by the Connell method. The patients all made good recoveries and the author suggests that perhaps the lack of a simple method of doing an intestinal anastomosis has been one of the causes of mortality in strangulated hernia and volvulus.—*Medical Record,* Feb. 4, 1905.

A. M. A. Portland and the Northwest is best reached by the Union Pacific and its connections. The trip is made in less than three days—200 miles of it being along the matchless Columbia river, a great part of the distance the train running so close to the river that one can look from the car window almost directly into the water. The superb equipment and splendid train service of the Union Pacific make the journey one of great pleasure as well as interest. This will be the popular route to the Lewis and Clarke Exposition. Before deciding on your vacation write for full information to any Union Pacific agent, or E. L. Lomax, G. P. & T. A., Omaha, Nebraska.—*Critique.*

SELECTIONS.

CHRONIC ABSCESS.—By L. H. Bewley, M.D., Atlantic City, N. J.—I have in the last few weeks had occasion to use Glyco-Thymoline a number of times as a surgical dressing and found it gave me excellent results.

One case in which I removed quite an area of skin in a chronic abscess case of the neck, I dressed the raw area first with Electrozone but found quite a pus formation on removing the dressing. I then used plain bichlorid solution with the same result, then sterile water, but with no better success, so I thought I would give Glyco-Thymoline a trial and was very much gratified with the result, as there was little or no pus on removing the dressings after twenty-four hours, so continued its use every day and found that the area skinned over and healed very kindly and rapidly.

I hope these few lines may help some other brother physician in such cases. I can't see why it would not be an excellent dressing in ulcers, chronic or acute, and I shall try it in the first case that comes under my care.

DR. PETTEY's RETREATS.—We take pleasure in directing attention to the work of Dr. Geo. E. Pettey, of Memphis, Tenn., who has recently completed the treatment of 800 cases of drug addiction at his Memphis retreat. He has also lately opened a branch of his work in this city and another at Oakland, Cal., each of which is under the care of one of his assistants. These institutions were opened and are being maintained solely for the purpose of treating the alcohol and narcotic drug addictions by methods based upon the original investigations of Dr. Pettey and first published to the profession by him in 1901. (See *Therapeutic, Gazette,* 1901.)

Itis stated upon good authority that the method of treatment introduced by Dr. Pettey removes these addictions from the list of almost incurable diseased and renders them the most certainly and readily curable of all the chronic ailments. In thus extending his work, the doctor is making an organized effort to rescue from the irregulars a class of patients who have been neglected by the profession generally until they have almost ceased to apply to

them for relief. These institutions are conducted upon strictly·
ethical lines and we bespeak for them the most hearty professional support.

TREATMENT OF MENSTRUAL DISORDERS, WITH SPECIAL·
REFERENCE TO CASES IN WOMEN SUFFERING FROM MENTAL
DISEASES.—Geo. S. Walker, M.D., Staunton, Va.—In an institution like the hospital with which I am connected, we naturally
come face to face frequently enough with the question of treating
the amenorrhea that is noted as an accompaniment of mental disease, and for a long time I have been experimenting with various
therapeutic agents recommended for the treatment of menstrual
disorders without obtaining perfect satisfaction from any, until I
tried the method of treatment which I am about to describe.   I
knew that Apiol, the active principle of Apium petroselinum,
Linne (Parsley), was a substance that had been long known to
possess marked emmenagogue properties but that had not been
used extensively in this country on account of certain unpleasant
after-effects connected with its administration.   The question was,
therefore, to obtain such a preparation of Apiol that eliminates
the impurities that do the harmful work of the ordinary preparation.   I selected a series of cases in the hospital, each of which
was characterized by a more or less pronounced menstrual disorder
of some standing, and administered no other medication for the
treatment of the disordered menstruation than Ergo-Apiol.   In
conclusion, I may note the fact that the treatment of amenorrhea
in the insane is always a matter of greater difficulty than in persons with normal minds, and that a remedy that produces perfect
therapeutic results, such as I have noted with Ergo-Apiol (Smith)
in insane women, may be expected to perform the same services
even more promptly in the average case of amenorrhea as met with
in ordinary family practice.   Ergo-Apiol in the shape of capsules
administered three times daily in doses of one of two, beginning
a little before the expected menses, and continuing through the
period, has proven the most efficient, prompt, safe, and pleasant
emmenagogue that I have ever employed.   My experience with
the drug was such as to lead me to adopt it as a routine treatment
in amenorrhea.

PHOSPHO-ALBUMEN AS A NERVE FOOD.—Phospho-Albumen is derived from the testes, spinal cords and brains of bulls. Its chemical constituents are di-oleyl-phosphoric acid, lecithin, spermin and nuclein. Phospho-Albumen renders possible the administration of 85 per cent. more phosphorus (organic) than is possible by any other method; it is absolutely without danger of intoxication or any undesirable after-effect. Gilbert and Lippman (Presse med., quoted by Jour. Amer. Med. Asso., Oct. 1, 1904) have pointed out the constant absence of mineral phosphates from, and the remarkable abundance of phospho-organic compounds in, the soft parts of the organism, and assert that the therapeutic use of mineral phosphates (which are found only in the excreta of the body, and represent the detritus of the organic compounds) is irrational while the organic phosphates, on the other hand, offer a promising field for therapeutic employment. Phospho-Albumen is, by reason of its derivation and chemical nature, the most trustworthy agent for the treatment of functional impotence, sexual atonicity, senile or pre-senile debility, seminal emissions, spermatorrhea, sterility, insomnia, alcoholism, etc., or as an adjuvant to other well-established measures for the treatment of epilepsy, locomotor ataxia, etc. As an aphrodisiac and general nerve tonic, the special formula, No. 33, of the Phospho-Albumen Co., of Chicago, has many advantages. The formula is as follows: Phospho-Albumen, grains 3; strychnine sulphate, grain 1-50th; zinc phosphate, grain 1-10th; gold chloride, grain 1-60th, in tablet form only.

QUININE WITHOUT EBRIETY.—When two such well-known drugs as antikamnia and quinine are offered to the profession it hardly seems necessary to indicate the special classes of affections which call for their use. Antikamnia is unquestionably a perfect substitute for morphine for internal administration. It has complete control over pain, while it is free from the undesirable after-effects of the alkaloid of opium. In cases of malarial fever the combination of antikamnia and quinine should be given as a prophylactic and cure. For all malarial conditions, quinine is the best remedy we have. But, associated with this condition, there is always more or less pain, and antikamnia will remove these unpleasant symptoms and place the system in the best condition for the quinine to do its work. There are a number of ailments, not closely defined, which are due to the presence of malarial poison. All such conditions are greatly benefited by the use of "Antikamnia and Quinine Tablets," each tablet containing 2½ gr. antikamnia and 2½ gr. sulph. quinine. The antikamnia in these tablets not only relieves the pain, but prevents the ebriety or ringing sensation produced when quinine is administered alone. In headache (hemicrania), in the neuralgias occurring in anaemic patients who have malarial cachexia, and in a large number of affections more or less dependent upon this cachectic condition, the regular administration of these tablets is indicated.—*Medical and Surgical News.*

That Acetozone is a valuable germicide is demonstrated by its effects upon typhoid bacilli and cholera vibrios in river water. In their experimental work Freer and Novy (Contributions to Medical Research, p. 107) made the following tests:

(a) A cylindrical glass-wool filter was prepared, and on it was placed a layer of Acetozone crystals, about 3 cm. thick. A bouillon suspension of typhoid bacilli *passed once through the filter yielded a sterile filtrate,* while control tubes gave the usual abundant growth.

(b) A liter of tap-water was sterilized by heat and, when cool, a suspension of cholera or typhoid germs was added, the experiment being repeated several times. Ten to twenty miligrams (1/6 to 1/3 grain) of Acetozone was added and, after thorough shaking, portions of the liquid were taken out and planted in bouillon and agar which was plated. In each instance the cholera germs were destroyed completely in five minutes, and the typhoid germs in fifteen minutes by the extremely small quantity of Acetozone used. It should be observed that the addition of 10 mg. of Acetozone to 1 liter of water represents a solution of 1 part to 100,000. Controls gave abundant growths, the plates yielding 600,000 to 800,000 colonies.

From the above experiments the authors draw the conclusion that pathogenic organisms are destroyed by extremely small amounts of Acetozone. They also suggest the practicability of this agent for the purification of contaminated waters, especially in connection with military operations. From other experiments rt was found that even sewage can be rendered almost sterile by the addition of relatively small amounts of Acetozone.

Therapeutically Acetozone is being very widely used in the treatment of typhoid fever, intestinal diseases, notably summer diarrheas in children, in gonorrhea, suppurating wounds and infectious processes generally. It is prescribed in the saturated aqueous solution which is prepared by adding 15 grains of Acetozone to a quart of water, shaking thoroughly and setting aside for a couple of hours to hydrolize. Messrs. Parke, Davis & Co., who prepare Acetozone, are sending out printed matter to physicians containing reports of very gratifying results from the use of this interesting compound. Any physician who has not received a brochure can obtain one on request.

PAUTABERGE'S SOLUTION.—The efficacy of the two principal constituents of Pautaberge's solution is a notable fact. The physiological action of hydrochloro-phosphate of lime is well known; it is to be preferred to the glycero-phosphate not only because it aids digestion but also on account of its invarying composition and stability in all climates. As for creosote, which is used in so many different ways and in various forms more or less efficacious, there is no doubt of its usefulness in bronch-pulmonary affections. As so many preparations which have not been tested are now being offered to the profession, we wish to declare that we use a creosote extracted from the pure beech-wood tar, concerning which Drs. Bouchard and Gimbert, after conclusive clinical tests, were able to make the following statement: "It gave good results in all cases of the first degree, in less than half of the second and in one-third of the cases of the third; it failed in two-thirds of the cases of the third degree, in less than half of the second, and in none of the first." The combination of hydrochloro-phosphate of lime with creosote facilitates the administration of the latter drug and increases its efficiency. The form if solution that we have adopted, which is capable of being greatly diluted, not only does not interfere with digestion but even improves it; now increased appetite is the earliest signs of improvement.

EDITORIAL ITEMS.— Continued.

Reflex Vomiting. This type of emesis is often apparently causeless, with prominent symptoms referable to other organs. The tongue is usually clear. By way of general remedies may be mentioned bromides and chloral; cerium oxalate; quinine, acids and minute doses of ipecac. For persistent cases Wm. F. Mitchell recommends the application to the epigastrium of ice-cold compresses changed every minute. For such obstinate cases Thornton employs a mustard-poultice over the abdomen, and gives a rectal injection of twenty grains of chloral hydrate and one drachm of potassium bromide in starch water. In hepatic attacks it is well to wash out the stomach freely with warm water.

For Post-Celiotomy Vomiting. Howard Kelly advises absolute rest for stomach, rectal alimentation; lime water in small quantities, or a few drops of spirit of chloroform at frequent intervals; a two per cent. solution of cocaine in ten to twenty minim doses; bismuth subnitrate, or morphine in small doses; iced champagne, two or three teaspoonfuls at a time; tincture of capsicum, two or three drops in a drachm of hot water; thorough evacuation of the bowels; lavage of stomach with weak boric acid solution in intractable cases; hot-water bag, ice bag or weak mustard plaster on epigastrium.

Intestinal Atony Without Indigestion. W. W. Johnston advises long vacation and travel; walking and riding; cold bathing or sponging with friction of whole body; warm baths and cold douches to abdomen; compresses of cold water to abdomen; compresses of cold water or of alcohol; cold douche to spine while in hot bath; massage for women, children and feeble persons; faradization with insulated cathode in rectum and anode moved along course of colon; Swedish movement course; easily digested diet with large amount of waste. Teach bowels to act at stated hours, using for this purpose a small enema of cool or cold water at same hour every day after breakfast. Administer a number of drugs in succession, rather than increasing dose of any one.

Abdominal Massage for Constipation. Brandt's method is as follows: The masseur stands on left side of recumbent patient

and places finger-tips of both hands (in opposite directions) over sigmoid flexure, forcing its contents into lower rectum by pressure and semi-circular stroking movements. Next place bands side by side, pointing upward, and go over whole colon from sigmoid upward, with deep downward pressure; next circular kneading with both hands, avoiding umbilical region. Both hands are now pressed deeply into lower abdomen, and entire contents are pressed up and gently shaken. In obstinate cases massage should be performed, patient standing, of both costoiliac spaces with the palms, and kneading of the colon from cecum toward sigmoid.

Constipation in Pregnant Women. Manna (one-half to one ounce) and compound licorice powder (a teaspoonful at bedtime) are useful remedies. Munde recommends a regular hour for going to closet; oatmeal wheaten grits, brown or graham bread, fruits, stewed prunes, figs or dates with a glass of water before going to bed and on rising. If those measures are not sufficient, use saline laxatives, compound licorice powder or cascara sagrada. In the later months it may be necessary to employ daily enemata or, in case of fecal impaction, mechanical means.

Cold Storage and Food Poisoning. Dr. Cavana, of Oneida, New York, contributes a timely article on exogenic toxicosis to the February number of the *International Journal of Surgery.* He claims that of 8,000 deaths yearly in New York state from diarrheal disorders, a large majority are due to food toxicosis, and of these eighty per cent. are from the consumption of poultry which has been kept in the undrawn state in cold storage for as long as two years. In order to bring up the weight and plumpness of the mummified fowls, it is the custom with the wholesale dealers to immerse them in fresh water just before shipment to their various patrons, thus rendering the distribution of ptomaines as complete as possible.

Hypertension. Under the title, "Early Recognition of Hypertension" (*American Medicine,* Jan. 14) Henry W. Cook calls attention to the growing importance relatively of cardiovascular factors in disease and death. The normal range of blood pressure is from 80 to 130 or 140 mm. of mercury. In chronic hypertension, with or without other signs and symptoms, it is important to

In all cases where the continued use of cod liver oil is necessary throughout the year, Scott's Emulsion will be found of greater service and of more direct benefit than any other form of cod liver oil. It guards the patient against the disorders that most cod liver oil preparations cause in weakened systems, especially during the summer months. The passage of Scott's Emulsion through the stomach and into the blood is so rapid that no tax is imposed upon any part of the system.

SCOTT & BOWNE, Chemists, 409 Pearl St., New York.

employ hygienic measures that correct overeating, gout, gastro-intestinal disease, toxemia, overwork, worry and anxiety. When such means fail, sodium nitrite is the most valuable remedy. Two to five drops of a saturated solution, may cause a drop in arterial tension of 30 mm. in 10 to 20 minutes, which may last several hours. Following the case with frequent sphygmomanometric observations, the blood pressure should be kept at the level which is most suitable for the individual.

Treatment of Hiccough. Try gargling with water, or excite sneezing, or give a hot infusion of capsicum, a teaspoonful of compound spirit of ether in cold water, or amyl nitrite inhalations. Christmas recommends two minims of nitro-glycerin solution in a drachm of chloroform and an ounce of water every hour. For typical singultus Thornton orders ten grains of musk by the mouth or in starch water per rectum. A few drops of beechwood creosote may be useful in the hiccough of drunkenness. For uremic hiccough Thornton recommends pilocarpine hydrochlorate, 1/6 to ¼ grain hypodermically in conjunction with the hot pack. Floyd M. Crandall states that hiccough in infants is often relieved promptly by putting a few grains of sugar into the baby's mouth.

For the Gastric Symptoms of Hepatic Cirhosis. Taylor mentions effervescing salines, bismuth and bitter tonics; a light, easily digested diet; no alcohol. Bruce directs a diet of milk, diluted essence of beef, eggs, farinaceous material, uncooked oysters, tripe, fish and game. If vomiting is urgent, he has the patient take at first only sips of hot water or small pieces of ice; later, milk (with soda or lime water) or koumiss in small quantities at short intervals. When intractable, champagne or brandy and soda must be given for a day or so. Calomel, four grains, and sugar of milk, two grains, may be given at night, followed by an effervescing saline aperient after six hours. Other remedies are bismuth subnitrate, gr. xx in one ounce of milk every three hours; dilute hydrocyanic acid, m. iii, tinct. cardamom. comp. m. xxx, spt. ammonii aromat. m. x, aquae chloroformi ℥ iv, aquam dest. ad ℥ i—avery three hours.

Vomiting of Pregnancy. E. P. Davis considers mild and prolonged epigastric counter-irritation the most useful single remedial measure. He also advises the removal of all pressure from the abdomen; avoidance of constipation; the free use of Apollinaris, Vichy or plain soda water for accompanying pyrosis; lavage of the bowels with physiologic salt solution, and use of stomach tube for mucous catarrh; sponging skin with hot water and soap or alcohol, followed by inunction with a mixture of two parts of olive oil and one part of alcohol; calomel and water for liver and kidneys. He directs to replace the uterus (under anesthesia, if congested), keeping it in place with sterile lint soaked in glycerin, to which tincture of belladonna may be added. Dilate the os uteri under anesthesia with finger or bougie or bladed dilator, if replacement fails. All these means failing to check hyperemesis, the uterus should be emptied at once.

Phthisical Vomiting. Matthieu directs to swallow small lumps of ice after eating. Knopf instructs to keep absolutely quiet after eating, and control approaching attacks of coughing. In the early stages Stevens has found small doses of calomel and soda useful for nausea. Oxygenated water may be of some service. Berthier applies to the fauces a two per cent solution of cocaine on lint or cotton-wool, twice daily just before expected attack, and Ferrand uses similarly a ten per cent. solution of potassium bromide in glycerine. Bruce gives bismuth subnitrate, twenty grains in a little milk or water t. i. d. three hours after meals. He has the patient gargle with a fresh effervescing soda water, and applies Spanish fly blister (1½ by 1½ inches) to the epigastrium.

Diet and Constipation. Foods containing little liquid or leaving little residue (starch, cereals, cheese, milk) or lacking in water are most liable to lead to constipation. A pint of fresh buttermilk daily is a reliable laxative. Ringer recommends one or two oranges before breakfast, or a glass of cold water before or soon after breakfast. Osler advises a light diet with plenty of fruit and vegetables, particularly salads and tomatoes, oatmeal and brown bread; a tumblerful of cold water taken slowly on rising, or a glass of hot water at night. For infants Jewett prescribes four to six per cent. of cream in their food; also sodium phosphate and sugar of milk, ten grains each at one dose in a little water.

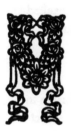

For nurslings we should secure more fat in the mother's milk, by means of a diet of fresh meat, vegetables and freshly cooked fruit, regular exercise and restriction of tea-drinking. Jacobi directs to give a lump of loaf sugar, dissolved in tepid water and given immediately before nursing, when the mother's milk is white and dense, containing a large amount of casein.

For Asthmatic Attacks. Apomorphine hypodermically in emetic dose is about the surest means of cutting short an attack. Paraldehyde (45 to 60 grains in simple elixir—giving another half dram in an hour or two if the first dose fails) may prove of service. Riegel asserts that a hypodermic injection of 1/120 to 1/60 grain of atropine during the attack is usually extremely prompt and gratifying. Boyland recommends terpin hydrate, two grains every fifteen minutes during the attack until ten grains are taken. Butler states that fluid extract of grindelia robusta is useful during paroxysms. The compound spirit of ether, a dram in cold water every 15 to 30 minutes, is an old and standard remedy. To cut short an attack Mays says: Break a perle of amyl nitrite into a handkerchief and inhale; or give two drops of one per cent. nitroglycerine in a dram of water, or a hypodermic of 1/20 grain each of strychnine and morphine. S. Solis-Cohen prescribes: R Morph. sulph. gr. ⅛ - ¼; strych. sulph. gr. 1/60 - 1/40; hyoscin. hydrobrom gr. 1/200: Give hypodermically at bed-time.

Dietetic Treatment of Constipation. Boas recommends foods that leave residue (bran, graham, rye and black breads, cabbage, turnips, carrots, asparagus, sauer kraut, spinach, salads, noodles, macaroni, farinaceae, potatoes, lentils, peas, fresh haricot beans); foods which produce marked transudation into intestines (stewed prunes, apples, aloes, plums, apricots, oranges); oils and fats; a large glass of water taken early in morning; cider, white wine, kephir; buttermilk, beaten milk, whey between meals or early in morning; honey, honey-cakes, spiced breads with honey or syrup; sugar of milk, two or three teaspoonfuls in a cup of milk early in morning, or a tablespoonful three or four times a day in milk or coffee. He forbids tea, red wines, fancy breads, biscuits, cakes, fillet of beef, rice, cocoa and also excess of meat, bread and potatoes.

Constipation of Infants. Goodhart and Starr advise adding oatmeal or more cream to the food; glycerine enemas (one-half dram to two drams of water at six months); massage along colon; regular habits and exercise of older children. They prescribe: ℞ Mannae out., magnes. carb. aa. gr. iiss.; ext. sennæ fl. m. viis.; syr. zingib. m. xx; aquam q.s.: A dessertspoonful once to three times daily for a child of two years.

Phthisical Emphysema. Knopf directs to use the pneumatic cabinet, inhaling outside air and exhaling into the rarefied atmosphere of cabinet; also respiratory exercises, prolonging expiratory effort and making pressure with palms of hands over chest during inspiration and expiration. Take moderate walks but avoid overexertion. Refrain from fermentative vegetables and over-eating, taking small, frequent meals and avoiding too much liquid.

Emphysema. Potter recommends terebene in chronic emphysema. H. C. Wood states that the grindelia is of great service when there is accompanying cough. Brunton gives a single large dose of chloral in the sudden, acute form ;small doses for long-continued dsypnea. For asthmatic cases Shoemaker prescribes: ℞ Tinct. euphorb. piluli. one part; ext. quebracho fl. seven parts: One-half to two teaspoonfuls in water every three or four hours.

Chronic Constipation of Infants and Children. J. Henry Fruitnight directs to correct diet or mother's milk; give a litttle molasses or melted sugar and butter, or sweet oil in teaspoonful doses; more water or oatmeal water if motions are dry and brittle; glycerine suppositories, well oiled and pushed up well into the internal sphincter; glycerine injections, 10-20 drops to 2 drams of water, or cold water injections (one or two drams for infants) containing a little table salt, t. i. d. at first, then twice and finally once daily; sodium phosphate (2 grains t. i. d. for a child under one year) in syrup of manna and anise water. Train older children to regular habits of evacuation; take most fruits and milk freely, but restrict farinaceous foods. Give pepsin with muriatic acid and cascara or taraxacum when indigestion complicates. When there is interference with the hepatic functions give podophyllum resin, 1/24 - 1/12 grain every morning, dissolved in alcohol and administered in syrup of raspberry. Employ gentle massage of the abdomen (especially of left side) for a few minutes two or three times a day, preferably before nursing or feeding— move the finger tips about with the skin over the intestines without rubbing.

DENVER MEDICAL TIMES

Volume XXIV.   JUNE, 1905   Number 12

PSAMMOMA OF THE MAXILLARY SINUS, WITH REPORT OF A CASE.*

By JOHN C. MUNRO, M.D.

Boston, Mass.

The formation of sand bodies may take place frequently in various portions of the central nervous system, such as the inner surface of the dura, the arachnoid, the pineal body, etc., without going on to the formation of a definite tumor. Virchow limits the term psammoma to tumors located in the central nervous system and its coverings, although the same type of sand bodies may be found in tumors of various sorts, such as fibroma, sarcoma, papilloma, carcinoma, etc. Ziegler describes the psammoma as "sarcoma or fibrosarcoma of the dura, inner meninges or pineal gland, which contains concretions of lime in greater or less abundance. Some of these concretions are similar in structure to the normal brain sand, the basis of their formation being a concentric mass of cells which have undergone hyaline degeneration. They usually form round nodules and may be of multiple occurrence." When, however, the sand bodies are found in tumors, the type of the latter must be determined partly from the sand bodies but essentially according to the constituent type of tissue (Virchow). Consonant with Virchow's theory of the origin of tumors he ascribes them to irritation or chronic inflammation. He has separated, moreover, from his great class of sarcomata this form of tumor under the name of psammoma, as it belongs, with respect to its histological construction in general, to the connective tissue type of growth (Steudener). Biegel has limited the term psammoma only to tumors in which there is slow growth with scarcely any tendency to multiply, and standing between the fibromata and the solid spindle-cell sarcomata, a sharp line of differentiation, however, being difficult of demonstration. In the carcinomata, including as well endotheliomata, we may infrequently find deposits of

*Read before the Rocky Mountain Inter-State Medical Association, Sept., 1904.

lime salts, mainly as concretion-like masses, just as we find them in psammoma. "These concretions may form either from the cells or in the connective tissue. They occur particularly in the papillary adenomata of the ovary and in cancer of the mammary glands." (Ziegler). The psammo-carcinomata, furthermore, form metastases of a type corresponding to that of the original growth, so that the secondary growths are found in organs of most varying types— in short, where a carcinoma may grow a psammo-carcinoma may also be found (Marben). The majority of these psammomata have been described as originating in the ovary, with metastases involving practically any of the intra-abdominal organs, but in addition to these there are a few psammo-carcinomata reported as primary in the liver, bones, skin, etc. (Marben). The case reported today apparently belongs to a similar type as found in the central nervous system and occasionally in distant organs such as the submaxillary glands, etc. As a careful examination of the literature has failed to unearth an analogous case, it has been deemed worth while to place this one on record.

Delia C., about twenty years old, servant girl, first consulted Dr. Allen Greenwood, who has kindly given me the following history: "Delia C. called at my office in December, 1902. Seven years prior to this she noticed that the left eye was a little more prominent than the right. Year by year this had become more marked, until at the time of her visit it had become so prominent that it was a source of annoyance on account of the resulting disfigurement. At no time had there been any pain and the vision of the eye had not been interfered with. She had never noticed diplopia.

Examination showed the following condition. The left eye was markedly proposed so that the lids could be closed with difficulty. The apex of the cornea was on a plane 2 cm. anterior to that of the other eye. The eye could be moved freely in all directions but the extent of motion was limited about 50 degrees less than normal, so that a diplopia could be produced by directing the vision as far from the line of central fixation as possible in any direction. The fundus was normal and the V.=20/20. The eye could not be pushed directly backward but could be pushed a little upward and backward. Palpation revealed a smooth rounded

mass in the lower part of the orbit beginning at the infra-orbital
ridge and running upward and backward as far as the eye would
allow the finger to go. How much farther it extended could not
be ascertained with the finger but it appeared from the feeling
that the bulk of the mass was back of the equator of the globe.
There was a sulcus between the mass and the ridge of the orbital
floor which admitted the finger nail, showing that while the mass
might be connected with the infra-orbital plate the ridge was not
involved. Laterally the mass could be felt to extend out to the
side walls of the orbit at the level of the canthi.

The slow development of the growth would count against its
being malignant and delay was advised as I thought it might be
an exostosis arising from the infra-orbital plate.

I saw her again in May of 1903 when it appeared that the
proptosis had slightly increased and I advised an exploratory
Krönlein's operation; sending her to Dr. J. C. Munro for that
purpose."

When the patient came to me in May 1903, I found the condition as described by Dr. Greenwood and advised operation, sup-
posing that we should find an intra-orbital bony growth. Under
ether a modified Krönlein's operation for exposing the orbit was
carried out. A curved incision at right angles to the line of the
external canthus was made and the outer wall of the orbit was
chiselled out in the form of a spherical triangle without stripping
the periosteum. The edges of the bone were bevelled so that when
replaced the fragment rested in practically normal position. The
bony, together with the undisturbed soft tissues overlying it, was
turned backward on a hinge of periosteum, skin, etc. A slightly
fluctuating tumor was found lying behind, below and to the outer
side of the globe; on chiselling the outer edges of the wall, which
proved to be soft bone of the thickness of blotting paper, a large
cyst-like tumor was encountered, full of reddish granular material,
feeling like a mixture of sand and putty. This was curetted out
in large quantity and lay for the most part below and behind the
globe, evidently having pushed upwards from the antrum, the bony
plate felt behind the orbital ridge before operation proving to be
the orbital floor forced upward like a trap-door by the invading
growth. A further opening was then made through the mouth into

the antrum. At first about a drachm of puriform mucus escaped, but above this, filling the antrum, was the same gritty material that had been found in the orbit. This was thoroughly curetted out, the inner surface of the walls feeling rough but not nodular. There was considerable venous oozing while the curetting was going on, but it was easily controlled by packing. The orbital floor was then pushed back into place and the antrum packed with iodoform gauze. In replacing the bone flap of the orbit the deep fascia was sutured with cat-gut and the skin closed with buried silk-worm gut. No shock followed the operation.

For some time following the operation there was marked edema and ecchymosis of the lids and conjunctiva as well as ecchymosis of the lids of the right eye. Some relief to the edema followed removal of the packing, and under irrigation and iced cloths no injury to the coma followed. Convalescence was not as satisfactory as had been anticipated. The pulse and temperature kept steadily above normal and in spite of persistent irrigation a foul discharge kept up and the exophthalmos did not subside satisfactorily. The patient had a poor appetitie and was in bed most of the time. The temporal wound healed per primam and left no deformity. The patient finally consented to a second operation with a view to removal of the upper jaw if necessary, as it did not seem unlikely that the growth was becoming malignant if it had not been so from the first.

Two months after the first operation the patient was again etherized, the left common carotid clamped with a Crile clamp, and the opening in the antrum enlarged for exploration. The latter, however, was found free of growth. As on examination with the finger fullness posterior to the upper jaw was found, an incision was made along the side of the nose and through the upper lid in order to turn the cheek back. The anterior wall of the upper jaw was removed up to the infra-orbital foramen. A hard tumor could be felt in the roof of the pharynx pushing the mucous membrane downwards, apparently having taken its origin from the antrum. This tumor proved to be psammomatous, exactly similar to that found at the first operation. On removing the pharyngeal portion more growth was found, so far as could be determined in the sphenoidal and ethmoidal cells of both sides and surrounding the left lateral wall of the nasal cavity, which was removed.

The vomer had been pushed far to the right but was not involved in the growth. The tumor lay also on the upper surface of the palate, but the latter itself appeared normal and did not require to be removed. Above, the growth extended to but did not involve the frontal sinuses. So far as could be told all of the tumor was removed. Exploration into the cavity of the orbit showed no sign of recurrence in any region. The resulting extensive cavity was packed with gauze and the wound closed with silk-worm gut and horsehair. Very little bleeding followed removal of the carotid compression and there was only a moderate degree of shock at the close of the operation.

The patient rapidly convalesced and was discharged in good condition at the end of a few weeks.

Examination of the growth removed at the first operation was made by Dr. J. H. Pratt and is as follows: "Tumor of orbit and antrum of Highmore.

MICROSCOPIC EXAMINATION.—The specimen consists of a mass about 15 c.c. in bulk. In appearance it does not look unlike fine sand soaked in blood. When a small portion of this substance was placed in a test tube and hydrochloric acid added, there was some effervescence, but the granules did not entirely dissolve. These sand-like particles were readily separated from one another.

MICROSCOPIC EXAMINATION.—Some of the material was decalcified in sulphuric acid and embedded in celloidine. It was found that the calcareous bodies were separated by tissue consisting of very closely-packed, long, spindle-cells with little or no intracellular fibrillar substance. The nodules varied in shape, averaging 50 to 70 mm. in size, and some had more or less concentric structure. They were in such close contact that the areas of tissue between them were very narrow.

DIAGNOSIS.—Psammoma of peculiar type, which possibly should be classed as a sarcoma."

Before the first operation there was no suspicion of any growth involving the respiratory tract, and no examination was made of the throat as everything pointed to a localized orbital lesion. After operation, however, although it was supposed that all the growth was removed, a poor general condition seemed to indicate that the tumor might be a malignant one, as examination of the throat did not suggest anything so extensive as was found at the second operation. Later, when operation was urged, consent was not obtained until it was apparent that something more radical must be undertaken. As to the origin taking place definitely in the maxillary sinus rather than in one of the deeper sinuses, an accurate determination could not be made. The invasion into the orbit must have been from below and must have dated back for seven or more years. The position and condition of the orbital floor seems to establish that definitely. The absence of nasal or throat symptoms would point to a slow-growing tumor of the max-illary sinus, gradually filling the cavity and pushing the lateral wall of the nose inward, invading the sinuses of the ethmoid and sphenoid latterly and possibly rapidly at the time of operation or thereabouts. Had the growth started originally in the ethmoid or sphenoid it hardly seems possible that it could have filled the antrum, and thence the orbit, without causing more nasal and throat symptoms. Origin from the dura was considered, but there were no indications of a basal fissure or other structural deformity.

The prognosis was doubtful, but, considering the cellular structure of the tumor, it seemed very possible that recurrence might take place at some time, even though the original course of the disease had been very slow.

Examination of the patient September 1, 1904, showed a temporal and facial scar barely visible except for a slight notch at the mucous border of the lip. The anterior wall of the upper jaw had reformed so that this part of the face was normal. Both nares were free and the septum was nearly back into its normal position. The sulcus between the alveolus and the cheek was fairly healed without any sinus. There was a slight varicosity of the lower lid and along the infra-orbital ridge could be felt a slight irregularity and thickening. Just above the inner cauthus a small bony prominence could be felt but not seen.

There was no paralysis of the palate. The voice sounds had only a faint trace of the hollow character that follows removal of the upper jaw.

The tears flowed normally through the duct instead of over the cheek as was the case before operation.

The eye was still prominent and turned outwards, but the globe was normally covered by the lids on closure. The globe could not be turned inwards beyond the median line. The sight was apparently normal though the right eye was commonly made use of.

The patient had been entirely relieved. of the headache that harassed her before operation and she had been at work steadily for some months, and gaining in weight. During the winter she felt the cold very much in the left side of the face.

There was no evidence of return of the growth, but the result in restoration of the globe to its normal position was a disappointment.

DISCUSSION OF DR. MUNRO'S PAPER.

DR. MOLEEN. This subject is something like an original research, so few cases of psammoma have been reported. I frankly admit the first time I saw the term and its meaning, I took it to be an outgrowth of the pituitary body. I was very much interested in the doctor's paper, in that he could not associate it with an outgrowth of this kind.

A great many inflammatory conditions of the glabellar, and more especially the sphenoidal sinus, are being found in post mortems. Rupture from them into the lateral sinus is being found very frequently. Why association between the mastoid cells and these bony sinuses should be the case is hard to understand, though oftimes there have been found inflammatory conditions of the sinuses associated with those of the mastoid cells. Such a tumor, whether it be sarcomatous, or deserving of the distinctive name of psammoma, or whether it be osteosarcomatous, or what not, we have fair reason to assume that it may result from inflammatory conditions in the lining periosteum of these sinuses. That may, however, remain for future cases to decide.

I have listened to this paper with a great deal of interest, though I should have expected some more ocular symptoms, but I could not hear the details very well from where I sat; I could not hear whether there were ocular symptoms. I understood this would break sometimes and extend to the membranes of the brain and give rise to meningitis, but in this case it was a case of tumor, as I understood it, and quite a rare case, to which I listened with considerable interest.

DR. POWERS. Some years ago I happened to drop in at a meeting of the New York Academy of Medicine. A subject new to me was being discussed, and there was a moderate amount of discussion following. I happened to have a seat next to a venerable medical friend, and during the discussion the doctor nudged me and said: "Get up and say something." I said I did not know anything about the subject. He said: "You don't have to know anything about the subject."

Now as I do not know anything about this subject, Mr. President, there is not much that I can say. Although I am not a member of this Association, I would like very much to express my sense of personal obligation to Dr. Munro for making such a long journey across the continent and giving us such a very excellent and valuable paper.

RHEUMATOID PAINS FOLLOWING INJURIES IN HIGH ALTITUDES.*

By MAJOR CHARLES F. KIEFFER
Surgeon U. S. Army.   Fort D. A. Russell, Wyo.

Rheumatism is so commonly associated in our minds with the low levels and damp atmosphere of the seaboard that we lose sight of its very great prevalence in our own regions. As a matter of fact, it is equally if not more prevalent in high, dry altitudes. Just why this should be so is not apparent, unless it be that the climatic conditions favor the spread of a virulent follicular tonsilitis, which must be considered as a very common precursor of acute articular rheumatism. Since Fort Russell was established as a military post in 1867, in 26,578 admissions for sickness there have been 1263 cases of acute articular rheumatism; amounting to 4.75% of all cases. In McCrae's review of the cases of acute rheumatism admitted to Johns Hopkins Hospital it is stated that the admissions for this disease amounted to 2% of all cases. In the report of the Montreal General Hospital the proportion is given as 3.8% and the figures from London range from 3.5 to 7%. The Montreal figures are considered very high for America and yet the

*Read before the Denver Academy of Medicine, April, 1906.

statistics I have just quoted from Fort Russell considerably exceed them. The altitude of Fort Russell is 6,195 feet.

I desire in this paper to call attention to a class of cases which I believe to be an expression of the increased rheumatic tendency seen in high altitudes. I refer to the very frequent development of severe rheumatoid pains after injuries of the most varied nature. These pains are sometimes very severe and harassing and may be out of all proportion to the severity of the original injury. They frequently are rebellious to treatment and may tax our therapeutic resources to the utmost. These post-traumatic pains are by no means to be confounded with the immediate painful reaction of joint, muscle or aponeurotic structure to the injury done them. They are on the contrary, markedly rheumatic in character, follow the injury at some considerable interval of time and have a distinct period of incubation.

It is very common indeed to observe in from two weeks to two months following, let us say, a Pott's fracture, a dislocation of the shoulder or a sprain of the ankle joint, that the patient develops a severe, crippling pain in the injured part and perhaps, in addition, in the articulations or muscles in its immediate vicinity. I have observed the condition in dislocations; it very frequently follows fractures and sprains; but it is most commonly observed after muscular contusions and in injuries involving severe stretching or even laceration of aponeurotic structures. A large proportion of our cases of lumbago may be traced to a direct contusion of the lumbar muscles or to a stretching of the muscles or the fibres of the lumbar fasciae received in falls or following violent muscular efforts. The pain also occurs in all sorts of scar tissue and is not infrequently seen in the scar of an abdominal incision .

The following may be related as a rather typical instance of of the condition under discussion. A woman, twenty-five years old, alighting from a carriage, stepped on a small stone and "turned her ankle." The sprain was not severe and thorough examination showed no tearing of the lateral ligaments. The immediate reaction to the injury was slight. There was moderate swelling of the peri-articular structures and some pain; all of which subsided in four or five days and the patient considered herself well. Twenty-three days after the injury, the joint became very painful with some local heat and swelling. The condition of the joint was now as the patient herself said, and as was apparent, much more painful and much worse than after the original injury. Seven days of active specific rheumatic treatment dissipated the symptoms. Most of the cases are not so pronounced as this. The pain is not so sharp but is rather dull and dragging and the evidences of local heat and swelling are less conspicuous. On the other hand some joints are seen in which the arthritis is of the most acute type.

I have records of thirty cases in which sharp rheumatoid pains with obvious objective symptoms, followed various injuries. Of these eleven were sprains; three of the knee, three of the ankle, two of the muscles of the back and one each of the wrist, elbow and shoulder. There were also eleven contusions; four of the muscles of the back, two of the thigh, two of the knee and one each of the hand, shoulder and foot. There were three cases of Pott's fracture, two cases of fracture of the forearm, one fracture of the thigh and two dislocations of the shoulder. The shortest time in which the symptoms appeared after the injury was five days, in one case, and the longest, seventy-three days. The average period of incubation in the thirty cases was twenty-four days.

In some cases, but not many, this painful condition arises in very old injuries. These cases occur in persons newly come to high altitudes, who are astonished to find a weary, harassing pain in an old fracture or in a joint which has frequently been sprained. The proximity of an attack of follicular tonsilitis to the time of injury increases the liability to the development of post traumatic rheumatism, even though an attack of acute articular rheumatism does not follow the angina.

It has already been said that these cases may prove very rebellious to treatment. Practically, they yield only to active antirheumatic treatment. And this I believe is a valuable corroborative point of their rheumatic nature. It cannot be held that the salicylates are specific anti-rheumatics; at the same time it cannot be denied that when prompt dispersal or abatement of arthritic or muscular pains follows their use, it is excellent diagnostic evidence of the purely rheumatic character of the affection. In these cases it will be found that the pain disappears with systematic salicylate saturation. For this purpose the sodium salt is probably the most generally useful. Yet in mild cases it would seem un-necessary to subject the patient to the very unpleasant by-effects attending large doses of the salicylates. The toxic manifestations are very readily produced in some persons and in these recourse must be had to some other salicylic compounds. When the pain is severe and the general aspect of the case is acute there is no better substitute for the salicylate of soda than Aspirin in doses of 15-20 grains every three or four hours. The advantages this drug possesses over the salicylate of soda are several. It is taste-less; it does not disturb the stomach and it does not produce the annoying head noises unless given in very much larger doses than those here indicated. In very large doses it will produce symptoms of salicylic intoxication and may act as a cardiac depressant. Its administration therefore requires some care and watching in en-feebled cardiac states. For the milder, muscular cases, salol and salophen are excellent remedies, but they cannot be depended on in the more acute types.

With respect to local treatment an important question comes up. Shall the joint or limb be immobilized or not? Whenever possible the part should be put at rest. Soothing lotions may be applied. In cases following fracture the symptoms may appear at the time when passive motion is necessary to restore function. These should also be put at rest. Because, in this way, with proper treatment, the acute condition will pass away in a very few days and the time will not be long enough, in any event, to jeopardize the restoration of function by prolonged immobilization.

Heat is especially grateful to these lesions, particularly in the form of dry, superheated air. The old-fashioned plan of ironing out a pain in the back is effective and has much to commend it.

When the pain is in the lumbar muscles, in selected cases, there is no remedy so good as acupuncture. For this purpose the punctures should be made in several places with a rather coarse needle. The needle should be thrust laterally into the lumbar mass and should penetrate deeply, say three or four inches. The relief which follows this procedure is very great.

In four cases of the series here reported, I had very excellent results from the use of the new local anti-rheumatic mesotan.

Mesotan is the methyl-oxy-methyl ester of salicylic acid. It is an oily liquid and is applied directly to the painful part; one-half to one or two drachms being used at a sitting, depending on the size of the painful area. This drug is rapidly absorbed through the skin and appears in the urine as salicylic acid in from one-half to one hour. It has not only a general action but also a local action probably on the sensory nerve ends in the diseased area, and therefore is especially valuable in these cases.

CONGENITAL ULCER OF STOMACH, WITH REPORT OF A CASE.

By J. N. HALL, M.D. and THOS. H. HAWKINS, M.D.
Denver, Colo.

While the diagnosis in this case is only a presumptive one, since the baby has recovered and we had no opportunity for an anatomical demonstration of the ulcer, it will be considered, we think, that there is sufficient ground for such a diagnosis, in view of the markedly acid character of the gastric juices, the gastric irritability, and the hemorrhages.

Dr. Hall saw baby L., female, 67 hours old, with Dr. Thos. H. Hawkins on January 5th, 1905. She was a well-developed baby of good parentage, and normal in appearance at birth, excepting for a moderate pallor. The delivery had been a normal one. Within 12 hours of birth the fluid regurgitated from the stomach, flowing over the right cheek and ear, excoriated these parts so that an almost continuous scab covered them on the second day. Careful questioning of the nurse showed that there had been no bile in this ejected fluid, and the cloths stained by it showed no color. The vomitus was strongly acid to litmus paper, when tested by Dr. Hawkins.

There was much vomiting during the first 4 days, black in color from the first. About 48 hours after birth a drachm or more of pure, bright red blood was ejected from the stomach. This occurred on 5 other occasions during the second 48 hours, probably two or more ounces being vomited in all.

The stools were black and tarry from the first, evidently from old blood clots. The early appearance of tarry stools indicates that hemorrhage had occurred in the alimentary tract before birth. No evidence of hemorrhage elsewhere was noted.

The temperature was subnormal, but the pulse was very weak, and the collapse severe. The abdomen was rather rigid, but no especially tender point was found.

A diagnosis of ulcer of the stomach was made. The treatment was: Bicarbonate of soda in half grain doses every hour, with bismuth. Soda was also given in the drinking water and lime water in the milk. This treatment was instituted within a few hours after birth of the child. Doses of 1/10 minim of the one-thousandth solution of adrenalin chloride were given every 15 minutes upon the occurrence of bleeding. There was no hemorrhage after the sixth day, and the baby has followed an entirely normal course since and at present is plump and well and in every respect a normal and healthy baby.

We have abundant support from the pathological side, for such a diagnosis, since many cases have been reported of ulcer found in babies less than a week old or even in those still-born. We know of no other condition which could produce the clinical picture here given, with recovery in such a manner.

Hematemesis could scarcely occur in a baby from cancer, hepatic cirrhosis, varices in the esophagus, aneurism, or the other causes occasionally noted in the adult. It appears to us that the case should not be classed as one of morbus maculosus neonatorum, since the bleeding was confined to the stomach to the best of our knowledge, and was accompanied by the marked gastric irritability, and hyperacidity so well known in connection with ulcer. In Townsend's cases the temperature was often elevated, while in this case it was depressed. "The general and not local nature of the affection, its self-limited character, the presence of fever, and the greater prevalence of the disease in hospitals, suggests an infectious origin" (for morbus maculous neonatorum) (Townsend). Says Dreschfeld: "The temperature (in ulcer) is normal, or even subnormal if the nutrition suffers much." The absence of jaundice and the recovery would also favor the probability of our proposed diagnosis, for but 19 out of 50 of Townsend's cases recovered.

Kundrat states that small ulcers are quite frequently found in children even only a few days old, but states that he has never known chronic ulcer to develop from these little ulcerations, probably because acid catarrh is rare in children. Henoch speaks of the occurrence of ulcer in the new-born, while Widerhofer denies its presence in childhood.

Dreschfeld states that "Before the age of puberty gastric ulcer is of very rare occurrence; yet it has been observed in infants, and occasionally soon after birth. The melena of the newly-born, though often due to erosions and small multiple ulcerations, has in some cases been found to be due to simple ulcers of the stomach with regular well-defined borders, varying in diameter from one to three centimeters, and situated in the stomach or duodenum. In other cases of melena neonatorum no lesion has been found in either the stomach or intestines."

Some of the American authors agree with the former authorities. The positive evidence is of much more value than the negative, here as elsewhere. The absence of history of pain and tenderness in so young a child, bearing in mind the difficulty of eliciting exact symptoms in a baby already nearly collapsed with frequent vomiting and loss of blood, could count but little in view of the presence of the severe vomiting, the hematemesis, and the corrosive action of the regurgitated fluids.

The prognosis seems to be better in children than in adults. Correction of the hyperacidity is looked upon as of great importance by most writers. We know of nothing promising better results than the adrenalin so far as the danger from hemorrhage is concerned. In cases of perforation attempt at operation might be justifiable, although the mortality would probably be excessive at this age.

INFECTION WITH FLY LARVAE.*

WM. C. MITCHELL, M.D.

When the female fly deposits its eggs in living tissue and the eggs develop into larvae, the diseased condition is known as myasis.

A study of the literature of this somewhat obscure subject shows that the condition is by no means so rare as one might sup-

*Read before the Denver Academy of Medicine, April, 1905.

pose. The eggs may be deposited on the mucous membrane of the eye, on the mucous membrane of the ear, on the mucous membrane of the nose, or in open wounds,—myiasis conjunctivae, myiasis aurium, myiasis narium and myiasis vulnerum.

It is a matter of common observation on the farm or on sheep ranches that at times wounds on cattle, horses or sheep may become the breeding places of maggots, so that the wound may teem with these pests. Such observations are also frequently met with by surgeons in open or exposed wounds.

In studying the natural history of the family *Muscidiae,* which embraces both the house flies and the blow flies, it develops that the mature house fly deposits her eggs chiefly in excrement, that of the horse being preferred, and after about 24 hours the eggs develop into larvae. The insects remain in this, the larval state, for about six or seven days. They then go into the pupal state and after from three to four days emerge as young flies. The blue bottle or blow fly prefers dead animal matter as a depository for its eggs, although in emergency it deposits them elsewhere, many cases being on record of the deposition of these eggs and their subsequent development on living animals. Lydekker in his chapter on diptera mentions that toads seem to be a particular object of attack by blow flies. In one instance nearly a whole colony of toads were exterminated by the larvae of these flies which chiefly infected the nostrils. As testifying to the most extraordinary vitality of these larvae may be mentioned the case of a lizard that dined on gravid blow flies. The eggs of these flies hatched out in the stomach of the lizard and promptly attacking the internal organs, killed the lizard. Other instances are also on record of the digestive tract of these animals being destroyed by fly larvae taken in as food.

A very different life-history is given by the bot flies of horses, of cattle and of sheep which form an entirely different family, the *oestridiae.* The larvae of these flies are forced from the very first to lead a parasitic existence in the bodies of their respective hosts. The horse fly deposits its eggs on the hide of the horse and when these eggs develop into larvae they irritate the skin. The horse licks the irritated part and swallows the maggots which promptly fasten to its mucous membrane. Here they live for about a year, when they pass out with the excrement, burrow into the ground and go into the pupal state. They remain as pupae for about six weeks and emerge as flies. The cattle flies lay their eggs on the hide of cattle, and the maggots as they develop burrow beneath the skin and form tumors with an opening externally. The larvae remain here for about eleven months and then, falling to the ground, go into the pupal state to emerge as flies after about one month. Sheep flies lay their eggs in the nostrils of sheep and the larvae migrating into the frontal sinuses remain here for about nine months, after which they drop to the ground and go into the pupal state, later to emerge as flies.

About August, 1900, Dr. E. P. Hershey brought me the larvae of a fly which he had taken from a boil on a child's neck. Child was one year old and had several boils on the right arm and neck. From this crop of boils Dr. Hershey obtained six maggots, four dead and two alive. Only one maggot was found in each boil. The child lived within half a block of the park at Twenty-eighth avenue and Gilpin street, where it was frequently taken for an airing. The child wore short sleeves and low-neck dresses. At my suggestion, as Dr. Hershey had met with failure in attempting to cultivate the larvae of another case to be described later, an attempt was made to cultivate this maggot by placing it in wet horse manure. When the larva was placed in this mixture, it moved in and out and was very lively like it had found a long-lost home. I can give no accurate description of this larva any more than to say that it presented the general appearance of fly maggots with which all are familiar. We had great hopes of raising a fly from this particular larva for the purpose of studying it, beliving that it would be much easier for inexperienced entymologists like ourselves to classify a fly than a larva. The janitor of the building, however, saved us all further trouble, as he threw the entire mass away after the larva had been developed nicely for two days.

Dr. Hershey informed me that ten years prior to the present case, he attended a child in the same neighborhood, afflicted with boils on the neck and back of the head, and that eight living maggots in all were taken from these boils. He attempted to cultivate the biggest of these on a piece of meat but the experiment was a failure.

In February, 1905, Dr. Thos. H. Hawkins brought me the larva of some insect taken from a patient ten years old, with the following history: Patient lives at Lamar, Colo., and was referred to Dr. Hawkins by Dr. Fewkes. The boy would complain of intense rheumatic pains, and a greenish-black spot varying in size from a nickel to a dollar would appear. Spots were seen on the legs, the arm, the thigh and the back. From three of these a living worm was extruded. One of those was sent to Dr. Hawkins preserved in alcohol, and this specimen, which I now present to you, was turned over to me. Following up to the greenish area from which this worm was extruded was a line about eight inches long extending in a tortuous path from one scapula to the other. This line was greenish black at first and gradually faded to a white line about one-eighth of an inch thick. With the extrusion of the worm in every case, the pain ceased and no further trouble was experienced. The boy lives on a farm and works around the horses, pigs, etc. There are no sheep on the place. No history of having been stung by any insect could be obtained.

The remarkable features about all three of these infections is first, their occurrence in this temperate climate, and, secondly, in the eggs of these flies being deposited in what was apparently the healthy unbroken skin and their developing to larvae. For it is by no means uncommon to have a development of maggots in an open wound or sore to which flies may have access to lay their eggs. Such boil-like infections as Dr. Hershey's two cases are apparently of frequent occurrence in tropical countries, due either to the blow of blue bottle fly, the dermatobia, the cayor fly or some similar species. Dr. Hawkins' case is a remarkable one, in view of the extraordinary length which the larva traveled under the skin, the distance as estimated by Dr. Hawkins being eight inches in route from one scalpula to the other.

As to the identification of the larvae of these two cases, in my opinion, they were the larvae of the blow flies.

This opinion may be entirely wrong. It is founded on what knowledge I could glean from a study of all the literature at my disposal in the city. Consultation with several local entomologists showed that they were as much in doubt as I was about the matter. I believe that the only other larva with which they could be confounded is the larvae of the sheep flies, and these larvae do not resemble the two specimens which were sent to me.

In appearance, the maggot from Dr. Hawkins' case is white, consists of nine segments, is five-eighths of an inch long by one-sixteenth of an inch in diameter. A distinct head and canal are visible.

Howslip reports the infection of two human beings with the larvae of the sheep bot, in this case called *oestrus humanus*. In both of these cases the larvae were removed from tumors on the infected individuals. Osler quotes Matas as reporting a case of similar infection in the gluteal region, and further states that in tropical countries the larvae of certain bot flies, dermatobia, are occasionally deposited in the skin, producing swellings not unlike the ordinary boil; and as mentioned before, the larvae of the cayor fly frequently deposits its eggs beneath the skin and gives rise to similar infection.

In concluding, it may be mentioned that *myiasis interna* is the term applied to the infection resulting from the swallowing of larvae. Many cases are on record of the vomiting of larvae. According to Osler, the cases in which the larvae are passed in the feces are very much less numerous.

MEDICAL ETHICS.

By B. B. FRANKLE, M.D.

MR. PRESIDENT AND GENTLEMEN: I make no apology for presenting for your consideration a subject which is so widely removed from more strictly medical themes, believing that whatever influences medical practice and medical standards for good is relevant, pertinent and seasonable. Neither do I assume the role of a teacher of ethics, nor do I pose as an example of the perfect ideal man from an ethical standpoint. I have selected the above subject in preference to others of a more conventional and scientific character, in the hope that this departure from well worn topics may prove a welcome and an interesting change. It is obviously impossible to consider every phase of the subject and I have in many instances only suggested and indicated the lines of thought to be followed. If the subject is one that has been previously dis-

*Read before the Pueblo County Medical Society, Jan. 15, 1905.

cussed at this society, I trust that the members of this honorable body will not consider its unintentional repetition to-night an intrusion. Medical ethics being only a part of that larger system of ethics in general, a brief reference to the latter will prove helpful in determining the dependence of one upon the other and the extent to which the greater influences the lesser.

Ethics in General.—Since the time of Aristotle, the subject of ethics has attracted the attention of philosophers all over the world and, though differing somewhat in their treatment of the subject and each having his own pet theory to advance, they agree on the more fundamental and basic principles which underlie our ethical system. Spencer in his "Data of Ethics" comments as follows:

"Ethics is conduct and in its full acceptation must be taken as comprehending all adjustments of acts to ends from the simplest to the most complex, whatever their special natures and whether considered separately or in their totality. Conduct is good or bad according as the acts are well or ill adjusted to ends."

Martineau, in his "Types of Ethical Theory," in a clear, concise and interesting manner, elucidates on the subject in this wise:

"In its broadest sense, ethics is the doctrine of human character and assume as their basis, the fact that men are prone to criticise themselves and others and can not help admiring traits in some and condemning others. This tendency displays itself actively in every aspect of life; giving pungency to the gossip of a village, interest to biography and fiction, the needful authority to law and the highest power to religion. All these take their origin from the consciousness of a better and a worse human beings and affairs and aspire with more or less distinctness to realize the good and exclude the ill. But while they all join in the confession that there is an interval between life as it is and life as it ought to be, they investigate no standard, they seek no ground for their own feeling but are content with reporting the estimates that rise spontaneously in the mind. These judgments constitute a body of ethical facts and it is the aim of ethical science to strip from them their accidental, impulsive and unreflecting character, to trace them to their ultimate seat in the constitution of our nature and the world and to exhibit not as a concrete picture but in its universal essence the ideal of an individual and social perfection, to interpret, vindicate and systematize the moral sentiments." The scope of ethics includes all conduct which furthers or hinders in either direct or indirect ways the welfare of self or others.

A code of personal conduct can never be made definite, as various types of men are adapted to various types of activities and may lead lives that are severally complete. In view of these facts, no specific statement of the activities universally required for personal well being is possible. So much for the philosophy of ethics.

The necessity for a Code of Ethics.—No one will deny the necessity for a code of medical ethics.

The intimate and confidential relation of physician and patient, the overcrowding of the ranks of the medical profession with its attendant evils, the encourgagement which the law, the laity and the press give to new cults and pathies and the increase of the number of medical charlatans who prey on the credulity of the public; all these are good and sufficient reasons for establishing certain principles for the guidance of physicians in their conduct toward themselves, their patients and the community at large. The members of the medical profession must stand together, they must co-operate with each other, they must unify their interests, they must protect one another from calumny and insult if they do not wish to see the the noblest calling in the gift of God and man relegated to the past, disgraced instead of honored, ridiculed instead of respected, and completely subordinated to fake systems of healing. There was a time when the word physician conveyed to the mind a combination of goodness, skill, sympathy, simplicity and greatness. The worship of the Golden Calf has largely replaced the worship of an ideal; the metallic tinkle of coin upon coin is a greater incentive to better work than the desire to excel and surpass. I do not wish to be understood as meaning that there are not many members of the medical profession who possess and practice the most ethical ideas and whom no amount of money, glory or prestige could cause to prostitute their profession; neither do I wish to be understood as prophesying the decadence of professional honor nor the destruction of the lofty ideals which have given the medical profession the high place it holds to-day among all classes and in all localities. What I do mean and emphasize is, that there is a strong tendency in the medical profession to ignore the many

' vital problems which face it, thereby seriously threatening its honor and its integrity.

The Principles of Medical Ethics.—Since we admit the importance of and the necessity for medical ethics, we must be guided in our conduct by certain principles which will be applicable to physicians everywhere.

The constitution and by-laws governing every medical society, be it county, state or national, technically constitute a code of medical ethics, in as much as the society demands that its members shall qualify up to certain standards of conduct.

Generally speaking, the principles of medical ethics comprise:

I.   The duties of physicians to their patients.

II.   The duties of physicians to each other and the profession.

III.   The duties of the profession to the public.

I.   The duties of physicians to their patients will fix the responsibility of the physician, will require the legitimate exercise of humanity, delicacy, secrecy, will demand honesty and wisdom in prognosis, will encourage the patient and will cause the physician to give the most judicious counsel at his command, thereby strengthing the good resolutions of patients suffering under the consequences of evil conduct.

II.   The duties of physicians to each other and to the profession at large, (a) duties for the support of professional character, (b) profesional services to each other, (c) duties of physicians in regard to consultation, (d) duties of physicians in cases of interference, (e) compensation.

III.   Duties of the profession to the public include, duties as to public hygiene—enlightenment of the public on sanitary matters—physicians as witnesses—enlightenment of the public as to charlatans—relations to the pharmacists.

(The above classification is that adopted by the American Medical Association, modified to suit the convenience and purpose of the writer.)

Observance of Medical Ethics.—Those portions of medical ethics which relate to the duties of physicians towards their patients and their duties toward the public, are usually observed in their entirety. Most physicians keenly realize the confidential relation existing between them and their patients, the broad human-

itarian lines of their life work, the necessity for the prompt relief'
of the sick and the injured, their unusual and unique position in
the social fabric, the necessity for gentleness and encouragement
in administering to the sick and strengthening the will of those
who wish to be emancipated from their evil habits and consequences. Similarly physicians thoroughly understand and fulfil
their duties towards the public at large by enlightening the people
on sanitary matters, by instructing them as to hygiene and prophylaxis by warning them against the wiles and dangers of the charla-
tan and by upholding the dignity and the honor of the profession.

There is practically no clash, nor quarrel, nor difference in
the observance of these principles of medical ethics. It is in the
physicians' relation to one another and to the profession at large
that the serious and flagrant infractions of ethics occur. It is
here that petty jealousies and rivalries flourish which tend to dis-
unite, disorganize and disrupt the medical fraternity.

Violation of Medical Ethics.—As already stated, the most frequent breach of the written and the unwritten laws of ethical conduct, so far as physicians are concerned, is that relating to their
treatment of each other in the course of their professional contact.
Sometimes, unintentionally, more often intentionally, occasionally
in ignorance of existing conditions, more frequently with a full
knowledge of conditions, often deliberately and actuated by no
other motive than a selfish one, some physicians will lose no opportunity to slander, malign and willingly attack the character and
standing of a brother physician.

There are some men in the world who are so bigoted and
prejudiced, so mean and selfish, so jealous and envious, that they
look upon a successful activity in a similar line of work as an
encroachment on their rights, a violation of their privilege, a harmful interference and pernicious influence. Such people hold the
olive branch of a false friendship in one hand and the assassin's
dagger in the other with which they murder reputation and character. This malevolent and jealous spirit is sometimes displayed
in the matter of consultation and frequently ends in the dismissal
of the attending physician, who has been faithful and conscientious
and in the retention and exaltation of the insinuating consultant.
Fortunately for the honor and the glory of the medical profession,

such instances are not very common but they occur sufficiently often to merit at least serious mention and criticism.

Consultation should be encouraged and promoted and the participants should not show in any manner that the treatment being pursued does not meet with their entire sanction and approval. The rights of the attending physician should at all times be scrupulously regarded and the position of the attendant should be strengthened in the eyes of the patient and family; fairness, justice, equity, should at all times prevail and then serious differences will be reduced to a minimum.

The Remedy for Existing Defects.—The remedy for existing defects and patent evils in our ethical system, does not depend on iron clad, written nor specific rules of conduct, nor upon the strict observance of such principles of ethics generally accepted as proper and necessary. We have at the outset accepted the philosophic statment, that a code of perfect personal conduct can never be made definite. This is easily accounted for by changing conditions, unusual exigencies and emergencies, the evolution of thought, action and ideas and the kaleidoscopic nature of our daily lives.

Character must be the foundation upon which ethical action is to be built. Proper conduct among men and affairs must be left to the man, his tact, his judgment, his education and his experience. The ranks of the medical profession must be recruited from men of broad minds, of high ideals, of lofty purposes, of enlightened thought, of charitable tendencies and of honest intentions.

This is the remedy for the defects in our ethical system and when this is accomplished, the medical profesison will be what it should be; a common brotherhood working harmoniously for the common welfare of humanity; dispensing charity to all, rendering pain less poignant, suffering less acute, encouraging the depressed and the despairing, making the world better and brighter and life more worth the living.

Pueblo, Colo., January 14, 1905.

NORMAL OBSTETRICS.

(CHAPTER THIRTEEN.)

THE MANAGEMENT OF THE SECOND STAGE OF LABOR.

By T. MITCHELL BURNS, M.D.

Denver, Colo.

Professor of Obstetrics, the Denver and Gross College of Medicine.

Antisepsis.—Cleanliness of the external parts, the obstetrician's hands, etc., should be continued. If not done before, the patient's gown should be rolled up and pinned at the waist. (The patient should not wear a wrapper after the second stage of labor has begun.) If the obstetrician has not sufficient time to thoroughly wash his hands, they should be moistened, sprinkled with boric acid, the rubber gloves removed from the pouch and put on without touching their exterior. If there are no gloves or not time enough to put them on, a sterile or clean towel should be taken in the hand and only the towel allowed to come in contact with the patient.. If several examinations have been made, or if the hand or forceps are to be introduced into the uterus, the vulva and vaginal orifice should be rewashed with soap, gauze and water and irrigated with bichlorid solution.

The Patient's Position.—As a rule, it is best that the parturient be in bed and upon her back or left side, according to the method used to preserve the perineum.

Vaginal Examinations.—These should not be more frequent than every half hour, until near the end of this stage.

Diagnosis of the Presence or Absence of the Membranes.—(See the first stage.)

Rupture of the Membranes.—If the membranes have not been ruptured, they should be ruptured according to the directions given in the first stage.

Diagnosis of Caput Succedaneum, Presentation and Position, Engagement, Complete Flexion, Descent and Rotation of the Head.—(See the first stage.) These should be ascertained after the rupture of the membranes, even if determined before, as mistakes in diagnosis are not rare before rupture of the membranes.

Bearing Down.—Bearing down should now be encouraged, i.

e., the patient should lie on her back, with her feet pressed firmly into the bed or against its foot, a sewing machine or other box; her shoulders should be raised by a pillow, and she should bend her head forward, grasp with her hands the hands of the nurse or a sheet tied to the foot of the bed, hold her breath and bear down as if she wished to move her bowels. Between pains she should extend her limbs to prevent them becoming cramped.

Perineal Pressure:—When the progress of descent is slow, pressure with two or more fingers, the whole hand or closed fist against the perineum, from above downward in the vagina, will often produce effective involuntary bearing down efforts.

Rectal Tenesmus.—This is usually due to the pressure of the presenting part upon the rectum, and therefore often causes the patient to think her bowels are about to move. If the patient wishes to get up, it is better to explain to her the cause of the tenesmus and to state that she should not remain more than five or ten minutes on the vessel and that if a pain occurs, she must not bear down.

Sacral Pain.—This can often be relieved by having the nurse place a hand firmly against the sacrum. A hot water bag, blanket or douche pan placed in this region will sometimes greatly relieve the pain. (Electricity ought to be of value):

Cramps in the Lower Limbs.—Cramps are usually relieved by pulling the foot sufficiently to completely extend the limb, or by rubbing.

When to Interfere.—When advancement ceases for one hour, the simple methods of increasing the contractions should be employed, i. e., change of posture, pressure on the perineum, quinin, etc., and as soon as two hours are up the forceps should be used. If the head is on the perineum, some use to good advantage abdominal pressure on the breech instead of using the forceps.

The Preservation of the Perineum.—The conditions which tend to prevent laceration are just the opposite of those which tend to cause laceration. (See chapter XII, Causes of Laceration.) The cause laceration. (See chapter XII, Causes of Laceration). The distensibility of the perineum is indicated by its thickness, tenseness and width. A tense and thick perineum does not generally tear, a tense and thin one generally does tear and a very tender perineum rarely escapes rupture. Numerous methods have been used to preserve the perineum, but the following are probably the best.

The Dorsal Multip Method: The patient, a multipara, with
a good perineum and whose last child is not more than two years
old, is left on her back and allowed to bear down, but if delivery
is rapid, bearing down is not permitted, no one is allowed to take
hold of her hands and she is directed to cry, "Oh! Oh!" continuously during each pain to prevent bearing down; the obsterician
places one hand toward the perineum, so that the fingers nearly
touch it; the hand forms a continuation of the perineal trough
and causes the head to pass along the palm in the curve of Carus.
If the exit is too rapid, the vertex is held back and flexion increased
by pressure of the fingers upon the frontal end of the head, just in
front of the perineum. No attempt is made to push the perineum
over the face, but if the vaginal orifice is tight, the anterior part
of the vulvar orifice is pushed over the head between and, at times,
during pains. After the head is born, the lower shoulder is allowed to follow along on the trough, care being used to allow it
to be fully born before the upper shoulder is allowed to exit. When
this method is used in cases as indicated above, lacerations are
rare. If this method is used with a primipara or when there is
considerable danger in a multipara, chloroform is used to the
surgical degree to prevent too rapid exit of the head.

The Lateral Primip Method: When the vulva is nearly half
dilated, the patient is turned upon her left side (to lessen bearing down), her hips are brought near the edge of the right side
of the bed, chloroform is given to control the progress of the
head, and, if necessary, to complete unconsciousness; the first two
fingers of the left hand are placed just behind the anus (which is
covered with cotton), the thumb touches the head just in front of
the perineum, the thumb of the right hand is carried just in front
of this, and the first two fingers are between the labia in contact
with the occiput. During a pain the head is held back, pushed
toward the pubic arch and kept flexed by pushing the sinciput
into the vulvar orifice. With each pain the head is allowed
to advance a little until the brow is about to be delivered, when
complete anesthesia is produced and no advancement allowed; between contractions the head is pushed out by the fingers of the
left hand, placed just behind the anus or partially in the rectum
and having the patient (if she is not unconscious) bear down
gently. As the head is born, it is flexed and guided, as before, up

against the subpubic ligament. The shoulders are managed as in the preceding method. In these methods, retarding the extension of the head until the occiput is well under the subpubic ligament, causes the neck, instead of the occiput, to be in contact with this ligament when extension occurs. As a result the diameters, which pivot on the subpubic ligament and pass the antero-posterior diameter of the vulvar orifice, are lessened.

Other Measures to Preserve the Perineum: Hot sitz baths and vaselin inunctions of the vulva during pregnancy and labor are of value. The free use of hot soap suds to the perineum is sometimes useful in cases where the perineum is rigid. *Episiotomy,* or cutting with the scalpel a half inch incision on each side of the perineum toward the side of the rectum, to prevent laceration, is rarely of value; as it is difficult to say when a perineum is likely to lacerate, and when a tear is expected, the indication is to slow the exit of the head, rather than to cut the perineum. (Many take half an hour to deliver the head in all primiparae). Episiotomy is indicated by the presence of a firm perineum preventing the exit of the head. (The author has performed episiotomy twice. In one of these cases, rather strong traction with the forceps had no effect, but cutting one incision was immediately followed by expulsion of the head between pains).

The Management of the Child as the Head is Being Born.— The Scalp Circulation.—As soon as the child's scalp can be seen, its circulation should be carefully noted. If sudden pressure of the finger upon the scalp causes the color of the skin to quickly disappear and reappear, the child is alive, and there is no hurry; but if the circulation does not respond quickly, the circulation is impeded locally from pressure on the head, or generally from asphyxia, and labor should be rapidly terminated, even if the heart sounds seem good, because there is no means of telling whether the cause is local or general, as frequently in the beginning the heart sounds are not markedly changed in frequency or force by asphyxia.

Cleansing of the Nose and the Mouth.—The exterior of the nose and mouth may be gently wiped to remove any mucus, but no attempt should be made to cleanse the interior of the mouth or nose of any mucus which may have entered from attempts at breathing, as the first good uterine contraction after birth of the head will compress the chest and expel all the mucus.

The Cord Around the Neck.—The cord should be slipped over the shoulders or pulled down and slipped over the head. If the cord is twice around the neck and cannot be slipped over the shoulders, it should be clamped twice and cut between the forceps (or cut without clamping) and delivery hastened.

The Delivery of the Shoulders.—Great care should be used to deliver the posterior shoulder before the anterior, so as to prevent converting a small perineal tear into a large one (an acromio-cervical diameter is smaller than a bis-acromial). If there is dangerous delay, a delay which prevents circulation in the scalp, the patient should be made to bear down, and assistance should be given by pressure of the hand on the fundus. Then if the shoulders are not born, a finger should be passed into the axilla of the child's posterior arm and by gentle traction the trunk delivered. Delay in delivery of the shoulders may cause fetal asphyxia from compression of the cord between the fetus and the bony pelvis or premature separation of the placenta.

The Delivery of the Trunk.—The head and shoulders are gently held up to keep them in the curve of Carus and to prevent loceration of the perineum. It is well to have an assistant place a hand on the fundus and follow the fetus down as it is delivered. This aids expulsion of the fetus and placenta, and retraction of the uterus and prevents hemorrhage.

The Care of the Child Just After It Is Born.—*Slight Asphyxia.*—If the child is slightly asphyxiated, its buttocks should be slapped several times with a quick movement of the hand. (The back of the child should never be slapped, unless gently to expel mucus from the lungs). If this is not effective, one hand should grasp the region of the axillaes, the other the buttocks, and the abdomen, flexed on the chest and extended several times to expel any mucus and to excite respiration. At the same time a little cold water should be forcibly sprinkled upon the chest. If these measures fail, there is considerable asphyxia, which calls for special treatment. (See Asphyxia Neonatorum under Abnormal Labor).

The Position of the Child and Its Covering.—The child should be laid in a warm diaper and blanket, on its right side, with its hips a little higher than the head (to aid expulsion of mucus and breathing), and so placed as not to pull the cord.

The Care of the Eyes.—The nurse should carefully wipe the eyes with boric acid solution.

Tying and Cutting of the Cord.—Five minutes after the child is born the cord should be clamped with hemostatic forceps or tied with silk ligatures one and two inches from the navel, and then the cord, resting upon two spread fingers, should be cut half-way between the clamps or ligatures. The writer ties the cord one inch from the navel, clamps it at two inches, cuts between the ligature and clamp, lifts the placental end of the cord with the hemostat, carries it off the blanket and then detaches the forceps. By waiting five minutes before tying the cord, the amount of blood is augmented four ounces, thus increasing the weight and strength of the child. Clamping the cord requires much less time than tying and should always be used when the mother or child's condition calls for immediate attention, but subsequently the cord must be tied. In tying the cord, the knot should be drawn tight enough to cause the suture to pass through Wharton's jelly and compress the blood vessels. After this knot is tied it is better to pass the ligature around the cord in the same place and tie mother. The placental end of the cord should be clamped and not again. When the cord is not properly tied hemorrhage may occur, and while rarely fatal or even harmful, greatly worries the mother. The placental end of the cord should be clamped and not tied, as the pressure is desired only long enough to carry this end of the cord off the blanket. Bleeding from the placental end of the cord does not harm, but lessens the size of the placenta, and thereby facilitates its delivery. If the cord is left one and a half inches long it will remain flat upon the abdomen, while if it is shorter, it may project directly outward and be rubbed when the child is moved. The scissors are blunt and are passed in between the obstetrician's fingers to prevent cutting a moving arm or leg. After the cord is tied and cut the child should be given to the nurse.

Lifting the Infant.—In lifting the infant to give it to the nurse it is best to grasp the chest with one hand so that the fingers are in one axilla and the thumb in the other. In this manner the infant may be lifted with one hand as easily as with two, and it allows the other hand to be kept on the fundus of the uterus.

THE MANAGEMENT OF THE THIRD STAGE OF LABOR.

There are four indications in this stage, viz: To empty the uterus, to prevent hemorrhage, to cause retraction of the uterus and to render the patient aseptic.

Ergot.—The ergot should be given as soon as the child is born, as some time is required before it takes effect. The majority say it should not be given until the uterus is empty, but it is more likely to aid the expulsion of the placenta than to retard it.

Crede's Method of Placental Delivery.—Crede's method, as used to-day, is as follows: As soon as the child is born, the fundus is gently held by the weight of the hand, the ulnar side being pressed into the abdomen sufficiently to prevent the cornua of the uterus relaxing, but care is used to use no more force than is necessary. When the first distinct pain occurs, generally twenty minutes after the birth of the child, the patient is told to bear down as at stool, and the nurse is asked to take hold of her hands. The fundus is grasped by placing the palm and thumb of the hand in front of it and the fingers behind; the fundus is then pressed backward a little to take the flexion out of the neck. If the placenta is not expelled with the first pain, the hand gently grasps the fundus until the next contraction occurs. With the next contraction *the fundus is pressed backward and also toward the pelvic inlet* to push the placenta into the vagina. If the placenta is not expelled, the same proceedure is carried out during each pain until the placenta is delivered or one hour is passed.

If the patient is not upon a Kelley pad, a bed-pan is placed under her to catch the placenta and blood. While waiting for the first pain the hand of the nurse, or even the patient herself, may hold the fundus. The right cornu frequently escapes the hand of the inexperienced, but too much irritation may retract the cervix before the placenta is expelled.

It is sometimes difficult to grasp the fundus during a contraction; if this is the case it is best to hold the hand in front of the fundus, push it back during a pain, and if, after repeated pains, the placenta does not come away, try to expel it between pains by grasping the fundus above, and having the patient bear down.

When all other external methods have failed, by placing one hand in front of the fundus and the other behind it, the uterus may be compressed from above downward between the two hands and the placenta gradually expressed into the vagina.

Delayed Delivery of the Placenta.—(While this really belongs to abnormal labor, it is given here because it is usually due to lack of skill in the use of the Crede method, and not to any abnormal condition). If, after an hour, the placenta is not delivered, an examination should be made. If most of the placenta is in the vagina, slight traction may be made upon the cord or placenta, but if the placenta is within the uterus, one or two fingers should be introduced to enlarge the cervix and to straighten the uterine canal during contractions. The squeezing of the fundus should be continued for three or four pains, then, if the placenta does not come, it is probably adherent and reujires the introduction of the hand into the uterus. (See Abnormal Labor).

Delivery of the Membrane.—As the placenta is expelled from the vulva, it is caught in the hand, the membrane brought together, twisted over the finger, and, by gentle traction and more twisting, delivered. If considerable traction is necessary, it is best to wait until the cervix has time to relax, as a clot of blood may be in the membrane within the cervix, preventing delivery.

The Examination of the Placenta and the Membranes.—The fundus is left in charge of the nurse or patient while the afterbirth is being examined. A careful examination should be made of the maternal surface of the placenta. Raw spots show that the placenta has been torn during delivery or handling, or that some of the maternal portion of the placenta has been retained. Marked unevenness indicates that more than the average amount of the maternal portion has been retained. This is due to improper Credeing, or to the irregular distribution of the weakest cells. Fissures may be present from separation of· cotyledons during expulsion, and not necessarily from loss of tissue. When any of the placenta is retained, it should be immediately removed by the finger. The membranes should be carefully examined. If the opening is no more than the size of the child's head, and there are two distinct layers (one of which, the combined decidua vera, reflexa and chorian, cannot be peeled from the surface of the placenta, but is continuous with the edge of the placenta), the mem-

branes have very probably all come away. If there is any doubt
as to the retention of a piece, the uterine cavity should be immediately examined. By using extreme care in regard to the after-
birth, many cases of sepsis are prevented.

The Treatment of the Placenta.—The placenta should be
placed in a paper and burned or buried, but, for sanitary reasons,
never put into a vault.

The Hand On the Fundus.—The hand of the accoucheur,
nurse or patient, should be kept on the fundus from the time the
head is born until the bandage is applied, or for one hour. This
prevents post-partum hemorrhage, aids involution and greatly
lessens the severity of after pains.

The Post-Partum Chill.—This is easily controlled by getting
the patient dry, well covered, and giving her a cup of hot milk.
It is always a good plan to give every patient a cup of hot milk
just as soon as she is covered. This prevents chilling and gives
strength. If the chill occurs, warm cloths next to the limbs, hot
whiskey, hot bottles, and more covering should be used.

Antisepsis.—The patient should be upon a Kelly pad or bed-
pan and near the edge of the bed, or, better, in the obstetric position. Then the vulva and vaginal orifice and adjacent soiled areas
should be carefully cleansed with gauze or cotton sponges and soap,
and then with bichlorid solution (1 to 2,000); next the perineum
should be carefully examined for tears, by sponging and spreading
the parts. Tears are often seemingly insignificant, until carefully
examined under good light, with the patient cross-wise on the bed.
If there is no tear, the vulvar pad should be applied.

The Repair of Lacerations of the Perineum.—All tears, however small, should be sutured at once. The patient should be
under chloroform to the stage of unconsciousness. The pan containing the sterilized instruments—two needles, needle holder, scissors, and ten silk and worm-gut sutures—should be brought in and
placed conveniently on a chair. The patient should be cross-wise
on the bed, in the forceps position (lithotomy position), or if a
slight tear, the feet on chairs. The Kelly pad should be under the
hips. The tear should be well opened to show its extent. The
needle should be introduced perpendicularly to the surface and
about a quarter of an inch from the edge of the tear, directed
back from the tear to take up more tissue and to include the

levator ani, then kept beneath the tissue by the guide of the left index finger until the middle of the tear is reached, when it should be brought to the surface, immediately reintroduced and carried beneath the tissues half an inch beyond the opposite edge of the tear, back to a quarter of an inch and then brought to the surface. Each suture should be tied at once. The vaginal sutures should be tied extra tight. The other sutures are introduced in the same way and near enough together to make the walls come in perfect apposition. The vaginal rent is closed without taking up the tissues belonging to the external tear. To prevent the ends from pricking the patient they are left long and tied together. The site of the wound is wiped dry and the vulvar pad applied. (The sutures should be removed on the tenth day. See Chapter XV, The Management of the Puerperal Period. (It is to be remembered that tears, apparently transverse, are usually longitudinal).

Changing Sheets and Pads.—If, for any reason, the bed sheets have become soiled and the patient's back and thighs are bloody, she is first turned on to her near side, her back exposed, washed and wiped. The soiled lower sheet and pads, which have not been removed, are rolled up to her back from the far side of the bed, a clean sheet, hip-pad and abdominal bandage are placed on the back part of the bed and their near half rolled so that it is next to the soiled one and just behind the patient's back. Then the patient is turned on to her back upon the clean bandage, pad and sheet, and the soiled upper sheet removed from the farther thigh, which is now washed, wiped and covered with the clean upper sheet, the soiled upper sheet removed from the bed and the nearer thigh washed and covered. After this the patient is turned on to her far side on the clean pad and sheet, her back rewashed, if necessary, and the soiled under sheet and pads removed from the bed and the clean roll brought forward into place and the patient turned on to her back.

Changing Gowns and Shirts.—If the patient's gown is soiled, it should be removed while she is on her back or side before placing her on the clean sheet. The best way to change the gown, if the bedding is changed, is to take the soiled gown from the upper arm and slip it over the head while the patient is on her near side, then slip the clean gown on her bare arm, and, when everything is ready, to turn the patient upon her opposite side, slip the soiled gown from the upper arm and the clean gown over the head and on this arm. (Extending the arm over the head often facilitates its introduction into the sleeve). When the bedding is not changed, it is best to roll the gown up to the armpits and, while the patient's back is held up from below the axillae, the gown drawn over the head and off the arms, which are extended over the head, and a clean gown slipped over the head and arms.

The Abdominal Binder.—(See Labor Directions under Hygiene of Pregnancy). (Two flour sacks make a very fair bandage. A bandage 18x40 inches is long enough to reach around the body at the trochanters, and wide enough to reach from the breasts to below the trochanters). Before applying the bandage, the gown should be rolled up to the breast, the vulva covered by the dressings or a sterilized towel, the sheet pushed down to the trochanters and the lower limbs extended. The binder should now be brought into place, if not done before, and pinned on the left side of the abdomen from below upwards with large safety pins. The left hand should hold the bandage taut while the right hand introduces and fastens the pins. The pins should be introduced parallel with the length of the patient and close together. The bandage should be made extra tight as far up as the crests of the ilia. Above this point the bandage should be snug, but not so tight as to predispose retroversion of the uterus. If it hurts the patient after it is pinned it is too tight and should be loosened at the tight points. Many do not use the bandage because of the belief that it tends to cause displacement of the uterus, but if properly applied it tends to prevent displacement and gives the patient much relief by stopping the "falling apart" sensation and allowing the patient to turn on her side without the uterus sagging. It also tends to keep the womb retracted and, therefore, lessens the danger of hemorrhage. Patients desire it, as they believe it preserves their shape.

The General Condition of the Mother.—The patient should be asked how she is feeling, and her pulse, the height, width and consistency of the fundus and the amount of flow determined. It is well to remember that the fundus should be below the navel and firmly retracted, but as an exception, it normally may be above the navel a finger's breadth or two, as the height of the fundus does not necessarily indicate the size of the uterus. The cervix may, if the fundus is above the navel, be opposite the brim, or if half way between the pubes and navel, be nearly on the perineum.

The Care of the Child's Eyes.—One or two drops of a two per cent. solution of protargol should be dropped into each eye as soon as the obstetrician has cared for the mother. This is used to prevent ophthalmia neonatorium.

The Umbilical Cord.—After the nurse has washed the baby, the cord should be dressed. If it is very thick, i. e., contains a large amount of Wharton's jelly, it should be cut just above the knot, stripped from the navel to expel the jelly and retied. Boric acid should be dusted about the cord. The cord shold be pushed through a small hole made in a three-inch square of gauze, sterilized cheese cloth or scorched soft linen, turned upwards, i. e., away from the genitals, to prevent soiling the gauze folded over it, a square of absorbent cotton applied—to prevent rubbing when the baby is lifted—and the belly-band put on and pinned sufficiently tight only to hold these dressings in place.

The Care of the Instruments and Other Articles.—All should be removed from the room as soon as possible; the obstetrician's hands should be washed with soap and water to remove blood or other stains; the instruments should be washed with soap or sapolio, wiped dry and put in their proper places. The Kelly pad should always be washed at once, as otherwise it will show the stain of blood and will indicate untidy habits on the part of its owner.

Directions as to the Subsequent Care of the Mother and Child. —These are directions regarding the care of the mother's vulva, breasts, nipples, hands, position, sleep, bladder, bowels, after pains, flow, tears, diet etc., and the child's nursing and navel. (These will be given under "The Management of the Puerperium).

The obstetrician should state the time he will make his first post-partum visit, and direct that if any abnormal condition appears he should be sent for at once, though it is near the appointed time of this visit, as he might be delayed because of other important cases or by loss of sleep.

Labor Records.—These are of much importance, but they should be brief. They may be kept on printed blanks, but one or two lines in the book, showing the names and addresses of obstetric cases, or on the back of the ante-partum record chart will do nearly as well. The date, character of the labor, the presentation or position, the sex of the child, abnormal conditions and any special management, are of importance in this record. (A sample of the labor blank used by the author may be secured for the asking).

Dissemination of Streptococci.—Alice Hamilton, Chicago (Journal A. M. A., April 8), reports the results of an investigation, conducted in the Memorial Institute for Infectious Diseases, Chicago, of the dissemination of streptococci through the breath, especially in scarlet fever and sepsis. She found that these organisms are expelled in invisible droplets of sputum in coughing, speaking, whispering, crying or breathing forcibly through the mouth, to a distance of at least thirty-six centimeters. This was observed in thirty-three out of fifty scarlet fever patients and in forty-two out of fifty normal individuals, and Dr. Hamilton concludes that when these germs are inhaled, or when they fall on exposed tissues, they may cause disease or suppuration. It is probable, also, that their virulence may be increased by passage from one individual to another, and this would explain the conversion of a simple case of scarlet fever into one of scarlatinal sepsis, and it also would explain the cases of surgical sepsis that occur and which otherwise cannot be accounted for. Dr. Hamilton suggests the isolation of cases of scarlet fever with streptococcal complications, and the employment of a mouth guard by surgeons and nurses during operations.

Still's Disease. This symptom-complex embraces arthritis and periarthritis, involving many joints, enlarged spleen and extreme enlargement of lymph-glands. It is probably of infectious origin.

Hooper's Pills. These old-fashioned pills contain in each one grain of ferrous sulphate and of powdered senna, 2/5 grain each of powdered jalap, cream of tartar and powdered ginger, and sufficient extract of gentian.

DENVER MEDICAL TIMES

THOMAS H. HAWKINS, A.M., M.D., EDITOR AND PUBLISHER.

COLLABORATORS:

Henry O. Marcy, M.D., Boston.
Thaddeus A. Reamy, M.D., Cincinnati.
Nicholas Senn, M.D., Chicago.
Joseph Price, M.D., Philadelphia.
Franklin H. Martin, M.D., Chicago.
William Oliver Moore, M.D.. New York.
L. S. McMurtry, M.D., Louisville.
Thomas B. Eastman, M.D., Indianapolis, Ind.
G. Law, M.D., Greeley, Colo.

S. H. Pinkerton, M.D., Salt Lake City
Flavel B. Tiffany, M.D., Kansas City.
Erskine M. Bates M.D., New York.
E. C. Gehrung, M.D., St. Louis.
Graeme M. Hammond, M.D.. New York.
James A. Lydston, M.D., Chicago.
Leonard Freeman, M.D., Denver.
Carey K. Fleming, M.D., Denver, Colo.

Subscriptions, $1.00 per year in advance; Single Copies. 10 cents.

Address all Communications to Denver Medical Times, 1740 Welton Street, Denver, Colo.
We will at all times be glad to give space to well written articles or items of interest to the
profession.
[Entered at the Postoffice of Denver, Colorado, as mail matter of the Second Class.]

EDITORIAL DEPARTMENT

A MEMORIAL MEETING TO THE MEMORY OF THE LATE DR. N. S. DAVIS.

The Society for the Study of Inebriety and Alcohol will hold a memorial service to the life and work of Dr. Davis, at Portland, Ore., on the evening of July 11, 1905, in the Atkinson Hall.

Dr. Davis will be remembered as one of the founders and presidents of the American Medical Association, and also as founder and president for fourteen years of the American Medical Temperance Association. His numerous friends and cotemporaries from both societies will unite on this occasion to commemorate his great services to both medicine and science.

The memorial address will be delivered by Dr. Henry O. Marcy, of Boston, Mass., ex-president of the American Medical Association. Other addresses will be delivered by Dr. G. W. Webster, president of the Illinois Board of Health, also by Dr. W. S. Hall of the Northwestern University, and Dr. T. D. Crothers of Hartford, Conn.; Dr. John Hollister of Chicago, Ill., and Dr. Henry D. Didama of Syracuse, N. Y.; also others will contribute memorial notes to the work and personal influence of Dr. Davis in American medicine.

Nasal Syphilis. Syphilis of the nose is nearly always secondary to specific disease elsewhere. The hereditary form appears in the first few months of life—purulent rhinitis not till the third or fourth year. Coryza is noted in from three weeks to six months after the appearance of the primary sores. The pain of gumma is deep and boring, extending to the side of the face, is more marked at night and disappears with ulceration, when begins a profuse sanguinopurulent discharge, forming putrid, repulsive casts. There is early venous engorgement and a brownish or grayish discharge in connection with the coryza. Mucous patches and superficial ulceration are rare. Later there may be gummatous turbinate swelling, resembling hypertrophy but more solid. Gummatous septal swellings are prominent, rounded, semi-elastic, usually sessile. Deep ulcers, arising from the gumma (particularly septal), are excavated, with overhanging, glistening, bright red edges; the surface is covered with dark, offensive crusts of blood, pus and black necrotic tissue; the probe shows denuded bone or a sequestrum. There is an accumulation of clear, white, cheesy mucus in the upper strait of the nasal cavity, and depression of the nasal bridge from necrosis.

Chronic Intestinal Indigestion of Children. Victor C. Vaughn says: Find cause and remove it; diminish amount of food as a rule. If the stools contain lumps of casein and masses of fat, or are acid from fermentation of milk sugar, discontinue milk for some days and feed child solely upon meat broths and egg albumen. If the stools are alkaline and putrid, use barley gruel, rice-water and solutions of dextrin obtained by roasting or boiling wheat flour. Other useful measures are removal, to better air of country or the mountains; port or sherry wine; cod-liver oil in protracted cases; a laxative dose of calomel, or two or three grains of calomel occasionally; large doses of bismuth subnitrate (gr. xv or more six to eight times a day) for lesions in small intestines. For lesions in large intestine use colon irrigations three or four times per week of three or four quarts of water, at body temperature, followed by an injection, to be retained, of one-half pint of water containing one or two drachms of bismuth subnitrate in suspension. Guard especially against relapse.

HOSPITALS.

The Cynosarge in Athens was a gymnasium transformed into an asylum for abandoned children. Several Grecian cities had retreats for meritorious citizens. The Buddhist Asoka, the most distinguished monarch of India who flourished a little later than Alexander the Great, filled India, says Wilder, with free hospitals, which were actively beneficial for more than a millenium. The first real almshouses and asylums in Europe were built by Christian charity, and about the end of the fourth century Saint Pauline, with other holy women, established a convalescent home in the suburbs of Jerusalem. The chief medico-religious orders of the Middle Ages were those of St. Mary, St. John, St. Lazarus and the Daughters of God. The head of the famous school of Salerno, situated on the highroad of the Crusades, gave to his patient, Robert of Normandy, son of the Conqueror, on his departure, a Latin poem entitled Regimen Sanitatis Salerni, which was very popular for many generations and is said to have passed through 240 different editions. The first hospital, or pest-house, was established in 1403 by the proveditors of Venice on an island near that city. According to Packard, the oldest institution solely for the care of the sick and wounded within the limits of what is now the United States is the Pennsylvania Hospital in Philadelphia, founded in 1752, largely through the efforts of Benjamin Franklin.

State hospitals, or rather penitentiaries, for the insane were first established at Feltro, Italy, and Seville, Spain, in 1409, with police jailers in charge. Up to the time of the French Revolution insane patients were fettered and caged, tortured and neglected and treated in general worse than if they had been wild beasts. To the humane fortitude of the pioneer reformer Pinel all lovers of mercy must render homage of true praise.

THE CARE OF THE EYES.

Whatever promotes general hygiene is beneficial to the eyes. One should avoid reading while lying down or when exhausted, and sudden changes from the dark to brilliant light. Unspaced type is injurious. Reading on the cars is bad for the eyes, by reason of the oscillating movements requiring the paper to be held too near, causing overwork of the muscles of accommodation. One should carry the head erect and avoid tight neckwear, which causes passive congestion of the head and eyes. Fox advises bathing the eyes twice daily with cold water up to 40 years; and after 50 with water as hot as possible, followed by the cold. The first symptoms of failing sight are hypersecretion of tears, burning of eyelids, loss of eyelashes and congestion of the mucosa.

Special care of the vision should be exercised by bookkeepers, typewriters, printers, proofreaders, etchers and engravers. All those engaged in near work should take short intervals of eye-rest. Fox suggests a thin piece of tin sheeting, colored green, blue or black, or a neutral-tinted blotting pad, to be placed under the glazed page while adding up accounts. A shade over the eyes to protect them from the direct rays of light, is very useful. Neutral (arundel) tinted glasses may be used by persons working under high pressure. If possible, the light should come over the left shoulder, and cross-lights are to be avoided. The pure white light of the Welsbach burner and electric bulb lacks diffusive power, and is not good for constant work. A pink or arundel shade should be used around the base. Reflectors cause eye-strain. Incandescent burners are generally not removed often enough. Blank walls strain the eyes; green discs on the wall and pastoral scenery give relief.

In the first six months of life we should guard the eyesight most carefully from the direct rays of the sun and from clouds of dust. During infancy and early childhood the predominating refractive anomalies are hypermetropia and astigmatism, alone or combined. In the early school years many of these cases pass from the hypermetropic into the myopic defect "through the turnstile of astigmatism." To prevent amblyopia ex anopsia in a squinting eye, proper glasses should be fitted as soon as the child begins to read. Ocular defects are a common cause of apparent mental dulness in children. Asthenopia, chorea and migraine may also depend on errors of refraction.

Myopia is a disease of civilization. Proper adjustment of glasses prevents increase of the defect, as well as headaches and other complications. Full correction for near and far vision should be obtained all the time. Frequent re-examination and, if need be, refitting of the patient should be insisted upon. Myopic persons should work only by daylight, with frequent rest to the eyes. Stringent restriction of near work is indicated in high, progressive myopia. To prevent myopia all books, sewing, etc., should be held at a distance of at least 25 c.m. from the eyes, the position of the body should be comfortable, and oblique positions of the head must be avoided. Plenty of sleep and outdoor exercise are of prophylactic consequence.

Although the staphylococcus pyogenes aureus is the predominating organism in acute catarrhal conjunctivitis, the primary cause is the conjunctival hyperemia, so common in large cities, arising from dust, smoke, bright lights, strong winds, exposure to cold and reflex ciliary strain. The sanguinous exudate furnishes a favorable nidus for the rapid propagation of the germs normally present in the conjunctival sac.

Workers in iron, steel and stone should protect their eyes by the use of large spectacles containing plane glasses, unless special lenses are required for ametropia. Snowblindness can be prevented by wearing smoked or tinted glasses, but the continued use of these increases the sensitiveness of the retina and makes asthenopic conditions worse.

The leucorrhea of pregnant women is infectious in from 20 to 40% of cases. To prevent ophthalmia neonatorum the woman's genitals should be bathed and syringed with antiseptic solutions before and during confinement. Trachoma is a strictly contagious disease, occurring generally in those who have no regard for the ordinary principles of cleanliness.

Treatment of Cardiac Asthma. According to J. Merklen *(International Clinics)* the three chief elements of these attacks are pulmonary stasis, spasmodic nervous dyspnea and cardiac asthenia. The first therapeutic indication is to resort to derivation or depletion by the use of mustard leaves, dry or wet cups, and in severe cases of actual bleeding. To calm the nervous factor small injections (1/24 to 1/12 grain) of morphin may be given, along with nitroglycerin, caffein, camphorated oil and ether (internally or freely by inhalation). The third indication is for the use of heart tonics, such as hypodermic inffiections of caffeine, ether or camphorated oil. These patients should avoid exposure to cold, fatigue, emotions and alimentary excesses of all kinds, and reduce the sodium chloride in the diet. They should be given theobromine ten to fifteen grains per dose, for long periods combined from time to time with digitalin.

EDITORIAL ITEMS

For Duodenal Atony. Hare prescribes: ℞ Ext. chiratae fl. gr. ii; ext. leptandrae gr. ii: One pill after each meal.

Intestinal Indigestion. W. W. Johnston recommends a milk diet, persisted in for some weeks.

For Myalgia. Herbert L. Burrell recommends the injection of 1/60 gr. of atropine into the body of the sore muscle.

Treatment of Trichinosis. Burrell gives pugatives, sedatives, ample nourishment and stimulants.

Maretin. This drug is a methylated acetanilid, recommended as an antipyretic in phthisis in the single dose of 7½ grains.

Narcyl. The chlorhydrate of ethyl narcein is a new nervous sedative used to allay pain and cough.

Whooping Cough. Koplik recommends full doses of digitalis (one or two minims of tincture) and antipyrine (one grain for each year, up to five grains).

Salit. This salicylic acid ester of borneol is an oily fluid which, when mixed with equal parts of olive oil, is painted on or rubbed into parts affected with rheumatic pains.

Rodagen. This preparation, obtained by precipitating with alcohol the milk of goats deprived of the thyroid gland, has been used, it is claimed, with success in treating exophthalmic goitre.

Ergot in Deafness. Schwabach *(International Medical Annual)* reports two cases of deafness with tinnitus and vertigo relieved by the administration of fluid extract of ergot.

Cardiac Insomnia. Colbeck affirms that insomnia due to high arterial tension is relieved by the administration of one or two grains of calomel at night.

Dyspnea of Pregnancy. Jewett recommends loose clothing and avoidance of excitement or much exertion; also to sleep with the head and shoulders elevated.

Stomach Flatulence. Shoemaker prescribes: ℞ Sodii bicarb. gr. vi; spt. ammon. arom., tinct. zingiberis aa. m. iv; spt. etheris comp. q.s.: A dessertspoonful in water, repeated as necessary.

For Gastric Fermentation. Hemmeter prescribes : ℞ Beta-napthol, bismuthi benzoatis, bismuthi salicylatis, magnesiae usta, menthol aa. gr. x; saccharini gr. v: One powder three times daily.

Post-Nasal Adenoids. Aside from surgical measures, Jacobi advises daily irrigation of the nasopharyngeal cavities with a physiologic salt solution.

Tubercular Laryngitis. Thornton directs to apply to each ulcer, with a brush or swab, lactic acid diluted with an equal amount of water, after applying four per cent. cocaine solution.

For Coryza. Lederman gives hydrastine sulphate, 1/10 grain every two or three hours, and he cleanses the nostrils and applies a two per cent. solution of menthol in benzoinol.

Cerebral Congestion. Hamilton gives at night one or two pills, containing four grains each of blue mass, extract of colocynth and fel bovis.

For Torpid Liver. Shoemaker prescribes: ℞ Fel bovis purif. gr. iii; ext. nucis vom. gr. 1/20; aloini gr. 1/20; olei cinnamomi m. 1/20: Two pills before meals.

Constipation of the Gouty Diathesis. Sodium phosphate or sulphate in plenty of water is a useful remedy, preferably taken cold and before breakfast.

Diabetic Insomnia. Hutchinson (Practical Medicine Series) gives twenty grains of stontium bromide and fifteen grains of antipyrin at night.

Pyrenol. This compound of sodium benzoylthymolate and benzoyloxybenzoic acid is a soluble aromatic powder recommended in asthma and neuralgic conditions in half-gramme tablets three times a day.

Mitral Stenosis. When digitalis disagrees in cases of mitral stenosis, says Colbeck, its place may be taken by a combination of strophanthus and convallaria majalis, which frequently gives surprisingly good results.

Pruritus Ani. Johns *(International Medical Annual)* has obtained good results by washing after each evacuation, drying with absorbent cotton and applying about twenty grains of calomel with the fingers. Epsom salt is given internally.

Pneumin. This is a light yellow powder prepared by the action of formaldehyde on creosote, and recommended as a stomachic tonic in phthisis in the dose of one-half gramme thrice daily.

Giving Digitalis. The administration of digitalis or any of its allies, says Colbeck, should always be preceded by a purge, preferably in the form of two or three grains of calomel or blue pill, with half a drachm or more of compound jalap powder.

Meteorism of Typhoid. Anders recommends turpentine stupes over the abdomen, or turpentine enemata, or the passage of a long rectal tube; also the change from milk diet to liquid peptonoids, meat juices and albumen water.

To Reduce Obesity. Von Basch advises graduated exercises and walking, short of exhaustion; restriction of carbohydrates and liquors; mineral waters containing Glauber's salts; and carbonated brine and vapor baths.

Syphilitic Dyspnea. Syphilitic cicatrices sometimes give rise to considerable difficulty in breathing. The diagnosis is made by the history and the presence of cutaneous eruptions or scars. By way of treatment Augagnew recommends bromides with iodides.

Spastic Constipation. Avoid cathartics and use warm oil enemata and belladonna suppositories. Lockwood employs hot fomentations to the abdomen at night, retained by means of a binder; also sodium bromide and belladonna internally.

Paralysis of Rectal Sphincters in Young Children. A. Jacobi prescribes: ℞ Ext. nucis vom. gr. xii; adipis ℨ iii-iv: Apply ointment after each defecation and use cold water injections twice daily..

Blood-Pressure and Kidney Disease. K. Sawoda (American Year-Book of Medicine) believes that a pressure above 160 mm. is sufficient to arouse a very strong suspicion of the presence of interstitial disease of the kidneys, even though albuminuria be absent.

Laryngeal Abscess. This lesion is manifested by dyspnea, dysphagia and constant pain. Levy thinks that some cases may be aborted by the use of ice internally and externally. If the case progresses without improvement, scarify, open abscess by the intralaryngeal method, or if necessary, perform tracheotomy.

Appendicular Albuminuria. Dieulafoy (*International Medical Annual*) gives this name to an infective inflammation of the kidneys resulting from the absorption of toxins. He thinks that in all cases of appendicitis the presence of albuminuria indicates toxic absorption.

Euguform. This preparation is methylene diguaiacol acetyl prepared from guaiacol and formalin acetylized by boiling with glacial acetic acid. The soluble form is a 50 per cent solution in acetone. The remedy is chiefly antipruritic, and has the same uses as liquor carbonis detergens.

Aortic Disease. Strophanthus, says Colbeck, though somewhat uncertain in its action, is sometimes of very great service in the treatment of aortic disease. It may be given in combination with iron, arsenic, strychnine, or with some other cardiac or general tonic.

Acute Laryngitis. Levy gives tincture of ferric chloride, a drachm to the ounce of glycerine—a teaspoonful every two hours. Thornton prescribes: ℞ Tinct. aconiti m. ss.; spt. etheris nit. m. xv; potass. citrat. m. x; syrupi m. x; aquam q.s.: A teaspoonful in water every two hours.

Laryngeal Spasms. These are commonly related to a neurotic diathesis, and may be excited by reflex irritation, as from nasal or nasopharyngeal growths. Other causes are locomotor ataxia, paralysis agitans, hydrophobia, tetany, tetanus, meningitis, brain syphilis or pressure on the medulla.

Phthisical Constipation. De Renzi gives two to four powders daily, each containing three grains of iodoform and three to six grains of naphthalin. In chronic cases Knopf recommends a wet pack over the abdominal cavity for a few hours, followed by gentle friction with alcohol.

Constipation With Skin Diseases. The mistura ferri acidi of Van Harlingen consists of the following ingredients: ℞ Magnes. sulph. ℨ i; ferri sulph. gr. ss.; sodii chloridi gr. iv; acidi sulph. dil. m. viiss; infusum quassiae q.s.: A tablespoonful in a goblet of water one-half hour before breakfast.

Portal Congestion of Valvular Cardiac Disease. Elaterium ½ grain and ext. hyoscyamus 4 grains in pill form make a good hydragogue cathartic. H. C. Wood recommends mercuric chloride gr. 1/100 - 1/50 for a long time, along with tinct. ferri chloridi; also mercurial purges occasionally.

Gastro-Intestinal Catarrh With Torpid Liver. E. P. Davis gives three times daily with food a powder of 1/12 grain rhubarb, 1/4 gr. sodium bicarbonate and 1/2 grain aromatic powder. In obstinate cases he gives t.i.d. with the food 1/8 drop creosote in five drops each of brandy and simple elixir and sufficient water.

Paresis of Phrenic Nerve or Diaphragm. If due to neuritis, Tyson tries to galvanize the nerve by pressing one pole over the epigastrium or the coresponding half of diaphragm. He also employs counter-irritation in the triangle of the neck outside of clavicular portion of the sternomastoid.

Constipation of Obesity. Falkin employs an India rubber ball 3½ inches in diameter filled about four-fifths full (3½ or 4 pounds) with shot and closed. The patient, lying supine, rolls the ball over the abdomen from right to left for four or five minutes night and morning.

Flatulence in Tuberculous Subjects. When flatulence is the prominent feature of the gastric or intestinal derangement, says Burton-Fanning, the most generally serviceable drug is creosote. The addition of one-eighth grain of menthol to one minim of creosote enhances the value of the latter.

Tuberculous Diarrhea. Burton-Fanning states that salicylate of bismuth is our best remedy here. It is convenient for the patient to get the pure powder and measure out a level teaspoonful (about twenty grains), which he takes along with his food at each meal.

Tuberculous Dyspepsia. F. W. Burton-Fanning says that the well known mixture of sodium bicarbonate gr. xv, tinct. nux vomica m. vii, tinct. gentian 3ss., aqua chloroformi to 3i, is particularly useful. It remedies flatulence and pyrosis, and increases appetite, and may be continued for long periods with advantage.

Editorial Items continued on page 686

BOOKS

WELCH & SCHAMBERG ON ACUTE CONTAGIOUS DISEASES.—A Treatise on Acute Contagious Diseases by William M. Welch, M.D., Consulting Physician to the Muncipal Hospital for Contagious and Infectious Diseases; Diagnostician to the Bureau of Health, etc., Philadelphia, and Jay F. Schamberg, A.B., M.D., Professor of Dermatology and of Infectious Eruptive Diseases, Philadelphia Polyclinic; Consulting Physician to the Muncipal Hospital for Contagious and Infectious Diseases, and Assistant Diagnostician to the Philadelphia Bureau of Health, etc. In one very handsome octavo volume of 781 pages, illustrated with 109 engravings and 61 full-page plates. Cloth, $5.00, net; leather, $6.00, net; half morocco, $6.50, net. Lea Brothers & Co., Publishers, Philadelphia and New York, 1905.

The text of this work is based upon a personal study of over 9,000 cases of smallpox, 9,000 cases of scarlet fever and 10,000 cases of diphtheria, in addition to a considerable number of cases of the other contagious diseases, treated in the Municipal Hospital of Philadelphia during the past thirty-five years. The relative infrequency nowadays of smallpox, renders the taking up of over one-third of the text with this disease a matter for congratulation, since its early diagnosis is of great importance to the community. The serial plates, showing the character of erruptions on different days, are very helpful. Altogether the book is one that commands attention by its thoroughness, reliability and general utility.

SURGICAL DIAGNOSIS.—A Manual for Practitioners of Medicine and Surgery by Otto G. T. Kiliani, M.D., Surgeon to the German Hospital; Member of the New York Surgical Society, and of the Surgical Society of Berlin, etc. Octavo, 466 pages. Illustrated by 59 full-page plates and by engravings in the text. Price, $4.50 in cloth; $5.50 in half morocco. Wm. Wood & Co., New York, 1905.

This is a very practical and timely work, equally helpful to the surgeon and the general practitioner, who in the great majority of instances makes the first diagnosis of surgical diseases. The author is master of his subject, and presents it in an impressive way, using side notes, heavy type for leading names and facts, and a large number of differential diagnostic tables. The plates are mostly skiagraphic representations. Dr. Kiliani's work is about the only modern one dealing exclusively with surgical diagnosis, and is to be commended from every point of view.

INTERNATIONAL CLINICS.—A Quarterly of Illustrated Clinical Lectures and Especially prepared Original Articles on Treatment, Medicine, Surgery, Neurology, Pediatrics, Obstetrics, Gynecology, Orthopedics, Pathology, Dermatology, Opthalmology, Otology, Rhinology, Laryngology, and Other Topics of Interest to Students and Practitioners. By Leading Members of the Medical Profession Throughout the World. Edited by A. O. J. Kelly, A.M., M.D. Vol. 1, Fifteenth Series. 1905. Price, $2.00. Philadelphia and London. J. B. Lippincott Co.

The latest volume of International Clinics is exceptionally rich in timely and practical information. Over one-third of the text is devoted to a resume of the progress of medicine during the year 1904, the part on treatment having been compiled by A. A. Stevens; that on Medicine, by David L. Edsall and Wm. B. Stanton; and that on Surgery, by Joseph C. Bloodgood. Among the original articles the one one on "The Eye and the Hand in the Diagnosis of Heart Diseases," by J. J. Walsh, is particularly noteworthy.

PRACTICAL PROBLEMS OF DIET AND NUTRITION.—By Max Einhorn, M.D., Professor of Medicine at the New York Post Graduate Medical School and Hospital, and Visiting Physician to the German Hospital, New York. Wm. Wood & Co., 1905.

This little volume will well repay a careful perusal. It treats of the titular subject in a strikingly original way. The author believes in strengthening the digestive functions by the diet, rather than weakening him. While we may not agree with all his propositions, we are certainly informed and benefited by reading his brochure.

A NURSE'S GUIDE FOR THE OPERATING ROOM.—Second Edition. Enlarged and Revised, by Nicholas Senn, M.D., Ph.D., LL. D., C.M., Professor of Surgery, Rush Medical College, Surgeon-in-Chief, St. Joseph's Hospital, Surgeon-General of the State of Illinois. Price, $1.75. W. T. Keener & Co., 90 Wabash Ave., Chicago.

The text of this little volume is made up largely of abstracts of lectures delivered by the author to the pupils of the Training School of St. Joseph's Hospital, Chicago. Asepsis is given especial

prominence, and formulas are furnished for the most reliable antiseptic solutions. The most important wound complications are
briefly described, so that the nurse may warn the surgeon in due
season. Sutures, dressing material and ligatures are explained,
a list of instruments is furnished for each important major operation and a large number of cuts of instruments, with names, are
appended to the text.

OPERATIVE SURGERY.—By Joseph D. Bryant, M.D., Professor of
the Principles and Practice of Surgery, Operative and Clinical Surgery, University and Bellevue Hospital Medical College. Fourth Edition, Printed from New Plates, Entirely
Revised and Largely Rewritten. New York and London. D.
Appleton & Co.

The two volumes comprised in this standard work contain
about 250 pages and 230 illustrations more than were in the third
edition. Altogether there are 1,793 illustrations, 100 of which are
colored. The text is written in a lucid and graphic style, and bears
the marks of the author's quarter-century of experience as a surgical teacher. General considerations are set forth forcibly, but
much the gerater portion of the text is devoted to the description
of special operative procedures. In this connection the author is
particularly clear and definite in his statements. He has taken
special pains to give due credit to fellow surgeons whose work
has been utilized in the pages of his books. This treatise on
operative surgery is more than ever worthy of the marked popularity which it has achieved.

Reflex Precordial Pain. Colbeck says that reflex disturbance
of the heart, often associated with pain in the precordial area, is
very commonly produced by sudden emotion or by prolonged grief
or anxiety. The pain over the heart that is so frequently found
in connection with conditions of nervous strain or exhaustion,
digestive derangements and uterine disorders, is also due to reflex
disturbance of the organ. Referred precordial pain is commonly
attended by headache and superficial tenderness of the scalp in the
supraorbital and temporal regions.

SELECTIONS

ANTIKAMNIA. Therapeutic Indications. Antikamnia is an American product, and conspicuous on this account and because of the immense popularity which it has achieved, it is to-day in greater use than any other of the synthetically produced antipyretics. The literature is voluminous, and clinical reports from prominent medical men in all parts of this country, with society proceedings and editorial references, attest its value in actual practice in an endless variety of diseases and symptomatic affections, such as the neuralgias, rheumatism, typhoid and other fevers, headaches, influenza and particularly in the pains due to irregularities of menstruation. Antikamnia has received more adverse criticism of a certain spiteful kind, particularly directed against its origin—and because of its success—than any other remedy known; critics have seemed personally aggrieved because of its American source, and that it did not emanate from the usual "color works," but their diatribes have fallen flat as do most persecutions and unreasonable and petty prejudices. The fact stands incontrovertible that antikamnia has proved an excellent and reliable remedy, and when a physician is satisfied with the effects achieved he usually holds fast to the product. That is the secret and mainspring of the antikamnia success. It is antipyretic, analgesic, and anodyne, and the dose is from 5 to 10 grains, in powder, tablets, or in konseals, taken with a swallow of water or wine. When prescribing Antikamnia, particularly in combination with other drugs, it is desirable to specify "in konseals," which are rice flour capsules, affording an unequalled vehicle for administering drugs of all kinds.

LIQUIZONE OR HYDROZONE. We are advised by excellent authority that various well authenticated instances have been reported where physicians have been using Liquozone on the supposition that it is practically of the same composition and therapeutic utility as Hydrozone and Glycozone.

The New York Sun recently described the experience of a confiding individual who actually gave up $50,000 to alleged wire tappers who posed as being philanthropic enough to give him inside information on the races. The characteristic editorial comment was that this confiding individual occupied the head of the list of a new class.

In view of the repeatedly published analyses of Liquozone, the doctor who is confiding enough to prescribe it in place of such old and reliable standard products as Hydrozone and Glycozone must also stand near the head of a new list.

ERGIAPOL (Smith) may be implicitly relied upon to promptly relieve the most intractable forms of amenorrhea, dysmenorrhea, menorrhagia, metrorrhagia, or, in fact, any disturbance of the menstrual function arising from a disordered condition of the organs of regeneration. It is an emmenagogue of incomparable excellence.

MENOPAUSE. Preceding and succeeding the final cessation of ovulation and menstruation, physical and psychical disturbances of a more or less serious character are frequently observed. Ergoapiol (Smith), because of its tonic effect upon the female generative system and its splendid antispasmodic influences, is of unsurpassed value in the treatment of the various disturbances incident to this period.

FOX'S EFFERVESCING SEIDLITZ SALT is a laxative, containing magnesium sulphate and sodium phosphate in effervescing combination. It relieves thirst, corrects acidity and relieves rement, producing a comfortable evacuation of the bowels. Pleasant to take as soda water. Every intelligent physician now recognizes the importance of keeping a clean aliamentary tract. There is no "saline laxative" on the market or combination of drugs that has had the efficacy in accomplishing this result as Seidlitz Salt. It should be used as a basis of treatment in all diseases. Indications: Hepatic torpor, constipation, obesity and gout; all fermentative condition of the stomach and bowels and diseases of the blood; rheumatism and diseases arising from rheumatic conditions. In all cases where there is a strong tendency to corpulency, it reduces to a minimum the tendency to apoplexy. In all diseases, because of its wonderful action on the liver and the valvulae conniventes of the intestines, it increases the action of all other drugs. Dose: One to three heaping teaspoonfuls in half tumbler of water, drank during effervescence and repeated as often as necessary. Price, per doz. 1/4 lbs., $3.00; per doz. 1-lbs., $8.50; 5-lbs. bulk, $2.50. Manufactured by The Fox Brumley Pharmaceutical Co., Denver, Colorado.

EDITORIAL ITEMS—Continued.

Surgical Treatment of Empyema. Senn advises preliminary aspiration, free incision under anasthesia, slow evacuation of the chest, and tubular drainage without irrigation at first. Free irrigation of the pleura should be employed during the subsequent treatment, using a double drain with the patient lying on his sound side.

Intestinal Perforation in Typhoid. Harte and Ashhurst (*Progressive Medicine*) state that pain is the most valuable symptom, though not pathognomonic. It is usually stabbing in character, and in the right lower quadrant, but may be located in the bladder or penis. It varies greatly in intensity, and a very apathetic patient may not complain at all.

Constipation in Psychoses. Butler recommends croton oil, one-fourth to two minims on a lump of sugar or with a little bland oil, on back of tongue in lunatics. In chronic mania Van der Kolk gives 1/4 grain aqueous extract of aloes and 1/12 grain tartar emetic, with some bitter extract—two to four pills four or five times a day. In coma Cushny advises a drop or two of croton oil on back of tongue, or colocynthin 1/12 grain hypodermically.

Edema Glottidis. Osler advises the use of an ice-bag on the larynx and ice to suck. If the symptoms are urgent, spray the throat with a strong solution of cocaine or adrenalin and scarify the swollen epiglottis. If relief does not follow, perform tracheotomy immediately. For edematous laryngitis due to the inhalations of irritating gases Waring recommends the repeated inhalation of five minims of ethyl water.

Psoas Abscesses. Says the *Medical Standard:* Never yield to the temptation to open and drain a psoas abscess about a tuberculous hip, or other cold abscess. Mixed infection will surely result and the patient will be afflicted with a chronic sinus and gradual deterioration of health. Such cases should be treated by immobilization in plaster with or without aseptic aspiration of the abscess and injection of iodoform emulsion.

Cardiac Hypertrophy. As Colbeck remarks, one of the chief desiderata in cases of cardiac hypertrophy is an adequate supply

If You Have
a Case of Anæmia

induced by defective nutrition—the result of a chronic digestive weakness, the first thing to do, of course, is to overcome the digestive trouble.

If the gastric juice is deficient in quantity and quality, the digestive glands must be stimulated and their proper functional activity restored. Iron, of course, is always demanded in these cases.

Ext. carnis fl. comp. (Colden) No. 1, is of great value in all secondary anæmias. In addition to the necessary iron, it contains three of the most potent digestive excitants. Administered twenty minutes before meals, it will stimulate the appetite, increase the gastric secretion, promote normal metabolism, and overcome the anæmia. Write for literature.

Sold by all druggists.

THE CHARLES N. CRITTENTON CO., Sole Agents,
115-117 FULTON STREET, NEW YORK.

PASSIFLORA

In Nerve-Starvation Daniel's Conct. Tinct. Passiflora Incarnata acts as a stimulating and invigorating food, as well as a sedative and hypnotic. Nerves are quieted and restored by nourishing and strengthening the depressed vital organs. In the hysteria of nervous women it regulates the heart action, urges composure and gives natural rest. Passiflora is unequaled in its power to control the nervous system.

Write for Literature.
Samples Supplied,
Physicians Paying Express Charges.

LABORATORY OF
JNO. B. DANIEL,
ATLANTA, GA.

—15—

of healthy blood to the myocardium. The drugs most useful for the purpose are iron and arsenic, which may be given separately or together, or with digitalis or strophanthus. Digestion should be attended to and the bowels kept open by mild saline and aloetic aperients.

Cardiac Failure. To relieve venous engorgement and cardiac distention, Colbeck recommends the application of eight or ten leeches over the hepatic region, and the administration of two or three grains of calomel with thirty or forty grains of compound jalap powder. When bowel action and diuresis fail to afford sufficient relief, direct removal of fluid from the edematous tissues, preferably by means of Southey's tubes, is indicated.

Diseases of Liver With Decrease of Bile. Butler recommends euonymin (dose 1/4 to 3 grains) for impaired functional activity of the liver, and lozenges of sulphur and cream of tartar for habitnal constipation due to disorders of the liver; also podophyllin (dose 1/4 to one grain) in hepatic cirrhosis and cancer. Shoemaker prescribes: ℞ Aloini gr. 1/10; ext. hyoscy. alc. gr. i; ext. ignatiae gr. 1/10; pulv. ipecac gr. 1/5: One pill t.i.d.

Meeting of Texas State Board of Medical Examiners. The Board of Medical Examiners for the State of Texas (Regular), will hold its next meeting in Austin, Texas, May 2nd, 3d. 4th and 5th, 1905, for the examination of applicants and transaction of other business. For further information address the secretary.

    J. T. WILSON, President, Austin, Texas.

    M. M. SMITH, Secretary, Austin, Texas.

Nasal Asthma. Insufflations of one part of cocaine, two parts of triturated camphor and sixteen parts of bismuth subnitrate are recommended. Kyle directs to correct any deformity and treat local inflammations. Pencil irritable area in parallel lines with a 10% solution of chromic acid applied on a probe tightly wrapped iwth cotton, excess of acid being carefully removed with another piece of cotton. For the paroxysm itself inject strychnine sulphate gr. 1/20, atropine sulphate gr. 1/150, and morphine sulphate gr. 1/4; also inhale the fumes of equal parts of saltpetre and stramonium leaves burned on a plate.

Whenever cod liver oil is indicated during the summer months' Scott's Emulsion can be used to better advantage than any other cod liver oil preparation. The quickness with which Scott's Emulsion passes into the blood is a guarantee that no fermentation occurs in the digestive tract. The uniformity of quality maintained in Scott's Emulsion and the absolute purity of its ingredients make it eminently superior to any other cod liver oil remedy.

SCOTT & BOWNE, Chemists, 409 Pearl St., New York.

Deficient Intestinal Secretion. Butler recommends small doses of jalap. Barthololow gave small doses of Fowler's solution, podophyllum and sulphurous and saline waters. When combined with torpor of the muscular layer of the intestines, he prescribed: ℞ Tinct. physostig. tinct. nucis vomicae, tinct. belladonnae aa. partes equales: Thirty drops in water morning and evening. Wm. Aitkin prescribes: ℞ Pulv. ipecac. gr. 2/3-i; ext. aloes gr. i; ferri sulph. gr. 1 1/3: One pill an hour before dinner and one before breakfast.

Spasmodic Croup. G. S. Marshall recommends trinitrin in the dose of 1/1000 to 1/600 grain for children five to ten months old. It may be repeated, if need be, in five or ten minutes and continued from time to time as indicated. Love gave turpeth mineral, one-half grain every hour till free emesis, for children over six months old. Dessar advises impregnating the air with one part each of carbolic acid and eucalyptol with six parts of turpentine— a drachm in a pint of water over a spirit lamp three or four times daily. Other useful measures are the hot bath; warm compresses around the neck; steam inhalations, and aconite in small doses every quarter or half hour.

Constipation of Neuropaths. Dubois advises regular rising from bed at a fixed hour; a tumblerful of cold water (or quassia infusion) just after getting up, followed at once by breakfast (including graham bread and butter), always at same hour; daily attempt at defecation at same hour (preferably after breakfast); abundant amounts of food, especially fruits and vegetables at each meal. De Holstein states that chloral is efficient in rebellious neuropathic cases. Asafetida is recommended in hypochondriasis. In hysteria Waring finds the official pill of aloes and asafetida most serviceable.

Treatment of Adenoids. Control intestinal irritation, says Kyle. Soft swellings in the very young can be scraped off with the aseptic finger nail, after carefully cleansing the nasopharynx with a warm solution of eight grains each of biborate and bicarbonate of sodium to the ounce of water, followed by equal parts of hydrogen peroxide and aqueous extract of hamamelis, and again by thorough cleansing with boric acid solution (eight grains to the ounce), as long as secretions are blood-stained. If the tissue is very sensitive, apply one-tenth of one per cent. formaldehyde in four per cent. cocaine—also eight grains of alum and four grains of tannin to the ounce of water as an astringent. Curettage under anasthesia should be employed in marked fibrous cases.

Weak Heart Sounds. Hoffman says (American Year Book of Medicine): If the aortic second sound becomes very weak, and the second pulmonary sound likewise, in infectious diseases, it indicates great weakness of the heart, and is, therefore, a bad sign. Marked weakness of the second pulmonary sound in mitral valvular disease indicates imperfect compensation. Marked weakness of the sounds at the base, as compared with those at the apex, indicates an alcoholic heart. Marked weakness of the sounds at the apex, as compared with those at the base, show a fatty heart.

Milk in Pulmonary Tuberculosis. When any dyspepsia arises from the use of milk, Burton-Fanning advises adding twenty grains (an eggspoonful) of sodium bicarbonate to each tumblerful. The milk may also be given warm, or thickened with some farinaceous food, or it may have a little spirit added. It should not be swallowed in bulk, but should be slowly sipped. With these modifications milk usually agrees, even when drunk at meals with other food. A great deal of milk can be administered in the form of junket or other pudding, to which cream may be added.

J. B. Lippincott Company announce that they will publish during the present year a translation by Dr. Albion Walter Hewlett of the third German edition of the "Principles of Clinical Pathology," by Dr. Ludolf Krehl, with an introduction by Dr. Wm. Osler, of Johns Hopkins University. The work is well known in this country and in Europe as an authority upon the subjects treated, and has been copyrighted in the United States under the Interim Copyright Act.

Diagnosis Between Functional Murmur and Organic Valvular Disease in Nephritis. It is well known that a systolic murmur is often heard at the apex in arteriosclerosis, and may be due to valvular lesion or to dilation. Syllaba (American Year-Book of Medicine) states that the above mentioned diagnosis depends chiefly upon whether the pulse is small and soft or tense; whether the right or the left heart is dilated; whether the pulmonary second sound or the aortic second is accentuated, and whether the blood-

The amily axative

alifornia ig Syrup ompany

an Francisco,
California.

Louisville, Ky.
New York, N. Y.

The ideal, safe, family laxative, known as "Syrup of Figs," is a product of the California Fig Syrup Co., and derives its laxative principles from senna, made pleasant to the taste and more acceptable to the stomach by being combined with pleasant aromatic syrups and the juice of figs. It is recommended by many of the most eminent physicians, and used by millions of families with entire satisfaction. It has gained its great reputation with the medical profession by reason of the acknowledged skill and care exercised by the California Fig Syrup Co. in securing the laxative principles of the senna by an original method of its own, and presenting them in the best and most convenient form. The California Fig Syrup Co. has special facilities for commanding the choicest qualities of Alexandria senna, and its chemists devote their entire attention to the manufacture of the one product. The name "Syrup of Figs" means to the medical profession "the family laxative, manufactured by the California Fig Syrup Co." and the name of the company is a guarantee of the excellence of its product. Informed of the above facts, the careful physician will know how to prevent the dispensing of worthless imitations when he recommends or prescribes the original and genuine "Syrup of Figs." It is well known to physicians that "Syrup of Figs" is a simple, safe and reliable laxative, which does not irritate or debilitate the organs on which it acts, and, being pleasant to the taste, it is especially adapted to ladies and children, although generally applicable in all cases. ✦ ✦ Special investigation of the profession invited.

"Syrup of Figs" is never sold in bulk. It retails at fifty cents per bottle, and the name "Syrup of Figs," as well as the name of the California Fig Syrup Co., is printed on the wrappers and labels of every bottle. ✦ ✦ ✦ ✦ ✦ ✦

REASON

Just cause for action.—Webster.

The high esteem in which **Ergoapiol (Smith)** is held by all calculating clinicians needs no speculative explanation. It is due to no other cause than that of **REASON.**

REASON guides the selection of each agent embraced in the remedy;

REASON dictates the mtehods by which their absolute purity is attained;

REASON prescribes the proportions in which they are presented, and

REASON appoints the cases in which the remedy may be employed with absolute certainty of satisfying results.

Amenorrhea yields, with almost incredible promptness, to the curative properties of **Ergoapiol (Smith)** for the **REASON** that the collaborative effects of its components at once institute functional activity.

Dysmenorrhea is releived by the administration of **Ergoapiol (Smith)** for the **REASON** that the remedy possesses marvelous tranquilizing properties despite the fact that it contains no narcotic drugs.

Menorrhagia invites the employment of **Ergoapiol (Smith)** for the **REASON** that the remedy restricts the flow to normal limits. Physicians prefer **Ergoapiol (Smith)** to all other agents of a similar character for the **REASON** that it is unquestionably the most dependable preparation ever designed for the relief of

Irregular Menstruation

DOSE:

One to two capsules 3 or 4 times a day.
    NOTE—To obviate substitution it is advisable to order in Original Packages only. Original Package contains 20 capsules.

MARTIN H. SMITH CO.
NEW YORK, N. Y.

pressure is increased or not; also upon the history and the microscopic examination of the urine.

The Museum in Medical Teaching. Maude E. Abbott, Montreal (Journal A. M. A., March 25), notices the great advance in laboratory methods in medical teaching, but considers that the adaptation of the medical museum to the didactic method of teaching is too little understood. When properly systematized the museum furnishes most valuable object lessons far more instructive than mere reading—a sort of observational study enabling the student more easily to fix the facts in his mind. She describes at length the methods employed in McGill University, the classification and general arrangement and the use of the specimens for direct teaching purposes in the way of examinations and quizzes on the specimens presented.

Arthritis Deformans. A characteristic deformity of the foot, says Billings, is a permanent hyperextension of the proximal phalanges, with flexion of the distal bones of the toes. The distal ends of the metatarsals become prominent and tender and make the foot tender, and in consequence walking is painful and awkward. In the majority of cases, says McCrae, the glands in association with the affected joints are enlarged. Heberden's nodes, at the terminal phalangeal joints of the fingers, may occur alone or with involvement of the larger joints. The joint (or joints) once attacked seldom clears up suddenly, and the disease, unlike acute articular rheumatism, rarely shifts from joint to joint. The pulse is nearly always above the normal. There is rapid muscular atrophy and exaggeration of reflexes. Chronicity, of course, is very suspicious of this disease. A highly nutritious diet, arsenic and syrup of iodide of iron are chiefly indicated.

Constipation in Anemic and Chlorotic Subjects. Sir Andrew Clarke recommended one-half grain each of aloin, ferri sulphas exsic., ext. belladonnae, ext. nucis vomicae, pulv. ipecac, pulv. myrrhae and soap: One pill one hour before last meal, should bowels not act during the day. Osler uses a sulphur confection in the morning and a pill of iron, rhubarb and aloes throughout day. Shoemaker prescribes: ℞ Aloes purif. gr. iii; massae ferri caro. gr. ii; pulv. aromat. gr. i: One or two pills at the bed hour. For anemic women Bushong advises exercise in fresh air; local and general massage and baths with frequent rubbing of the skin. He prescribes: ℞ Pulv. ipecac gr. 1/4; tinct. nucis vom. m. viiss; ext. cascarae fl. m. viss-xiiss; mist. rhei t. sodae q.s.: A dessertspoonful before each meal in a half tumblerful of water. Anemic children with constipation, says Earle, are well treatel with a mixture of sulphate of iron, sulphate of magnesium and tincture of nux vomica.

The Colon Bacillus Toxin. Sybil May Wheeler, Ann Arbor, Mich. (Journal A. M. A., April), describes in detail the methods of extracting the intracellular toxin of the colon bacillus by treatment with 2 per cent. solution of sodium hydrate and absolute alcohol, leaving a water—soluble and non-toxic residue. The toxin is obtained from cultures either on agar or on Frankel's modified Uschinsky's medium, showing that it is an integral part of the cell. The use of the modified Uschinsky's medium also shows that the organism is able to build the toxin synthetically from chemical compounds. The toxic substance, freely soluble in water and perfectly in absolute alcohol, gives all the ordinary proteid color reactions, but its alkaloidal nature. It may be broken up by concentrated acid and a toxic crystallizable body precipitated with mercuric chlorid. The cell substance of typhoid and anthrax bacilli, like that of the colon bacillus, is broken up by dilute alkali in alcohol at 78 F. into portions A and B, the former being in solution in the alcohol, while the latter forms an insoluble residue. Both A and B are soluble in water, and aqueous solutions of A are poisonous, while similar solutions of B are inert or relatively so. Portion A from the colon bacillus at least (the others not having been so thoroughly studied as yet), can be divided into two portions a and a' by precipitation with platinum chlorid. Portion a constitutes from 10 to 15 per cent. of A, and is poisonous, while a' is inert. The proteid color reactions follow the poisonous portion in these separations. By breaking up portion A with concentrated hydrochloric acid a crystalline toxic body is obtained.

NORMAL OBSTETRICS.

CHAPTER ELEVEN.

THE HYGIENE OF PREGNANCY AND LABOR DIRECTIONS.

By T. MITCHELL BURNS, M.D.,

Denver, Colorado,

Professor of Obstetrics, The Denver and Gross College of Medicine.

THE HYGIENE OF PREGNANCY.

Examinations.—If any abnormal symptoms, especially those of uterine disease, abortion or kidney disorder, occur, a thorough, gentle examination should be made at once. In all cases the regular obstetric examination of pregnancy should be made at about the end of the eighth month, but it should be made at the end of the seventh month if there is a probability of contracted pelvis.

The Teeth.—The teeth should be kept clean and acidity prevented by the use of a brush and a solution of bicarbonate of sodium. For toughening the gums and preventing toothache, one or two drops of tincture of myrrh on the wet tooth brush, well rubbed into the gums after each meal, is of great value. Toothache is caused by an acid condition of the stomach, malnutrition, and increased irritability of the nervous system, which predisposes to neuralgia. Decayed teeth should be filled, and if the treatment does not stop their aching, they should be extracted under an anæsthetic, preferably chloroform. There is more danger of abortion from severe toothache than from the shock of an extraction under an anæsthetic. (The author has seen premature labor induced by severe toothache, and then stopped by chloroform and extraction).

Food.—The amount of food need not be restricted as long as the general health is good. Often in the first and last months the amount has to be lessened—in the first month from weak digestion and in the last month from lack of room. Any kind of food may be eaten, but preference should be given to easily digested and nutritious foods. Vegetables, fruits and milk are especially indicated. The use of meat should never be excessive, and often nature prevents this by changing the taste so that there is no desire for it. Sugar and starch should be avoided, especially potatoes, as there is a natural tendency to acidity of the stomach, heart-burn, flatulence and colic. A milk diet is of great value in lessening the complications of pregnancy and the duration and severity of labor. "Longings," if within reason, should be satisfied, as the constant refusal is likely to result in more harm than the gratification. Water should be drunk freely, as it aids elimination. Tea, coffee and chocolate may be continued, but they should be taken weak and in small amounts. Alcoholic drinks are not indicated as a beverage, as instead of stimulation, there is generally need of mental and physical rest, and in some there is a tendency to form the habit during pregnancy. In those who have been used to drinking beer or wine it probably would not be best to prohibit these entirely.

A vegetarian diet and the use of distilled water is supposed by some to lessen the amount of bone material, and therefore, to make an easier labor by the bones of the head being softer, but it is more probable that nature will take from the mother all the bone material required, and that the vegetarian diet by causing a more healthy parturient, lessens considerably the severity of labor.

Clothing.—The clothing should not be too light or too warm. In the latter half of pregnancy a little warmer and probably part woolen underwear should be worn, as then the increase in the size of the abdomen removes the skirts from close contact with the lower limbs. Corsets should not be worn unless specially made with elastic sides. The improper use of the corset is said to have stunted and even killed children by interfering with the growth of the uterus.

The Abdominal Bandage.—When the abdominal walls are relaxed, an elastic or other bandage is of great value, if fitted so as to hold up the abdomen without pressing upon the fundus of the uterus.

Bathing.—A general bath should be taken at least once a week during the whole nine months, and during the last month a sitzbath every other night keeps the external genitals clean, and tends to relax the soft parts and the pelvic joints and thereby lessen the duration and suffering of labor. The water should be neither too hot nor too cold, as either extreme tends to excite uterine contractions. (During pregnancy, although hot water may

Full No. 282.

ESTABLISHED 1882.

VOL. XXIV. No. 12.

JUNE, 1

Denver Medical Tim

THOMAS HAYDEN HAWKINS, A.M., M.D., Editor.

Contents, Page 21.

Index to Advertisers,

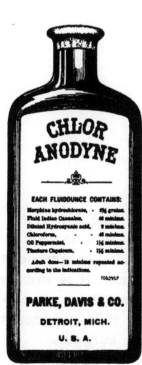

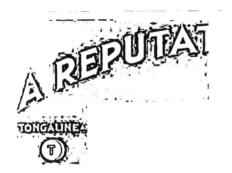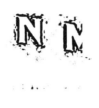

TONGALINE
(T)

Every physician wishes to establish a reputation for curing his patients prom

For over twenty five years Tongaline has been recognized by the

medical·profession as the standard prescription for

RHEUMATISM , NEURALGIA , GRIPPE , SCIATICA , LUMBAGO and GO

In every instance where Tongaline is used a physician secu

certain results *from* certain doses *in a* certain time .

All the salicylic acid in Tongaline is from the purest natural oil of winter

CAL
(TRADE MA
THE PER
DENTIFR
U.S. PATENT ALLOW
ENGLISH

The Standard Antiseptic
LISTERINE

A non-toxic antiseptic of known and definite power, prepared in a form convenient for immediate use, of ready dilution, sightly, pleasant, and sufficiently powerful for all purposes of asepsis: these are advantages which Listerine embodies.

The success of Listerine is based upon merit, and the best advertisement of Listerine is—Listerine.

LISTERINE
DERMATIC SOAP

An antiseptic detergent for use in the antiseptic treatment of diseases of the skin.

Listerine "Dermatic" Soap contains the essential antiseptic constituents of eucalyptus (1%), mentha, gaultheria and thyme (each ½%), which enter into the composition of the well known antiseptic preparation, Listerine, while the quality of excellence of the soap-stock employed as the vehicle for this medication, will be readily apparent when used upon the most delicate skin, and upon the scalp. Listerine "Dermatic" Soap contains no animal fats, and none but the very best vegetable oils; after its manufacture, and before it is "milled" and pressed into cakes a high percentage of an emollient oil is incorporated with the soap, and the smooth, elastic condition of the skin secured by using Listerine "Dermatic" Soap is largely due to the presence of this ingredient. Unusual care is exercised in the preparation of Listerine "Dermatic" Soap, and as the antiseptic constituents of Listerine are added to the soap after it has received its surplus of unsaponified emollient oil, they retain their peculiar antiseptic virtues and fragrance.

A sample of Listerine Dermatic Soap may be had upon application to the Manufacturers—

Lambert Pharmacal Company
St. Louis, U. S. A.

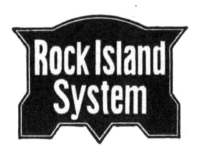

Tonsillitis Scarlet Fever Diphtheria

Infection in these diseases enters through an inflamed throat. The neighboring lymph glands guard against the passage of toxines into the circulation. But just at this critical time they become engorged and need assistance.

ANTIPHLOGISTINE

permits of the continuous application of moist heat, the physical principle of osmosis and the continuous stimulation of cutaneous reflexes, all of which tend to maintain the blood and lymph circulation in the affected part and to hasten the elimination of toxines.

The enlarged glands are depleted and the liability to Mastoiditis, Middle-ear and Laryngeal complications is lessened. Pain and sense of oppression are overcome, the patient experiences decided comfort and convalescence is materially hastened.

Directions: Always heat Antiphlogistine in the can (never on cloth) by placing it in hot water. Do not allow water to get into the preparation. When as hot as can be borne, take a suitable knife and spread the Antiphlogistine as quickly as possible on the skin *from ear to ear*, at least an eighth of an inch thick. Cover with a liberal supply of absorbent cotton and hold in place with a suitable compress. Change the dressing every 12 hours

The seamless, air-tight original containers of Antiphlogistine not only insure its delivery in perfect condition, but are economical for the patient; therefore always order an original package and specify the size required—Small, Medium, Large or Hospital Size.

(Never sold in bulk.)

The Denver Chemical Mfg. Co., New York.

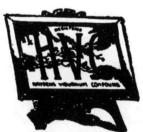

—6—

THE PREPARATION OF A PHYSIOLOGICAL IMITATION OF MOTHERS' MILK BY MEANS OF

Peptogenic Milk Powder

FIRST: A milk-mixture adjusted to the normal percentage composition of mothers' milk.

SECOND: The submission of this milk-mixture to heat, under which the Peptogenic Powder (its enzyme) converts the caseine into a form remarkably approximating to the soluble, diffusible proteids of human milk.

This milk is then Pasteurised or sterilised 160° F. or boiling—and the enzyme thus instantly destroyed.

In consequence of this proteid conversion, the milk takes on a striking, visible resemblance to human milk; likewise corresponds to it in behavior (with rennet, acid, etc.) and in susceptibility to digestion. The original milk-mixture does not even look like mothers' milk—coagulates with acid just like all percentage modifications. In this we have confirmation of the fact that the "pivotal", radical difference between cows' and human milk lies in the nature of their proteids, not in any quantitative detail, a fact moreover highly significant of the futility of mere percentage modifications.

N. B. The food, by the "Fairchild" method, contains no digestive ferment, no "aid to digestion"--has simply the digestibility of mothers' milk.

FAIRCHILD BROS. & FOSTER

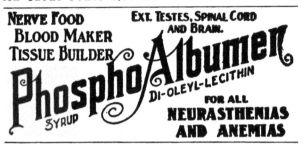
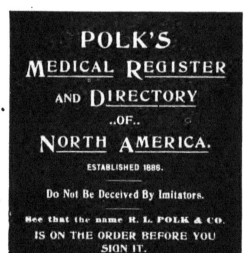

Chicago Policlinic and Hospital

PIONEER POST-GRADUATE SCHOOL OF THE WEST

SUMMER COURSE begins June 1st. Abundance of clinical material and excellent Hospital facilities. Finely equipped Pathological and Anatomical Laboratories.

For schedule, announcement and full information, address

M. L. Harris, M.D., Secretary

174-176 East Chicago Ave., Chicago,

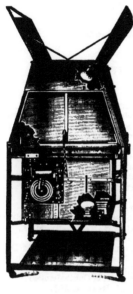
CONTENTS.

INDEX TO ADVERTISERS.

J. B. STOTT, PRINTER, DENVER, COLO.

Denver and Gross College of Medic

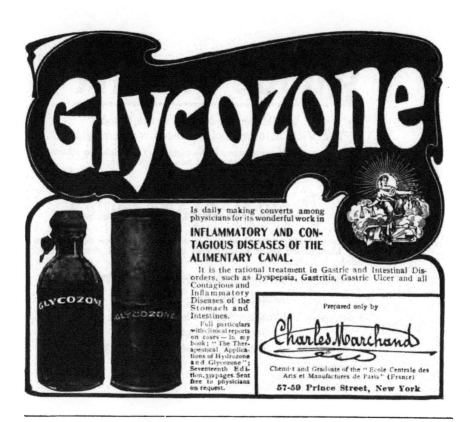

—14—

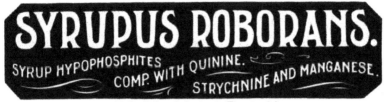

SYRUPUS ROBORANS.
SYRUP HYPOPHOSPHITES COMP. WITH QUININE. STRYCHNINE AND MANGANESE.

1-125 Grain Strychnine to the Teaspoonful.

he pharmaceutical skill displayed in making this favorite compound more stable and agreeable deserves th approbation of the profession.

Syrupus Roborans as a Tonic During Convalescence Has No Equal.

As a nerve stimulant and restorative in wasting and debilitating diseases, as a constructive agent in Insom ia, Pneumonia, Tuberculosis, Bronchial Asthma, Marasmus, Strumous Diseases and General Debility, this com pound has no superior. Owing to the solubility of the salts, addition can be made of Fowler's Solution, Syru Iod. Iron, Iod. Potass., etc., giving the advantages of those remedies without interfering with the stability of th reparations. **SYRUPUS ROBORANS** is a perfect solution and will keep in any climate.

DR. W. O. ROBERTS says: "In cases convalescing from 'La Grippe' Syrupus Roborans has no equal."

Messrs. Arthur Peter & Co., Louisville, Ky. Gentlemen—The excellence of your preparations—"SYRUPU ROBORANS" and "PEPTIC ESSENCE COMP."—cannot be questioned. I use both in my practice, and have alway been pleased with the effect of each. Respectfully, J. M. MATHEWS, A.M., M.D., Prof. of Surg. and Diseases Rectum, Hospital College of Medicine, Ex-President Am. Medical Association and Mississippi Valley Medi Association; President Kentucky State Board of Health.

Messrs Arthur Peter & Co
Louisville Ky

Gentlemen, The excellence of your preparation
'Syrupus Roborans" and Peptic Essence
compound" cannot be questioned.
I use both in my practice and
have always been pleased with the
effect of Each. Respectfully
Jm Mathews. M.D. L.S.D.

Prof. of Surgery, and diseases of Rectum, Hos. Col. of Med.; **EX-PRES. AM. MED.**
ASS'N. and Miss. Valley Med. Ass'n.; Ky. State Board of Health.

PETER'S PEPTIC ESSENCE COMP.
A POWERFUL DIGESTIVE FLUID IN PALATABLE FORM.

Please note that Essence and Elixir Pepsin contains only Pepsin, while in **Peter's Peptic Essence** we hav ll the digestive ferments. These are preserved in solution wit h C. P. Glycerine in a manner retaining their ful therapeutic value, which is exerted in and beyond the stomach.

It is a Stomachic Tonic, and relieves Indigestion, Flatulency, and has the remarkable property of arres vomiting during pregnancy. It is a remedy of great value in Gastralgia, Enteralgia, Cholera Infantum, an intestinal derangements, especially those of an inflammatory character. For nursing mothers and teething chil dren it has no superior. Besides mere digestive properties, Pepsin and Pancreatine have powerful soothing an sedative effects, and are therefore indicated in all gastric and intestinal derangements, and especially in inflam matory conditions. It is perfectly miscible with any appropriate medium. In certain cases the addition of Ti Nux Vomica gives much satisfaction. Please write for Peter's Peptic Essence, and you will not be disappointed These preparations are held strictly in the hands of the medical profession, never having been advertised as popu lar remedies, nor put up with wrappers and circulars expatiating on the use of the Hypophosphites or Digestives thus educating the public in the use of these valuable compounds.

Samples Sent upon application.
Express Charges at Your Expense
For Sale by all Wholesale Druggists.

ARTHUR PETER & CO.
LOUISVILLE, KENTUCKY.

Lightning Source UK Ltd.
Milton Keynes UK
UKHW021346100219

336936UK00006B/324/P